The Vulnerable Atherosclerotic Plaque

Strategies for Diagnosis and Management

EDITED BY

Renu Virmani, MD
Medical Director, CVPath
International Registry of Pathology
Gaithersburg MD, USA

Jagat Narula, MD, PhD
Professor of Medicine
Chief, Division of Cardiology
Associate Dean
University of California, Irvine
School of Medicine
Irvine CA, USA

Martin B. Leon, MD
Professor of Medicine
Center for Interventional Vascular Therapy
Columbia, University Medical Center
NewYork NY, USA

James T. Willerson, MD
President
The University of Texas Health Science Center at Houston
President and Medical Director
Texas Heart Institute
Houston TX, USA

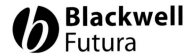

Blackwell Publishing, Inc., 350 Main Street, Malden, Massachusetts 02148-5020, USA
Blackwell Publishing Ltd, 9600 Garsington Road, Oxford OX4 2DQ, UK
Blackwell Science Asia Pty Ltd, 550 Swanston Street, Carlton, Victoria 3053, Australia

First published 2007

1   2007

ISBN-13: 9781405158596
ISBN-10: 140515859X

Library of Congress Cataloging-in-Publication Data

The vulnerable atherosclerotic plaque : strategies for diagnosis and management / edited by
R. Virmani . . . [et al.].
        p.;   cm.
   Includes bibliographical references and index.
   ISBN-13: 978-1-4051-5859-6 (alk. paper)
   ISBN-10: 1-4051-5859-X (alk. paper)
   1. Atherosclerosis.   2. Heart – Diseases – Prevention.   I. Virmani, Renu.
   [DNLM: 1. Atherosclerosis – diagnosis.   2. Atherosclerosis – therapy.
   3. Atherosclerosis – physiopathology.   4. Diagnostic Imaging. WG 550 V991 2007]

   RC692.V85 2007
   616.1′36-dc22

                                                              2006017667

A catalogue record for this title is available from the British Library

Acquisitions: Gina Almond
Production: Charlie Hamlyn
Set in 9.5/12pt Minion by Graphicraft Limited, Hong Kong
Printed and bound by COS Printers Pte Ltd, Singapore

For further information on Blackwell Publishing, visit our website:
www.blackwellfutura.com

The publisher's policy is to use permanent paper from mills that operate a sustainable forestry
policy, and which has been manufactured from pulp processed using acid-free and elementary
chlorine-free practices. Furthermore, the publisher ensures that the text paper and cover board
used have met acceptable environmental accreditation standards.

Contents

iii

Contributors

Ibrahim Aboshady, MD
University of Texas Health Science Center at Houston
Texas Heart Institute
Houston, TX

Chowdhury Ahsan, MD
University of California, Irvine
Irvine, CA

Allen P Burke, MD
CV Path
International Registry of Pathology
Gaithsburg, MD

Samuel Ward Casscells, MD
University of Texas Health Science Center at Houston
Texas Heart Institute
Houston, TX

Pim de Feyter, MD, PHD
Thoraxcenter
Erasmus Medical Center
Rotterdam
The Netherlands

Chris L de Korte, PHD
Thoraxcenter
Erasmus Medical Center
Rotterdam
The Netherlands

Chunming Dong, MD
Duke University Medical Center
Durham, NC

Andrew Farb, MD
US Food and Drug Administration
Rockville, MD

Irwin M Feuerstein, MD
Walter Reed Army Medical Center
Washington, DC

Aloke V Finn, MD
Massachusetts General Hospital
Boston, MA

David R Fowler, MD
Office of the Chief Medical Examiner
Baltimore, MD

Zorina S Galis, PHD
Lilly Research Laboratories
Lilly Corporate Center
Indianapolis, IN

Yong-Jian Geng, MD, PHD
University of Texas-Houston Health Science Center
Texas Heart Institute
Houston, TX

Herman K Gold, MD
Massachusetts General Hospital
Boston, MA

Pascal J Goldschmidt-Clermont, MD, FACC
Miller School of Medicine
University of Miami
Miami, FL

Mark M Kockx, MD
AZ-Middelheim
The Netherlands

Frank D Kolodgie, PHD
CV Path
International Registry of Pathology
Gaithersburg, MD

Michiel Knaapen, PHD
AZ-Middelheim
The Netherlands

Robert Kutys, MS
CV Path
International Registry of Pathology
Gaithersburg, MD

Birendra N Lal, MD
University of Texas Health Science Center at Houston
Texas Heart Institute
Houston, TX

Richard T Lee, MD
Harvard Medical School and
Brigham and Women's Hospital
Boston, MA

Martin B Leon, MD
Center for Interventional Vascular Therapy
Columbia
University Medical Center
New York, NY

Susan M Lessner, PHD
University of South Carolina School of Medicine
Columbia, SC

Silvio Litovsky, MD
University of Alabama at Birmingham
Birmingnam, AL

Mohammad Madjid, MD
University of Texas Health Science Center at Houston
Texas Heart Institute
Houston, TX

Paul Magnin, PHD
Lightlab Imaging Inc
Westford, MA

Barbara Marshik, PHD
Cardiovascular Institute
Mount Sinai Medical Center
New York

Wim Martinet, PHD
University of Antwerp
Belgium

Frits Mastik, PHD
Thoraxcenter
Erasmus Medical Center
Rotterdam
The Netherlands

Pauline E McEwan, PHD
Miravant Medical Technologies
Santa Barbara, CA

Pedro R Moreno, MD
Mount Sinai Medical Center
New York, NY

James E Muller, MD
Harvard Medical School
Boston, MA

Morteza Naghavi, MD
University of Texas–Houston Health Science Center
Houston, TX

Anuja Nair, PHD
Volcano Corporation
Cleveland, OH

Jagat Narula, MD, PHD
University of California, Irvine
Irvine, CA

Artiom Petrov, PHD
University of California, Irvine
Irvine, CA

Evelyn Regar, MD, PHD
Thoraxcenter
Erasmus Medical Center
Rotterdam
The Netherlands

Luis E Rohde, MD
Hospital de Clinicas de Porto Alegre
Medical School of Rio Grande do Sol Federal University
Porto Alegre, Brazil

Michael E Rosenfeld, PHD
School of Public Health and Community Medicine
University of Washington
Seattle, WA

Johannes A Schaar, MD, PHD
Thoraxcenter
Erasmus Medical Center
Rotterdam
The Netherlands

Jacob Schneiderman, MD
Sheba Medical Center
Israel

Stephen M Schwartz, MD, PHD
University of Washington
Seattle, WA

Patrick W Serruys, MD, PHD
Thoraxcenter
Erasmus Medical Center
Rotterdam
The Netherlands

Cornelis J Slager, PHD
Thoraxcenter
Erasmus Medical Center
Rotterdam
The Netherlands

Hee Kwon Song, PHD
University of Pennsylvania School of Medicine
Philadelphia, PA

Allen J Taylor, MD
Walter Reed Army Medical Center
Washington, DC

Tarun Tewatia, MD
University of Texas Health Science Center at Houston
Texas Heart Institute
Houston, TX

Sotirios Tsimikas, MD, FACC, FAHA, FSCAI
University of California, San Diego
La Jolla, CA

Anton FW van der Steen, PHD
Thoraxcenter
Erasmus Medical Center
Rotterdam
The Netherlands

Mani A Vannan, MBBS
University of California, Irvine
Irvine, CA

Deborah Vela, MD
University of Texas Health Science Center at Houston
Texas Heart Institute
Houston, TX

Johan Verjans, MS
University of California, Irvine
Irvine, CA

D Geoffrey Vince, PHD
Volcano Corporation
Cleveland, Ohio

Renu Virmani, MD
CV Path
International Registry of Pathology
Gaithersburg, MD

Ron Waksman, MD
Cardiovascular Research Institute
Washington Hospital Center
Washington, DC

Thomas N Wight, MD
The Hope Heart Institute
Seattle, WA

Robert L Wilensky, MD
University of Pennsylvania Medical Center
Philadelphia, PA

James T Willerson, MD
University of Texas Health Science Center at Houston
Texas Heart Institute
Houston, TX

Ronald L Wolf, MD, PHD
University of Pennsylvania Medical Center
Philadelphia, PA

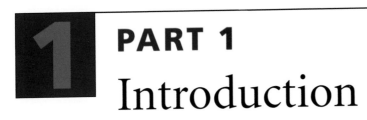

PART 1

Introduction

CHAPTER 1

History of atherosclerosis and vulnerable plaque research

Mohammad Madjid, Ibrahim Aboshady, Samuel Ward Casscells, Renu Virmani & James T Willerson

If I Have Seen Further, It Is by Standing on the Shoulders of Giants

Sir Isaac Newton, 1676

The history of atherosclerosis research is a fascinating one. A disease as old as mankind, coronary heart disease came into the spotlight as it transformed from a rare and sporadic disease in the beginning of the 20th century to a disease of pandemic dimensions by the mid-century, and remains the leading cause of death in the Western world. The main underlying mechanism of heart attacks is atherosclerosis. The term "atherosclerosis" implies the two main components of the lesion, "athero" the Greek word for gruel, corresponding to the necrotic core area at the base of the atherosclerotic plaque, and "sclerosis" from the Greek for hardening or induration, matching the fibrotic cap at the luminal edge of the plaque.[1,2]

Atherosclerosis: an ancient disease

Atherosclerosis and its clinical correlates date back to ancient times. Documentation of these lesions dates back more than 3500 years[3] and lesions have been found in Egyptian mummies dating from 1580 BC.[3] Atherosclerosis existed in ancient Egyptians and showed the same pathologic features as in modern times.[4]

Hippocrates (460–377 BC) described sudden death probably due to acute myocardial infarction.[5] **Erasistratos**, an Egyptian physician in 300 BC, described the arteries, veins, and nerves as the three main pathways in the human body.

In 1852, **Czermak** was the first to ascribe calcification of the aorta in mummies.[4] In 42 pages, he described microscopic examinations of two Egyptian mummies. The first was a boy 15 years of age and the other was an elderly woman.[4] In the latter, he reported several calcareous deposits on the anterior wall of the descending part of the aortic arch.

In the 1970s, members of the US Paleopathology Association studied a number of mummies from Egypt[6-9] and North America[10-12] which were received through the Smithsonian Institution. Cockburn and his colleague published their detailed autopsies of Pum II (170 ± 70 BC based on carbon 14 measurements) in *Science*. They reported: "Large and small atherosclerotic plaques were present in the portions of aorta. . . . In other organs found within the viscera, large and small arterioles and arteries also had areas of intimal fibrosis, typical of arteriolar sclerosis."[6]

They examined a mummy found in a cave in the Aleutian Islands and observed pleural adhesions, possible pneumonia or bronchiectasis, and aortic atherosclerosis.[13]

At the beginning of this century, the graves of Pharaohs in the Egyptian pyramids were found and opened. Sclerotic changes were found at autopsy of **Pharaoh Menephtah**, who lived at the time of the Jewish exodus from Egypt.[3] These findings are important as they prove that arteriosclerotic disease did not originate after the industrial revolution, but has affected mankind with the same histopathologic features for at least several thousand years.

Galenic medicine

Claudius Galen (AD 129–200), the prominent physician of the Roman Empire had more influence in medicine than any other individual until the Renaissance.[14] He demonstrated that the heart is made up of muscle and described the presence and movement of blood in the arteries.[14] Galen believed that veins contain blood, that the heart was more than a "circulation junction", and that blood flows throughout the body. He believed that blood ebbs and flows with the heartbeat.[15] Galen's ideas shaped medical teachings for centuries afterwards.

Erasistratus (304–250 BC) described intermittent claudication, showing that peripheral artery disease was present in the antiquity.[16] He believed that arteries contained a substance called "pneuma" which is replaced each time a person breathes. Pneuma was believed to be identical with air spirit, or soul. He believed that veins carried blood to nourish the tissues and that arteries contained pneuma only during life. When the artery was cut, blood rushed in as the pneuma escaped.[17]

Medicine in the Renaissance

It was not until the Renaissance that Galen's teachings came under scrutiny. The Swiss physician **Paracelsus** (1493–1541) was one of the first to reject Galen's thoughts and spoke against the tendency to accept Galen's beliefs as facts.[18] **Paracelsus** believed that the liver was the central organ of the circulation with the heart playing an important role. He could not determine how blood could move from the right side to the left side, and hypothesized that that there were pores in the heart allowing blood to move from right to left.[19,20]

Leonardo da Vinci's artistic description of atherosclerosis

Leonardo da Vinci (1452–1519) made one of the earliest descriptions of atherosclerosis and hardening of the arteries.[20] He wrote, "Vessels in the elderly, through the thickenings of the tunics, restrict the transit of blood," and "the artery and vein in the aged which extend between the spleen and the liver, acquires so thick a covering that it contracts the passage of blood." His description is one of the earliest reports of the atherosclerotic changes.[21]

Leonardo admirably described atherosclerosis as a "debility through lack of blood and deficiency of

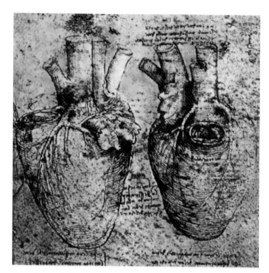

Figure 1.1 Anatomy of coronary artery by Leonardo da Vinci. (Reprinted with permission from The Royal Collection, Her Majesty Queen Elizabeth II.)

the artery which nourishes the heart and other lower members." His drawings of coronary arteries are very accurate (Figure 1.1).[20] He wrote about his problem in drawing the coronary vessels since "they are surrounded by waxy fat." This may explain the failure of the earlier anatomists to observe and describe the coronary arteries.[22]

Modern anatomy and physiology of circulatory system

Andreas Vesalius (1514–1564) challenged Galen's school of thought.[23] He compiled the completeanatomy of the human body and discovered hundreds of errors by Galen which led to his forced retirement from academic pursuits.[24] *De Humani Corpus Fabrica Libri System* was a collection published in 1555 by Vesalius. His studies greatly contributed to understanding vascular anatomy.[14]

William Harvey (1578–1657) was the first to accurately and correctly describe the physiology of blood circulation. He described the presence of left and right circulation systems and showed correctly how blood flows through the heart. He believed that the heart, lungs, and blood vessels are interdependent and that the diseases of the heart may actually originate in organs other than the heart, especially in the circulatory systems.[25]

Table 1.1 Descriptions of chest pain before the term "angina pectoris" was introduced. (Adapted from Hanke H, et al. Acta Chir Belg 2001;101:162–9.[29])

Poterius: "Opera omnia et chymica," 1645

T. Bonetus: "Sepulchretum sive anatomia practica ex cadaveribus morbo denatis," Geneve 1700

M. Lancisi: "De subitaneis mortibus libri duo," Roma 1709

G. Ballonius: "Consilia medicinalia," Venice 1735

F. Petraglia: "De cordis affectionibus," Roma 1778

Angina pectoris

Cardiac pain was described by Hippocrates in the Corpus Hippocraticum, the fundamental text of medicine.[26] In the early years of the 16th century, the Florentine physician Benivieni wrote about a woman who "was sometimes troubled with pain at her heart."[27]

In one of the earliest descriptions of cardiac symptoms, **Andreas Vesalius** wrote about a "sad feeling and pain in the heart" of one of his patients and ascribed them to heart disease.[22] One of the earliest detailed descriptions of chest pain was actually written by Edward Earl of Clarendon (1609–1674) who was not a physician.[28] He described bouts of chest and arm pain in his father.

In the 17th and 18th century, there were a few descriptions of what seems to be pains of cardiac origin (Table 1.1).[29] However, it was in 1772 when **William Heberden** (1710–1781) introduced the term "angina pectoris" for the first time.[30] His description of chest pain is still one of the most accurate ever written.

Coronary origin of angina pectoris

In 1812, **John Warren**, in the first issue of the *New England Journal of Medicine*, wrote his view on the contemporary knowledge on angina pectoris.[31] He described cases of angina pectoris reported by **Fothergill** in 1744, two of whom were dissected after death (one by the famous **John Hunter**). He stated that "the heart must have been principally, if not altogether, the seat of the complaint." Considering these reports, **Caleb Hillier Parry** was the first to relate symptoms of angina pectoris to presence of coronary sclerosis in 1799.[31] Parry reported that the ossification of the coronary arteries is the

predisposing cause of this disease. Decades later in 1880, **A. Potain** described angina pectoris as a result of myocardial ischemia.[29]

In 1786, **Edward Jenner** (1749–1823) was the first to link angina pectoris with disease of the coronary arteries.[32] William Heberden used to ascribe chest pain to cramping of the myocardium. The Scottish anatomist **Allan Burns** claimed that angina pectoris is caused by the spasm of the coronary arteries. Jenner, in a series of five autopsies, correctly related angina pectoris to coronary atherosclerosis.[33] In 1776, he was able to diagnose angina pectoris in his famous mentor **John Hunter** and shared it with Heberden, but didn't inform Hunter as there was no treatment available at that time and he feared upsetting him.[34] Postmortem examination of Hunter, who perished after an argument at a meeting of the Board of Governors of St George's Hospital, demonstrated coronary atherosclerotic disease.[a]

In 1852, Sir **Richard Quain** in his paper "On fatty diseases of the heart," records his observation of the deposition of fatty material in the blood vessels, which he attributed to ". . . local modification of nutrition." He linked the fatty heart to a number of effects, including, "languid and feeble circulation, a sense of uneasiness and oppression in the chest, embarrassment and distress in breathing, coma, syncope, angina pectoris, sudden death. . . ."

It was Danielpolu who, in 1924, stated that angina is due to a disproportion between coronary flow and work of heart.[35] In 1928, Chester Keefer and William Resnik published their landmark paper "Angina pectoris: a syndrome caused by anoxemia of the myocardium."[36] In their detailed review, they discussed anoxemia as the cause of angina, and discussed its diverse causes (including coronary artery disease, vasospasm, and decreased oxygen delivery), silent myocardial infarction, sudden cardiac

---

[a] John Hunter (1728–1793) was a celebrated anatomist and surgeon. He believed in scientific experiments, and in a famous experiment inoculated himself with pus to prove his theory that gonorrhea is different from syphilis. Unfortunately the source patient was afflicted with both and he got both diseases. Sensing the impending doom from his paroxysms of chest pain, he once mentioned that his life "is in the hands of any rascal who chooses to annoy him." This was a prophecy which unfortunately came true.[34]

death, the role of ventricular fibrillation, and collateral formation.[36]

Coronary spasm

The conception of spasmodic constriction of coronary artery was suggested to account for the cases of angina in the absence of coronary disease. This notion was first advocated by **Latham** and supported by **von Neusser** and many others, including **Gallavardin** and **Kohn**.[37–40] **Prinzmetal** and **Massumi** in 1955 introduced "anterior chest wall syndrome," later referred to as Prinzmetal–Massumi syndrome.[41] They described a "symptom complex consisting of somatic involvement of the anterior chest wall leading to pain and tenderness." In their experience, this syndrome was commonly seen after myocardial infarction (MI), but in many cases was not associated with coronary artery disease.[41] **Attilio Maseri** in 1978 proved the existence of coronary spasm in angiographic studies in unstable angina patients.[42]

Histopathologic description of atherosclerosis

An early gross description of atherosclerosis is ascribed to **Caleb Hillier Parry** who, in 1799, during an autopsy, discovered something hard and gritty in the coronary arteries and "well remembered looking up to the ceiling which was old and crumbling, conceiving that some plaster (sic) had fallen down."[43] From his discovery of hardened, "ossified" vessels, he suggested that the cause of the "syncope anginosa" should be sought in the coronary arteries.[43]

The first use of the term "arteriosclerosis" can possibly be traced back to **Johannes Friedrich Lobstein** (1777–1835), who as a professor at the Medical University Clinic Strasurg, in "Lehrbuch der pathologischen Anatomie"[44] reported sclerotic changes of the arterial wall, writing "von der Verdikhung der arterien, oder der Arteriosklerose." The term "atherosclerosis" was proposed and justified in 1904 by **Felix Merchand** of Leipzig to characterize the lesions in the arterial wall with increased lipid content.

In 1740, **Krell** published a dissertation on hardening of coronary arteries which were not bony but had a tophaceous nature, derived from atheromatous material.[32] **Morgagni**[45] reported in his opus "De sedibus, et causis morborum" on an old patient who had been taken to his Nosocomium in Padova in 1743 in a moribund state: "Already with inspection of the heart from the outside, the coronaria sinistra attracts attention which has changed to an 'osseous channel' from its beginning over a distance of several crossfingers." He also correctly described atheromatous lesions as a predisposing factor for aneurysms.[46]

In 1755, **Albert von Haller**, a Swiss physiologist (1708–1777), illustrated atherosclerotic changes in arteries of aged people.[47] During an autopsy, he hurt his finger on sharp calcified lesions in the abdominal aorta of his father-in-law. **Jean Cruveilheir**, the French pathologist (1829–1846), showed atherosclerotic changes in arteries and the related cerebral and cardiac complications in his atlas.[48]

Gmelin[49] and **Tiedmann**[50] found by chemical analysis that the "earthy" substances in atherosclerotic plaques are composed of calcium phosphate and carbonate and cannot be detected in healthy arteries, but were to a great extent present in diseased arteries. **Teidmann** also pointed to the narrowing and the occlusion of the arteries and regarded the disease pathogenetically as an inflammatory disease. **Bürger** continued the chemical analysis of the sclerotically altered arterial wall after Virchow in Berlin had already drawn attention to the deposition of lipids in the vascular wall in 1852 and had designated arteriosclerosis as vessel wall inflammation.[29]

Early theories of atherogenesis

In the early 19th century, **Rokitansky**[51] and **Virchow**[52,53] described the main components of atherosclerosis. They observed crystals of cholesterol, foam cells, and necroses. Virchow[54] compared the rupture of an atherosclerotic plaque to the perforation of an abscess. At that time, there were two prevailing theories for atherosclerosis.

Karl Rokitansky (1894–1878), the celebrated Viennese pathologist, believed in humoral disease theory concerning "crases and stases": the doctrine of bodily fluids. This view stated that phlebitis causes most of the diseases. Rokitansky previously endorsed the "encrustation" theory of atherosclerosis (i.e. mural thrombi are formed over the arterial surface and once fibrin is incorporated into the vessel wall, it causes atherosclerosis[b]). This theory was brutally attacked by **Rudolf Virchow** (1821–1902) whose influence in the medical world was growing fast. He rejected the views of Rokitansky on the pathogenesis of arteriosclerosis.[52] After Virchow's attacks, Rokitansky removed all references to the humor and crases doctrine in his second textbook (see footnote c).

Virchow used a microscope to a great extent and showed that the intimal thickening is located in the subendothelial layer, and therefore could not be derived from surface deposits (as opposed to Rokitansky's theory).[52]

In 1840s, Virchow described his famous triad explaining the factors leading to the formation of clots. Virchow hypothesized that thrombosis (a term he coined along with ischemia) occurs in the presence of: (i) changes in the vessel wall; (ii) changes in the blood flow (stasis); and (iii) changes in the constituents of blood (hypercoagulability). He described the relationship between deep vein thrombosis and pulmonary embolism.

Atherosclerosis as an inflammatory disease

In 1815 **Joseph Hodgson** published a monograph on vascular disease in which he claimed that inflammation is the underlying cause of atherosclerosis and is not a simple degenerative manifestation of the aging process. He also identified that the disease process occurred in the intima.[47]

---

[b] Rokitansky's theory was not completely devoid of truth. Fuster and others have indicated that asymptomatic plaque ruptures may heal and superimposed clots may become organized in the plaque. Also, there is a strong interaction between inflammation and the coagulation system.[55,56]

[c] Virchow was a passionate and outspoken scientist[57] whose stubbornness once led to his being called to a duel by the "Iron Chancellor" Bismarck. He wisely declined the challenge. Despite all his extraordinary achievements in medicine, anthropology, politics, and social work, his stifling dogmatism caused him to stubbornly antagonize views of Koch, Behring, and Charles Darwin. He opposed the prophylactic handwashings of Semmelweiss, while Rokitansky, with his extraordinary pleasant and charming manners, stood by him when he was being viciously attacked by the medical establishment.[57]

Virchow considered arteriosclerosis an inflammatory process, and gave an extensive description of the various stages of atherosclerotic disease that he named "endarteritis deformans."[53] He believed that the atheroma was a product of an inflammatory process within the intima, and that the fibrous thickening evolved as a consequence of a reactive fibrosis induced by proliferating connective tissue cells followed by the fatty changes. He noted that cholesterol was present in atheromas, but considered it secondary. He observed that lesions tended to form where there was pressure from blood flow, and hypothesized that the mechanical forces initiated the irritant stimulus to the artery and that the endarteritis was part of a repair mechanism.

In 1907, **Aschoff** discovered that fatty material in diseased portions of arteries consisted largely of cholesterol esters.[58] A few years later, **Anitschkow**[59] in breakthrough experiments demonstrated that lipid deposits could be induced in rabbit arteries by feeding the animals a diet high in cholesterol or egg yolk. These studies originated the lipid hypothesis and in a few decades the inflammatory origin of the atherosclerosis was sent to oblivion. In 1967, Saphir[60] noted that references to inflammation as a component of atherosclerosis had almost disappeared from the literature.

It was in 1976 when **Russell Ross** (1929–1999), a dentist with a PhD in experimental pathology, following extensive research on wound healing and the role of smooth muscle cells in the process, unified the current concepts of atherogenesis in the **response-to-injury theory** and revived the inflammation theory,[61,62] and during the following years extended and completed it (Figure 1.2).[63] In 1993, in light of new findings (especially by Steinberg and Witztum),[64,65] he put emphasis on the role of lipid oxidation in causation of atherosclerosis,[66] and in 1999 he declared atherosclerosis an inflammatory disease.[67]

Role of thrombosis in myocardial infarction

Though thrombus has often been noticed in autopsies, its role in pathogenesis of myocardial infarction has been under debate for a long time. In 1912, **John B. Herrick** wrote his classic paper in the *Journal of the American Medical Association* in which he

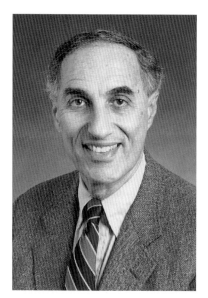

Figure 1.2 Russell Ross (1929–1999). (Picture courtesy of the University of Washington.)

described effects of coronary obstruction and the role of coronary thrombosis in clinical settings. He also demonstrated that thrombosis and occlusion are not necessarily fatal, thus differentiating between ischemia and infarction.[68]

Charles Friedberg in1949 in his textbook *Diseases of the Heart* put emphasis on the role of coronary thrombosis in acute myocardial infarction.[69]

In the 1940s, **Duguid** continued to champion Rokitansky's theory of encrustation and claimed a role for thrombosis in formation and progression of atherosclerotic plaques and claimed that thrombosis in the coronary arteries was a key feature in coronary heart disease (CHD).[70,71] He recommended studying factors which "govern fibrin formation in the circulating blood" and suggested that thrombi are initiated on the arterial intima by platelet clumping or local failure of fibrinolysis. In 1951, **Crawford** and **Levene** (London) showed that fibrin is actually incorporated into aortic intima[72] and Meade and Chakrabarti demonstrated that raised fibrinogen level is an independent predictor of CHD.[73]

In 1960s and 1970s, there was a debate over whether thrombosis followed myocardial infarction (AMI) or preceded it. The skepticism regarding the role of thrombosis in AMI originated mainly from the inconsistent reporting of thrombi in fatal MIs. As **William Roberts** outlined in 1972, reported incidence of thrombi varied from 21% to 91% in AMI.[74] He, and many others at that time, believed that "the virtual absence of coronary arterial thrombi in patients dying suddenly of cardiac disease, and their presence in only about one half of those with myocardial necrosis supported the concept that coronary artery thrombi were *consequences* rather than *causes* of AMI."[74] Though lysis of antemortem thrombosis or platelet aggregates was suggested as an explanation, it was not accepted due to a lack of evidence.

The role of thrombus in vascular occlusion and MI was not confirmed until 1980 when **Marcus De Wood** provided the angiographic evidence that intracoronary thrombi have causal roles in the development of AMI.[75] **Fulton** used pre-mortem injections of ^{125}I-labeled fibrinogen to show that thrombosis often preceded MI.[76]

In 1941, **Blumgart** et al. used transient coronary occlusion in dogs and showed that the extent of MI was affected by the duration of occlusion.[77] This study and subsequent confirmatory ones[77–79] heralded the clinical importance of a patent as opposed to an occluded infarct-related artery and led to "open infarct-related artery theory" championed by **Eugene Braunwald** and others.[80] This theory encouraged scientists to develop new thrombolytic agents to reperfuse the occluded coronary arteries and use them in megatrials, such as GUSTO, GISSI, ISIS, and TIMI series.[80] The development of recombinant tissue plasminogen activator for use in AMI, established the place of thrombolysis in the treatment of acute ST elevation myocardial infarct.[81]

Atherosclerosis: a disease of "everyone"

It has been known for a long time that atherosclerosis is a widespread disease. In the early years of the last century, Osler mentioned that "atheroma of the aorta is not in all cases senile; it was exceptional to find no patches of arterial degeneration in any body post mortem, and even children might show some slight foci of fatty degeneration."[82]

It was the report by **William F. Enos** et al. in 1953 that reminded scientists of this fact. They demonstrated the presence of coronary artery disease among young US soldiers killed in Korea.[83] Enos' findings were replicated by **McNamara** in autopsies of young soldiers killed in the Vietnam War.[84] These findings were later re-confirmed by **Renu Virmani** and her colleagues who examined previously uncut coronary arteries from the hearts of 94 American male combat casualties from the Korean War. Using computerized planimetry and microscopic evaluation, they found a prevalence similar to that reported previously (5%).[85] Systematic histopathologic studies in Pathobiological Determinants of Atherosclerosis in Youth (PDAY) and Bogalusa study, showed that atherosclerosis originates in childhood and is related to the presence of risk factors.[86,87] In fact, oxidation of LDL cholesterol and fatty streaks formation have even been reported in the fetal stage.[88]

Increased awareness about the widespread nature of atherosclerosis in the population and its often multifocal distribution in individuals prompted researchers to look for the causes which lead to thrombosis/myocardial infarction in certain patients at specific arterial locations.

Plaque rupture and role of vulnerable plaques

Plaque rupture was first reported at the autopsy of **Bertel Thorvaldsen**, the celebrated neoclassical Danish artist and sculptor who died of sudden cardiac death in the Royal Theater in Copenhagen in 1844.[68] On autopsy, his death was attributed to the rupture of an atherosclerotic plaque in the left coronary artery. It was stated that the vessel wall contained "several atheromatous plaques, one of which quite clearly had ulcerated, pouring the atheromatous mass into the arterial lumen."[89]

In the 1930 and 1940s, researchers focused on the pathologic features of culprit lesions leading to thrombotic events and sudden cardiac death. **Clark, Koch, Friedman,** and **Constantinides** were among the first to describe fissures and erosions on the intimal surface of the coronary arteries and held them responsible for initiation of the thrombotic process.[90-92] Others concluded that an intramural hemorrhage usually initiates the process leading to thrombosis.[93,94] **Leary** was among the first to introduce the rupture of an intramural atheromatous "abscess" as the main cause of coronary throm-

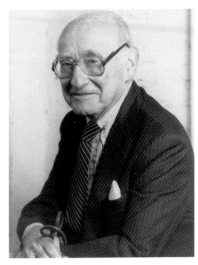

Figure 1.3 Meyer Friedman (1911–2001). (Reprinted with permission Circulation 2001;104:2758.)

bosis.[93,94] The idea of an "intramural atheromatous abscess" probably goes back to **Virchow** who described the inflammatory nature of atheromas.[95] **Paris Constantinides** at the same time described association of fissures and cracks in the plaque with thrombus formation.[92] **Chapman** reported formation of thrombus over a tear on atherosclerotic plaques and in connection with plaque debris.[96]

A great deal of research on this subject was done by **Meyer Friedman**, who systematically studied coronary arteries by doing serial sections (Figure 1.3).[97] Friedman's descriptions are impressively accurate and sophisticated even by today's standards.[d] He described many of the findings that form the basis of today's knowledge of plaque inflammation and rupture. He described, in detail, "intramural atheromatous abscesses" – first reported by Leary[94] – in the atherosclerotic plaques in almost all patients who had died with coronary thrombus.[97] These "atheromatous abscesses" were degenerative or necrotic areas consisting of a pultaceous mixture of cholesterol crystals, lipid, cellular

---

[d] A prolific scientist, Meyer Friedman conducted many original studies and is credited with discovery of the type A behavior and its role as a coronary risk factor. He coined the term "hurry sickness" and was the first to show that cholesterol is absorbed by the lymphatic vessels of the distal ileum and was the first to perform coronary angiograms in dogs.[98]

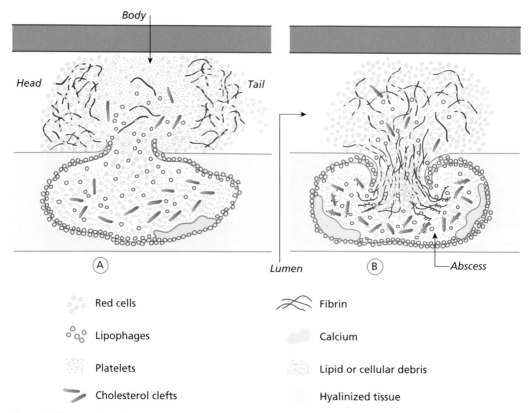

Red cells

Lipophages

Platelets

Cholesterol clefts

Fibrin

Calcium

Lipid or cellular debris

Hyalinized tissue

Figure 1.4 Rupture of an atheromatous abscess depicted by Meyer Friedman. (Reprinted from Am J Pathol 1966;48:19–44 with permission from the American Society for Investigative Pathology.)

debris, and a considerable number of macrophages (Figure 1.4). He believed that macrophages are derived from the adventitia. He described a direct communication between the occluding thrombi and the atheromatous abscesses in 39 of the 40 arteries he studied, and concluded that this rupture exposed the highly thrombogenic contents of the abscess to the blood leading to clot formation.[97] His careful pathologic examinations demonstrated that the rupture of these abscesses was almost always preceded by or associated with its invasion by lipophages. He wrote that "the cells not only advanced toward the lumen but also frequently toward the tunica media and adventitia as well." This finding was recently confirmed by **Pedro Moreno** and **Valentin Fuster**.[99]

Michael Davies (1937–2002) was another pioneer scientist who extensively studied plaque rupture and its associated features.[100] He exquisitely described the pathologic features of plaque disruption and the role of inflammation in the development of plaque instability. His invited address to the American Heart Association in 1995 "Stability and Instability: Two Faces of Coronary Atherosclerosis: The Paul Dudley White Lecture, 1995" summarized his findings.[101] Davies and Thomas[100] convincingly demonstrated the role of thrombosis in sudden cardiac death.

In 1987, **Seymour Glagov** introduced the "vascular remodeling phenomenon".[102] He demonstrated that human coronary arteries enlarge as the plaque grows. He showed that hemodynamically significant lumen stenosis may be delayed until the lesion occupies 40% of the internal elastic lamina area.[e] One year later, several research teams[105–108] showed that approximately 70% of MIs involve nonobstructive lesions that are not hemodynamically

---

[e] These remodeled lesions were later shown by Varnava and Davies to have a higher lipid content and macrophage count and high temperature heterogeneity, factors associated with plaque vulnerability.[103,104]

significant. These findings were of great clinical relevance, as in 1974 **V. Lance Gould** and his colleagues showed that resting coronary blood flow doesn't decrease until coronary arterial diameter is reduced by 85%,[109] which explains why many acute coronary events happen in the absence of previous chest pain or other clinical symptoms. The scientific community understood that the majority of the life-threatening lesions could not be detected by the available techniques and major research was begun to delineate the nature of these lesions and to find ways to detect and treat them.

During the 1980s and 1990s, numerous studies were performed to determine the mechanism leading to the development of atherosclerosis and its acute complications. **Erling Falk**, in a series of seminal studies, demonstrated the pivotal role of plaque disruptions and ruptures in sudden coronary death.[110–112]

In 1993, **Arbustini** demonstrated that in victims of sudden cardiac death, plaque erosion plays a significant role in addition to plaque rupture.[113] **Van der Wal, Farb**, and **Virmani** later carefully described the lesions and showed their importance especially in young women who smoke.[114,115]

Nomenclature

It was **James E. Muller**[f] who in 1989 named these hemodynamically insignificant, albeit dangerous, plaques "vulnerable plaques."[118] In 2001, **Renu Virmani** and her colleagues, **Kolodgie, Farb**, and **Burke** took into account the diverse etiology of coronary thrombi and described the type of precursor lesion associated with rupture as "thin-cap fibroatheroma (TCFA)".[119] **Valentin Fuster** proposed the nomenclature "high risk plaque" to acknowledge the role of plaques other than those with a large lipid content and thin fibrous cap (i.e. the classic vulnerable plaques) in the development of acute coronary syndromes.[120]

---

[f] Dr. James E. Muller is one of the founders of the International Physicians for the Prevention of Nuclear War (IPPNW), an organization which was awarded the 1985 Nobel Peace Prize. He compared the inflamed plaques to the nuclear silos which were vulnerable to attacks and coined the term "vulnerable plaque." In addition to researching the triggers of acute coronary syndromes,[116] he has been developing near infrared imaging tools for detection of vulnerable plaques.[117]

Biology of vulnerable plaques

Gerald Pasterkamp from the Netherlands illustrated the remodeling phenomenon in extensive pathologic studies and also showed the role of inflammation and macrophage infiltration in the development of plaque rupture and subsequent coronary thrombosis.[121,122] **PK Shah** and **Peter Libby** showed that a paucity of smooth muscle cells coupled with accumulation of macrophages, cause a decrease in collagen formation, hence weakening the fibrous cap.[123,124] Libby's lab illustrated that inflammation and the subsequent production of cytokines increase the expression of proteases and at the same time diminish the effect of proteolytic inhibitors.[125,126] **Zorina Galis** from Libby's lab described the importance of several matrix metalloproteinases in developing unstable lesions.[127] Libby's lab also showed the role of cytokine expression in initiation and progression of atherosclerosis.[128] **Yong-Jian Geng** described the importance of smooth muscle cell apoptosis in plaque instability, and **Mark Rekhter** detailed the balance of collagen synthesis and degradation and effect of inflammation in tipping the balance unfavorably.[129,130]

Valentin Fuster demonstrated the importance of platelets and blood coagulation diathesis in the development of thrombosis.[131] He and **Badimon** showed that a "vulnerable blood" state is important in thrombogenesis and that fast thrombosis is heavily affected by tissue factor production both in blood and in plaques.[132] In the 1990s, **Goran Hansson** from Sweden and **George Wick** from Austria pioneered the research illustrating the role of the immune system in the development of atherosclerosis and plaque formation. **Hansson** emphasized that specific antigens may elicit T-cell activation in plaques, and **Wick** described the role of heat shock proteins as important antigens in atherogenesis.[133,134]

James T Willerson and his colleagues, in an effort to explain the transition of stable lesions to unstable ones in the late 1970s, suggested that the changes in atherosclerotic plaques cause platelet adhesion and aggregation, release of thromboxane A_2, and dynamic vasoconstriction.[135,136] They subsequently showed the importance of several different platelet and nonplatelet derived mediators in leading to thrombosis and vasoconstriction in injured arteries, including thromboxane A_2, serotonin, adenosine diphosphate (ADP), thrombin, oxygen-derived free radicals, platelet activating factor, and endothelin.[135,137–140] They also demonstrated a relative absence of prostacyclin in injured arteries in contributing to thrombosis, vasoconstriction, and inflammation.[136] Subsequently, others have demonstrated a relative deficiency of tissue plasminogen activator and nitric oxide at similar locations.[141] This work emphasizes the "prothrom-

botic, proinflammatory and provasoconstrictive environment" that exists at sites of arterial injury. Willerson et al further suggested that at sites of arterial injury, transient thrombosis and vasoconstriction lead to unstable angina and more prolonged thrombosis and vasoconstriction to MI (Figure 1.5).[142] In 1996, **Ward Casscells** and **James T Willerson** showed that vulnerable plaques with a thin cap and a high macrophage content give off

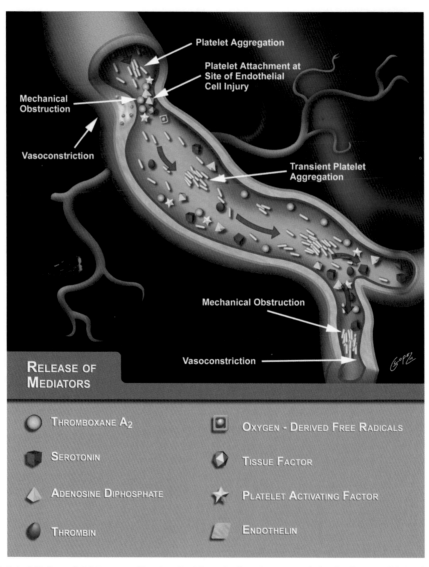

Figure 1.5 Arterial injury, platelet aggregation, transient thrombosis and vasoconstriction lead to unstable angina and myocardial infarction. (Adapted from Willerson JT, Cohn JN. Cardiovascular Medicine. Philadelphia: Churchill Livingstone, 2000.)

more heat and demonstrate temperature heterogeneity. This description was one of the first to suggest a method for "functional" assessment of plaque vulnerability.[143] Following a lecture by Dr Willerson in Athens, Greece in 1997, **Christodoulos Stefanadis** et al in 1999 demonstrated the presence of temperature heterogeneity in patients with unstable angina and AMI who underwent intravascular thermography.[144]

Conclusions

We have witnessed a rapid and extensive increase in atherosclerosis research in the past few decades. Pathologic studies have been the mainstay of studies for hundreds of years and have founded the majority of our current knowledge of this disease. New developments in imaging techniques and access to animal models of atherosclerosis through genetic modulations are enabling insight into both anatomy and physiology of the disease and the study of the disease in *in vivo* conditions.

Acknowledgment

Supported in part by DOD Grant #DAMD 17-01-2-0047.

References

1. Davies MJ, Woolf N. Atherosclerosis: what is it and why does it occur? Br Heart J 1993;69:S3–11.
2. Woolf N. Pathology of atherosclerosis. Br Med Bull 1990;46:960–85.
3. Ruffer MA. On arterial lesions found in Egyptian mummies. J Pathol Bacteriol 1911;15:453.
4. Moodie RL. Paleopathology: an introduction to the study of Ancient Evidences of Disease. Urbana: University of Illinois Press, 1923.
5. Graul EH. Environtologie – Fakten und Spekulationen. Medicef 1985;1:1–24.
6. Cockburn A, Barraco RA, Reyman TA, Peck WH. Autopsy of an Egyptian mummy. Science 1975;187:1155–60.
7. Hart GD, Cockburn A, Millet NB, Scott JW. Lessons learned from the autopsy of an Egyptian mummy. Can Med Assoc J 1977;117:415–18.
8. Zimmermann MR. The mummies of the Tomb of Nebwenenef: paleopathology and archeology. J Am Res Center Egypt 1977;14:33–6.
9. Zimmerman MR, Clark WH Jr. A possible case of subcorneal pustular dermatosis in an Egyptian mummy. Arch Dermatol 1976;112:204–5.
10. Zimmerman MR, Yeatman GW, Sprinz H, Titterington WP. Examination of an Aleutian mummy. Bull NY Acad Med 1971;47:80–103.
11. El-Najjar MY, Benitez J, Fry G, et al. Autopsies on two native American Mummies. Am J Phys Anthropol 1980;53:197–202.
12. Zimmerman MR, Smith GS. A probable case of accidental inhumation of 1600 years ago. Bull NY Acad Med 1975;51:828–37.
13. Zimmerman MR, Trinkaus E, LeMay M, et al. The paleopathology of an Aleutian mummy. Arch Pathol Lab Med 1981;105:638–41.
14. Dunn PM. Andreas Vesalius (1514–1564), Padua, and the fetal "shunts". Arch Dis Child Fetal Neonatal Ed 2003;88:F157–9.
15. Van der Eijk PJ. [Heart and brains, blood and pneuma. Hippocrates, Aristotle en Diocles on the localization of cognitive functions.] Gewina 1995;18:8–23.
16. Kohn H. Zur Geschichte der Angina pectoris. Zsahr Klin Med 1927:106.
17. Wilson LG. Erasistratus, Galen and the pneuma. Bull Hist Med 1959;33:293.
18. Tan SY, Yeow ME. Medicine in stamps. Paracelsus (1493–1541): the man who dared. Singapore Med J 2003;44:5–7.
19. Willius FA, Dry TJ. A history of heart and the circulation. Philadelphia: WB Saunders, 1948.
20. Leibowitz JO. The history of coronary heart disease. In: Berkely, ed: University of California, 1970 (cited in Gotto 1985[22]).
21. Keele KD. Leonardo da Vinci's views on arteriosclerosis. Med Hist 1973;17:304–8 (cited in Gotto 1985[22]).
22. Gotto AM Jr. Some reflections on arteriosclerosis: past, present, and future. Circulation 1985;72:8–17.
23. Bing RJ. Atherosclerosis. In: Bing RJ, ed. Cardiology: the evolution of science and the art. Philadelphia: Harwood Academic Publishers, 1992:127–143.
24. Long ER. Development of our knowledge of arteriosclerosis. In: Blumenthal HT, ed. Cowdry's Atherosclerosis. Springfield, IL: Charles C Thomas, 1967:5–20.
25. Harvey W. Exercitation Anatomica. De Motu Cordis et Sanguinis in Animalibus: Springfield, IL: Charles C Thomas, 1928.
26. Pascucci G. Storia della Letteratura Greca. Firenze: Sansoni, 1948.
27. Benivieni A. De Abditis nonnulis ac mirandis morborum et sanatorium causis. Springfield: Charles C Thomas, 1507.
28. Eslick GD. Chest pain: a historical perspective. Int J Cardiol 2001;77:5–11.

29. Hanke H, Lenz C, Finking G. The discovery of the pathophysiological aspects of atherosclerosis – a review. Acta Chir Belg 2001;101:162–9.

30. Silverman ME. Angina pectoris two hundred years later. J Med Assoc Ga 1970;59:464–5.

31. Warren J. Remarks on angina pectoris. N Engl J Med 1812;1:1–11.

32. Moriyama IM, Krueger DE, Stamler J. Cardiovascular disease in the United States. Harvard: Harvard University Press, 1971.

33. Manders EC, Manders EK. Academic surgeons, take heart: the story of a student, his mentor, and the discovery of the etiology of angina pectoris. Am Surg 1996;62:1076–9.

34. Osler W. Lectures on angina pectoris and allied states (1897). In: Fye BF, ed. William Osler's collected papers on the cardiovascular system. New York: Adams L B, 1985:239–57.

35. Danielopolu D. The pathology and surgical treatment of angina pectoris. Br Med J 1924;2:553.

36. Keefer CS, Resnik WH. Angina pectoris: a syndrome caused by anoxemia of the myocardium. Arch Intern Med 1928;41:769–807.

37. Latham PM. Diseases of the heart. London, 1845 (cited in Keefer 1928[36]).

38. Von Neusser E. Angina Pectoris. New York: EB Treat, 1909.

39. Gallavardin L. Les Angines de Poitrine. Paris: Masson & Cie, 1925.

40. Kohn H. Angina Pectoris, Aorten oder Koronarhypothese. Med Klin 1926;22:983.

41. Prinzmetal M, Massumi RA. The anterior chest wall syndrome: chest pain resembling pain of cardiac origin. J Am Med Assoc 1955;159:177–84.

42. Maseri A, L'Abbate A, Baroldi G, et al. Coronary vasospasm as a possible cause of myocardial infarction. A conclusion derived from the study of "preinfarction" angina. N Engl J Med 1978;299:1271–7.

43. Parry CH. An Inquiry into the Symptoms and Causes of the Syncope Angionosa, Commonly Called Angina Pectoris; illustrated by dissections. London: Candel & Davis, 1799:43–4.

44. Lobstein JF. Lehrbuch der pathologischen Anatomie. 2 Bd. Stuttgart: Fr. Brodhag'sche Buchhandlung, 1835.

45. Morgagni JOB. De sedibus, et causis morborum per anatomen indagatis libri quinque. In: Ventiis, ed. Ex Typographia Remondiniana, 1761.

46. Enzi G, Busetto L, Inelmen EM, Coin A, Sergi G. Historical perspective: visceral obesity and related comorbidity in Joannes Baptista Morgagni's "De sedibus et causis morborum per anatomen indagata." Int J Obes Relat Metab Disord 2003;27:534–5.

47. Acierno LJ. Atherosclerosis (arteriosclerosis). The history of cardiology. New York: Parthenon Publishing Group, 1994.

48. Cruveilhier J, Pattison GS, Madden WH. The anatomy of the human body. New York: Harper & Brothers, 1844.

49. Gmelin L. Von der Verengung und Schliessung der Pulsadern in Krankheiten. In: Tiedmann F, ed. Heidelberg/Leipzig: Druck und Velag von Karl Groose, 1843.

50. Tiedmann F. Von der Verengung und Schliessung der Pulsadern in Krankeiten. Heidelberg/Leipzig: Druck und Verlag von Karl Groos, 1843.

51. Rokitansky C. Lehrbuch der Pathologischen Anatomie. 3. umgearbeitete Aufl., Bd I. Wien: Braumüller und Seidel, 1855.

52. Virchow R. Preßische Medicinal-Zeitung XV. 1846:137 und 243.

53. Virchow R. Phlogose und Thrombose im Gefass-system. Gesammelte Abhandlungen zur Wissenschaftlichen. Medizin. Frankfurt: F, Meidinger, 1856.

54. Virchow R. Die Cellularpathologie in ihrer Begründung auf physiologische und pathologische Gewerbelehre.1. Aufl. Berlin: Hirschwald, 1858.

55. Burke AP, Kolodgie FD, Farb A, et al. Healed plaque ruptures and sudden coronary death: evidence that subclinical rupture has a role in plaque progression. Circulation 2001;103:934–40.

56. Libby P, Simon DI. Inflammation and thrombosis: the clot thickens. Circulation 2001;103:1718–20.

57. Kleinert R, Reichenhall B. Rudolf Ludwig Karl Virchow: http://www.whonamedit.com/doctor.cfm/912.html, 2001.

58. Aschoff L. Verh Dtsch Pathol Gesellsch 1907;10:106.

59. Anitschkow N, Chalatow S. On experimental cholesterin steatosis and its significance in the origin of some pathologic processes. Central Allg Pathol Pathol Anat 1913;24.

60. Saphir O. In: Bluementhal HT, ed. Inflammatory factors in arteriosclerosis. Springfield, IL: Charles C Thomas: 1967:415.

61. Ross R, Glomset JA. The pathogenesis of atherosclerosis (first of two parts). N Engl J Med 1976;295:369–77.

62. Ross R, Glomset JA. The pathogenesis of atherosclerosis (second of two parts). N Engl J Med 1976;295:420–5.

63. Ross R. The pathogenesis of atherosclerosis. N Engl J Med 1986;314:488.

64. Steinberg D, Parthasarathy S, Carew TE, Khoo JC, Witztum JL. Beyond cholesterol. Modifications of low-density lipoprotein that increase its atherogenicity. N Engl J Med 1989;320:915–24.

65. Steinberg D, Witztum JL. Lipoproteins and atherogenesis. Current concepts. JAMA 1990;264:3047–52.

66. Ross R. The pathogenesis of atherosclerosis: a perspective for the 1990s. Nature 1993;362:801–9.

67. Ross R. Atherosclerosis – an inflammatory disease. N Engl J Med 1999;340:115–26.

68. Herrick JB. Clinical features of sudden obstruction of the coronary arteries. JAMA 1912;23:2015.

69. Friedberg CK. Diseases of the Heart. Philadelphia, PA: WB Saunders, 1949:401–2.

70. Duguid JB. Thrombosis as a factor in pathogenesis of atherosclerosis. J Path Bact 1946;58:207.

71. Duguid JB. Pathogenesis of atherosclerosis. Lancet 1949;2:925.

72. Crawford T, Levene CI. Incorporation of fibrin in the aortic intima. J Path Bact 1952;64:523–8.

73. Meade TW, Mellows S, Brozovic M, et al. Haemostatic function and ischaemic heart disease: principal results of the Northwick Park Heart Study. Lancet 1986;2:533–7.

74. Roberts WC. Relationship between coronary thrombosis and myocardial infarction. Mod Concepts Cardiovasc Dis 1972;41:7–10.

75. DeWood MA, Spores J, Notske R, et al. Prevalence of total coronary occlusion during the early hours of transmural myocardial infarction. N Engl J Med 1980;303:897–902.

76. Fulton WFM. Does coronary thrombosis cause myocardial infarction or vice versa? In: Weatherall D, ed. Advanced Medicine. London: Pitman Medical, 1978:138–47.

77. Blumgart HL, Gilligan RMS. Experimental studies on the effect of temporary occlusion of coronary arteries. II. The production of myocardial infarction. Am Heart J 1941;22:374–89.

78. Maroko PR, Braunwald E. Modification of myocardial infarction size after coronary occlusion. Ann Intern Med 1973;79:720–33.

79. Reimer KA, Lowe JE, Rasmussen MM, Jennings RB. The wavefront phenomenon of ischemic cell death. 1. Myocardial infarct size vs duration of coronary occlusion in dogs. Circulation 1977;56:786–94.

80. Braunwald E. The open-artery theory is alive and well – again. N Engl J Med 1993;329:1650–2.

81. Loscalzo J, Braunwald E. Tissue plasminogen activator. N Engl J Med 1988;319:925–31.

82. Arteriosclerosis. Br Med J 1909:1800.

83. Enos WF, Holmes RH, Beyer J. Landmark article, July 18, 1953: Coronary disease among United States soldiers killed in action in Korea. Preliminary report. By William F. Enos, Robert H. Holmes and James Beyer. JAMA 1986;256:2859–62.

84. McNamara JJ, Molot MA, Stremple JF, Cutting RT. Coronary artery disease in combat casualties in Vietnam. JAMA 1971;216:1185–7.

85. Virmani R, Robinowitz M, Geer JC, Breslin PP, Beyer JC, McAllister HA. Coronary artery atherosclerosis revisited in Korean war combat casualties. Arch Pathol Lab Med 1987;111:972–6.

86. Berenson GS, Srinivasan SR, Bao W, Newman WP 3rd, Tracy RE, Wattigney WA. Association between multiple cardiovascular risk factors and atherosclerosis in children and young adults. The Bogalusa Heart Study. N Engl J Med 1998;338:1650–6.

87. Natural history of aortic and coronary atherosclerotic lesions in youth. Findings from the PDAY Study. Pathobiological Determinants of Atherosclerosis in Youth (PDAY) Research Group. Arterioscler Thromb 1993;13:1291–8.

88. Napoli C, D'Armiento FP, Mancini FP, et al. Fatty streak formation occurs in human fetal aortas and is greatly enhanced by maternal hypercholesterolemia. Intimal accumulation of low density lipoprotein and its oxidation precede monocyte recruitment into early atherosclerotic lesions. J Clin Invest 1997;100:2680–90.

89. Faergeman O. The atherosclerosis epidemic: methodology, nosology, and clinical practice. Am J Cardiol 2001;88:4–7.

90. Clark E, Graef I, Chasis H. Thrombosis of the aorta and coronary arteries with special reference to the "fibrinoid" lesions. Arch Pathol (Chicago) 1936;22:183–212.

91. Koch W, Kong LC. Über die formen des coronarverschlusses, die anderungen im coronarkreislauf und die beziehungen zur angina pectoris. Beitr Path Anat 1932/33;90:21–84.

92. Constantinides P. Plaque fissures in human coronary thrombosis. (Abstract). Fed Proc 1964;23:443.

93. Leary T. Pathology of coronary sclerosis. Am Heart J 1934;10:328–37.

94. Leary T. Coronary spasm as a possible factor in producing sudden death. Am Heart J 1934/35;10:338–44.

95. Yee KO, Ikari Y, Schwartz SM. An update of the Grutzbalg hypothesis: the role of thrombosis and coagulation in atherosclerotic progression. Thromb Haemost 2001;85:207–17.

96. Chapman I. Morphogenesis of occluding coronary artery thrombosis. Arch Pathol 1965;80:256–61.

97. Friedman M, Van den Bovenkamp GJ. The pathogenesis of a coronary thrombus. Am J Pathol 1966;48:19–44.

98. Friedland GW. Meyer Friedman, MD. Circulation 2001;104:2758.

99. Moreno PR, Purushothaman KR, Fuster V, O'Connor WN. Intimomedial interface damage and adventitial inflammation is increased beneath disrupted atherosclerosis in the aorta: implications for plaque vulnerability. Circulation 2002;105:2504–11.

100. Davies MJ, Thomas A. Thrombosis and acute coronary artery lesions in sudden cardiac ischemic death. N Engl J Med 1984;310:1137–40.

101. Davies MJ. Stability and instability: two faces of coronary atherosclerosis. The Paul Dudley White Lecture 1995. Circulation 1996;94:2013–20.

102. Glagov S, Weisenberg E, Zarins CK, Stankunavicius R, Kolettis GJ. Compensatory enlargement of human atherosclerotic coronary arteries. N Engl J Med 1987;316:1371–5.

103. Varnava AM, Mills PG, Davies MJ. Relationship between coronary artery remodeling and plaque vulnerability. Circulation 2002;105:939–43.

104. Toutouzas MK, Stefanadis CM, Vavuranakis MM, et al. Arterial remodeling in acute coronary syndromes: correlation of IVUS characteristics with temperature of the culprit lesion. Circulation 2000;102:II-707.

105. Ambrose JA, Tannenbaum MA, Alexopoulos D, et al. Angiographic progression of coronary artery disease and the development of myocardial infarction. J Am Coll Cardiol 1988;12:56–62.

106. Haft JI, Haik BJ, Goldstein JE, Brodyn NE. Development of significant coronary artery lesions in areas of minimal disease. A common mechanism for coronary disease progression. Chest 1988;94:731–6.

107. Hackett D, Davies G, Maseri A. Pre-existing coronary stenoses in patients with first myocardial infarction are not necessarily severe. Eur Heart J 1988;9:1317–23.

108. Little WC, Constantinescu M, Applegate RJ, et al. Can coronary angiography predict the site of a subsequent myocardial infarction in patients with mild-to-moderate coronary artery disease? Circulation 1988;78:1157–66.

109. Gould KL, Lipscomb K, Hamilton GW. Physiologic basis for assessing critical coronary stenosis. Instantaneous flow response and regional distribution during coronary hyperemia as measures of coronary flow reserve. Am J Cardiol 1974;33:87–94.

110. Falk E. Plaque rupture with severe pre-existing stenosis precipitating coronary thrombosis. Characteristics of coronary atherosclerotic plaques underlying fatal occlusive thrombi. Br Heart J 1983;50:127–34.

111. Falk E. Why do plaques rupture? Circulation 1992;86:III30–42.

112. Falk E, Shah PK, Fuster V. Coronary plaque disruption. Circulation 1995;92:657–71.

113. Arbustini E, Grasso M, Diegoli M, et al. Coronary thrombosis in non-cardiac death. Coron Artery Dis 1993;4:751–9.

114. van der Wal A, Becker A, van der Loos C, Das P. Site of intimal rupture or erosion of thrombosed coronary atherosclerotic plaques is characterized by an inflammatory process irrespective of the dominant plaque morphology. Circulation 1994;89:36–44.

115. Farb A, Burke AP, Tang AL, et al. Coronary plaque erosion without rupture into a lipid core: a frequent cause of coronary thrombosis in sudden coronary death. Circulation 1996;93:1354–63.

116. Tofler GH, Muller JE. Prevention and practical aspects of triggering of cardiovascular events. Cardiol Clin 1996;14:309–12.

117. Moreno PR, Muller JE. Detection of high-risk atherosclerotic coronary plaques by intravascular spectroscopy. J Interv Cardiol 2003;16:243–52.

118. Muller JE, Tofler GH, Stone PH. Circadian variation and triggers of onset of acute cardiovascular disease. Circulation 1989;79:733–43.

119. Kolodgie FD, Burke AP, Farb A, et al. The thin-cap fibroatheroma: a type of vulnerable plaque: the major precursor lesion to acute coronary syndromes. Curr Opin Cardiol 2001;16:285–92.

120. Fayad ZA, Fuster V. The human high-risk plaque and its detection by magnetic resonance imaging. Am J Cardiol 2001;88:42E–45E.

121. Pasterkamp G, Schoneveld AH, van der Wal AC, et al. Inflammation of the atherosclerotic cap and shoulder of the plaque is a common and locally observed feature in unruptured plaques of femoral and coronary arteries. Arterioscler Thromb Vasc Biol 1999;19:54–8.

122. Pasterkamp G, Wensing PJW, Post MJ, Hillen B, Mali WPTM, Borst C. Paradoxical arterial wall shrinkage may contribute to luminal narrowing of human atherosclerotic femoral arteries. Circulation 1995;91:1444–9.

123. Shah PK, Falk E, Badimon JJ, et al. Human monocyte-derived macrophages induce collagen breakdown in fibrous caps of atherosclerotic plaques. Potential role of matrix-degrading metalloproteinases and implications for plaque rupture. Circulation 1995;92:1565–9.

124. Libby P, Geng YJ, Aikawa M, et al. Macrophages and atherosclerotic plaque stability. Curr Opin Lipidol 1996;7:330–5.

125. Shi G-P, Sukhova GK, Grubb A, et al. Cystatin C deficiency in human atherosclerosis and aortic aneurysms. J Clin Invest 1999;104:1191–7.

126. Dollery CM, Owen CA, Sukhova GK, Krettek A, Shapiro SD, Libby P. Neutrophil elastase in human atherosclerotic plaques: production by macrophages. Circulation 2003;107:2829–36.

127. Galis ZS, Sukhova GK, Lark MW, Libby P. Increased expression of matrix metalloproteinases and matrix degrading activity in vulnerable regions of human atherosclerotic plaques. J Clin Invest 1994;94:2493–503.

128. Libby P. Molecular bases of the acute coronary syndromes. Circulation 1995;91:2844–50.

129. Geng Y-J, Libby P. Progression of atheroma: a struggle between death and procreation. Arterioscler Thromb Vasc Biol 2002;22:1370–80.

130. Rekhter MD. Collagen synthesis in atherosclerosis: too much and not enough. Cardiovascular Research 1999;41:376–84.

131. Fuster V, Steele PM, Chesebro JH. Role of platelets and thrombosis in coronary atherosclerotic disease and sudden death. J Am Coll Cardiol 1985;5:175B–184B.

132. Badimon L, Badimon JJ, Galvez A, Chesebro JH, Fuster V. Influence of arterial damage and wall shear rate on platelet deposition. Ex vivo study in a swine model. Arteriosclerosis 1986;6:312–20.

133. Hansson GK, Jonasson L, Seifert PS, Stemme S. Immune mechanisms in atherosclerosis. Arteriosclerosis 1989;9: 567–78.

134. Wick G, Schett G, Amberger A, Kleindienst R, Xu Q. Is atherosclerosis an immunologically mediated disease? Immunol Today 1995;16:27–33.

135. Hirsh PD, Hillis LD, Campbell WB, Firth BG, Willerson JT. Release of prostaglandins and thromboxane into the coronary circulation in patients with ischemic heart disease. N Engl J Med 1981;304:685–91.

136. Hirsh PD, Campbell WB, Willerson JT, Hillis LD. Prostaglandins and ischemic heart disease. Am J Med 1981;71:1009–26.

137. Fujise K, Stacy L, Beck P, et al. Differential effects of endothelin receptor activation on cyclic flow variations in rat mesenteric arteries. Circulation 1997;96:3641–6.

138. Apprill P, Schmitz JM, Campbell WB, et al. Cyclic blood flow variations induced by platelet-activating factor in stenosed canine coronary arteries despite inhibition of thromboxane synthetase, serotonin receptors, and alpha-adrenergic receptors. Circulation 1985;72:397–405.

139. Guyton JR, Willerson JT. Peripheral venous platelet aggregates in patients with unstable angina pectoris and acute myocardial infarction. Angiology 1977;28: 695–701.

140. Willerson JT. Conversion from chronic to acute coronary heart disease syndromes. Role of platelets and platelet products. Tex Heart Inst J 1995;22:13–19.

141. Folts JD, Stamler J, Loscalzo J. Intravenous nitroglycerin infusion inhibits cyclic blood flow responses caused by periodic platelet thrombus formation in stenosed canine coronary arteries. Circulation 1991;83:2122–7.

142. Willerson JT, Campbell WB, Winniford MD, et al. Conversion from chronic to acute coronary artery disease: speculation regarding mechanisms. Am J Cardiol 1984;54:1349–54.

143. Casscells W, Hathorn B, David M, et al. Thermal detection of cellular infiltrates in living atherosclerotic plaques: possible implications for plaque rupture and thrombosis. Lancet 1996;347:1447–51.

144. Stefanadis C, Diamantopoulos L, Vlachopoulos C, et al. Thermal heterogeneity within human atherosclerotic coronary arteries detected *in vivo*: a new method of detection by application of a special thermography catheter. Circulation 1999;99:1965–71.

PART 2

Pathology

CHAPTER 2

The pathology of vulnerable plaque

Renu Virmani, Allen P Burke, James T Willerson, Andrew Farb,
Jagat Narula & Frank D Kolodgie

Although cellular and molecular biology studies have greatly advanced our knowledge of the pathophysiology of cardiovascular disease, our laboratory has gathered insight into the mechanisms responsible for coronary thrombosis by meticulous analysis of the underlying plaque morphology in autopsy specimens from sudden coronary death victims with severe coronary artery atherosclerosis.[1,2] In approximately 50–60% of these cases, the culprit lesion (fatal plaque) exhibits an acute coronary thrombus whereas the remainder include stable coronary plaques with >75% cross-sectional area luminal narrowing.[3] More than half of patients without acute coronary thrombi have healed myocardial infarcts that could be responsible for sudden death, and in 15–20% of cases there is no myocardial pathology to point to a terminal arrhythmia.[4] In this overview, we will discuss what characterizes an arterial plaque that is vulnerable to rupture in addition to how plaque progression leads to severe stenosis. These critical issues may help define the causes of sudden coronary death and assist in the development of treatment options targeting the unstable plaque.

Luminal thrombosis and acute coronary syndromes

Patients with acute coronary syndromes typically present with unstable angina, acute myocardial infarction, and sudden coronary death. Most acute coronary syndromes are precipitated by luminal thrombi, which arise from three different plaque morphologies: rupture, erosion, and calcified nodules.[4] Plaque rupture is defined as a lesion consisting of a necrotic core with an overlying thin disrupted fibrous cap heavily infiltrated by macrophages and T-lymphocytes; a luminal thrombus develops because of physical contact between platelets and the thrombogenic necrotic core. By contrast, erosions present with a luminal thrombus superimposed on a smooth muscle cell and proteoglycan-rich plaque with few inflammatory cells. Most eroded lesions are devoid of a necrotic core, but when present, there is no communication of the thrombus with the necrotic core because of a thick intact fibrous cap. Finally, the calcified nodule is the least common of all lesions that cause coronary thrombi. These lesions typically contain calcified plates along with bony nodules that erupt into a lumen devoid of endothelial cells.

The frequency of the coronary lesions with thrombi is 55–60% for ruptures, 30–35% for erosions, and 3–7% along with calcified nodules. Both ruptured and eroded lesions appear similar by angiography (Figure 2.1).[5] Although lesions with rupture occur in men of all ages (this is consistent for all plaque morphologies with thrombi), the frequency of sudden coronary death decreases with advancing age. Approximately 80% of coronary thrombi in women greater than 50 years old occur from plaque rupture and there is a strong association with circulating cholesterol. In acute myocardial infarction or sudden coronary death, plaque erosion occurs primarily in patients under the age of 50 years, and represents the majority of acute coronary thrombi in premenopausal women.[6] Further, 20–25% of acute myocardial infarcts occurring in hospitalized patients are due to plaque erosion.[7] In elderly patients, nonthrombotic substrates for sudden

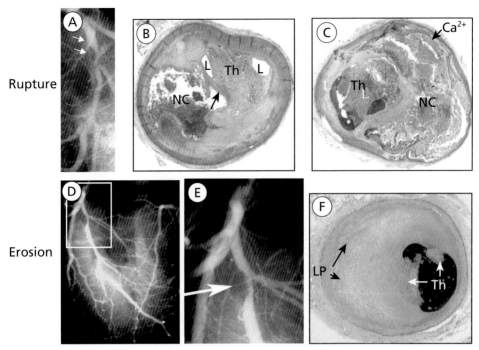

Figure 2.1 Angiographic and histologic representation of plaque rupture and erosion. A 43-year-old white male with no known history of risk factors was found unresponsive in the bathroom where he was last seen alive 20 minutes earlier. A, Postmortem angiogram shows the LAD at the origin of the left diagonal with a near total occlusion. Sections taken from these sites show a plaque rupture (arrow, B) with an underlying necrotic core (NC). The occluded artery shows an organizing thrombus with small lumens (L). In C, the fibrous cap is intact with a large underlying necrotic core with peripheral calcification (Ca²⁺) and the lumen shows organizing thrombus (Th) with small lumens (L). At autopsy there was a healing transmural myocardial infarction present in the distribution of the LAD. Postmortem angiogram (D, E) and corresponding photomicrograph (F) from a 38-year-old man who was last seen alive 8 hours antemortem, who died from sudden coronary death. A focal stenosis is present in the left anterior coronary artery (boxed area), which is highlighted in E and an arrow points to the area of narrowing at the take off of the left diagonal. F, Acute nonocclusive luminal thrombus (Th) is present on the surface of an erosive plaque rich in proteoglycans (green), and the underlying plaque shows pathologic intimal thickening with lipid pools (LP). (Reproduced in part from figure 4, Farb A, et al., Circulation 1995;92:1701–1709.)

cardiac death, such as cardiomegaly and myocardial scarring, are more frequent.

Plaque rupture and its precursor lesion – the thin cap fibroatheroma

The morphology of plaque rupture consists of a relatively large necrotic core with an overlying thin disrupted fibrous cap infiltrated by macrophages. The smooth muscle cells component within the cap is absent or sparse. The thickness of the fibrous cap near the rupture site is 23 ± 19 μm, with 95% of the caps measuring less than 64 μm.[1] Those plaques that closely resemble ruptures but lack a luminal

thrombus have been designated by our laboratory as thin-cap fibroatheromas (TCFA), or more traditionally, vulnerable plaques (Figures 2.2, 2.3).[4] In a more conservative sense, however, the term "vulnerable" should be reserved for lesions that underlie all causes of coronary thrombi, including pathologic intimal thickening, thick- and thin-cap fibroatheromas, and calcified plaques with nodules.

Although there are similarities, TCFAs differ from ruptured plaques based on a trend towards a smaller necrotic core, fewer macrophages within the fibrous cap, and generally less calcification (Table 2.1). We have quantified several morphologic

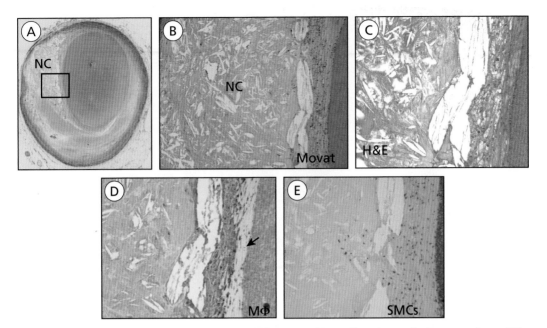

Figure 2.2 A nonhemodynamically limiting thin-cap fibroatheroma. A thin-cap fibroatheroma having a necrotic core (NC) and an overlying thin fibrous cap (<65 μm) is shown in A. B, High-power view of the boxed area in A. Note an advanced necrotic core with a large number of cholesterol clefts with surrounding loss of matrix, and no cellular infiltration is seen. The fibrous cap is infiltrated by macrophages, better seen in C when stained by H&E. D and E show macrophage infiltration (CD68+) and rare staining of smooth muscle cells (α-actin positive) in the fibrous cap. (Reproduced with permission from Kolodgie F, et al., Heart 2004;90:1385–1391.)

Table 2.1 Morphologic characteristics of plaque rupture and thin-cap fibroatheroma. (Reproduced with permission from Kolodgie FD et al., Curr Opin Cardiol 2001;16:286–290.)

Plaque type	Necrotic core (%)	Fibrous cap thickness (μm)	Mφs (%)	SMCs (%)	T-lymph	Calcification score
Rupture	34 ± 17	23 ± 19	26 ± 20	0.002 ± 0.004	4.9 ± 4.3	1.53 ± 1.03
TCFA	23 ± 17	<65	14 ± 10	6.6 ± 10.4	6.6 ± 10.4	0.97 ± 1.1
P value	NS		0.005		NS	0.014

Mean values ± standard deviation are given. Abbreviations: Mφs = macrophages; SMCs = smooth muscle cells; T-lymph = T-lymphocytes; TCFA = thin-cap fibroatheroma.

parameters in various human coronary plaque types, including culprit lesions (Table 2.2). The number of cholesterol clefts in the necrotic core, vasa vasorum, and hemosiderin-laden macrophages are significantly greater in ruptured plaques than in erosions or stable plaques with >75% cross-sectional-luminal narrowing. Significant differences in cellular infiltration between TCFAs and ruptures were found only for macrophages as well as a greater

accumulation of hemosiderin. Hemorrhagic events at other sites of the coronary vasculature are more common in rupture cases than in those with severe coronary disease without luminal thrombi. The mean number of hemorrhages in lesions from patients with plaque rupture was 2.5 ± 1.3 versus zero in erosion ($P = 0.0001$) and 0.05 ± 0.6 in stable plaques ($P = 0.04$).[4] Evidence of prior hemorrhages in TCFAs, when analyzed by anti-glycophorin

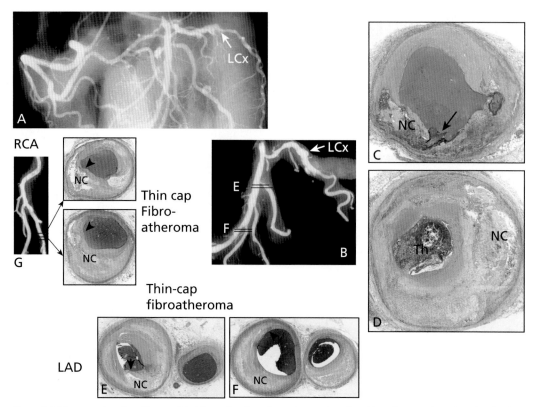

Figure 2.3 Plaque rupture in a 43-year-old white male who collapsed at work and could not be resuscitated. Patient had recent complaints of shoulder pain and headache but no known medical history or risk factor. At autopsy there was hemopericardium with 500 ml of blood and a long vertical tear on the posterolateral surface of the left ventricle. There was an acute transmural myocardial infarction lateral wall of the left ventricle and a hemorrhagic tract in the area of the rupture, which was located in the middle of the infarct. Coagulation necrosis with prominent neutrophilic inflammatory infiltrate was noted, consistent with a 2–3-day-old infarct. A postmortem angiogram showed total occlusion of the left circumflex (LCx) artery (arrow in A and B) and the sections showed the site of fibrous cap rupture (arrow in C) and an underlying hemorrhagic necrosis (NC), just distal to the site of rupture the coronary artery showed underlying atherosclerosis with a 70% diameter stenosis and an overlying occlusive thrombus (Th) (D). Sections taken from the first diagonal and left anterior descending (LAD) (E) and another from the third diagonal and LAD (F) show areas of thin cap fibroatheroma (vulnerable plaque) with mild insignificant luminal narrowing of the LAD with positive remodeling. G, Angiogram of the distal right coronary artery (RCA) and the PDA, shows mild irregularities and at the site of sectioning, shown in white lines. Note in these two sections the sites of thin cap fibroatheroma (vulnerable plaque; arrow) with thin fibrous cap and underlying necrotic core (NC). (Reproduced with permission from Kolodgie F. et al., Heart 2004;90:1385–1391.)

A staining (a protein specific to the erythrocyte membrane), is significantly greater than in fibroatheromas with early or late necrosis or lesions with pathologic intimal thickening and correlates with both necrotic core size and extent of macrophage infiltration.[8]

Healed plaque ruptures

Morphologic studies suggest that plaque progression beyond 40–50% cross-sectional-luminal narrowing occurs secondary to repeated ruptures, which may or may not be clinically silent. Ruptured lesions with healed repair sites are called healed plaque ruptures (HPR) and as shown by Davies et al., these plaques are easily detected microscopically by the identification of breaks in the fibrous cap with an overlying repair reaction consisting of a proteoglycan-rich mass or a collagen-rich scar tissue, depending on the duration of healing (Figure 2.4).[9]

Table 2.2 Comparison of necrotic core size, number of cholesterol clefts, macrophage infiltration, number of vasa vasorum, and hemosiderin-laden macrophages in culprit plaques. (Reproduced with permission from Virmani R et al., Arterioscler Thromb Vasc Biol 2000;20:1262–1275.)

Plaque type	Necrotic core (%)	Cholesterol clefts (%)	Macrophage infiltration of fibrous cap (%)	Mean no. vasa vasorum	Mean no. hemosiderin-laden macrophages
Rupture	$34 \pm 17^{\Omega,\ni}$	$12 \pm 12^{*,\wedge}$	$26 \pm 20^{\psi,\tau,\varpi}$	$44 \pm 22^{\varphi,\perp,\partial}$	$18.9 \pm 11^{\delta,\lambda,\in}$
TCFA	24 ± 17	8 ± 9	$14 \pm 10^{\psi}$	$26 \pm 23^{\varphi}$	$4.4 \pm 3.6^{\sigma}$
Erosion	$14 \pm 14^{\Omega}$	$2 \pm 5^{*}$	$10 \pm 12^{\tau}$	$28 \pm 18^{\perp}$	$4.3 \pm 4.7^{\lambda}$
Stable	$12 \pm 25^{\ni}$	$4 \pm 6^{\wedge}$	$3 \pm 0.7^{\varpi}$	$13 \pm 9^{\partial}$	$5.0 \pm 9.3^{\in}$
P value	$\Omega\,0.003$	$*0.002$	$\psi\,0.005$	$\varphi\,0.07$	$\delta\,0.001$
	$\ni\,0.01$	$\wedge\,0.04$	$\tau < 0.0001$	$\perp\,0.02$	$\lambda < 0.0001$
			$\varpi\,0.0001$	$\partial\,0.01$	$\in\,0.03$

Abbreviation: TCFA = thin-cap fibroatheroma.
The Greek notations are for comparison.

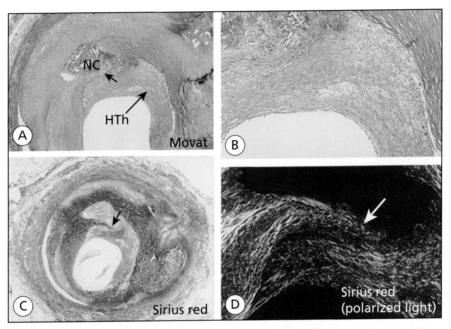

Figure 2.4 Healed plaque rupture. A and B, Movat pentachrome. A, Areas of intraintimal lipid-rich core with hemorrhage and cholesterol clefts; an old area of necrosis (NC) is seen underlying a healed thrombus (HTh). B, Higher magnification showing extensive smooth muscle cells within a collagenous proteoglycan-rich neointima (healed thrombus) with clear demarcation from the fibrous region of old plaque to right. C and D, Layers of collagen by Sirius red staining. C, Note area of dense, dark-red collagen surrounding lipid hemorrhagic cores seen in corresponding view in A. D, Image taken with polarized light. Dense collagen (type 1) that forms fibrous cap is reddish-yellow and is disrupted (arrow), with newer greenish type III collagen on right and above rupture site. (Reproduced with permission from Burke et al., Circulation 2001;103:934–940.)

Early-healed lesions are rich in proteoglycans, which is eventually replaced by type I collagen.

The prevalence of silent ruptures in the clinical population is unknown. Few angiographic studies have demonstrated plaque progression and short-term studies have suggested that thrombosis is the likely cause. Davies showed that the frequency of HPRs increases along with lumen narrowing.[9] In

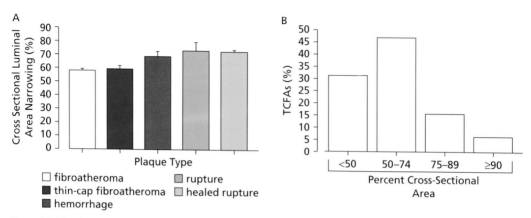

Figure 2.5 Morphometric analysis of thin-cap fibroatheromas. A, The percentage cross-sectional area luminal narrowing by type of plaque. The thin-cap fibroatheromas and fibroatheromas are less narrowed than plaque rupture and healed plaque rupture. B, Over 80% of thin-cap atheromas have <75% cross-sectional area luminal narrowing.

plaques with 0–20% diameter stenosis, the incidence of HPRs was 16%, and in lesions with 21–50% stenosis the incidence was 19% and in plaques with >50% narrowing, the incidence was 73%. In our laboratory, 61% of hearts from sudden coronary death victims show HRPs; this incidence is highest in stable plaques (80% HPRs), followed by acute plaque rupture (75% HPRs) and plaque erosions (9% HPRs).[10] Multiple healed ruptures with layering were common in segments with acute and healed ruptures and the percent cross-sectional-luminal narrowing was dependent on the number of healed repair sites. The underlying percent luminal narrowing for acute ruptures exceeds that for healed ruptures (79 ± 15% vs. 66 ± 14%, $P = 0.0001$).

Thin-cap fibroatheroma – location, extent of luminal narrowing, length and percent area of the plaque occupied by necrotic core

The extent of luminal narrowing varies with lesion morphology (Figure 2.5A). TCFAs and fibroatheromas have the least luminal narrowing while lesions with acute plaque rupture, hemorrhage, or healed repair sites show the most stenosis. The vast majority of TCFAs (over 80%) have <75% cross-sectional-area luminal narrowing (i.e. <50% diameter stenosis, Figure 2.5B). Healed and acute plaque ruptures show the severest narrowing with 46% and 43%, respectively showing less than 70%

cross-sectional-area narrowing. By contrast, only 27% of TCFAs show severe luminal narrowing (Figure 2.6). In a population whose first manifestation of coronary disease is sudden death, these findings are consistent with the hypothesis that TCFAs are precursor lesions to ruptures and that healed plaque ruptures are mostly clinically silent.[10]

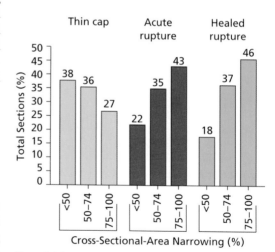

Figure 2.6 Percent cross-sectional area narrowing by plaque morphology. Severe narrowing (>75% cross-sectional area luminal narrowing) was more frequently seen in plaque ruptures and healed plaque ruptures than thin-cap fibroatheroma. Note 74% of thin-cap fibroatheromas were ≤74% narrowed in cross-sectional area. (Reproduced with permission from Virmani R, et al., J Interv Cardiol 2002;15:439–446.)

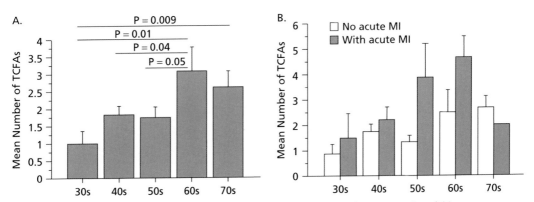

Figure 2.7 Frequency of thin-cap fibroatheromas by decades. A, Bar graph shows the mean number of thin-cap fibroatheromas (TCFAs) in individuals with sudden coronary death stratified by decades. Note, the majority of TCFAs are found in individuals in their sixties and seventies. B, Bar plot illustrating the mean number of TCFA (purple bars) in individuals with or without acute myocardial infarction (AMI). Patients with an AMI have a greater frequency of TCFA then those without and the difference are greater in those in their fifties and sixties.

Table 2.3 Approximate size of the necrotic core in advanced plaques. (Reproduced with permission from Virmani R et al., J Interv Cardiol 2002;15:439–46.)

| | Plaque type | | |
Dimension	Fibrous cap atheroma	Thin-cap fibroatheroma	Acute plaque rupture
Length (mm)			
Mean	6	8 mm	9 mm
Range	1–18 mm	2–17 mm	2.5–22 mm
Necrotic core area (mm²)	1.2 ± 2.2	1.7 ± 1.1	3.8 ± 5.5
Necrotic core (%)	15 ± 20	23 ± 17	34 ± 17

Values of the necrotic core represent mean $\pm$ SD.

In sudden coronary deaths, the number of TCFAs is least in individuals dying in their thirties versus their sixties or seventies. Although the incidence of TCFAs occurring in the thirties, forties or fifties is similar, there is a sudden rise in the sixties and seventies (Figure 2.7A). Moreover, the incidence in each decade is highest in individuals dying with an acute myocardial infarction versus those without a history of infarction (Figure 2.7B).

The mean necrotic core size in lesions from sudden coronary death victims is independent of luminal narrowing and greatest in plaque ruptures, followed by TCFAs, and is least in fibroatheromas (Table 2.3). In a detailed morphometric analysis of ruptured plaques, 80% of necrotic cores were larger than 1.0 mm² and comprised >10% of the plaque area in nearly 90% of lesions (Figure 2.8). In 65% of ruptures, the necrotic core occupies >25% of the plaque. By contrast, only 75% of TCFAs have necrotic cores >10% of the plaque area. The mean cross-section-luminal narrowing in TCFAs is 71% with the necrotic core representing 10–25% of the lesion. On the other hand, the length of the necrotic core in ruptures and TCFAs is similar, varying from 2 to 22.5 mm, with a mean of 8 and 9 mm, respectively (Table 2.3).[11] In plaque vulnerability, it may be critical whether the necrotic core is circumferential and what percentage of the artery is affected. We have measured the circumference of necrotic cores in cross-sections of coronary arteries and

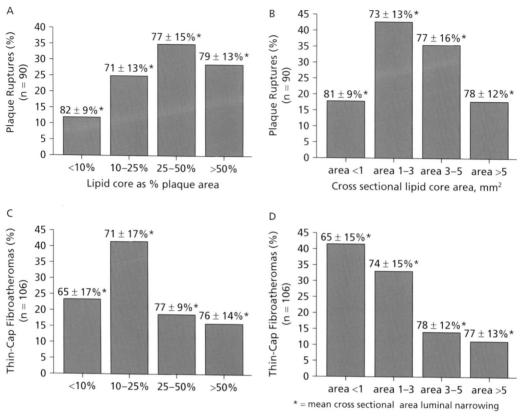

Figure 2.8 The distribution frequency of plaque ruptures (A, B) and thin-cap fibroatheromas (C, D) by size of lipid core or lipid core as a percent of plaque area. The majority of plaque ruptures occur when the lipid core area forms 25–50% of plaque area, or 1–3 mm² lipid core area. In the case of thin-cap fibroatheromas, the degree of cross-sectional area luminal narrowing and area of necrotic core is shifted to the left (lesser or smaller) as compared to plaque ruptures. (Reproduced with permission from Burke AP, et al., J Am Cardiol 2003;41:1874–1886.)

have determined that on average 75% of TCFAs have >120 degrees of the intima affected by necrosis (Figures 2.9, 2.10).

In 38 hearts with severe stenosis, in which the coronary arteries had been serially cut from the ostium to a distal intramyocardial location, the mean cross-sectional narrowing was least in lesions with TCFAs (59.6%), intermediate for those lesions with hemorrhage into a plaque (68.8%), and greatest in ruptures (73.3%) or healed plaque rupture (72.8%).[11] Overall, approximately 80% of TCFAs show <75% cross-sectional-luminal narrowing (Figure 2.5A), indicating that sites with <50% diameter stenosis are the most useful for the detection of vulnerable plaque. Moreover, acute and healed ruptures, lesions with intramural hemorrhage, and TCFAs

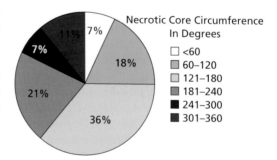

Figure 2.9 Circumferential presence of the necrotic core in each section measured in degrees. The majority of necrotic cores in thin-cap fibroatheromas are between 121 and 180 degrees in circumference; approximately 75% of these lesions have necrotic cores >120 degrees in circumference.

Insignificant plaque burden	Large eccentric necrotic core	Large concentric necrotic core	Healed rupture(s)

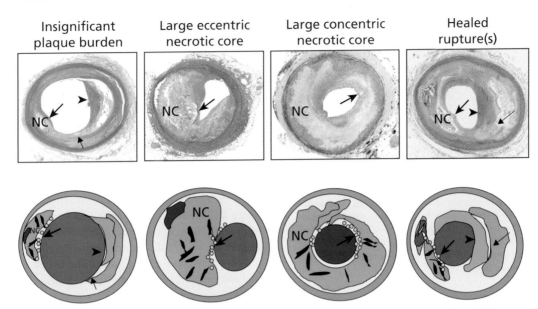

Figure 2.10 Photomicrographs with corresponding cartoon illustrations demonstrating morphologic variants of the thin-cap fibroatheroma. An attenuated fibrous cap infiltrated by macrophages, and sparsely populated by α-actin positive smooth muscle cells, characterizes this lesion. The underlying necrotic core may be calcified with areas of hemorrhage. The lesion in the left panel is an example of insignificant plaque burden; there is marked fibrous cap thinning (arrow) with a relatively small necrotic core (NC). A healed plaque rupture repair site is seen on the right (arrowhead) and the small arrow highlights the suspected point of rupture. The lesion on the extreme right shows a previous site of plaque rupture and an area of fibrous cap thinning (arrow) in a plaque with severe luminal narrowing. Stenotic lesions with previous healed repair sites and cap thinning are the most common variant of the thin-cap fibroatheroma. The two lesions in the middle panels are examples of plaques containing large eccentric or concentric necrotic cores with fibrous cap thinning (arrows). Note these lesions are an uncommon cause of sudden death in the presence of plaque rupture. In a large series of 142 cases only 11% of acute ruptures show rupture of a virgin plaque without evidence of prior rupture. Key: yellow = collagen; red = lumen/hemorrhage; green = new collagen; purple = calcification, orange = necrotic core, blue = macrophages, and white = cholesterol crystals. (Reproduced with permission from Kolodgie FD, et al., Curr Opin Cardiol 2001;16:286–290.)

are associated with positive remodeling, while stable plaques (fibrous-rich lesions), total occlusions, and erosions all show negative remodeling.

Incidence of thin-cap fibroatheroma in various coronary syndromes and its distribution in the coronary arteries

In patients with an acute myocardial infarction, the incidence of TCFAs is highest in males with a mean of three per heart with half as many in women (Figure 2.11). In patients dying suddenly, however, the incidence is similar between both sexes. Incidental deaths or those from plaque erosion show the fewest number of TCFAs. The number of TCFAs by plaque morphology shows the highest

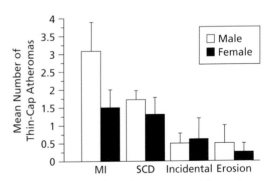

Figure 2.11 Thin-cap fibroatheromas are most frequent in patients dying with acute myocardial infarction (MI), followed by sudden coronary death (SCD) victims and incidental disease. Fibroatheromas and thin-cap fibroatheromas are uncommon in patients dying with plaque erosion. (Reproduced with permission from Burke AP, et al., J Am Coll Cardiol 2003;41:1874–86.)

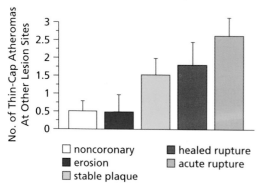

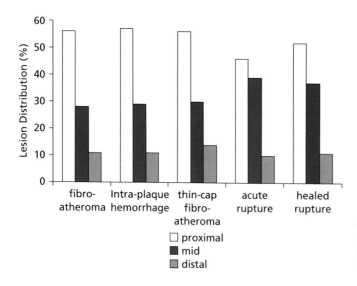

Figure 2.12 Number of thin-cap atheromas by cause of sudden coronary death. Bar graph showing the number of thin-cap fibroatheromas by cause of sudden coronary death. On average, each case of acute rupture shows at least two thin-cap fibroatheromas at other sites of coronary tree.

in cases of plaque rupture followed by healed plaque rupture, and stable plaques; the incidence is least in erosion and noncoronary deaths (Figure 2.12).[12]

Location and distribution of thin-cap fibroatheromas

The majority of TCFAs, acute and healed ruptures, lesion with intraplaque hemorrhage, and fibroatheromas occur predominantly in the proximal portion of the three major coronary arteries and about half arise in the mid-portion of these arteries (Figure 2.13). These lesions are few in the distal coronary circulation. By far the proximal portion

of the left anterior descending coronary artery is the most frequent location with sites in the proximal right and left circumflex coronary arteries about half as common. Other locations of significant lesion development are infrequent (Figure 2.14).

Inflammation and causation of occlusive thrombi

We have shown that fibrous cap thickness is dependent on the amount of macrophage infiltrate; the thicker the fibrous cap the fewer the macrophages (Figure 2.15). Serial sections of TCFAs have show that necrotic cores may begin deep within the plaque but over a relatively short distance of <1.4 cm the lipid core may approach the lumen, and therefore serial sectioning may help identify the presence of TCFAs (Figure 2.16).

Many investigators believe that inflammation is predominantly responsible for acute coronary syndromes, in particular ruptured plaques.[13] Fibrous cap rupture allows platelets and inflammatory cells to come into contact with the thrombogenic necrotic core. Before the innovative studies of Nemerson et al., demonstrating circulating tissue factor, the necrotic core was thought to be its major source.[14] It is now thought that circulating monocytes rather than plaque macrophages support the development of acute thrombi in unstable coronary plaques.

In a preliminary study, monocyte infiltration of the thrombus correlated with the severity of

Figure 2.13 Distribution of various unstable plaques from the coronary ostium. Coronary locations were divided into proximal, middle, and distal.

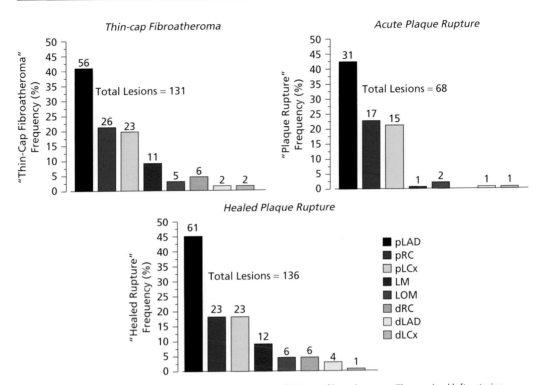

Thin-cap Fibroatheroma

Acute Plaque Rupture

Healed Plaque Rupture

Figure 2.14 Bar graphs illustrating the frequency and location of thin-cap fibroatheromas. The proximal left anterior descending coronary artery (pLAD) represents the first 0.5 cm of the artery measured to the second diagonal branch. The proximal right coronary artery (pRC) includes the distance to the right marginal branch of the right coronary artery (first 5 cm). The proximal left circumflex (pLCx) is the level to the first left obtuse marginal (LOM) origin and is the most variable in length. LM = left main; dRC = distal right coronary; dLAD = distal left anterior descending; dLCx = distal left circumflex artery. Note, the majority of thin-cap fibroatheromas, ruptures, and healed ruptures occur in the pLAD. (Reproduced with permission from Kolodgie FD, et al., Curr Opin Cardiol 2001;16:286–290.)

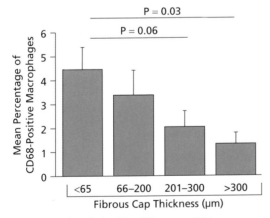

Figure 2.15 The relationship of fibrous cap thickness to macrophage infiltration. Bar graphs plotting the percentage of CD68-positive macrophages with fibrous cap thickness stratified into caps <65 μm, 66–200 μm, 201–300 μm, and >300 μm in thickness. The amount of macrophage infiltrate increases with decreased fibrous cap thickness.

thrombosis.[15] Occlusive thrombi showed a greater density of CD68-positive macrophage ($15.7 \pm 12.5\%$ vs. $3.0 \pm 2.7\%$, $P = 0.05$) and myeloperoxidase (MPO)-positive monocytes ($12.2 \pm 7.5\%$ vs. $5.0 \pm 2.7\%$, $P = 0.006$) and neutrophils ($2.9 \pm 3.4\%$ vs. 0.36 ± 0.50, $P = 0.03$) than nonocclusive thrombi. Similarly, the length of the thrombus showed a positive correlation with the density of macrophages ($P = 0.004$) and MPO positive cells ($P = 0.04$) within the thrombus. In the disrupted fibrous cap, the density of MPO-positive cells was greater in occlusive (5.5%) than nonocclusive (0.9%) thrombi; although this association was similar for neutrophils (0.7% vs. 0.4%), this was not apparent for macrophages (13% vs. 20%). The precise role of MPO in triggering acute coronary thrombosis is unclear, in addition to providing a pro-oxidant milieu, the production of hypochlorous acid may cause breakdown of the fibrous cap.[16–18]

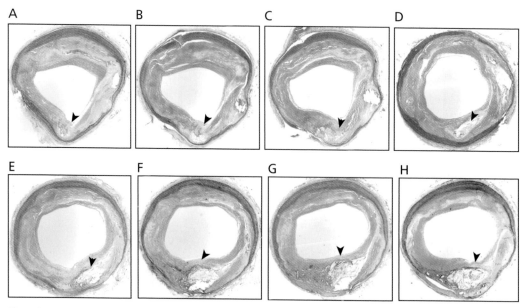

Figure 2.16 Serial sections of a thin-cap fibroatheroma. Photomicrographs to show a vulnerable plaque with sections taken at every 200-μm interval in the coronary artery of a patient dying suddenly with acute thrombus with underlying plaque rupture. Note the gradual increase in the necrotic core size (arrowhead) from A to E and thereafter the necrotic core is large with a thin fibrous cap that is infiltrated with macrophages. The necrotic core is rich in free cholesterol and there is extensive inflammatory reaction with giant cell formation. (Reproduced with permission from Virmani R, et al., J Interv Cardiol 2002;15:439–446.)

Plaque erosion

Plaque erosion is defined as an acute thrombus in direct contact with the intima in an area of absent endothelium. The underlying plaque in erosion is rich in smooth muscle cells and proteoglycan matrix.[6] We speculate that coronary vasospasm may be involved in its pathophysiology since macrophages and lymphocytes are typically absent. Further, eroded lesions tend to be eccentric and are infrequently calcified. The underlying lesion morphology tends to be that of pathologic intimal thickening or fibroatheroma. As with rupture, the most frequent location for erosion is the proximal left anterior descending (LAD; 66%) followed by the right (18%) and the left circumflex (14%) coronary arteries. Single vessel disease is approximately twice as frequent (56%) as double vessel (26%) disease. Finally, in comparison to ruptures, preliminary data suggests that erosions tend to embolize more frequently (74% vs. 40%), respectively.[19]

Plaque erosion accounts for 20% of all sudden deaths or 40% of coronary thrombi in patients dying suddenly with coronary artery thrombosis.[1,4,6] The risk factors for erosion are poorly understood and are different from those of rupture. Consistently plaque erosion is associated with smoking, especially in women; plaque erosions account for over 80% of thrombi occurring in women less than 50 years old. On average, individuals with erosion are younger than those with rupture, and there is less severe narrowing at the thrombus site.

Calcified nodules

The least frequent lesion associated with coronary thrombosis is the calcified nodule. These lesions consist of heavily calcified plates and fibrous tissue in lesions with or without a necrotic core. The luminal surface of the plaque shows fractured calcified plates with nodules of calcium and/or bone formation. Calcified nodules appear to erupt from the plaque into a lumen obstructed by a superimposed thrombus. There is often fibrin surrounding bony spicules along with osteoblasts and osteoclasts, and inflammatory cells.[4] Calcified nodules are more common in older male individuals than women. These lesions are more frequent in carotid than coronary arteries and may be related to repeated intraplaque hemorrhage.

Role of calcification in the detection of the thin-cap atheroma

Coronary calcification correlates highly with plaque burden, but its effect on plaque instability is less obvious. The earliest calcification in coronary lesions occurs in apoptotic smooth muscle cells in lesions with pathologic intimal thickening where the formation of remnant membrane vesicles shows active calcification. The coalescence of microscopic calcium deposits forms larger granules and plates that can be visualized by standard imaging techniques. In a series of sudden death cases, over 50% of TCFAs showed an absence or only speckled calcification on postmortem radiographs.[20] In the remaining segments, calcification was almost equally divided into fragmented or diffuse patterns, suggesting a large variation in the degree of calcification within these lesions. By contrast, 65% of acute ruptures show speckled calcification, with the remainder showing a fragmented or diffuse pattern. Plaque erosions are almost devoid of calcification or, when present, it is only speckled. Calcified nodules contain massive amounts of calcium relative to plaque area and in some instances even show bone formation. This type of lesion, however, only rarely triggers thrombosis and tends to occur in the right or left anterior descending coronary artery of older individuals.[4] It has been reported that calcification is greatest in sudden coronary death victims than those dying with acute myocardial infarction or unstable angina in arteries with 76–100% cross-sectional luminal narrowing.[21,22] However, in our experience in sudden coronary death victims, calcification is dependent on the age of the patient; radiographic coronary calcification is present in 46% of men and women under the age of 40 years, 79% of men and women aged 50–60 years, and 100% in individuals older than 60 years.[12] The amount of calcification within a coronary artery increases with age; however, women generally show a 10-year lag compared to men, with equalization by the eighth decade.

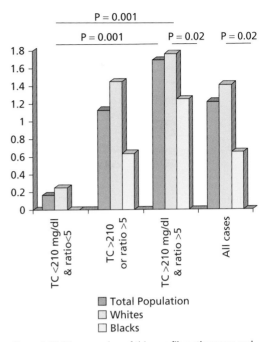

Figure 2.17 Mean number of thin-cap fibroatheromas and serum cholesterol in men. The bar plot is based on total population and race. The mean numbers of thin-cap fibroatheromas (TCFAs) are plotted against total cholesterol (TC) or total cholesterol/high-density lipoprotein cholesterol ratio (TC/HDL-C). The number of TCFAs are greatest in individuals with TC >210 and ratio >5. Whites generally demonstrated an increased incidence of TCFAs over blacks.

Role of risk factors in predicting thin-cap atheromas

Thin-cap fibroatheromas are a frequent finding in men dying suddenly with coronary thrombosis, in particular in individuals with a high total cholesterol (TC) and TC/high density lipoprotein (HDL) ratio (>210 mg/dl and TC/HDL-C ratio >5) (Figure 2.17).[1] The incidence of TCFAs in women is most frequent in those over 50 years with total cholesterol levels >210 mg/dl (Figure 2.18).[2] In sudden coronary deaths, smoking shows a positive correlation with thrombosis, and is more common in women with plaque erosion as compared to rupture.[2] Plaques of premenopausal women demonstrate relatively little necrotic core and calcification compared to those of postmenopausal status and men, possibly reflected by the high rate of plaque erosion in young women.[2] Another risk factor

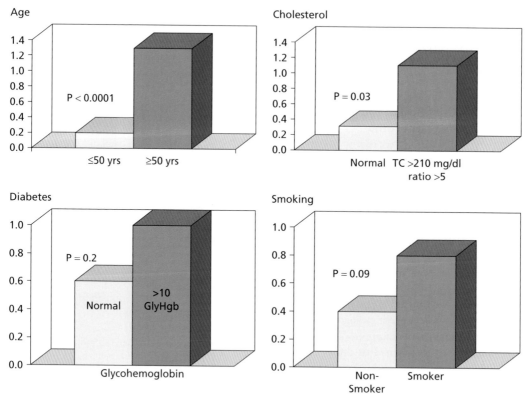

Figure 2.18 Mean number of thin-cap fibroatheromas in 51 women with sudden coronary death (SCD) and severe coronary disease. Traditional risk factors of age, cholesterol, diabetes, and smoking are plotted. In women, predictive factors of TCFAs include age, serum cholesterol, and smoking; diabetes as measured by glycohemoglobin was not. (Reproduced in part with permission from Burke AP, et al., Am Heart J 2001;141(2 Suppl):S58–62.)

reported to predict the development of acute coronary syndromes is high sensitivity C-reactive protein (hs-CRP, lower limit of normal is equal or less than 3 mg/ml).[23] The increased relative risk of sudden cardiac death associated with hs-CRP is seen only in the highest quartile, who were at a 2.78-fold increased risk of sudden cardiac death (95% CI 1.35–5.72) compared to men in the lowest quartile.[24] We have shown that the median hs-CRP was significantly higher in sudden coronary death victims dying of plaque rupture, erosion, or stable plaque than controls dying of noncoronary conditions (control hs-CRP 1.4 µg/dl versus sudden death 2.7 µg/dl, $P < 0.0001$).[25] By multivariate analysis, log-transformed hs-CRP levels were associated with greater plaque burden ($P = 0.03$), independent of age, gender, smoking, and body mass index. Antibody staining demonstrated hs-CRP

localized to the necrotic core and surrounding macrophages and was strongest in patients with high serum hs-CRP levels. In addition, the mean number of TCFAs was most frequent in patients with high hs-CRP than in those with lower hs-CRP values (Table 2.4).[25]

Conclusions

The majority of acute coronary syndromes are the result of plaque rupture, followed by erosion, and least frequently eruptive calcified nodules. The lesion that mostly resembles acute rupture is the thin-cap fibroatheroma, which is characterized by a necrotic core with an overlying fibrous cap measuring <65 µm, containing rare smooth muscle cells and numerous macrophages. These lesions are mostly found in patients dying with acute

Table 2.4 Correlation of serum hs-CRP with immunohistochemical staining intensity of plaques with thin-cap fibroatheromas. (Reproduced with permission from Burke AP et al., Circulation 2002;105:2019–23.)

CRP	CRP staining intensity of plaques*	Mean no. thin-cap fibroatheromas
Low hs-CRP group (<1.0 mg/ml)	2.9 ± 0.5	0.95 ± 0.22
High hs-CRP group (>3.2 mg/ml)	6.2 ± 0.6	3.0 ± 0.3

*Staining intensity was assessed for macrophages and lipid core. A semiquantitative score of 0–4 was assigned to each section. A sum of the two scores resulted in an overall grading system of 0–8.
Abbreviation: hs-CRP = high sensitivity C-reactive protein.

myocardial infarction and are least common in plaque erosions or incidental noncoronary deaths. They are often located in the proximal coronary arteries, less frequent in the mid, and rarely present in the distal vessels. The average necrotic core length is ~2–17 mm (mean 8 mm) and the underlying cross-sectional area narrowing in the majority of lesions is <75%. The total necrotic core area in at least 75% of cases is 1 mm^2. Thin-cap fibroatheromas usually do not show severe luminal narrowing but are associated with positive remodeling and are generally less calcified than ruptures. Coronary risk factors such as high TC and high TC/HDL-C ratio, women >50 years, and patients with elevated levels of hs-CRP are predictive of thin-cap fibroatheromas. Because of its clinical significance, identification of the thin-cap fibroatheroma is a pivotal step towards reducing the morbidity and mortality of coronary artery disease. Newer imaging modalities and treatments are being developed, which will eventually play a significant role in the prevention and treatment of fatal cardiovascular events.

References

1. Burke AP, Farb A, Malcom GT, et al. Coronary risk factors and plaque morphology in men with coronary disease who died suddenly. N Engl J Med 1997;336: 1276–82.
2. Burke AP, Farb A, Malcom GT, et al. Effect of risk factors on the mechanism of acute thrombosis and sudden coronary death in women. Circulation. 1998;97:2110–16.
3. Farb A, Tang AL, Burke AP, et al. Sudden coronary death. Frequency of active coronary lesions, inactive coronary lesions, and myocardial infarction. Circulation. 1995;92:1701–9.
4. Virmani R, Kolodgie FD, Burke AP, Farb A, Schwartz SM. Lessons from sudden coronary death: a comprehensive morphological classification scheme for atherosclerotic lesions. Arterioscler Thromb Vasc Biol. 2000;20:1262–75.
5. Kolodgie FD, Burke AP, Farb A, et al. The thin-cap fibroatheroma: a type of vulnerable plaque: the major precursor lesion to acute coronary syndromes. Curr Opin Cardiol 2001;16:285–92.
6. Farb A, Burke AP, Tang AL, et al. Coronary plaque erosion without rupture into a lipid core. A frequent cause of coronary thrombosis in sudden coronary death. Circulation 1996;93:1354–63.
7. Arbustini E, Dal Bello B, Morbini P, et al. Plaque erosion is a major substrate for coronary thrombosis in acute myocardial infarction. Heart 1999;82:269–72.
8. Kolodgie FD, Gold HK, Burke AP, et al. Intraplaque hemorrhage and progression of coronary atheroma. N Engl J Med 2003;349:2316–25.
9. Mann J, Davies MJ. Mechanisms of progression in native coronary artery disease: role of healed plaque disruption. Heart 1999;82:265–8.
10. Burke AP, Kolodgie FD, Farb A, et al. Healed plaque ruptures and sudden coronary death: evidence that subclinical rupture has a role in plaque progression. Circulation 2001;103:934–40.
11. Virmani R, Burke AP, Kolodgie FD, Farb A. Vulnerable plaque: the pathology of unstable coronary lesions. J Interv Cardiol 2002;15:439–46.
12. Burke AP, Virmani R, Galis Z, Haudenschild CC, Muller JE. 34th Bethesda Conference: Task force #2 – What is the pathologic basis for new atherosclerosis imaging techniques? J Am Coll Cardiol 2003;41:1874–86.
13. Ross R. Atherosclerosis – an inflammatory disease. N Engl J Med 1999;340:115–26.
14. Nemerson Y. A simple experiment and a weakening paradigm: the contribution of blood to propensity for thrombus formation. Arterioscler Thromb Vasc Biol 2002;22:1369.
15. Burke AP, Kolodgie FD, Farb A, Weber DK, Virmani R. Role of circulating myeloperoxidase positive monocytes and neutrophils in occlusive coronary thrombi. J Am Coll Cardiol 2002;39:256A.

16. Sugiyama S, Okada Y, Sukhova GK, et al. Macrophage myeloperoxidase regulation by granulocyte macrophage colony-stimulating factor in human atherosclerosis and implications in acute coronary syndromes. Am J Pathol 2001;158:879–91.

17. Woods AA, Davies MJ. Fragmentation of extracellular matrix by hypochlorous acid. Biochem J 2003;376:219–27.

18. Woods AA, Linton SM, Davies MJ. Detection of HOCl-mediated protein oxidation products in the extracellular matrix of human atherosclerotic plaques. Biochem J 2003;370:729–35.

19. Farb A, Burke AP, Kolodgie FD, et al. Platelet-rich intramyocardial thromboemboli are frequent in acute coronary thrombosis, especially plaque erosions. Circulation 2000;102:II-774.

20. Burke AP, Weber DK, Kolodgie FD, et al. Pathophysiology of calcium deposition in coronary arteries. Herz 2001;26:239–44.

21. Kragel AH, Reddy SG, Wittes JT, Roberts WC. Morphometric analysis of the composition of coronary arterial plaques in isolated unstable angina pectoris with pain at rest. Am J Cardiol 1990;66:562–7.

22. Kragel AH, Gertz SD, Roberts WC. Morphologic comparison of frequency and types of acute lesions in the major epicardial coronary arteries in unstable angina pectoris, sudden coronary death and acute myocardial infarction. J Am Coll Cardiol 1991;18:801–8.

23. Torres JL, Ridker PM. Clinical use of high sensitivity C-reactive protein for the prediction of adverse cardiovascular events. Curr Opin Cardiol 2003;18:471–8.

24. Albert CM, Ma J, Rifai N, Stampfer MJ, Ridker PM. Prospective study of C-reactive protein, homocysteine, and plasma lipid levels as predictors of sudden cardiac death. Circulation 2002;105:2595–9.

25. Burke AP, Tracy RP, Kolodgie F, et al. Elevated C-reactive protein values and atherosclerosis in sudden coronary death: association with different pathologies. Circulation 2002;105:2019–23.

CHAPTER 3

Plaque rupture

Renu Virmani, Allen P Burke, Andrew Farb, Herman K Gold,
Aloke V Finn & Frank D Kolodgie

Atheromatous ulcer commences as a small hole in the internal coat, through which the thick, viscus contents of the atheromatous dépôt are squeezed out on to the surface

Cellular Pathology, Rudolph Virchow 1858[1]

The above statement by Virchow describing an atheromatous ulcer is not that different from what we today call "plaque rupture." Plaque rupture is defined as a lesion with a necrotic core and an overlying thin fibrous cap, with sparse smooth muscle cells but infiltrated by macrophages and lymphocytes, which has focal discontinuity and an overlying thrombus.[2,3] This is the lesion that over the last century has taken more lives than any other disease in the Western world. It is a major cause of acute coronary syndromes and is responsible for a large share of the economic burden in both underdeveloped and developed countries. A new or a recurrent myocardial infarction afflicts approximately 1.1 million people in the USA per year, of which 40% are fatal; 220 000 of these deaths occur without hospitalization.[4] Approximately 650 000 acute myocardial infarcts are initial attacks and 450 000 are recurrent myocardial infarction. About 400 000 cases of stable angina and about 150 000 new cases of unstable angina are diagnosed each year. Sudden coronary death as a first manifestation of the atherosclerotic process occurs in >450 000 individuals annually.[4] Therefore, a better understanding of the atherosclerotic process that leads to plaque rupture is vital.

Approximately 60% of sudden coronary deaths result from luminal thrombi and the vast majority of acute myocardial infarctions (~75%) occur from plaque rupture; other causes of coronary thrombosis include erosion and calcified nodules.[3,5] Ruptured plaques have a large necrotic core, which on average occupies 34–50% of the plaque area,[6,7] this is significantly greater than lipid cores found in erosion or fibrocalcific stable plaques with >75% cross-sectional area luminal narrowing (Table 3.1, Figure 3.1).[3] Before discussing the details of plaque rupture it is essential to understand the underlying processes that proceed to form a plaque that will ultimately rupture. The American Heart Association classification of atherosclerosis and the stages of the progression along with our modification of the classification are helpful in understanding what factors may determine the processes involved in plaque rupture.[8,9] Moreover, development of a practical animal model of plaque rupture would not only help understand how and why plaques rupture but perhaps also eventually help design new therapies for treatment and prevention.[10]

Classification of atherosclerosis

The cellular and acellular components of atherosclerosis and ultimately plaque rupture are those that reside in the vessel wall and circulating blood. Those integral to the vessel wall include endothelial and smooth muscle cells, along with the extracellular matrix that is secreted by these cells such as proteoglycans, collagen, and elastic fibers. Active circulating components consist of plasma lipoproteins, fibrinogen, clotting factors, and cells: platelets, red blood cells, monocytes, lymphocytes, mast cells, and neutrophils.[11]

Table 3.1 Morphological characteristics of culprit and rupture-prone plaques in 241 cases of sudden coronary death. (Reproduced with permission from Virman R, et al., Arterioscler Thromb Vasc Biol 2000;20:1262–1275.)

Plaque type	Necrotic core (%)	Cholesterol clefts (%)	Macrophages (%)	Mean no. of sections with intraplaque hemorrhage
Rupture	34 ± 17*	12 ± 12**	26 ± 20†	2.5 ± 1.3††
Thin fibrous cap atheroma	23 ± 17	8 ± 9	14 ± 10	–
Erosion	14 ± 14	2 ± 5	10 ± 12	0
Fibrocalcific	15 ± 20	4 ± 6	6 ± 8	0.05 ± 0.6
P value	0.003 vs. erosion, 0.01 vs. fibrocalcific*	0.002 vs. erosion, 0.04 vs. fibrocalcific**	<0.001 vs. erosion and stable plaque, 0.03 vs. atrophic fibrous cap atheroma†	<0.01 vs. erosion and fibrocalcific plaque††

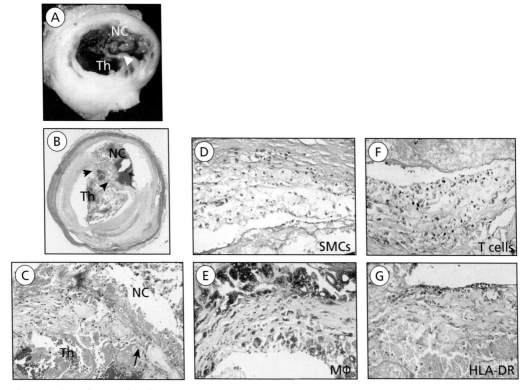

Figure 3.1 Gross photograph and composition in plaque rupture. A, Gross photograph of a coronary artery cut in cross-section showing site of plaque rupture (arrow) with an underlying necrotic core (NC) and luminal thrombus (Th). B, Histologic section of the artery in A showing rupture site, necrotic core, and luminal thrombus (Movat ×20). C, High power view of the area of the fibrous cap disruption (arrow) and there is communication of the thrombus (Th) with the underlying necrotic core (NC) (×200). D, High power view of the thin fibrous cap showing a paucity of smooth muscle cells (α-actin, ×200). E and F, The fibrous cap is heavily infiltrated by macrophages and T-lymphocytes (CD68 and CD45Ro, respectively) (×200). G, Shows the strong expression of HLA-DR antigens, particularly in macrophages and T-cells of the fibrous cap. (Reproduced with permission from Farb A, et al., Circulation 1996;93:1354–63.[68])

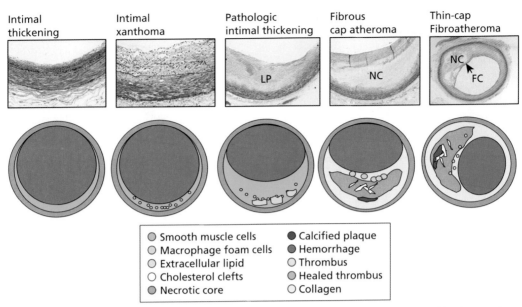

| Intimal thickening | Intimal xanthoma | Pathologic intimal thickening | Fibrous cap atheroma | Thin-cap Fibroatheroma |

○ Smooth muscle cells
○ Macrophage foam cells
○ Extracellular lipid
○ Cholesterol clefts
● Necrotic core

● Calcified plaque
● Hemorrhage
○ Thrombus
◐ Healed thrombus
○ Collagen

Figure 3.2 Intimal thickening and intimal xanthoma: preatherosclerotic coronary lesions. Lesions are uniformly present in all populations, although intimal xanthomas (fatty streaks) are more prevalent with exposure to a Western diet. Both lesions occur soon after birth; the intimal xanthoma (fatty streak) is known to regress. Intimal thickening consists mainly of SMCs in a proteoglycan matrix, whereas intimal xanthomas primarily contain macrophage-derived foam cell, T-lymphocytes, and varying degrees of SMCs. Pathologic intimal thickening versus atheroma: pathologic intimal thickening (PIT) is a poorly defined entity, refered to in the literature as "intermediate" lesion. True necrosis is not apparent, and there is no evidence of cellular debris; lipid pools (LP) are seen deep in the lesion. The tissue over the lipid pools is rich in SMCs and proteoglycans, some scattered macrophages, and lymphocytes may also be present. The more definitive lesions, of fibrous cap atheroma, classically shows a true necrotic core (NC) containing cholesterol esters, free cholesterol, phospholipids, and triglycerides. The fibrous cap consists of SMCs in a proteoglycan–collagen matrix, with a variable number of macrophages and lymphocytes. The thin-cap fibroatheroma (VULNERABLE PLAQUE): thin-cap fibroathomas are lesions with large necrotic cores containing numerous cholesterol clefts. The overlying fibrous cap (FC) is thin (<65 μm) and heavily infiltrated by macrophages; SMCs are rare and microvessels are generally present in the adventitia. (Reproduced with permission from Virmani R, et al., Arteriosclero Thromb Vasc Biol 2000;20:1262–75.[3])

The first atherogenic change that occurs in the vessel wall is termed **adaptive intimal thickening**. This condition usually occurs at branch points and lesions are predominantly composed primarily of smooth muscle cells and proteoglycan matrix (Figure 3.2). Lesions of adaptive intimal thickening are found in 30% of infants at birth and the distribution and development of intimal masses correlates with the presence of atherosclerotic plaques later in life.[12] It has been shown that cell replication is low at these sites and the plaques that develop later in life may be clonal in origin.[12] Tabas et al. have proposed that the extracellular matrix in early lesions contain enzymes capable of retaining lipids, a step towards early necrotic core formation.[13] However, there are few published studies on the

early evolution of intimal masses in humans and these do not clarify the precise pathologic mechanism(s) of development.

Intimal xanthomas or "fatty streaks" in the AHA classification correspond to a lesion with fat-laden macrophages (Figure 3.2).[9] In humans, these lesions are common in the thoracic aorta of young individuals while advanced lesions in the thoracic aorta of the adult are usually absent.[14] Therefore, it is our understanding that fatty streaks are not part of the atherosclerotic process since the vast majority regress with age.[3]

Pathologic intimal thickening or type III lesions in the AHA classification are thought to constitute the morphologic and chemical basis representing the progression from the intimal mass lesion

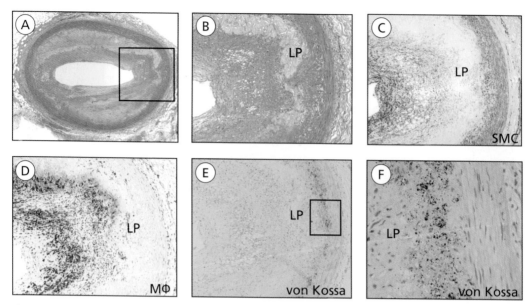

Figure 3.3 Pathologic intimal thickening (PIT). A, Low power micrograph of a coronary lesion with pathologic intimal thickening (hematoxlyin and eosion, ×20). B, Higher power view represented by the black box in A shows lipid pools (LP) in the deep intima. C, Smooth muscle cells are found deep in the intima and dispersed in the superficial layers of the plaque (α-actin, ×200). D, CD68+ macrophages are predominantly confined to the upper perimeter of the lipid pools and in the superficial neointima (×200). E and F, Calcification is typically found deep within the lesions in the lipid pools and, when present, is mostly speckled (×200 and ×400, respectively). F is higher power view of the boxed in area in E.

(Figure 3.3).[9] These plaques are characterized by layers of smooth muscle cells often located near the medial layer surrounded by extracellular lipid droplets and lipid pools.[3] Localized to the lipid pool is proteoglycan matrix with a few viable smooth muscle cells among empty shells, identified by PAS staining representing the basement membranes of earlier "viable" smooth muscle cells.[15] By electron microscopy, sites of attenuated smooth muscle cells contain plasma membrane remnants and apoptotic bodies. Areas of lipid pools may also contain free cholesterol appearing as cholesterol clefts in a paraffin section.[16] Specific stains reveal speckled granular calcification, which is underappreciated by hematoxylin and eosin staining (Figure 3.3). The proteoglycan matrix, rich in sulfated glycosaminoglycans, can effectively bind apolipoprotein B; additional intimal proteoglycans including dermatan sulfate proteoglycan (decorin and biglycan) also accumulate during this phase.[17] Other negatively charged proteoglycans such as chondroitin sulfate function in the retention of apo B-100.[18] The lesion area above the lipid pool often shows scattered intact lipid-laden macrophages in addition to T-lymphocytes.[19] By contrast, B-lymphocytes are restricted mostly to the adventitia; only a few are found within the developing plaque. Similarly mast cells may also be present, but these cells are far fewer than other cell types.[20] No true necrosis is present at this stage although these lesions do contain free cholesterol, fatty acid, sphingomyelin, lysolecithin, and triglycerides.[21]

The **fibroatheroma** has a distinct layer of superficial fibrous tissue confining an area of necrosis (Figure 3.2). The fibrous cap consists of smooth muscle cells and proteoglycan–collagen matrix, with varying degrees of inflammatory cells, mostly macrophages and lymphocytes. The fibrous cap thickness primarily distinguishes the fibroatheroma from the thin fibrous cap atheroma (classic "vulnerable" plaque).[3] Moreover, we have recently subtyped fibroatheromas with "early" and "late" necrosis.[22] The "early fibroatheroma" is a lesion with a lipid-rich matrix containing proteoglycans, versican, hyaluronan, and type III collagen interspersed with intact foamy macrophages (Figures 3.4–3.6). Early necrotic cores are recognized by special proteoglycan and macrophage stains. On

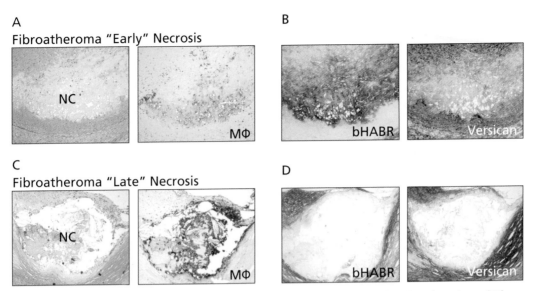

A
Fibroatheroma "Early" Necrosis

C
Fibroatheroma "Late" Necrosis

Figure 3.4 Fibroatheroma with early (upper panel A, B) and late (lower panel C, D) necrosis. A, Note the early core (NC) shows an area of acellularity containing proteoglycans (Movat pentachrome, blue-green) and small cholesterol clefts interspersed with CD68+ macrophages (Mφ). B, This same area shows intense staining for hyaluronan with moderate expression of versican. C, The late necrotic core consists of a well-defined area of cellular and acellular debris surrounded by CD68+ macrophages. D, The late core shows a virtual absence of hyaluronan and versican. (Matrix staining courtesy of Dr Tom Wight, Hope Heart Institute, WA.)

the other hand, necrotic cores with late necrosis show numerous cholesterol clefts, cellular debris, and an absence of extracellular matrix (especially versican and hyaluronan).[22] Within the center and perimeter of necrosis, ghosts of macrophages identified by anti-CD68 staining with ill-defined cell membranes are found and picrosirius red staining for collagen is negative.

The **thin-cap fibroatheroma** (TCFA) is identified based on a fibrous cap <65 μm thick, which is heavily infiltrated by macrophages, lymphocytes, and rare smooth muscle cells (Table 3.1, Figures 3.2, 3.7).[7,23] It is important to classify this lesion as a distinct entity from plaque rupture because its early diagnosis as a precursor lesion to rupture may help reduce the incidence of sudden coronary death and the morbidity associated with coronary heart disease.

Biologic markers of plaque progression

Intimal thickening of coronary arteries is an early phenomenon and is present in newborn infants. Smooth muscle cells in the intima may originate from dividing and migrating cells of the media, although recent data suggests that up to 10% of smooth muscle cells may arise from bone marrow-derived circulating progenitor cells.[24] Medial smooth muscle cells proliferate and migrate into the intima by first converting from a contractile to a synthetic state.[25,26] Further, a monoclonal population of smooth muscle cells in the intima itself may also constitute an atherogenic process.[12] Intimal smooth muscle cells secret proteoglycans that attract lipoproteins into the intima through a "leaky" endothelium. The amount of lipoproteins present in the arterial wall are far less than in the circulation; the precise mechanism(s) of lipoprotein accumulation in the human intima remains unknown.[27]

Atherosclerosis is considered for the most part an inflammatory disease, with monocyte infiltration being one of the early steps in its development.[20] The presence of intimal lipoproteins causes an increase in the expression of adhesion molecules on the endothelial surface. The initiation of adhesion involves selectins, which facilitate the rolling of monocytes followed by their firm attachment by endothelial integrins.[28] The

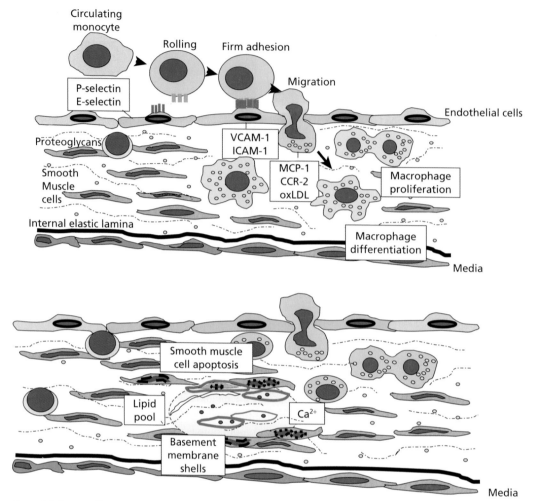

Figure 3.5 Cartoon illustration of early atherosclerosis and pathological thickening. Early atherosclerosis is characterized by the retention of modified lipoproteins by proteoglycans. The rolling of monocytes is facilitated by selectins while the expression of adhesion molecules on the luminal endothelium aids in the attachment and migration of circulating monocytes into the plaque. Conversion of macrophages into foam cells involved phagocytosis of lipids, which are likely first oxidized and via scavenger and nonscavenger receptors, the macrophages take up lipid. Pathologic intimal thickening represents a transitional lesion with an accumulated lipid pool within the deep intima. The lipid pool shows the presence of matrix but the smooth muscle cells have largely disappeared from apoptotic death and may be represented at this stage only by the basement membrane. Also, within the lipid pools is seen scattered small areas of microcalcification. This lesion is thought to give rise to more complex lesions and is the substrate in plaque erosion. Abbreviations: VCAM-1 = vascular cell adhesion molecule 1; ICAM-1 = intercellular adhesion molecule 1; MCP-1 = macrophage chemoattractant protein 1; oxLDL = oxidized low density lipoprotein. Also refer to separate identification key to Figures 3.5–3.7 on page 44.

oxidation of LDL is critical for atherosclerosis development and is promoted by macrophages, endothelial cells, and smooth muscle cells.[29,30] LDL oxidation has been shown to occur as a result of lipoxygenases, myeloperoxidases, inducible nitric oxide synthase, and NADPH oxidase.[27,31] Oxidized LDL is a potent chemoattractant and induces the secretion of macrophage-chemotactic protein 1 (MCP-1) by endothelial cells (Figure 3.5).[31,32] Moreover, macrophages express several scavenger receptors (scavenger receptors A and B1, CD36, CD68) which can bind a broad spectrum of ligands, including modified lipoproteins, native lipoproteins, and anionic phospholipids, many of which

Early
Necrosis

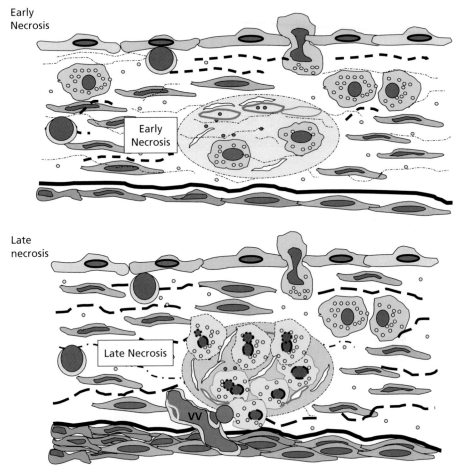

Early
Necrosis

Late
necrosis

Late Necrosis

vv

Figure 3.6 Cartoon illustration of the fibroatheroma. Fibroatheromas have areas of "true" necrosis surrounded by a fibrous cap predominantly consisting of smooth muscle cells and proteoglycan/collagen matrix; inflammatory infiltrate is variable. Both "early" and "late" stages of necrosis are recognized. Areas of "early" necrosis typically show some free cholesterol with mostly intact macrophages and extracellular matrix made up of proteoglycans but not collagen type 1. "Late" stages of necrosis consist of increased macrophage debris with mostly dead or dying macrophages with prominent cholesterol clefts with the absence of tissue matrix. There are usually red cells or red cell membrane present. Abbreviation: vv = vasa vasorum. Also refer to separate identification key to Figures 3.5–3.7 on page 44.

facilitate the massive accumulation of intracellular cholesterol.[27]

Although immune reactions involve many cell types, mononuclear cells are critical to the atherosclerosis processes. Macrophages express receptors that recognize molecular patterns foreign to the body like bacterial pathogens. These receptors include the various scavengers as stated above, in addition to Toll-like receptors (TLRs), which are being recognized in many cardiovascular pathologies.[33] Recent studies have closely linked infections to atherosclerosis, and while the ligation of

scavenger receptors leads to endocytosis and lysosomal degradation, those that activate TLRs participate in transmembrane signaling.[34] TLRs activate the proinflammatory transcription factor nuclear factor kappa-B (NF-κB) on endothelial cells and macrophages and the mitogen-activated protein kinase (MAPK) pathway resulting in the production of cytokines that augment local inflammation and smooth muscle cell proliferation.[35,36] TLR-4 has been identified as the signaling receptor for endotoxins and is expressed by macrophages in murine and human lipid-rich

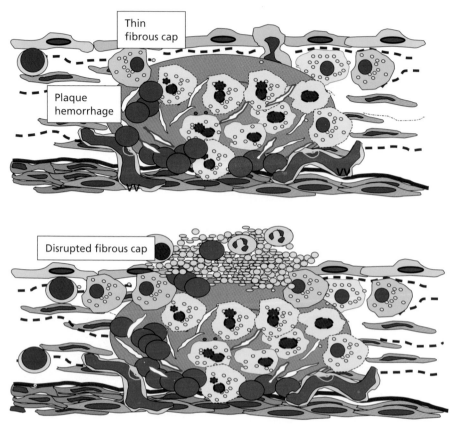

Figure 3.7 Cartoon illustration of the thin-cap fibroatheroma and plaque rupture. Thin-cap fibroatheromas are lesions with a relatively large necrotic core confined by an attenuated fibrous cap heavily infiltrated by macrophages. These lesions frequently contain accumulated erythrocytes (intraplaque hemorrhage) within the necrotic core. Plaque ruptures are lesions with luminal thrombus, which is in communication with the necrotic core. The morphology of ruptures is very similar to thin-cap fibroatheromas, except the thin fibrous cap is discontinuous and as in thin-cap fibroatheroma the fibrous cap is infiltrated by macrophages. The macrophages often are myeloperoxidase positive and a few neutrophils may also be present in some ruptures. The thrombus is rich in platelets. Also refer to separate identification key below.

Identification Key for Figures 3.5 to 3.7

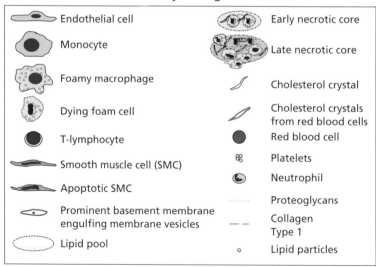

atherosclerotic plaques.[37] In vitro studies have shown basal expression of TLR-4 by macrophages with upregulation by oxidized LDL.[37] The uptake of oxidized LDL transforms macrophages into foam cells. These cells proliferate in the presence of MCP-1 and macrophage colony stimulating factor (MCSF) and play a critical function in the formation of the atherosclerotic plaque.[20]

Macrophages elaborate many cytokines that regulate the function of various cells involved in the initiation, progression, and complications of atherosclerosis. The initial activation of T-cells requires a hearty stimulus delivered by dendritic cells (a specialized macrophage), while memory T-cells have a lower activation threshold and require reduced amounts of antigen.[19] Endothelial cells play an important role in the inflammatory response that leads to leukocyte recruitment, increased permeability, edema, and many other processes involved in atherosclerosis.[27] T-cells respond by secreting interferon gamma (IFN-γ), which lowers the threshold for Toll-like receptor activation on the macrophages. Moreover, T-cell activation leads to the expression of CD40 ligand (CD40L/CD154), which binds to CD40 receptors on the macrophage, B-lymphocytes, and others cells including endothelial and smooth muscle cells.[10,19,20,38] Ligation of CD40 on endothelial cells triggers the expression of leukocyte adhesion molecules such as VCAM-1, E-selectin, and ICAM-1, whereas activation of CD40 on monocytes leads to the expression of LFA-1 and ICAM-1 (Figure 3.5).[10,39] Furthermore, CD40/CD40L interactions also pose a stimulus along with IFN-γ for the activation of Th1 responses, which lead to cytokine-driven enhancement of inflammation within the atherosclerotic plaque. In LDLr-deficient mice, anti-CD40L antibody treatment results in decreased plaque progression.[19,39,40] Several investigators have shown activation of endothelial cells and angiogenesis by CD40L and release of several matrix metalloproteinases (MMPs) and expression of vascular endothelial growth factor (VEGF), Cox-2, and FGF.[10,19,39,40] The loss of fibrillar collagen by active MMPs is thought to be responsible for fibrous cap thinning. CD40 and CD40L have been shown to co-localize with MMPs-1, -8, and -13 in human atheroma and therefore may contribute to disruption of the fibrous cap.[20,39] Lastly, but importantly, CD40/CD40L interactions in endothelial cells, smooth muscle cells, and macrophages induces the expression of tissue factor in vitro; this together with diminished expression of thrombomodulin may activate critical procoagulant pathways involved in thrombosis.[10,40]

Necrotic core and its enlargement are critical for plaque rupture

Necrotic core formation has been attributed to the death of macrophages.[41,42] It has been shown that macrophage infiltration is the first step towards the eventual formation of an atherosclerotic plaque.[3,8] In vitro studies have shown that LDL oxidation facilitates its uptake by the macrophage.[43,44] This two-step process begins with mild oxidation of lipid followed by apolipoprotein B oxidation, a modification required for its recognition by the scavenger receptor, which is unaffected by the cholesterol content of the cell.[31] Foam cells contain cholesterol esters and free cholesterol, no different from a nonfoamy macrophage.[27] However, as the plaque progresses the free cholesterol content of the lesion increases while the cholesteryl esters decrease.[21] In a study by Felton et al. in human aortic atherosclerotic plaques, the progression from a nondisrupted to a disrupted lesion was associated with an increase in free cholesterol, cholesterol esters, and the ratio of free-to-esterified cholesterol with no change in triglyceride content.[21] Further, the percentage of cholesterol clefts was greater in lesions that have ruptured than in fibrocalcific plaques.[3,7]

In the first half of the 20th century Wartmen, Winternitz, and Patterson put forth the hypothesis that intraplaque hemorrhage is a major contributor to the progression of coronary atherosclerosis; however, the precise nature of this relationship was not well defined (Figure 3.8).[45–47] In an effort to further understand the influence of intraplaque hemorrhage on lesion progression, we examined various types of human coronary plaques for hemorrhagic events.[22] It became of interest to us that areas of extravasated erythrocytes outside the vasculature such as those found in atrial hemangioma, hemorrhagic pericarditis, and pulmonary hemorrhage showed atherogenic changes with the accumulation of free cholesterol, foamy macrophages, and iron with fibrosis (Figure 3.9).[48–50]

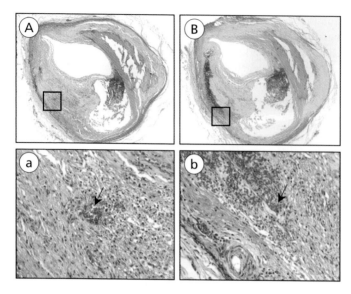

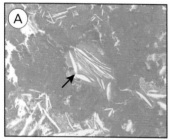

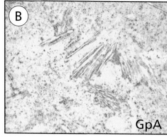

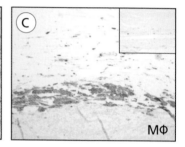

Figure 3.8 Recent intraplaque hemorrhage in the thin-cap fibroatheroma. A, Low (×20) and high power (×200) views, respectively, of a thin-cap fibroatheroma with recent hemorrhage. Note, in (a) there is spillage of erythrocytes from surrounding intraplaque vasa vasorum (arrow). B, Serial section of the lesion in A shows a large pool of extravasated erythrocytes with proximate microvessels (arrow). Panel b is a high power view of boxed area in B.

Figure 3.9 Atherogenic change associated with extravasated red blood cells in a case of hemorrhagic pericarditis. A, Section of pericardium (acute hemorrhagic pericarditis) with erythrocytes and cholesterol clefts (arrow, ×100). B, GpA staining in a similar region as in A; note the co-localization of erythrocyte membranes with crystalline cholesterol and the absence of macrophages. C, Macrophage staining at the periphery of accumulated erythrocytes; iron staining (inset, ×400) was also noted. (Reproduced with permission from Kolodgie FD, et al. New Engl J Med 2003:349;2316–25[22])

Interestingly, the cholesterol content of erythrocyte membrane exceeds that of all other cells in the body, with lipid constituting 40% of the weight, and therefore the accumulation of free cholesterol in plaque may be in part derived from erythrocyte membrane.[51,52] Further, the red blood cell membrane cholesterol is elevated in patients with hypercholesterolemia and decreases with short-term treatment with statins.[53,54]

Using an antibody directed against glycophorin A, a protein specific to erythrocyte membranes, a greater frequency of previous hemorrhages in coronary atherosclerotic lesions with late cores and those prone to rupture were found relative to lesions with early cores or pathologic intimal thickening.[22] The degree of reactivity of glycophorin A and the level of iron deposits in the plaque corresponded to the size of the necrotic core, and changes in these variables paralleled an increase in macrophage density, suggesting that hemorrhage itself serves as an inflammatory stimulus (Table 3.2, Figures 3.6, 3.7 to 3.10).[22] Intraplaque hemorrhage is believed to occur from the disruption of thin-walled microvessels that are lined by a discontinuous endothelium without supporting smooth muscle cells (Figure 3.8).[55] Many investigators, including some from our laboratory, have suggested that intraplaque hemorrhage and plaque rupture is associated with an increased density of microvessels.[2,56,57] The precise mechanism of how

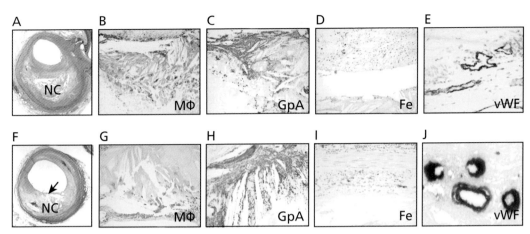

Figure 3.10 Late core (A–E) and thin fibrous cap atheroma (F–J) showing intraplaque hemorrhage. A, Shows a low power view of a fibrous cap atheroma with a late necrotic core (NC) (Movat Pentachrome ×20). B, Intense staining of CD68+ macrophages (MΦ) is seen within the necrotic core). C, Shows extensive glycophorin A (GpA) positive erythrocyte membranes co-localized with numerous cholesterol clefts within the necrotic core (×200). D, Iron deposits (blue) are seen within macrophage foam cells (×200). E, Microvessels bordering the necrotic core show perivascular von Willebrand factor (vWF) deposition (×400). F, A low power view of a fibroatheroma with a thin fibrous cap (arrow) overlying a relatively large necrotic core (Movat Pentachrome, ×20). G, The fibrous cap is devoid of smooth muscle cells (not shown) and is heavily infiltrated by CD68+ macrophages (MΦ, ×200). H, Intense glycophorin (GpA) staining of erythrocyte membranes within the necrotic core co-localized with cholesterol clefts (×100). I, Adjacent coronary segment with accumulated iron (blue pigment) in a macrophage-rich region deep within the plaque (×200). J, Perivascular diffuse deposits of von Willebrand factor (vWF) in microvessels, indicates leaky vessels bordering the necrotic core (×400). (Reproduced with permission from Kolodgie, et al., N Engl J Med 2003;349:2316–325[22].)

Table 3.2 Morphometric analysis of plaque and hemorrhagic events in human coronary arteries from sudden death victims. (Reproduced with permission from Kolodgie FD, et al., N Engl J Med 2003;349:2316–2325.)

Plaque type	GpA Score	Iron	Necrotic core (mm²)	MΦ (mm²)
Pathologic intimal thickening "no" core (n = 129)	0.09 ± 0.04	0.07 ± 0.05	0.0	0.002 ± 0.001
Fibrous cap atheroma "early" core (n = 79)	0.23 ± 0.07	0.17 ± 0.08	0.06 ± 0.02	0.018 ± 0.004
Fibrous cap atheroma "late" core (n = 105)	0.94 ± 0.11*	0.41 ± 0.09*	0.84 ± 0.08*	0.059 ± 0.007*
Thin fibrous cap atheroma (n = 52)	1.60 ± 0.20*	1.24 ± 0.24*	1.95 ± 0.30*	0.142 ± 0.016*

Values are reported as the means ± SEM, *$P < 0.001$ vs. early core. The number in parentheses represent the number of lesions examined; the total number = 365.
Abbreviations: GpA = glycophorin A; MΦ = macrophages.

red blood cells leak into the necrotic core is poorly understood. We have shown diffuse perivascular staining of von Willebrand factor of intraplaque vasa vasorum and evidence of erythrocyte membranes within necrotic cores, which point to microvascular disruption or leakiness as a source of erythrocyte-derived cholesterol (Figure 3.10).[22] Plaque fissures could also account for the accumulation of erythrocytes; however, fissures are often accompanied by luminal thrombi, which we did not find in any lesions in this series.[58]

Arterial remodeling in coronary atherosclerosis with and without thrombosis

In the late 1980s Glagov et al. reported that plaque burden compromised lumen size only when 40%

or greater cross-sectional luminal narrowing had occurred.[59] The absence of a loss of lumen was because of compensatory enlargement of the vessel.[59,60] The relationship between atherosclerotic plaque size and compensatory enlargement is now well established by both postmortem and intravascular ultrasound studies.[61,62] We and others have shown that there is a wide variation in expansion of the internal elastic lamina (IEL) that is dependent on both the type of plaque and its components.[63,64] In general, lesions with hemorrhage and inflammation, characterized by large necrotic cores, macrophage infiltration, and calcification, are more likely to exhibit vessel expansion than plaques without these features (Figure 3.11). In addition, vessel enlargement is also dependent on the plaque morphology related to the underlying luminal thrombus such that plaque rupture is associated with severe IEL expansion while erosion results in arterial shrinkage.

Healing plaque ruptures do not show as much positive remodeling as fibroatheromas without healed rupture sites and arteries with total occlusion show negative remodeling. In a multivariate analysis adjusting for age, sex, and distance from coronary ostium, the plaque components most strongly associated with remodeling are macrophage infiltration, the percentage of calcium, and lipid core (all $P < 0.0001$). Increased fibrous tissue is strongly associated with negative remodeling ($P < 0.0001$). A calcified lipid core and medial atrophy were less strongly associated with remodeling ($P = 0.002$ and $P = 0.05$, respectively).[63]

The expression of activated MMPs likely influences the extent of arterial remodeling and in human atherectomy specimens, macrophages and smooth muscle cells have been shown to actively synthesize MMP-9. Peripheral blood levels of MMPs-2 and -9 are increased in patients with acute coronary syndromes.[65] Further, the genetic manipulation of

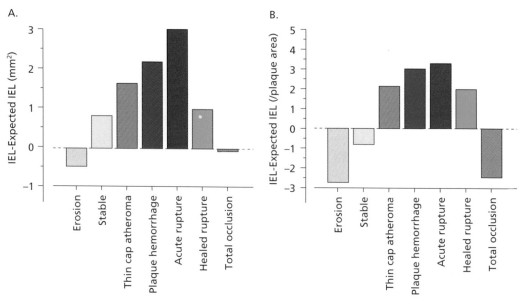

Figure 3.11 Bar graph representing remodeling by type of plaque. Relating atheromatous segments to proximal references segments adjusted for tapering assessed remodeling.[21] In this way, an expected internal elastic lamina (IEL) was calculated for each segment, and IEL expansion calculated by the formula (IEL area – expected IEL area). Because remodeling is a function of plaque size, IEL expansion was also adjusted for plaque area by the formula (IEL area – expected IEL area/plaque area). Using the latter formula, remodeling that allows no reduction in lumen with increasing plaque size would result in a value of 1. In general, those plaques with hemorrhage and inflammation, characterized by large lipid cores, infiltrates of macrophages, and calcific deposits, are much more likely to undergo plaque expansion than plaques without these features. Notably, severe IEL expansion was noted in plaque ruptures, whereas plaque erosion results in arterial shrinkage. (Reproduced with permission from Burke AP, et al., Circulation 2002;105:297–303.[63])

individual MMPs has lead to evidence that MMP-9 may be the dominant MMP in vascular remodeling along with MMPs-1, -2, -3, -8, and -14.[66]

Mechanisms of plaque rupture

Although the precise mechanism(s) of plaque rupture are poorly understood, most researchers agree that disruption of a fibrous cap rich in macrophages and T-lymphocytes in addition to the necrotic core coming in contact with circulating blood are events that lead to the development of thrombi in fatal plaques.[3,20] It has only recently been appreciated, however, that plaque ruptures are likely episodic and may develop without causing symptoms.[67] Further, it is now established that at least 50% of plaque ruptures occur at lesion sites with less than 50% diameter stenosis.[68] In our laboratory, the frequency of coronary thrombosis at sites of insignificant narrowing was 70% in patients dying with plaque erosion and 50% in plaque ruptures.[68] Mann and Davies reported that in plaques causing <20% diameter stenosis, healed plaque rupture (HPR) was observed in 16% of lesions, while in 21–50% diameter stenosis HPR was observed in 19% and in those with ≥51% HPR were seen in 73% of plaques.[69] We have shown that 61% of patients dying from sudden coronary death have HPRs, and as the number of HPR in a specific lesion site increases so does the extent of luminal narrowing. De novo plaques (i.e. plaques without a previous rupture) are uncommon and found only in 11% of patients dying suddenly.[67]

Over the last decade, much interest focused on the role of MMPs as the main cause of fibrous cap disruption in plaque rupture. Fibrillar collagens, especially type I, provide most of the tensile strength to the fibrous cap and certain proinflammatory cytokines, such as INF-γ, inhibit collagen synthesis by smooth muscle cells.[70] The initial proteolytic nick in the collagen chain is provided by MMPs-1, -8, and 13 while the gelatinases MMP-2, and -9 support collagen breakdown.[20,71–74] However, the artery also possesses endogenous antagonists to MMPs, the tissue inhibitors of metalloproteinases (TIMPS).[28] It has been shown that atheromatous rather than fibrous plaques preferentially exhibit type I collagen cleavage occuring at sites that are rich in macrophages expressing both MMP-1 and

-13.[74] Other proteinases capable of degrading extracellular matrix include the cathepsin family (cathepsins S and K) and the inhibitor cystatin C.[75] However, these possess potent elastolytic activity and have been implicated more with matrix remodeling and migration and proliferation of cells.[72] While elastolysis may be more important in aneurysm formation, collagenolysis may be a major determinant of plaque rupture.[66] Although we believe that both collagenolysis and elastolysis are important in the atherosclerosis process, the actual rupture event may reflect greater local factors related to blood flow dynamics and vasospasm.

Apoptosis may also play a critical role in the development of plaque rupture.[76] Macrophage and smooth muscle cell apoptosis have been observed in both progression and regression of the atherosclerotic plaque.[77] Plaque rupture sites typically shows very few smooth muscle cells, which are required for synthesis of extracellular matrix proteins and maintenance of the fibrous cap (Figure 3.1).[7] Geng et al. have shown in vitro that various mediators secreted by macrophages and T-lymphocytes including IFN-γ, FasL, TNF-α, IL-1, and reactive oxygen species, can promote smooth muscle cell apoptosis.[78] These upstream effectors can activate caspases causing mitochondrial dysfunction and death via the release of cytochrome c.[76] Apoptosis is thought to account for the decrease in smooth muscle cells seen in thin cap fibroatheroma and ruptured plaques.[79]

In advanced atherosclerotic plaques, macrophage apoptosis is frequently observed and we have shown excessive macrophage cell death at sites of plaque rupture (Figures 3.12, 3.13).[80] Although our results show an association between macrophage apoptosis and plaque rupture, it is unresolved whether apoptosis triggers a primary event. In vitro studies have suggested that oxidized LDL is capable of inducing macrophage apoptosis.[76] In addition to smooth muscle cells, INF-γ has also been shown to induce apoptotic cell death of THP-1 macrophages.[77] Moreover, INF-γ, while inducing apoptosis in macrophages, also leads to overgeneration of MCP-1, which may further promote an inflammatory response. INF-γ regulates the mRNA expression of pro-apoptotic molecules like TNF-α and caspase-8,[77] and treatment with TNF-α antibodies completely neutralizes the inhibition of DNA

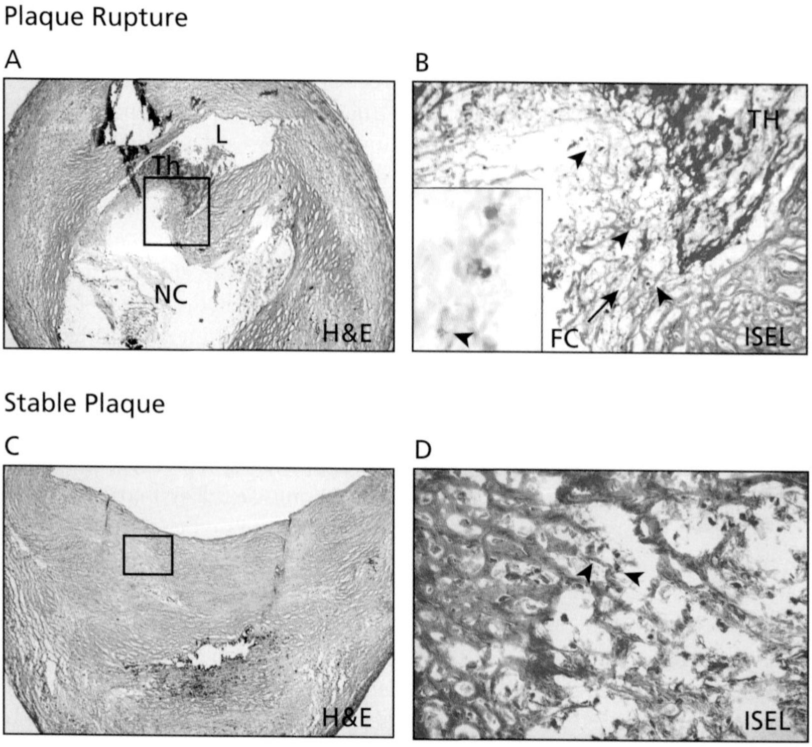

Plaque Rupture

Stable Plaque

Figure 3.12 Apoptosis in culprit plaques. A, Micrograph of a cross-section of an epicardial coronary artery shows a plaque rupture with an acute luminal thrombus (Th); note the thin fibrous cap, boxed area (H&E stain, ×30). B, Serial section of A after DNA fragmentation staining by in-situ end-labeling (ISEL, see methods). Numerous apoptotic cells (blue nuclear staining, arrowheads) are identified at the plaque rupture site (eosin counterstain, ×150). The inset shows a high power view illustrating the nuclear detail; note the fragmented nucleus (arrowhead; ×1000). C, Micrograph of a cross-section of an epicardial coronary artery shows an eccentric stable plaque. The lesion is characterized by dense fibrous cap, boxed area, overlying a calcified region (H&E, ×30). D, Serial section of C after DNA fragmentation staining, there is a paucity of apoptotic cells (arrowheads) relative to rupture site in B (eosin counterstain, ×150). Abbreviations: L = lumen; NC = necrotic core. (Reproduced from Kolodgie FD, Am J Pathol 2000;157:1259–68 with permission from the American Society for Investigative Pathology.[80])

synthesis as well as apoptosis of macrophages induced by IFN-γ.[81] We have demonstrated caspase-1 cleavage in plaque ruptures but not in stable plaques.[80] Immunohistochemical studies showed caspase-1 localized to rupture sites heavily infiltrated by macrophages, although reactivity for caspase-3 in these areas was weak.

The precise etiology of macrophage apoptosis at rupture site is speculative; experimental evidence suggests that dissolution of extracellular matrix (as occurs in the fibrous cap) may threaten cell survival.[82] This process, termed "anoikis," is defined as a process of programmed cell death induced by the loss of cell/matrix interactions.[82] As mentioned, active proteases either secreted directly by inflammatory cells, such as elastase and cathepsin G

by polymorphonuclear leukocytes, chymases and tryptase by mast cells, and granzymes by lymphocytes, or those generated from circulating zymogens may promote matrix degradation.[20]

Alternatively, thin-cap fibroatheromas may form de novo and protease activation accompanies all stages of atherosclerosis including plaque rupture. This possibility arises from the finding that ruptured lesions in some cases form at superficial sites (i.e. close to the lumen) and that leaky vasa vasorum or plaque fissures are responsible for intraplaque hemorrhage, which induces excessive macrophage infiltration. Moreover, atherosclerotic plaques typically form near branch points and repeated rupture and thrombosis propagation is a likely cause of diffuse coronary disease.

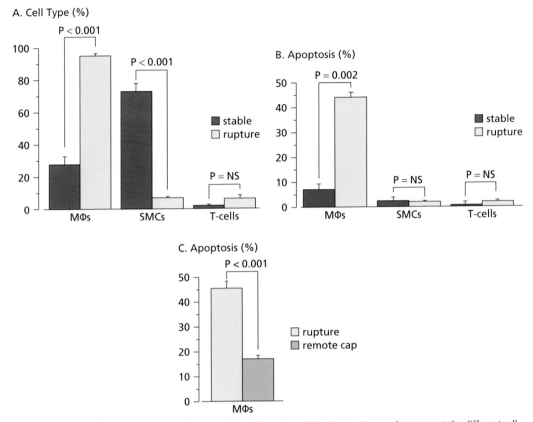

Figure 3.13 Comparision of apotosis relative to specific cell types in culprit plaques. Bar graphs represent the different cell populations and apoptotic index in the fibrous cap of ruptured and stable plaques. The cells were quantified after double labeling experiments using serial frozen sections. Not all cells undergoing apoptosis were positive by antibody staining. The results are expressed as the mean ± SE of 21 ruptures and 11 stable plaques. A, Overall, cell populations expressed as a percentage of the total number of nuclei; note the predominance of macrophages and paucity of SMCs at the rupture site. B, Apoptotic cells as represented as a percentage of cell type; almost 45% of macrophages were recognized as apoptotic. C, Macrophage apoptosis compared with a remote region of the fibrous cap. Abbreviations: MΦs = macrophages; SMC = smooth muscle cells. (Reproduced with permission from Kolodgie FD, Am J Pathol 2000;157:1259–68.[80])

Distribution of plaque rupture in sudden coronary death

Differences by sex and race

We have shown that the incidence of thrombosis in sudden coronary death is 50% and that plaque rupture (60%) is the major cause of thrombosis, while erosion accounts for a third of the cases (Table 3.3). The incidence of rupture varies with each decade and the highest incidence of plaque rupture is seen in the fourties in men while in women the incidence increased beyond the age of 50 years (Figure 3.14). In a cohort of 457 cases of sudden coronary deaths (327 whites and 130 blacks), no racial differences in the rate of acute thrombi were observed but ruptures were more frequent in whites (Figure 3.14). The frequency of thrombi decreased with advancing age (60% in the 4th decade, 70% in the 5th decade, 50% in the 6th decade, and 35% in the 7th decade). Whites tend to have more thrombi in the younger decades than blacks. Women older than 50 years tend to die from plaque rupture while women <50 years died more frequently from erosion.

Type of thrombus

Characteristically, most acute thrombi at rupture sites are platelet-rich ("white" thrombi). The stimulus for platelet aggregation involves many factors

Table 3.3 Distribution of culprit plaques by sex and age in 241 cases of sudden coronary death. (Reproduced with permission from Virmani R, et al., Arterioscler Thromb Vasc Biol 2000;20:1262–1275.)

	Acute thrombi					
	Rupture	Erosion	Calcified nodule	Organized thrombi	No thrombi: fibro-calcific plaque	Totals
Men						
<50 yr	45(46%)	17(17%)	2(2%)	15(15%)	20(20%)	99
>50 yr	19(23%)	8(10%)	3(4%)	27(33%)	26(31%)	83
Women						
<50 yr	1(3%)	24(42%)	0	5(15%)	13(40%)	33
>50 yr	9(35%)	6(23%)	1(4%)	5(19%)	5(19%)	26
Totals	74(31%)	45(19%)	6(2%)	52(22%)*	64(26%)†	241

*Organized thrombi with healed myocardial infarction (HMI) = 46/52(89%).

†No thrombi (stable plaque) with HMI = 32/64(50%), thus, 32/241 or (13%) of sudden deaths have stable plaque without HMI or AMI.

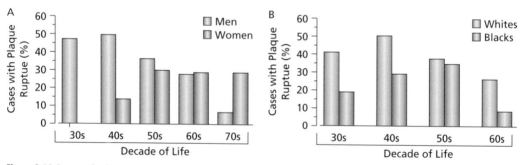

Figure 3.14 Bar graphs showing number of sudden coronary death cases dying from plaque rupture distributed by decade and split by sex (A) and race (B). Note in men as age advances so does the incidence of plaque rupture decrease, whereas in women the incidence increases with age. There is a greater incidence of plaque rupture in white men in the younger decades as compared to black men.

including calcium, platelet surface receptors for fibrinogen, and von Willebrand factor. The proximal propagated thrombus, however, forms mostly a fibrin-rich ("red") thrombus secondary to the absence of flow at the site of rupture. The propagated thrombus occurs from the repeated layering of fibrin interspersed with red blood cells, platelets, and inflammatory cells; however, fibrin is the dominant component (Figure 3.15). Usually, the red thrombus will propagate to the closest side branch, which allows blood to reflow. The nature of thrombus is clinically important since it may predict the effectiveness of thrombolytic therapy in patients presenting with acute myocardial infarction. The

duration of the thrombus determines its consistency; a short duration forms a predominantly platelet-rich thrombus while older thrombi are likely to be longer in length and contain layered fibrin and are therefore more difficult to lyse.

Association of risk factors with the development of fatal plaques

Traditional risk factors

Although risk factors such as hyperlipidemia, smoking, diabetes mellitus, and hypertension are associated with accelerated atherosclerosis, their relationship to thrombi with different plaque

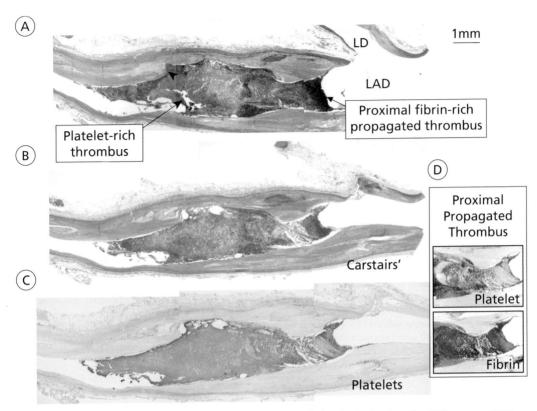

Figure 3.15 Thrombus propagation in plaque rupture. A, Composite of a longitudinal section of an LAD coronary artery with plaque rupture; the rupture site is marked by the arrowhead (Movat pentachrome, original magnification ×20). B, The same longitudinal section as in A stained with Carstairs' method for the detection of fibrin (dark red) and platelets (blue-grey). The proximal thrombus consists predominantly of fibrin while the more distal portion at the rupture site is platelet-rich. C, Platelets were further confirmed using an antibody directed against glycoprotein IIIa. D, Proximal propagated portion of the thrombus showing mostly fibrin; mild layered reactivity is seen for platelets.

etiologies has only recently been investigated.[2,83–85] In an autopsy study from our laboratory, we assessed risk factors in 113 males with sudden coronary death. Serum analysis of total cholesterol (TC), HDL-C, TC/HDL ratio, and serum thiocyanate, a surrogate marker for smoking, were assessed; red blood cell glycosylated hemoglobin was used to determine presence of glucose intolerance. Overall, these risk factors were present in 96.5% of sudden coronary death. Smoking was a predictor of acute thrombosis regardless of plaque etiology, and plaque rupture correlated with high total cholesterol, low HDL-cholesterol, and an elevated TC/HDL-cholesterol ratio.[23] Further, a rise in levels of total cholesterol correlated with an increase in the number of thin cap fibroatheromas.[2] As age advances the incidence of stable plaques increases and healed plaque ruptures being more often associated with diabetes mellitus.

In women, the incidence of plaque erosion correlates highly with smoking and is found with a greater frequency in individuals <50 years. By contrast, plaque rupture is more prevalent in women >50 years and is associated with elevated total cholesterol and an increased incidence of thin-cap fibroatheromas.[86] Stable plaques with healed myocardial infarction are seen more frequently in women with ≥10% glycohemoglobin.[87]

Inflammatory markers that have been associated with future events or plaque rupture are high sensitivity C-reactive protein (hs-CRP), P-selectin, soluble intercellular cell adhesion molecule 1

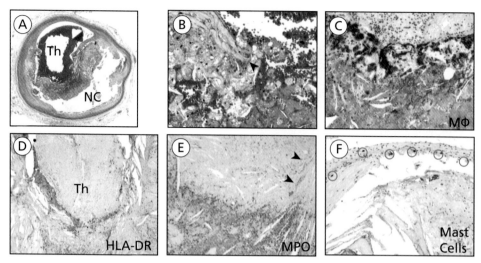

Figure 3.16 Plaque ruptures represent highly active lesions. A, Low power view of a coronary section with plaque rupture, note the relatively large necrotic core (NC, Movat pentachrome, ×20); some of the thrombus (Th) was lost during processing. B, Higher power view of the lesion in A showing a disrupted thin fibrous cap (arrowhead, ×200). C, The thin fibrous cap is heavily infiltrated by CD68+ macrophages (×200). D, Strong reactivity to HLA-DR is noted in the area of the fibrous cap corresponding with the site of accumulated macrophages (×100). E, Myeloperoxidase (MPO) staining; the majority of reactivity is within the necrotic core. Some MPO positive cells, however, are located in the disrupted fibrous cap (arrowheads, ×200). F, In addition to macrophages, mast cells (anti-tryptase, red circles) are also seen within the cap (×200).

(ICAM-1), soluble vascular cell adhesion molecule 1 (VCAM-1), IL-6, TNF-α, IL-18, and soluble CD40L.[10,88] Inflammation consisting of neutrophils and macrophages is more prevalent in ruptured than nonruptured plaques (Figure 3.16).[89] Myeloperoxidase (MPO), an enzyme that generates reactive oxygen species, is released from leukocytes on activation, and plasma levels of MPO may also serve as a marker of inflammation. Brennan et al. have shown plasma MPO levels in patients presenting to the emergency room with chest pain to be predictive of myocardial infarction, as well as the risk of major adverse events in the ensuing 30-day and 6-month periods.[90] In a preliminary study, we have shown that MPO-positive staining within the thrombus may be predictive of an occlusive or a nonocclusive thrombus.

C-reactive protein and unstable coronary syndromes

CRP is an acute phase reactant and has been suggested to contribute directly to the inflammatory process. CRP may stimulate monocyte release of cytokines IL-1, IL-6, and TNF-α and cause expression of ICAM-1 and VCAM-1 by endothelial cells. In large epidemiologic studies carried out in individuals without history of prior cardiovascular disease, a single CRP measure is a strong predictor of future cardiovascular risk.[88] Cardiovascular event-free survival among healthy individuals according to baseline CRP levels, when divided into <1, 1–3, and >3 mg/dl, represent low, moderate, and high risk of future events, respectively.[91] It has also been shown that CRP does not supplant lipid values but has an additive value to lipid screening for coronary risk prediction and adds prognostic information at all levels of the Framingham Risk Score.[92]

We have shown that hs-CRP is significantly elevated in patients dying suddenly with severe coronary artery disease with or without thrombosis. High serum hs-CRP shows a positive correlation with its presence in plaques and is a predictor of the number of thin-cap fibroatheromas.[84] The percentage of patients with hs-CRP >3.0 μg/mL was significantly greater in patients dying with stable plaque (epicardial lesions with >75% cross-sectional area luminal narrowing) (35%), ruptured plaque (53%), and erosion (39%) compared to controls dying of noncoronary causes (21%). Elevated hs-CRP is associated with age, body mass index, and smoking and was independent of risk factors in our cases of sudden coronary death. Although we noted the association of hs-CRP with plaque burden and acute thrombosis, this relationship was lessened when covariates of glycohemoglobin and HDL cholesterol were considered. This was expected as both hs-CRP and glycohemoglobin are strongly associated with metabolic syndrome and hs-CRP and HDL (negatively) are sensitive to inflammatory status.[84]

Hyperhomocysteinemia and unstable coronary syndromes

Homocysteine is a rare inborn error of metabolism that is a result of cystathionine β-synthase deficiency and results in a high (>100 μmol/L) plasma homocysteine and premature mortality from thromboembolism.[93,94] By contrast, modest elevations of total homocysteine between 10 and 100 μmol/L are due to variation in vitamin B intake and genetic factors, especially 5,10-methylenetetrahydrofolate reductase polymorphism.[95] There has been a link between modest elevations of total homocysteine with acute myocardial infarction, stroke, aortic atherosclerosis, and mortality in patients with known coronary artery disease.[95–98] We have shown that men dying with severe coronary atherosclerosis had higher homocysteine levels as compared to individuals dying of noncoronary causes (10.5 vs.9.8 μmol/L, $P = 0.05$). Autopsy patients with severe coronary disease without thrombosis had the highest serum homocysteine 15.6 μmol/L compared to those with thrombi (10.8) and controls 9.8 μmol/L ($P = 0.007$). The number of fibrous plaques was associated with log-normalized homocysteine ($P = 0.004$), independent of age, albumin, smoking, hypertension, and serum cholesterol. Homocysteine levels in the upper tertile (>15 μmol/L) were associated with sudden death without acute or organized thrombus (odds ratio 3.8, $P = 0.03$) independent of age and

other risk factors; the coexistance of diabetes increased the association (odds ratio 25.1, $P = 0.009$, versus lowest tertile ≤8.5 μmol/L).[83]

Conclusions

Plaque rupture involves a lesion with a necrotic core and a thin disrupted fibrous cap heavily infiltrated by macrophages, lymphocytes, and occasional smooth muscle cells. The fibrous cap is focally discontinuous and the luminal thrombus is in communication with the necrotic core. Ruptured plaques are associated with positive remodeling and ~50% of sudden coronary deaths attributed to plaque rupture occur in lesions with <50% diameter stenosis. Repeated ruptures, which may or may not be silent, are likely responsible for plaque progression. Necrotic core expansion may occur from intraplaque hemorrhage through the accumulation of free cholesterol derived from erythrocyte membranes and the recruitment of macrophages. While the precise etiology of rupture is poorly understood, the destruction of extracellular matrix by matrix metalloproteinases together with local rheological forces and vasospasm are likely involved. Risk factors closely associated with rupture are hypercholesterolemia, smoking, age, and high serum levels of hs-CRP.

Acknowledgments

The work in Dr Virmani's laboratory was supported through grants from the National Institutes of Health Heart and Lung Blood Institute RO1 HL61799–02 and R01 HL71148–01.

References

1. Virchow R. Cellular Pathology. In: Virchow R, ed. Cellular Pathology as Based Upon Physiological and Pathological Histology. Birmingham, Alabama: The Classics of Medicine Library, 1858:362.

2. Burke AP, Farb A, Malcom GT, et al. Plaque rupture and sudden death related to exertion in men with coronary artery disease. JAMA 1999;281:921–6.

3. Virmani R, Kolodgie FD, Burke AP, Farb A, Schwartz SM. Lessons from sudden coronary death: a comprehensive morphological classification scheme for atheroscle-

rotic lesions. Arterioscler Thromb Vasc Biol 2000;20: 1262–75.

4. 2001 Heart and Stroke Statistical Update. Dallas, TX: American Heart Association, 2001.

5. Arbustini E, Dal Bello B, Morbini P, et al. Plaque erosion is a major substrate for coronary thrombosis in acute myocardial infarction. Heart 1999;82:269–72.

6. Davies MJ. Stability and instability: two faces of coronary atherosclerosis. The Paul Dudley White Lecture 1995. Circulation 1996;94:2013–20.

7. Kolodgie FD, Burke AP, Farb A, et al. The thin-cap fibroatheroma: a type of vulnerable plaque: the major precursor lesion to acute coronary syndromes. Curr Opin Cardiol 2001;16:285–92.

8. Stary HC, Chandler AB, Dinsmore RE, et al. A definition of advanced types of atherosclerotic lesions and a histological classification of atherosclerosis. A report from the Committee on Vascular Lesions of the Council on Arteriosclerosis, American Heart Association. Circulation 1995;92:1355–74.

9. Stary HC, Chandler AB, Glagov S, et al. A definition of initial, fatty streak, and intermediate lesions of atherosclerosis. A report from the Committee on Vascular Lesions of the Council on Arteriosclerosis, American Heart Association. Circulation 1994;89:2462–78.

10. Lutgens E, Suylen R-J, Faber BC, et al. Atherosclerotic plaque rupture: local or systemic process? Atheroscler Thromb Vasc Biol 2003;23:2123–30.

11. Burke AP, Virmani R, Galis Z, Haudenschild CC, Muller JE. 34th Bethesda Conference: Task force #2 – What is the pathologic basis for new atherosclerosis imaging techniques? J Am Coll Cardiol 2003;41:1874–86.

12. Schwartz SM, deBlois D, O'Brien ER. The intima. Soil for atherosclerosis and restenosis. Circ Res 1995;77:445–65.

13. Tabas I, Marathe S, Keesler GA, Beatini N, Shiratori Y. Evidence that the initial up-regulation of phosphatidylcholine biosynthesis in free cholesterol-loaded macrophages is an adaptive response that prevents cholesterol-induced cellular necrosis. Proposed role of an eventual failure of this response in foam cell necrosis in advanced atherosclerosis. J Biol Chem 1996;271: 22773–81.

14. McGill HC, Jr, McMahan CA, Herderick EE, et al. Origin of atherosclerosis in childhood and adolescence. Am J Clin Nutr 2000;72:1307S–15S.

15. Kockx MM, De Meyer GR, Bortier H, et al. Luminal foam cell accumulation is associated with smooth muscle cell death in the intimal thickening of human saphenous vein grafts. Circulation 1996;94:1255–62.

16. Tanimura A, McGregor DH, Anderson HC. Calcification in atherosclerosis. I. Human studies. J Exp Pathol 1986;2:261–73.

17. Hoff HF, Heideman CL, Gaubatz JW, et al. Correlation of apolipoprotein B retention with the structure of atherosclerotic plaques from human aortas in the grossly normal and atherosclerotic human aorta. Lab Invest 1978;38:560–7.

18. Radhakrishnamurthy B, Tracy RE, Dalferes ER, Jr, Berenson GS. Proteoglycans in human coronary arteriosclerotic lesions. Exp Mol Pathol 1998;65:1–8.

19. Hansson GK. Immune mechanisms in atherosclerosis. Arterioscler Thromb Vasc Biol 2001;21:1876–90.

20. Libby P, Hansson GK, Schonbeck U, Yan ZQ. Inflammation in atherosclerosis. Nature 2002;420:868–74.

21. Felton CV, Crook D, Davies MJ, Oliver MF. Relation of plaque lipid composition and morphology to the stability of human aortic plaques. Arterioscler Thromb Vasc Biol 1997;17:1337–45.

22. Kolodgie FD, Gold HK, Burke AP, et al. Intraplaque hemorrhage and progression of coronary atheroma. N Engl J Med 2003;349:2316–25.

23. Burke AP, Farb A, Malcom GT, et al. Coronary risk factors and plaque morphology in men with coronary disease who died suddenly. N Engl J Med 1997;336: 1276–82.

24. Simper D, Wang S, Deb A, et al. Endothelial progenitor cells are decreased in blood of cardiac allograft patients with vasculopathy and endothelial cells of noncardiac origin are enriched in transplant atherosclerosis. Circulation 2003;108:143–9.

25. Campbell JH, Campbell GR. The role of smooth muscle cells in atherosclerosis. Curr Opin Lipidol 1994;5:323–30.

26. Schwartz SM, Virmani R, Rosenfeld ME. The good smooth muscle cells in atherosclerosis. Curr Atheroscler Rep 2000;2:422–9.

27. Li AC, Glass CK. The macrophage foam cell as a target for therapeutic intervention. Nat Med 2002;8:1235–42.

28. Libby P. Changing concepts of atherogenesis. J Intern Med 2000;247:349–58.

29. Babior BM. Phagocytes and oxidative stress. Am J Med 2000;109:33–44.

30. Endemann G, Stanton LW, Madden KS, et al. CD36 is a receptor for oxidized low density lipoprotein. J Biol Chem 1993;268:11811–16.

31. Steinberg D. Atherogenesis in perspective: hypercholesterolemia and inflammation as partners in crime. Nat Med 2002;8:1211–17.

32. Witztum JL, Steinberg D. The oxidative modification hypothesis of atherosclerosis: does it hold for humans? Trends Cardiovasc Med 2001;11:93–102.

33. Krieger M. The other side of scavenger receptors: pattern recognition for host defense. Curr Opin Lipidol 1997;8:275–80.

34. Pearson AM. Scavenger receptors in innate immunity. Curr Opin Immunol 1996;8:20–8.

35. Muzio M, Mantovani A. Toll-like receptors (TLRs) signalling and expression pattern. J Endotoxin Res 2001;7:297–300.

36. Faure E, Thomas L, Xu H, et al. Bacterial lipopolysaccharide and IFN-gamma induce Toll-like receptor 2 and Toll-like receptor 4 expression in human endothelial cells: role of NF-kappa B activation. J Immunol 2001;166:2018–24.

37. Xu XH, Shah PK, Faure E, et al. Toll-like receptor-4 is expressed by macrophages in murine and human lipid-rich atherosclerotic plaques and upregulated by oxidized LDL. Circulation 2001;104:3103–8.

38. Hansson GK, Libby P, Schonbeck U, Yan ZQ. Innate and adaptive immunity in the pathogenesis of atherosclerosis. Circ Res 2002;91:281–91.

39. Schonbeck U, Libby P. CD40 signaling and plaque instability. Circ Res 2001;89:1092–103.

40. Lutgens E, Daemen MJ. CD40–CD40L interactions in atherosclerosis. Trends Cardiovasc Med 2002;12:27–32.

41. Kruth HS. Localization of unesterified cholesterol in human atherosclerotic lesions. Demonstration of filipin-positive, oil-red-O-negative particles. Am J Pathol 1984;114:201–8.

42. Guyton JR, Klemp KF. Development of the lipid-rich core in human atherosclerosis. Arterioscler Thromb Vasc Biol 1996;16:4–11.

43. Yuan XM, Brunk UT, Olsson AG. Effects of iron- and hemoglobin-loaded human monocyte-derived macrophages on oxidation and uptake of LDL. Arterioscler Thromb Vasc Biol 1995;15:1345–51.

44. Coffey MD, Cole RA, Colles SM, Chisolm GM. In vitro cell injury by oxidized low density lipoprotein involves lipid hydroperoxide-induced formation of alkoxyl, lipid, and peroxyl radicals. J Clin Invest 1995;96:1866–73.

45. Wartman WB, Laipply TC. The fate of blood injected into the arterial wall. Am J Path 1949;25:383–8.

46. Winternitz MC, Thomas RM, Le Compte PM. Thrombosis. In: Thomas CC, ed. The Biology of Atherosclerosis. Springfield, IL/Baltimore, MD: CC Thomas, 1938:94–103.

47. Patterson JC. The reaction of the arterial wall to intramural hemorrhage. In: Symposium of Atherosclerosis. Washington DC: National Academy of Sciences, 1954:65–73.

48. Virmani R, Roberts WC. Pulmonary arteries in congenital heart disease: a structure–function analysis. In: Roberts WC, ed. Adult Congenital Heart Disease. Philadelphia: FA Davis, 1987:77–130.

49. Virmani R, Burke AP, Farb A. Non-neoplastic diseases of the pericardium. In: Atlas of Cardiovascular Pathology. Philadelphia: WB Saunders, 1996:103–10.

50. Arbustini E, Morbini P, D'Armini AM, et al. Plaque composition in plexogenic and thromboembolic pulmonary hypertension: the critical role of thrombotic material in pultaceous core formation. Heart 2002;88:177–82.

51. Bloch K. Cholesterol: evolution of structure and function. In: Vance DE, Vance JE, eds. Biochemistry of Lipids, Lipoproteins and Membranes. Amsterdam: Elsevier Science, 1991:363–81.

52. Yeagle PL. Cholesterol and the cell membrane. Biochim Biophys Acta 1985;822:267–87.

53. Balkan J, Oztezcan S, Aykac-Toker G, Uysal M. Effects of added dietary taurine on erythrocyte lipids and oxidative stress in rabbits fed a high cholesterol diet. Biosci Biotechnol Biochem 2002;66:2701–5.

54. Koter M, Broncel M, Chojnowska-Jezierska J, Klikczynska K, Franiak I. The effect of atorvastatin on erythrocyte membranes and serum lipids in patients with type-2 hypercholesterolemia. Eur J Clin Pharmacol 2002;58:501–6.

55. Virmani R, Narula J, Farb A. When neoangiogenesis ricochets. Am Heart J 1998;136:937–9.

56. McCarthy MJ, Loftus IM, Thompson MM, et al. Angiogenesis and the atherosclerotic carotid plaque: an association between symptomatology and plaque morphology. J Vasc Surg 1999;30:261–8.

57. Mofidi R, Crotty TB, McCarthy P, et al. Association between plaque instability, angiogenesis and symptomatic carotid occlusive disease. Br J Surg 2001;88:945–50.

58. Davies MJ, Woolf N, Rowles P, Richardson PD. Lipid and cellular constituents of unstable human aortic plaques. Basic Res Cardiol 1994;89:33–9.

59. Glagov S, Weisenberg E, Zarins CK, Stankunavicius R, Kolettis GJ. Compensatory enlargement of human atherosclerotic coronary arteries. N Engl J Med 1987;316:1371–5.

60. Clarkson TB, Prichard RW, Morgan TM, Petrick GS, Klein KP. Remodeling of coronary arteries in human and nonhuman primates. JAMA 1994;271:289–94.

61. McPherson DD, Sirna SJ, Hiratzka LF, et al. Coronary arterial remodeling studied by high-frequency epicardial echocardiography: an early compensatory mechanism in patients with obstructive coronary atherosclerosis. J Am Coll Cardiol 1991;17:79–86.

62. Shiran A, Mintz GS, Leiboff B, et al. Serial volumetric intravascular ultrasound assessment of arterial remodeling in left main coronary artery disease. Am J Cardiol 1999;83:1427–32.

63. Burke AP, Kolodgie FD, Farb A, Weber D, Virmani R. Morphological predictors of arterial remodeling in coronary atherosclerosis. Circulation 2002;105:297–303.

64. Varnava AM, Mills PG, Davies MJ. Relationship between coronary artery remodeling and plaque vulnerability. Circulation 2002;105:939–43.

65. Kai H, Ikeda H, Yasukawa H, et al. Peripheral blood levels of matrix metalloproteases-2 and -9 are elevated

in patients with acute coronary syndromes. J Am Coll Cardiol 1998;32:368–72.

66. Galis ZS, Khatri JJ. Matrix metalloproteinases in vascular remodeling and atherogenesis: the good, the bad, and the ugly. Circ Res 2002;90:251–62.

67. Burke AP, Kolodgie FD, Farb A, et al. Healed plaque ruptures and sudden coronary death: evidence that subclinical rupture has a role in plaque progression. Circulation 2001;103:934–40.

68. Farb A, Burke AP, Tang AL, et al. Coronary plaque erosion without rupture into a lipid core. A frequent cause of coronary thrombosis in sudden coronary death. Circulation 1996;93:1354–63.

69. Mann J, Davies MJ. Mechanisms of progression in native coronary artery disease: role of healed plaque disruption. Heart 1999;82:265–8.

70. Libby P. Molecular bases of the acute coronary syndromes. Circulation 1995;91:2844–50.

71. Libby P. Coronary artery injury and the biology of atherosclerosis: inflammation, thrombosis, and stabilization. Am J Cardiol 2000;86:3J–8J; discussion 8J–9J.

72. Dollery CM, Owen CA, Sukhova GK, et al. Neutrophil elastase in human atherosclerotic plaques: production by macrophages. Circulation 2003;107:2829–36.

73. Herman MP, Sukhova GK, Libby P, et al. Expression of neutrophil collagenase (matrix metalloproteinase-8) in human atheroma: a novel collagenolytic pathway suggested by transcriptional profiling. Circulation 2001;104:1899–904.

74. Sukhova GK, Schonbeck U, Rabkin E, et al. Evidence for increased collagenolysis by interstitial collagenases-1 and -3 in vulnerable human atheromatous plaques. Circulation 1999;99:2503–9.

75. Sukhova GK, Shi GP, Simon DI, Chapman HA, Libby P. Expression of the elastolytic cathepsins S and K in human atheroma and regulation of their production in smooth muscle cells. J Clin Invest 1998;102:576–83.

76. Kolodgie FD, Narula J, Guillo P, Virmani R. Apoptosis in human atherosclerotic plaques. Apoptosis 1999;4:5–10.

77. Geng YJ, Libby P. Progression of atheroma: a struggle between death and procreation. Arterioscler Thromb Vasc Biol 2002;22:1370–80.

78. Geng YJ, Henderson LE, Levesque EB, Muszynski M, Libby P. Fas is expressed in human atherosclerotic intima and promotes apoptosis of cytokine-primed human vascular smooth muscle cells. Arterioscler Thromb Vasc Biol 1997;17:2200–8.

79. Bennett MR, Evan GI, Schwartz SM. Apoptosis of human vascular smooth muscle cells derived from normal vessels and coronary atherosclerotic plaques. J Clin Invest 1995;95:2266–74.

80. Kolodgie FD, Narula J, Burke AP, et al. Localization of apoptotic macrophages at the site of plaque rupture in sudden coronary death. Am J Pathol 2000;157:1259–68.

81. Kolodgie FD, Narula J, Haider N, Virmani R. Apoptosis in atherosclerosis. Does it contribute to plaque instability? Cardiol Clin 2001;19:127–39, ix.

82. Michel JB. Anoikis in the cardiovascular system: known and unknown extracellular mediators. Arterioscler Thromb Vasc Biol 2003;23:2146–54.

83. Burke AP, Fonseca V, Kolodgie F, et al. Increased serum homocysteine and sudden death resulting from coronary atherosclerosis with fibrous plaques. Arterioscler Thromb Vasc Biol 2002;22:1936–41.

84. Burke AP, Tracy RP, Kolodgie F, et al. Elevated C-reactive protein values and atherosclerosis in sudden coronary death: association with different pathologies. Circulation 2002;105:2019–23.

85. Burke AP, Farb A, Pestaner J, et al. Traditional risk factors and the incidence of sudden coronary death with and without coronary thrombosis in blacks. Circulation 2002;105:419–24.

86. Burke AP, Farb A, Malcom GT, et al. Effect of risk factors on the mechanism of acute thrombosis and sudden coronary death in women. Circulation 1998;97:2110–16.

87. Burke AP, Farb A, Malcom G, Virmani R. Effect of menopause on plaque morphologic characteristics in coronary atherosclerosis. Am Heart J 2001;141:S58–62.

88. Blake GJ, Ridker PM. Novel clinical markers of vascular wall inflammation. Circ Res 2001;89:763–71.

89. Burke A, Kolodgie F, Farb A, Weber D, Virmani R. Role of circulating myeloperoxidase postive monocytes and neutrophils in occlusive coronary thrombi. J Am Coll Cardiol 2002;39:256A.

90. Brennan ML, Penn MS, Van Lente F, et al. Prognostic value of myeloperoxidase in patients with chest pain. N Engl J Med 2003;349:1595–604.

91. Ridker PM. Clinical application of C-reactive protein for cardiovascular disease detection and prevention. Circulation 2003;107:363–9.

92. Ridker PM, Rifai N, Rose L, Buring JE, Cook NR. Comparison of C-reactive protein and low-density lipoprotein cholesterol levels in the prediction of first cardiovascular events. N Engl J Med 2002;347:1557–65.

93. Mudd SH, Skovby F, Levy HL, et al. The natural history of homocystinuria due to cystathionine beta-synthase deficiency. Am J Hum Genet 1985;37:1–31.

94. Tyagi SC, Smiley LM, Mujumdar VS, Clonts B, Parker JL. Reduction-oxidation (Redox) and vascular tissue level of homocyst(e)ine in human coronary atherosclerotic lesions and role in extracellular matrix remodeling and vascular tone. Mol Cell Biochem 1998;181:107–16.

95. Ma J, Stampfer MJ, Hennekens CH, et al. Methylenetetrahydrofolate reductase polymorphism, plasma folate, homocysteine, and risk of myocardial infarction in US physicians. Circulation 1996;94:2410–16.

96. Perry IJ, Refsum H, Morris RW, et al. Prospective study of serum total homocysteine concentration and risk of stroke in middle-aged British men. Lancet 1995;346:1395–8.

97. Tribouilloy CM, Peltier M, Iannetta Peltier MC, et al. Plasma homocysteine and severity of thoracic aortic atherosclerosis. Chest 2000;118:1685–9.

98. Israelsson B, Brattstrom LE, Hultberg BL. Homocysteine and myocardial infarction. Atherosclerosis 1988;71: 227–33.

CHAPTER 4

Plaque erosion

Frank D Kolodgie, Allen P Burke, Andrew Farb, David R Fowler,
Robert Kutys, Thomas N Wight & Renu Virmani

Approximately 1.1 million patients annually experience a myocardial infarction in the USA with about half this number seen in emergency rooms.[1] An estimated 2–8% of patients who present to the ER with acute myocardial infarction (AMI) are sent home from the hospital, representing approximately 11 000 missed diagnoses of myocardial infarction (MI) per year.[2,3] Multivariate analysis confirms that patients who presented to the ER with cardiac ischemia are more likely not to be hospitalized if they were women <55 years of age, nonwhite, reported shortness of breath as their chief complaint, or had a normal or nondiagnostic electrocardiogram.[3] For many years, the perception that cardiac ischemia occurs primarily in men caused the exclusion of women in clinical trials.[4] Since the identification of cardiovascular disease as the number one killer of women in the USA, it has been recognized that women have a higher mortality from AMI than men (10.3% versus 7.4%) which may be partly explained by older age, greater frequency of diabetes, and higher Killip class on presentation.[5,6]

Plaque erosion: a case history

A 33-year-old female complaining of chest pain at rest for 2 weeks was admitted to the emergency room. Her ECG was normal. Analysis of hematology/ chemistry and tests for cardiac markers was unremarkable; troponin I levels were within normal limits (<0.2 ng/ml). The patient had a history of hypercholesterolemia and was taking methylprednisone. She was diagnosed with anxiety and released from the hospital. Early next morning, the family witnessed her having a seizure. An emergency response team called to the scene found the patient in cardiac arrest.

Autopsy examination showed a right dominant heart with normal ostia. There was focal severe atherosclerosis with total occlusion of the proximal left anterior descending coronary artery by a fibrin- and platelet-rich thrombus, and underlying fibroatheroma with 80% cross-sectional area luminal – narrowing consistent with plaque erosion (Figure 4.1). There was no evidence of plaque rupture or any myocardial injury and the remaining major coronary arteries were unremarkable.

The development of coronary thrombi in the absence of rupture

Until recently, rupture of an atherosclerotic plaque was uniformly accepted as the leading event in sudden coronary death.[7] This widely held paradigm was predicated on morphologic data from autopsy as well as angiographic studies in which the presence of surface irregularities was interpreted as plaque rupture.[8,9] Precursor lesions to rupture usually contain relatively large areas of necrosis encapsulated by a thin fibrous cap heavily infiltrated by macrophages. Early studies on the incidence of sudden death report that plaque rupture is the primary cause of coronary thrombosis in 73% of cases, while 8% consist of plaque fissures with intraplaque fibrin deposition and hemorrhage, and 19% of lesions fail to show evidence of thrombi.[10]

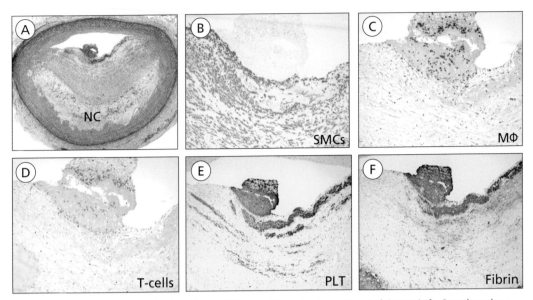

Figure 4.1 Case study: plaque erosion in a 33-year-old female. The patient complained of chest pain for 2 weeks and was discharged from the emergency room with a diagnosis of anxiety. A, The left anterior descending coronary artery contains a luminal thrombus (Th) with >80% cross-sectional area luminal narrowing by atherosclerotic plaque. The underlying lesion shows a necrotic core (NC) consistent with a fibroatheroma (Movat pentachrome, ×20). B, The eroded surface contains α-actin positive smooth muscle cells (×200). C and D, Note macrophages (anti-CD68) and T-cells (anti-CD45Ro) are mostly limited to the thrombus and those within the plaque are few (×200). E and F, Platelet (PLT, anti-CD61) and fibrin (anti-fibrin II) staining show partial organization of the thrombus (×100).

More recent data indicate that acute coronary syndromes resulting from thrombi may occur in the absence of plaque rupture. In a series of 20 patients who died with AMI, van der Wal et al. found plaque ruptures in 60% of lesions with thrombi while the remaining 40% demonstrated what was termed "superficial erosion."[11] In these lesions, the thrombus was confined to the most luminal portion of the plaque and there was an absence of fissures or ruptures after serial sectioning. The term "erosion" was chosen because the luminal surface beneath the thrombus lacked endothelial cells.

At the same time, erosion data became available from our own laboratory of nearly 100 cases of sudden coronary death (Figures 4.2, 4.3). Our definition of sudden coronary death included luminal thrombi in one or more arteries or at least one major coronary artery with >75% cross-sectional area luminal narrowing. In data remarkably similar to those of van der Wal, 60% of all thrombi could be attributed to plaque rupture while 40% were erosions.[12] Notably, 69% of coronary thrombi in erosions occurred in patients <50 years of age and

with a far greater frequency in women than men (Figure 4.4).

The prevalence of plaque erosion in patients dying from AMIs not treated with thrombolysis or percutaneous coronary interventions was reported by Arbustini et al.[13] Acute coronary thrombi were found in 291 coronary arteries, and in 74 of these plaques the lesion underlying the thrombus was defined as erosion. Thus in this series, 25% of thrombi in patients with AMI occurred from plaque erosion, while 75% were associated with rupture. Consistent with previous studies, erosion was more common in women; 40 of the 107 women with coronary thrombosis (37.4%) and 34 of the 184 men (18.5%) showed features of erosion ($P = 0.0004$). In addition, cardiac rupture was more common in women (22%; 24 of 107) than in men (10.9%; 20 of 184, $P = 0.01$). The site of cardiac rupture, however, was not significantly associated with the type of plaque lesion underlying the thrombus. Overall, these data emphasize that plaque erosion is an important substrate for coronary thrombosis in patients dying with AMIs, and

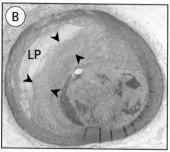

→: Occlusive thrombus

↓: Left anterior descending artery

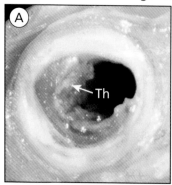

↓: Eroded intima with thrombus

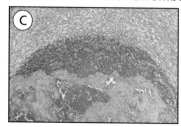

Figure 4.2 Coronary thrombosis in plaque erosion. A, Gross micrograph showing a nonocclusive thrombus (Th) in the left anterior descending coronary artery; plaque burden is minimal. B, Low power view of an eroded plaque with an occlusive thrombus (Movat pentachrome, ×20). The underlying lesion shows an eccentric lesion containing a lipid pool (LP) consistent with pathologic intimal thickening or the American Heart Association type III plaque. Above the LP is a collagen-rich layer (yellow staining) representing old plaque (arrowheads) covered by proteoglycan matrix (bluish-green), which is in contact with the fresh thrombus. This layered appearance is suggest of repetitive episodes of injury and healing. C, High power view of an eroded plaque shows details of the thrombus and the adjacent plaque surface. The thrombus shows partial organization with invading smooth muscle cells and proteoglycan matrix (bluish-green staining within the thrombus, Movat pentachrome staining ×200).

PROXIMAL LEFT ANTERIOR DESCENDING ⟶

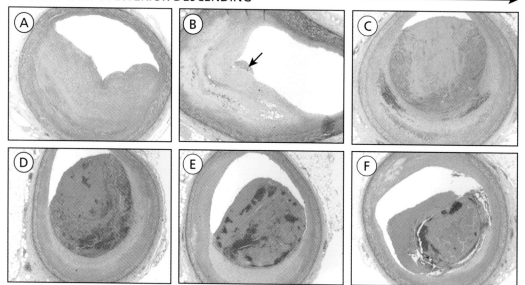

DISTAL

Figure 4.3 Plaque erosion in serial sections. A–F, Serial cross-sections of plaque erosion from a 38-year-old female sudden coronary death victim (Movat pentachrome, ×20). A, An eccentric lesion consisting predominantly of smooth muscle cells and proteoglycan matrix (bluish-green) producing approximately 60% cross-sectional luminal narrowing of the lumen; no areas of necrosis are present. B, A small surface thrombus is noted (arrow). C, A large nonocclusive thrombus is seen in the lumen. There is obvious layering of platelets/fibrin extending into the deeper layers of the plaque. D–F, Continuation of plaque and thrombus; the lesion size is insignificant and notably less, there is no evidence of plaque disruption, and a consistent base of smooth muscle cells is seen throughout.

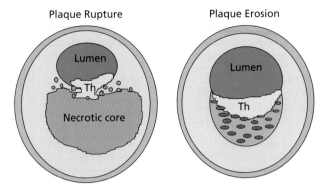

Figure 4.4 Clinical and morphologic differences in plaque erosion and rupture. Approximately 55–60% of all sudden coronary deaths occur from plaque rupture. This entity is more common in men than in women and it usually occurs in older individuals. Ruptured coronary arteries frequently show calcification and the lesions are equally concentric and eccentric. Cross-sectional luminal narrowing is greater in ruptures than in erosions and the fibrous cap of ruptured plaques is rich in macrophages and T-lymphocytes. While the inflammatory component of erosions is typically minimal, both lesions show a strong positive reaction for HLA-DR at the rupture or eroded site. Erosions account for 35–40% of coronary thrombi and the incidence is similar in males and females. Eroded lesions are usually eccentric and show less severe luminal narrowing than ruptures. Unlike ruptured plaque which contain few smooth muscle cells and matrix at the disrupted site, erosions show an abundance of smooth muscle cells and proteoglycans, specifically versican and hyaluronan matrix.

as with sudden coronary death, the occurrence is more frequent in women than men.

Comparison of plaque ruptures and erosions

Both clinical and morphologic differences are widely apparent between ruptures and erosion (Tables 4.1, 4.2). Beginning with age, patients with plaque rupture tend to be significantly older than those with erosion (53 ± 10 vs. 44 ± 7 years, $P < 0.02$). Survival is also a critical factor since an estimation of fatal ruptures in the fifth decade of life is 17 per 100 000 per year compared with 6 per 100 000 for plaque erosion.[14] Although the relationship between risk factors and culprit plaques is similar between

Table 4.1 Coronary thrombosis with rupture into a lipid core compared with thrombosis associated with plaque erosion. Macrophages, T-cells, smooth muscle cells, and HLA-DR+ refer to cellular collections at the sites of rupture or erosion. (Reproduced with permission from Farb A et al., Circulation. 1996;93:1354–1363.)

	Plaque rupture (n = 28)	Plaque erosion (n = 22)	P value
Male : female	23 : 5	11 : 11	0.03
Age (yr)	53 ± 10	44 ± 7	< 0.02
% Stenosis	78 ± 12	70 ± 11	< 0.03
Calcified plaque	19 (69%)	5 (23%)	0.002
Occlusive : nonocclusive thrombus	12 : 16 (43% : 57%)	4 : 18 (18% : 82%)	0.08
Concentric : eccentric	13 : 15 (46% : 54%)	4 : 18 (18% : 82%)	0.07
Macrophages	28 (100%)	11 (50%)	< 0.0001
T-cells	21 (75%)	7 (32%)	< 0.004
Smooth muscle cells	11 (33%)	21 (95%)	< 0.0001
HLA-DR+	25 (89%)	8 (36%)	0.0002

Table 4.2 Frequency distribution of percent cross-sectional area stenosis by plaque in coronary thrombosis attributed to rupture or erosion. (Reproduced with permission from Farb A et al., Circulation. 1996;93:1354–1363.)

Stenosis (%)	Mean age	Cases (no. (%))	Ruptures (no. (%))	Erosions (no. (%))
50–59	42 ± 5	4 (8)	1 (4)	3 (14)
60–69	46 ± 7	9 (18)	4 (14)	5 (23)
70–79	49 ± 10	21 (42)	11 (39)	10 (45)
80–89	50 ± 5	8 (16)	5 (18)	3 (14)
90–99	52 ± 16	8 (16)	7 (25)	1 (5)
Total	49 ± 10	50 (100)	28 (100)	22 (100)

women and men, the proportion of women dying suddenly with plaque erosion is remarkably higher, in particular in deaths under the age of 50. Plaque burden expressed as the percentage of cross-sectional area stenosis excluding the thrombus is greater in ruptures (78 ± 12%) than erosions (70 ± 11%, $P < 0.03$) while eccentric plaques are more common in erosions (Tables 4.1, 4.2). Unlike the prominent fibrous cap inflammation described in ruptures, eroded surfaces contain few macrophages (rupture 100% vs. erosion 50%, $P < 0.0001$) and T-lymphocytes (rupture 75% vs. erosion 32%, $P < 0.004$).[12,15] Cell activation, indicated by HLA-DR staining, was identified in macrophages and T-cells in 25 (89%) plaque ruptures and in 8 (36%) plaque erosions ($P = 0.0002$). The incidence of calcification is also less common in erosion than ruptures. Taken together, eroded plaques tend to be eccentric lesions rich in smooth muscle cells (SMCs) and proteoglycans with very little inflammation or calcification.

Absence of a role for inflammation in plaque erosion

Major differences exist in the cellular composition of plaques with rupture or erosion (Figure 4.4). In ruptures, macrophages typically infiltrate the thin fibrous cap and are present at the margins of the rupture site. In eroded plaques, macrophages are sparsely distributed in the upper layers of the lesion near the plaque/thrombus interface. Clusters of spindle-shaped α-actin positive SMCs are typically found beneath the thrombus in erosions, while SMCs in the fibrous cap at ruptures sites are generally sparse or nonexistent. The relationship of plaque calcification to culprit lesion morphology is also of interest; plaque erosions frequently show areas with speckled or no calcification while ruptures additionally contain areas with diffuse or fragmented clacification.[16] In a quantitative analysis of culprit lesions from our laboratory, plaque erosions were far richer in SMCs (794 ± 334 cells/mm^2) than were plaque ruptures (164 ± 177 cells/mm^2, $P < 0.0001$). Conversely, the area occupied by macrophages was significantly greater in rupture than in erosion (585 ± 219 cells/mm^2 vs. 251 ± 159 cells/mm^2, $P = 0.0007$), while T-lymphocytes are the least represented cell type and are significantly more frequently seen in rupture (6.4 ± 1.3 cells/mm^2) than erosion (1.3 ± 0.8 cells/mm^2, $P = 0.008$).

The lack of inflammation in eroded plaques conflicts with reports from other laboratories. In the original paper by van der Wal, plaque erosions identified from eight of 20 patients who had died of AMI divided into three different morphologic subtypes consisting of lipid-rich plaques without a substantial fibrous cap ($n = 2$), solid fibrous caps with an overlying atheroma ($n = 3$), and fibrous plaques ($n = 3$).[11] The inflammatory cells (macrophages and T-lymphocytes) were the predominant cell types in all erosion cases with lipid-rich plaques with or without an overlying fibrous cap and in two of the three lesions with fibrous plaques; one case showed a mixture of both macrophages and T-cells and SMCs/collagen. In a small series of culprit plaques from another laboratory, Sugiyama et al. found an increased number of myeloperoxidase-expressing macrophages in both ruptures ($n = 8$) and erosions ($n = 7$) relative to fibroatheromas or atheromatous plaques.[17] Although a semiquantitative analysis of myeloperoxidase (MPO)-positive cells showed the greatest numbers in ruptures (118 ± 25 MPO-positive cells/low power field (LPF)), those found in erosions (69 ± 26 cells/LPF) were not significantly different from atheromatous plaques (45 ± 5 cells/LPF).

We believe the notion that inflammation is indispensable to the development of plaque erosion is misleading. From our extensive examination of over 70 cases of sudden coronary death attributed to plaque erosion, no underlying lesions with thin fibrous caps were identified. To our knowledge the thin-cap fibroatheroma is an exclusive precursor lesion to rupture.[18] In some cases, rupture sites are inconspicuous and we suspect that the erosions described by van der Wal, in particular those with thin fibrous caps, were indeed ruptures.[11] Further one must be vigilant in estimating macrophages in culprit plaques since there may be confusion with boundaries separating the thrombus from the actual plaque. This limitation may have particular significance in the paper by Sugiyama et al., since some of the MPO-positive cells may be associated with the thrombus itself.[17] Finally, small subsets of erosions actually do display a relatively high degree of inflammation; however, these lesions are fairly atypical (Figure 4.5). The identification of inflammatory erosions would generate a selection bias, particularly if the study consisted of small sample observations.

Does plaque erosion represent an atherosclerotic process?

The lack of an obvious inflammatory response in plaque erosion is perplexing and raises the provocative question of whether these lesions truly represent an atherosclerotic process. The SMCs near the erosion site appear "activated" often displaying bizarre shapes with hyperchromatic nuclei and prominent nucleoli (Figure 4.6).[18] Moreover, besides the thrombus, the most striking aspect is the absence of endothelium at the plaque/thrombus interface (Figure 4.6). Direct pathologic evidence of endothelial injury in eroded plaques, however, is difficult to establish due to the obscuring nature of the thrombus, which is often in varying stages of organization.

The incidence of coronary thrombosis stratified by age

In both men and women, the frequency of various culprit plaque morphologies varies with age (Figure 4.7). While ruptures are more common in men <50 years old, erosions are more prevalent in women of this age group. The incidence of ruptures in men and women >50 years old, however, is similar. In a large series of over 400 sudden coronary death cases we report that the frequency of acute

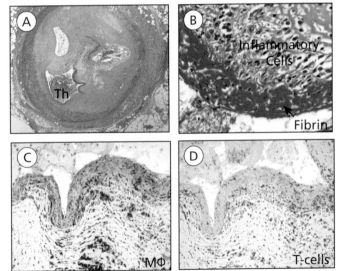

Figure 4.5 Atypical "inflamed" erosion. A, Low power view shows a plaque erosion in the mid-right coronary artery from a 32-year-old male with a history of diabetes and hypertension. The lesion shows significant stenosis and areas of hemorrhage and necrosis are seen deep within the plaque (hematoxylin and eosin, ×20). B, Higher power view of the erosion site in A showing accumulated surface fibrin with numerous inflammatory cells in the thrombus and superficial layers of the plaque (×400). C and D, Numerous macrophages (CD68 stain) and T-cells (CD45Ro), respectively, are seen invading the plaque.

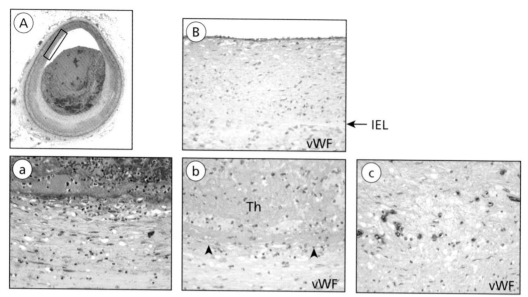

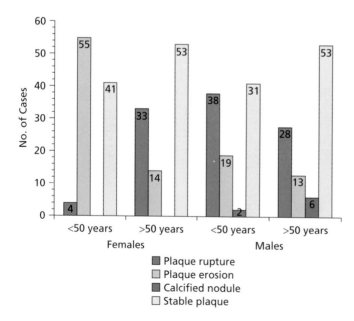

Figure 4.6 The endothelium in plaque erosion. A, Lower power magnification of plaque erosion in the left circumflex coronary artery of a 33-year-old female (Movat pentachrome, ×20). A nonocclusive thrombus is noted superimposed on an eccentric plaque of no clinical significance. The lower panel (a) represents a higher power view of the erosion site (×400). B, Identification of endothelium in plaque erosion using an antibody directed against von Willebrand factor (vWF) antigen. B, The area outlined by the black box in A, showing a normal endothelialized surface overlying a thickened intima at a remote site from the erosion. b, The surface at the plaque/thrombus interface, however, is de-endothelialized (vWf, ×400). C, A coronary lesion from a different patient with plaque erosion demonstrating numerous microvessels deep within the plaque (vWF, ×400).

Figure 4.7 Bar graph representing influence of age on coronary thrombosis in men and women. The frequency of culprit lesions in males and females is greater in patients <50 years of age. Plaque erosion is most prevalent in females <50 years of age, while males in this group show a greater frequency of ruptures. By contrast, ruptures are a common cause of coronary thrombosis in both men and women >50 years of age.

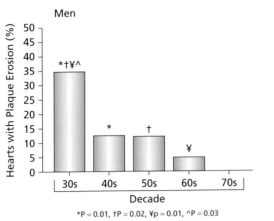
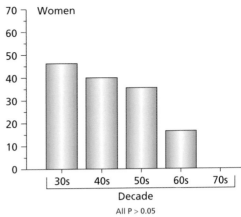

*P = 0.01, †P = 0.02, ¥p = 0.01, ^P = 0.03

All P > 0.05

Figure 4.8 Bar graph representing plaque erosions in men and women stratified by decades. Erosions are more prevalent in men and women in their thirties and forties. Although the frequency of erosions declines with age, this response is more gradual in women than in men.

thrombosis decreases with advancing age (60% in the fourth decade, 60% in the fifth decade, 45% in the sixth decade, and 30% in the seventh decade).[14] Of 224 patients with coronary thrombi, 69% were attributed to rupture while 31% had erosion. As with previous studies, a greater frequency of erosions occurs in women than men; however, this incidence rapidly decreases in men after the thirties, whereas in women, the age-dependent incidence of erosion decreases more gradually (Figure 4.8).

Erosion in patients <40 years old

Registry data at the Armed Forces Institute of Pathology (AFIP) was searched for patients <40 years old who had died suddenly with acute coron-

ary thrombosis; 32 men and five women were identified.[19] Of the individuals, 23 (62%) showed plaque erosion while ruptures were found in only 14 (38%) cases. Of the 23 erosions, 21 contained few inflammatory cells at the plaque/thrombus interface while the remaining two showed intense inflammatory infiltrate (Table 4.3). Of major interest, deep thrombus organization was noted in 13 of 23 eroded plaques. These data are in agreement with a study by Henriques de Gouveia et al. of acute coronary thrombi in 11 patients <35 years old with a diagnosis of sudden coronary death.[20] All patients died within 1 hour of the onset of symptoms, and of the 11 culprit plaques with thrombi, nine showed plaque erosion of which four were women; only one patient had hypercholesterolemia and four were

Table 4.3 Characterization of luminal thrombi associated with plaque rupture or erosion in patients <40 years old.

Plaque type	Underlying lesion	Thrombus organization	Lesions with inflammation (no.)	Lymphocyte density (cells/mm²)	Mφ density (cells/mm²)
Erosion (n = 23)	Fibrous = 1 LP = 17 NC = 1	Org = 11 Focally org at base = 12	2	147 ± 28	97 ± 11
Rupture (n = 14)	Large NC = 8 Small NC = 4 Ulcerated = 2	Org = 7 No Org = 7	12	121 ± 18	368 ± 57

Values of cells/mm² represent the means ± SEM.
Abbreviations: LP = lipid pool; NC = necrotic core; Org = organization.

smokers. Notably, eight of the total nine erosion cases showed a thrombus with signs of organization, characterized by smooth muscle cell ingrowth at the base of the thrombus. Taken together, these studies indicate the initiation of thrombus formation days or even weeks before the onset of death and suggest that erosions, like ruptures, may occur while being clinically silent.

The fatal thrombus

The nature of the thrombus itself, and the frequency of myocardial infarction, is not significantly different between the ruptures and erosions. In ruptures, however, thrombi tend to be more occlusive than in erosions. Thrombi are predominately composed of platelets in 13 (48%) plaque rupture cases and fibrin in 15 (52%); a similar distribution to the eroded plaque group in which 14 (64%) were predominately composed of platelets and 8 (36%) were predominately fibrin ($P = 0.35$).[12] Increased fibrin content may represent propagation of the thrombus or early organization of the thrombus progressing from initial platelet deposition to infiltration and stabilization by fibrin. However, evidence

of acute infarction is equivalent in plaque erosion lesions but healed myocardial infarcts are more frequent in plaque rupture and stable plaques.

Organization and healing

Plaque erosions contain thrombi which may show either no evidence of healing or demonstrate varying degrees of organization (Figures 4.9, 4.10, 4.11). Typically, erosions without organization contain platelet-rich thrombi overlying a plaque rich in SMCs, proteoglycans, and type III collagen (Figure 4.9). Early evidence of healing shows a thin mural thrombus invaded by α-actin positive SMCs and proteoglycan matrix (Figure 4.10). Late stages of organization are accompanied by greater numbers of SMCs and accumulated proteoglycan with residual platelet/fibrin layering (Figure 4.11). The resolution of thrombi in plaque erosion is often accompanied by an ingrowth of capillaries, in particular in the mid to deep layers of the neointima which appears to be analogous to angiogenesis in other tissues (Figure 4.6C).

This pattern of thrombus organization seen with erosion in many ways is analogous to that of healing wounds and these pathologic observations

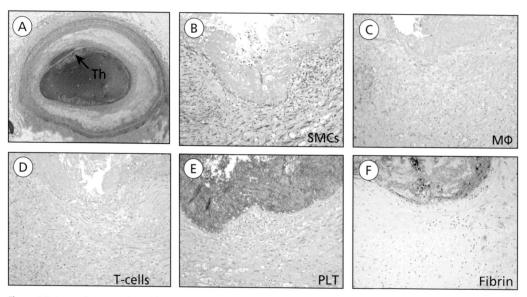

Figure 4.9 Acute plaque erosion without thrombus organization. A, Coronary artery with a concentric and almost circumferentially eroded atherosclerotic lesion with a recent thrombus (Th, arrow); the artery was injected postmortem with barium gelatin (dark gray). B, α-actin staining shows an eroded surface rich in smooth muscle cells. C and D, Few macrophages and T-cells are present. E and F, Platelet (PLT) and fibrin stains are localized to the area of the thrombus, no layering within the plaque is observed.

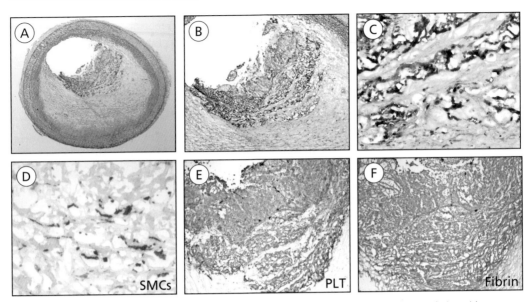

Figure 4.10 Plaque erosion with early thrombus organization. A, Cryosection of an eccentric coronary lesion with a superimposed nonocclusive thrombus (Movat pentachrome, ×20). B and C, Higher power views of the erosion site in A showing layering of platelets/fibrin (red stain) and proteoglycan matrix (bluish-green) (×100 and ×400, respectively). D, Smooth muscle cells (α-actin stain) are seen invading the provisional matrix provided by the thrombus (×400). E and F, Immunohistochemical localization of platelets (CD61) and fibrin are shown, respectively.

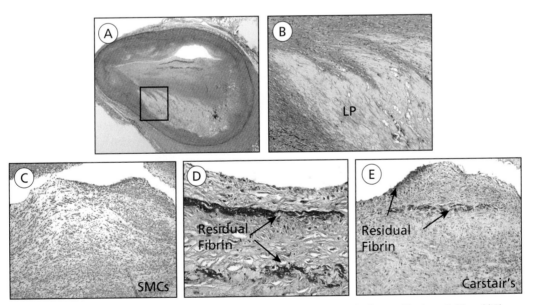

Figure 4.11 Plaque erosion with a healed organized thrombus. A and B, An eccentric plaque with a large lipid pool (LP) consistent with pathologic intimal thickening (Movat pentachrome, ×20 and ×200, respectively). C, Accumulated smooth muscle cells in the area of the healed thrombus (α-actin stain). D and E, Small bands of fibrin (red stain) remain in the superficial layers of the plaque (Movat pentachrome and Carstairs', respectively, ×400).

suggest that tissue contraction may play a role in lumen narrowing. As a consequence, recent evidence from our laboratory suggests a wide variation in expansion of the IEL that is dependent on plaque type and components.[21] In general, those plaques with hemorrhage and inflammation, characterized by large lipid cores, infiltrates of macrophages, and calcific deposits, are more likely to undergo plaque expansion than plaques without these features. Arterial expansion may occur through the release of macrophage-derived matrix metalloproteinase, which may participate in IEL destruction. By contrast, IEL measurements in a relatively large series of erosions demonstrate significant negative remodeling to the extent found in total occlusions and fibrous plaques.

The prognosis following coronary thrombosis is dependent on the extent of myocardial perfusion, and differences in the nature of the thrombus in ruptures and erosions may influence the propensity for distal embolization. In a preliminary study from our laboratory, the frequency of intramyocardial emboli and their association with plaque morphology in coronary thrombosis was examined in sudden coronary death victims where revascularization procedures were not perfomed.[22] In 27 cases of acute coronary thrombosis (24 men, 3 women, mean age 52 years), nearly 60% of hearts had at least one intramyocardial embolus. In addition, the incidence of intracoronary emboli was significantly greater in plaque erosion than ruptures. These preliminary investigations were extended to a larger population of women with coronary artery disease as a potential explanation of why women with coronary artery disease have relatively higher rates of morbidity and mortality.[23] In a series of 64 women and 238 men dying suddenly with severe coronary artery disease, 26% of women had erosions versus 12% of men, while 40% of men had ruptures versus 20% of women ($P < 0.005$). In hearts with acute coronary thrombi, evidence of distal embolization was more frequent in erosion than ruptures (74% vs. 40%, $P = 0.03$) as determined by multifocal sampling and immunohistochemical staining for platelet glycoprotein IIIa. While women had less plaque burden independent of age and diabetes, overall lumen size was equivalent to men. Since erosions are more frequent in women and cause an increased frequency of distal embolization, small vessel thromboembolism may account for increased coronary morbidity in women.

Erosion presents a plaque substrate rich in proteoglycan and hyaluronan

Proteoglycans (versican, biglycan, and decorin) and hyaluronan are extracellular matrix molecules that have been shown to accumulate in topographically distinct patterns within the developing atherosclerotic plaque.[24] The mechanically active environment of the artery can sense mechanical stimuli that result in the regulation of extracellular matrix synthesis by the smooth muscle cells. Lee et al have shown that versican-hyaluronan aggregation is enhanced but the hydrodynamic size of proteoglycans is not altered by mechanical smooth muscle cell deformation.[25] In addition, a fourfold increase in steady state mRNA for the hyaluronan binding protein, TSG6 expression, was observed following deformation. Although early observations demonstrated that plaque erosions were rich in proteoglycans, the extensive nature of the extracellular matrix in culprit plaques with or without coronary thrombi was unknown. A recent study from our laboratory explored the possibility of whether the accumulation of specific types of proteoglycans discriminate among lesions types associated with sudden coronary events. Plaque erosions demonstrated a selective increase in hyaluronan and versican content at the plaque/thrombus interface compared with the fibrous caps of ruptures or stable plaques (Figures 4.12, 4.13).[15] These differences occurred despite similarities in SMC phenotype between erosion and stable plaques. In fact, plaque rupture sites contain very little proteoglycan content relative to stable or eroded lesions.

The appearance of increased hyaluronan at the plaque/thrombus interface is unique, and therefore we postulated that hyaluronan might provide a high-risk substrate for the development of thrombosis in erosion. Indirect support for this notion comes from culture models demonstrating a decreased potential for endothelial cell adherence, growth and survival on hyaluronan substrates.[26] Further, the major cell surface receptor for hyaluronan (CD44) was found highly localized to a

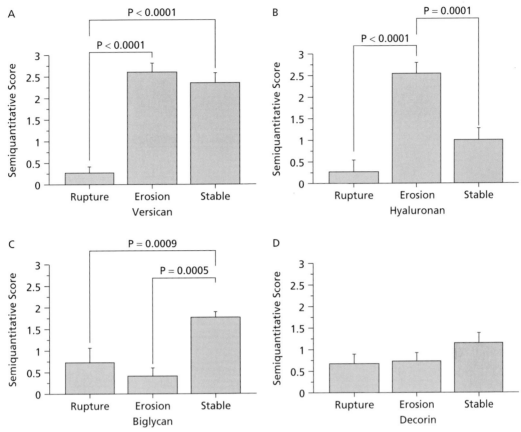

Figure 4.12 Bar graphs representing the semiquantitative analysis of the proteoglycans versican (A), hyaluronan (B), biglycan (C), and decorin (D) in culprit plaques. Note the reciprocal relationship between hyaluronan and biglycan in stable and eroded lesions. (Reproduced with permission from Kolodgie FD et al., Arterioscler Thromb Vasc Biol 2002;22:1642–8.[15])

subset of SMCs at the plaque/thrombus interface as well as in some platelets and inflammatory cells within the thrombus (Figure 4.14). Hyaluronan binds to the specific receptors, such as CD44, and the receptor for hyaluronan-mediated motility, RHAMM, as well as other proteins, such as TSG-6, collagen, and proteoglycans. CD44 has been shown to mediate the adhesion of platelets to hyaluronan.[27] The de-endothelialized surface of erosion exposes hyaluronan to the flowing blood, thereby promoting platelet attachment via a CD44-dependent mechanism.[28] Moreover, the expression of CD44 in erosion may also promote vascular cell activation and migration of SMCs to the wounded edge represented by the loss of endothelium. Consistent with a wounding hypothesis, acute erosions are often superimposed on what appears to be repeated

episodes of thrombosis and healing such that layers of platelets and fibrin are commonly found deep within the plaque.[18] The increase in hyaluronan/versican may be secondary to mechanical deformation of SMCs in vivo because vessel vasospasm has previously been reported to be more common in women presenting with acute coronary syndromes.[29]

Apoptosis of endothelial cells: contribution to plaque erosion

Despite the lack of direct evidence of endothelial cells apoptosis in eroded plaques, emerging studies suggest its potential role in acute coronary syndromes. The contribution of endothelial cell apoptosis to plaque thrombogenicity comes from initial studies by Mallat and coworkers, who demonstrated

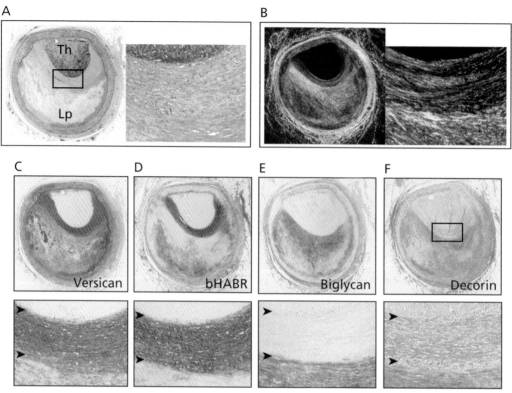

Figure 4.13 Plaque erosion: picrosirius red staining and identification of proteoglycans. A, Low (×20) and high power micrographs (×200) of an eroded plaque (Movat pentachrome stain); the black box outlines a region at the plaque/thrombus interface. A SMC–proteoglycan-rich (blue-green) surface is seen adjacent to the thrombus. Abbreviations: Lp = lipid pool; Th = thrombus. B, Corresponding picrosirius red staining showing a plaque surface rich in collagen type III. C–F, Immunohistochemical identification of the extracellular matrix molecules versican, hyaluronan, biglycan, and decorin, respectively. Note the intense staining for versican and hyaluronan at the plaque/thrombus interface whereas the staining for decorin was weak and that for biglycan was negative. (Reproduced with permission from Kolodgie FD et al., Arterioscler Thromb Vasc Biol 2002;22:1642–8.[15])

that shed microparticles, derived from apoptotic cells, are elevated in patients with recent clinical signs of plaque disruption and thrombosis.[30] Approximately one-third of the microparticles detected in these patients were shown to express endothelial marker proteins. Similarly, other studies of an increase in circulating endothelial cells in myocardial infarction and unstable angina have been reported.[31,32] Moreover, apoptotic endothelial cells are shown to be procoagulant. Tissue factor is said to be operational on the surface of cell membranes, and its activity is highly dependent on the presence of anionic phospholipids, especially phosphatidylserine (PS). Because apoptosis is associated with significant PS exposure on the cell surface and leads to the shedding of PS-containing membrane

particles, it is not surprising that tissue factor expression has been found on apoptotic bodies.[33] Thus, apoptosis induction in endothelial cells stimulates the binding of platelets and tissue factor to the endothelium and further induces activation of platelets and thrombosis. Likewise, the residual membrane particles of apoptosis or activated cells are procoagulant.[34,35]

Atherosclerotic plaques from carotid endarterectomy specimens demonstrated endothelial cell apoptosis.[36] Luminal endothelial cell apoptosis has been observed in 60% of atherosclerotic plaques and flow exerts a direct influence on the extent of cells death; endothelial apoptosis preferentially occurs in the downstream parts of the plaque where low flow and low shear stress prevail. These data

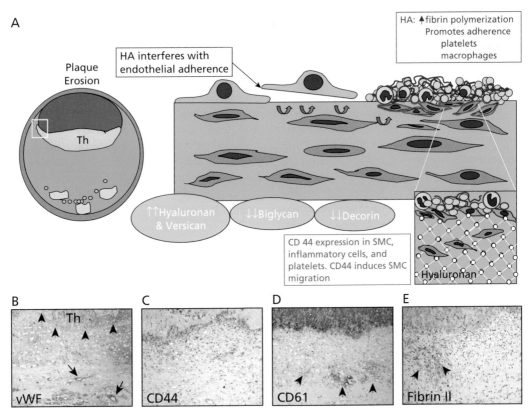

Figure 4.14 Role of hyaluronan and its CD44 ligand in plaque erosion. A, Cartoon illustration suggesting a functional role of hyaluronan (HA) in promoting plaque erosion. The upper right panel is a magnified view of the boxed area of the thrombus/plaque interface. Green = hyaluronan and versican; yellow = lipid pools; blue circles = macrophages; Th = thrombus. The red border represents CD44 receptors and the white circles in the insert depict the CD44 ligand on hyaluronan. The selective accumulation of hyaluronan near the luminal surface may promote de-endothelialization resulting in CD44-dependent platelet adhesion. Further, the presence of CD44 on activated SMCs may stimulate proliferation and migration. Hyaluronan can directly promote the polymerization of fibrin, which may also facilitate SMC migration. B, Immunohistochemical identification of endothelium by von Willebrand factor (vWF) demonstrating the loss of surface endothelium (arrowheads). Note the positive reaction of the intraplaque capillaries in the deeper layers of the lesion (arrows). C, Intense reaction to CD44 localized to the plaque/thrombus interface. D and E, Thrombus showing CD61+ platelets and fibrin staining, respectively. The layering (arrowheads) of both platelets and fibrin is suggestive of ongoing thrombosis. (B–E, original magnification ×200.) (Reproduced with permission from Kolodgie FD et al., Arterioscler Thromb Vasc Biol 2002;22:1642–8.[15])

would suggest that the acute induction of endothelial cell apoptosis may not only expose the matrix and thereby stimulate thrombus formation, but may also actively participate in stimulating platelet aggregation.

Animal model of plaque erosion

The natural history of erosion precludes its study in humans since currently there are no means for its diagnosis in a live patient. Further, because erosions like ruptures are generally episodic, it is exceedingly difficult to identify trigger factors and it is equally as challenging to investigate effective treatments. An acceptable animal model would not only help in the understanding of how erosion occurs but also assist with the design of test strategies to prevent it from happening. There is no doubt that luminal surface defects most likely account for the increased thrombogenicity of the plaque. In this respect, targeting the endothelium would constitute a rational approach when developing an animal model of erosion. Evidence of this comes from one intriguing study by Abela et al, in a model introduced by Constantinides and Chakravarti using cholesterol-fed rabbits challenged pharmacologically with Russell's viper venom, a proteolytic procoagulant, and histamine, a potent vasoconstrictor.[37] Notably, a high frequency of arterial thrombosis was observed after triggering agents were delivered in rabbits with previous balloon arterial injury with or without pulse high cholesterol feeding. Although the goal of the study was to develop a model of plaque rupture, most if not all the lesions did not show disruption of the fibrous cap and were more consistent with features of plaque erosion. Therefore, further development of a similar animal model or others may expand our investigation into the pathology of plaque erosion.

Clinical risk factors in culprit plaques

In men and women, traditional risk factors appear to play a critical role in culprit plaque morphology and the frequency of vulnerable plaques in patients dying suddenly. Vulnerable plaques or thin-cap fibroatheromas are defined as lesions with a large necrotic core and a thin fibrous cap ($<65\,\mu m$) heavily infiltrated by macrophages.[38] In patients dying from plaque erosion, we have infrequently observed thin-cap fibroatheromas whereas they are exceedingly frequently observed in patients dying with plaque rupture.

In a series of men dying suddenly with severe coronary atherosclerosis, we observed that traditional risk factors were present in 96.5% of patients. Smoking was a predictor of acute thrombosis, and thrombi from plaque rupture correlated with high total cholesterol (TC) (262 ± 58 mg/dl), low HDL-cholesterol (35.8 ± 13.5 mg/dl), and a high TC/HDL-cholesterol ratio (8.5 ± 4.0). Moreover, an increase in levels of total cholesterol correlated with an increased incidence in the number of thin-cap fibroatheromas.[38]

In women, we have observed that plaque erosion is highly correlated with smoking and is generally seen in women <50 years. By contrast, plaque rupture is more frequent in women >50 years and correlated with elevated total cholesterol (270 ± 55 mg/dl). Vulnerable plaques are more frequently seen in

women >50 years than those <50 years. Stable plaque with healed myocardial infarction is seen more frequently in diabetic women with ≥10% glycohemoglobin.[39]

It appears, therefore, that in both men and women, cigarette smoking demonstrates an association with acute thrombosis, but elevated levels of cholesterol are associated exclusively with plaque rupture. Furthermore, the hormonal status of the patient appears to influence the morphology of the atherosclerotic plaque, as vulnerable plaques and acute plaque ruptures are infrequent in premenopausal women.[39]

Conclusions

Plaque erosion is a fatal lesion that accounts for an estimated 35% of all thrombi in sudden coronary deaths. Erosions occur principally in younger individuals, especially women with a smoking history. The plaque substrate consists of either pathological intimal thickening or fibroatheroma with early necrosis, and therefore these lesions typically do not show advanced disease. The plaque/thrombus interface in erosion is unique, consisting of proteoglycans (specifically versican) and hyaluronan; there are often aberrant SMCs with little or no inflammatory cells. The lack of a significant inflammatory response raises the possibility that erosions represent chronic wounding and tissue repair rather than a direct atherogenic process. The loss of surface endothelium together with other procoagulant factors likely causes the development of platelet-rich thrombi, which are prone to distal embolization.

Acknowledgments

The work in Dr Virmani's laboratory was supported through grants from the National Institutes of Health Heart and Lung Blood Institute RO1 HL61799-02 and R01 HL71148-01.

References

1. Cardiovascular disease statistics, heart and stroke A to Z guide. In. Dallas: American Heart Association; 1995:1–2.
2. Pope JH, Ruthazer R, Beshansky JR, Griffith JL, Selker HP. Clinical Features of Emergency Department Patients Presenting with Symptoms Suggestive of Acute

Cardiac Ischemia: A Multicenter Study. *J Thromb Thrombolysis*. 1998;6:63–74.

3. Pope JH, Aufderheide TP, Ruthazer R, et al. Missed diagnoses of acute cardiac ischemia in the emergency department. *N Engl J Med*. 2000;342:1163–70.

4. Wegner NK. Coronary heart disease in women: an overview. In: Wegner NK, Speroff L, Packard B, eds. *Proceedings of a National Heart, Lung and Blood Institute conference*. Greenwich (CT): Le Jacq Communications; 1993.

5. U.S. Bureau of the Census. Statistical Abstracts of the United States. In: *US Bureau of the Census*. 110th ed. Washington (DC); 1990.

6. Coronado BE, Griffith JL, Beshansky JR, Selker HP. Hospital mortality in women and men with acute cardiac ischemia: a prospective multicenter study. *J Am Coll Cardiol*. 1997;29:1490–6.

7. Falk E, Shah PK, Fuster V. Coronary plaque disruption. *Circulation*. 1995;92:657–71.

8. Davies MJ, Thomas A. Thrombosis and acute coronary-artery lesions in sudden cardiac ischemic death. *N Engl J Med*. 1984;310:1137–40.

9. Ambrose JA, Winters SL, Stern A, et al. Angiographic morphology and the pathogenesis of unstable angina pectoris. *J Am Coll Cardiol*. 1985;5:609–16.

10. Davies MJ, Thomas AC. Plaque fissuring – the cause of acute myocardial infarction, sudden ischaemic death, and crescendo angina. *Br Heart J*. 1985;53:363–73.

11. van der Wal AC, Becker AE, van der Loos CM, Das PK. Site of intimal rupture or erosion of thrombosed coronary atherosclerotic plaques is characterized by an inflammatory process irrespective of the dominant plaque morphology. *Circulation*. 1994;89:36–44.

12. Farb A, Burke AP, Tang AL, et al. Coronary plaque erosion without rupture into a lipid core. A frequent cause of coronary thrombosis in sudden coronary death. *Circulation*. 1996;93:1354–63.

13. Arbustini E, Dal Bello B, Morbini P, et al. Plaque erosion is a major substrate for coronary thrombosis in acute myocardial infarction. *Heart*. 1999;82:269–72.

14. Burke AP, Farb A, Pestaner J, et al. Traditional risk factors and the incidence of sudden coronary death with and without coronary thrombosis in blacks. *Circulation*. 2002;105:419–24.

15. Kolodgie FD, Burke AP, Farb A, et al. Differential accumulation of proteoglycans and hyaluronan in culprit lesions: insights into plaque erosion. *Arterioscler Thromb Vasc Biol*. 2002;22:1642–8.

16. Burke AP, Virmani R, Galis Z, Haudenschild CC, Muller JE. 34th Bethesda Conference: Task force #2 – What is the pathologic basis for new atherosclerosis imaging techniques? *J Am Coll Cardiol*. 2003;41:1874–86.

17. Sugiyama S, Okada Y, Sukhova GK, et al. Macrophage myeloperoxidase regulation by granulocyte macrophage colony-stimulating factor in human atherosclerosis and implications in acute coronary syndromes. *Am J Pathol*. 2001;158:879–91.

18. Virmani R, Kolodgie FD, Burke AP, Farb A, Schwartz SM. Lessons from sudden coronary death: a comprehensive morphological classification scheme for atherosclerotic lesions. *Arterioscler Thromb Vasc Biol*. 2000;20:1262–75.

19. Burke A, Kolodgie F, Virmani R. Organization and inflammation in fatal coronary thrombi in men and women younger than 40 years. *Atheroscler Thromb Vasc Biol*. 2003;23:a-72.

20. Henriques de Gouveia R, van der Wal AC, van der Loos CM, Becker AE. Sudden unexpected death in young adults. Discrepancies between initiation of acute plaque complications and the onset of acute coronary death. *Eur Heart J*. 2002;23:1433–40.

21. Burke AP, Kolodgie FD, Farb A, Weber D, Virmani R. Morphological predictors of arterial remodeling in coronary atherosclerosis. *Circulation*. 2002;105:297–303.

22. Farb A, Burke AP, Kolodgie FD, et al. Platelet-rich intramyocardial thromboemboli are frequent in acute coronary thrombosis, especially plaque erosions. *Circulation*. 2000;102:II-774.

23. Burke A, Kolodgie F, Farb A, Virmani R. Gender differences in coronary plaque morphology in sudden coronary death. *Circulation*. 2003;108:IV-165.

24. Toole BP, Wight TN, Tammi MI. Hyaluronan-cell interactions in cancer and vascular disease. *J Biol Chem*. 2002;277:4593–6.

25. Lee RT, Yamamoto C, Feng Y, et al. Mechanical strain induces specific changes in the synthesis and organization of proteoglycans by vascular smooth muscle cells. *J Biol Chem*. 2001;276:13847–51.

26. Relou IA, Damen CA, van der Schaft DW, Groenewegen G, Griffioen AW. Effect of culture conditions on endothelial cell growth and responsiveness. *Tissue Cell*. 1998;30:525–30.

27. Day AJ. The structure and regulation of hyaluronan-binding proteins. *Biochem Soc Trans*. 1999;27:115–21.

28. Koshiishi I, Shizari M, Underhill CB. CD44 can mediate the adhesion of platelets to hyaluronan. *Blood*. 1994;84:390–6.

29. Mosca L, Manson JE, Sutherland SE, et al. Cardiovascular disease in women: a statement for healthcare professionals from the American Heart Association. Writing Group. *Circulation*. 1997;96:2468–82.

30. Mallat Z, Benamer H, Hugel B, et al. Elevated levels of shed membrane microparticles with procoagulant potential in the peripheral circulating blood of patients with acute coronary syndromes. *Circulation*. 2000;101:841–3.

31. Hladovec J, Prerovsky I, Stanek V, Fabian J. Circulating endothelial cells in acute myocardial infarction and angina pectoris. *Klin Wochenschr*. 1978;56:1033–6.

32. Mutin M, Canavy I, Blann A, et al. Direct evidence of endothelial injury in acute myocardial infarction and unstable angina by demonstration of circulating endothelial cells. *Blood*. 1999;93:2951–8.

33. Mallat Z, Hugel B, Ohan J, et al. Shed membrane microparticles with procoagulant potential in human atherosclerotic plaques: a role for apoptosis in plaque thrombogenicity. *Circulation*. 1999;99:348–53.

34. Bombeli T, Karsan A, Tait JF, Harlan JM. Apoptotic vascular endothelial cells become procoagulant. *Blood*. 1997;89:2429–42.

35. Bombeli T, Schwartz BR, Harlan JM. Endothelial cells undergoing apoptosis become proadhesive for non-activated platelets. *Blood*. 1999;93:3831–8.

36. Tricot O, Mallat Z, Heymes C, et al. Relation between endothelial cell apoptosis and blood flow direction in human atherosclerotic plaques. *Circulation*. 2000;101: 2450–3.

37. Abela GS, Picon PD, Friedl SE, et al. Triggering of plaque disruption and arterial thrombosis in an atherosclerotic rabbit model. *Circulation*. 1995;91:776–84.

38. Burke AP, Farb A, Malcom GT, et al. Coronary risk factors and plaque morphology in men with coronary disease who died suddenly. *N Engl J Med*. 1997;336:1276–82.

39. Burke AP, Farb A, Malcom GT, et al. Effect of risk factors on the mechanism of acute thrombosis and sudden coronary death in women. *Circulation*. 1998;97:2110–6.

CHAPTER 5

Pathogenesis and significance of calcification in coronary atherosclerosis

Allen P Burke, Frank D Kolodgie, Andrew Farb & Renu Virmani

Calcification is an invariable component of advanced coronary artery atherosclerosis. Local factors involved in calcification include smooth muscle cell apoptosis and inflammation. Systemic factors strongly moderate the degree of coronary artery calcification, as well as poorly understood genetic influences. Calcification is a reasonable reflection of the degree of plaque burden, but does not reliably predict sites of plaque instability.

Pathogenesis

Local factors

Atherosclerosis is characterized by the accumulation of smooth muscle cells and inflammatory cells in the intima of muscular and elastic arteries. Smooth muscle cells and macrophages that are sequestered in the plaque undergo degeneration, largely via apoptosis. Although the triggers for apoptosis within the atherosclerotic plaque are unclear, it is thought that cell death leads to calcification of the extracellular matrix within the intima. Prior to the stage of cell death, however, microscopic calcifications may appear solely in association with extracellular lipid.

Plaque classification, early stages

An understanding of the heterogeneity of the atherosclerotic plaque is essential before a meaningful description of atherosclerotic calcification can

take place. Lesion development begins with an increase in smooth muscle cells (adaptive intimal thickening), accumulation of extracellular lipid without significant inflammation (pathologic intimal thickening), and accumulation of lipid-laden foamy macrophages and smooth muscle cells (fatty streak). These stages of plaque are not associated with significant cell death, and are therefore largely devoid of calcium. However, cases of pathologic intimal thickening may have areas of punctate microscopic calcification as seen with von Kossa calcium stains, even in the absence of obvious cell death (Figure 5.1).

Intermediate stages of the plaque are generally grouped together as "fibroatheromas," which contain apoptotic/necrotic cores surrounded by smooth muscle cells and/or macrophages. The calcium deposits in these plaques are morphologically heterogeneous (Table 5.1). The earliest cores form as a result of smooth muscle cell death before digestion of proteoglycan ground substance (Figure 5.2). These lesions do not show matrix breakdown, but contain small, delicate cholesterol clefts with extracellular lipid and few if any macrophages. The dying smooth muscle cells are identified only by a prominent basement membrane, which stains strongly with periodic acid-Schiff reagent (PAS) (Figures 5.3, 5.4). Alternatively, "necrotic" cores are characterized by an early influx of macrophages which typically

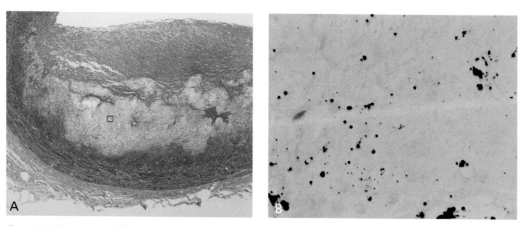

Figure 5.1 Microscopic calcifications, pathologic intimal thickening. A periodic-acid Schiff (PAS) stain (A) demonstrates a relatively acellular area with accumulation of extracellular lipid. A von Kossa stain (B) demonstrates at higher magnification punctate microcalcifications.

Table 5.1 Histologic types of coronary plaque calcification.

| Type of calcification | Type of atherosclerotic lesion | | | | |
	Pathologic intimal thickening	Fibroatheroma	Plaque rupture	Fibrocalcific plaque	Calcified nodule
Microscopic, punctate	+	+/–	+/–	+/–	+/–
Microscopic, blocky	0	+	+/–	+/–	+/–
Calcified plates	0	+/–	+/–	++	+/+
Calcified nodules	0	0	0	+/–	++
Ossification	0	0	0	+/–	+/–

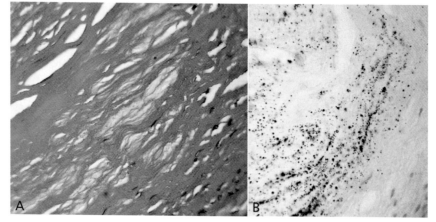

Figure 5.2 Smooth muscle cell calcification: microscopic calcifications, pathologic intimal thickening. There is loss of smooth muscle cells, is seen in A. When stained for calcium (von Kossa), there are multiple microscopic calcifications identified within the region, as seen in B.

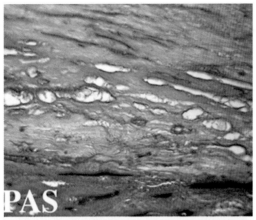

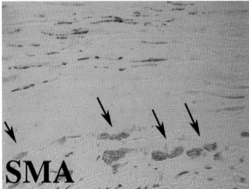

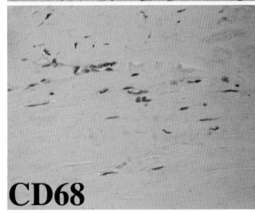

Figure 5.3 Histologic features of pathologic intimal thickening. A PAS stain shows an early core, with apoptotic smooth muscle cells characterized by prominent PAS-positive basement membranes. An immunohistochemical stain for smooth muscle actin (SMA) shows occasional spindled cells remaining in the early core. Note also amorphous small calcium deposits, which stain with blue hematoxylin counterstain (arrows). An immunohistochemical stain for macrophages (CD68) shows an absence of macrophages. Residual smooth muscle cell nuclei are blue.

localize to the luminal side of the core region. These macrophage-rich cores are characterized by a loss of proteoglycan matrix, large cholesterol clefts, hemorrhage, and masses of degenerated macrophages. Grossly, these cores are often described as a necrotic "gruel." These cores differ from fibrous cores in that they stain diffusely immunohistochemically with anti-macrophage markers. It is unclear if macrophage-rich cores arise spontaneously, or evolve secondarily from early cores. The calcification process, then, likely differs depending on the type of core. In summary, the "early fibroatheroma" has a lipid-rich matrix containing proteoglycans, versican, hyaluronan, and type III collagen interspersed with intact foamy macrophages. By contrast, late (necrotic) cores have numerous cholesterol clefts and cellular debris, and an absence of extracellular matrix (especially versican, hyaluronan, and collagen).

Calcification in early plaques

If one analyzes microscopic calcifications in early and intermediate coronary atherosclerotic plaques using von Kossa stains, there is little if any calcium in intimal thickening or fatty streaks. However, the majority of pathologic intimal thickening (Figure 5.1) and early cores contain extracellular calcifications, which are microscopic and only identifiable by calcium stains, such as von Kossa. In later cores with cellular breakdown and intense macrophage cell death, approximately 50% of macrophage cores contain extracellular calcifications. The nature of the calcifications differ, in that early cores contain finely granular calcifications, often coalescing into masses (Figure 5.4), whereas macrophage "necrotic" cores often contain larger crystalline deposits (Figures 5.5–5.9). Extensive calcification may occur in the absence of rupture or thrombosis; therefore, marked degrees of calcification may be present in arteries that show only mild degrees of luminal narrowing (Figure 5.10). Terms such as fibrocalcific plaque have been used for predominantly fibrous plaques, in which the apoptotic smooth muscle cells have been transformed into plates of calcified collagen matrix, and in which the stimulus for macrophage ingress did not occur. Rarely, true ossification may occur in atherosclerotic plaques, with the formation of

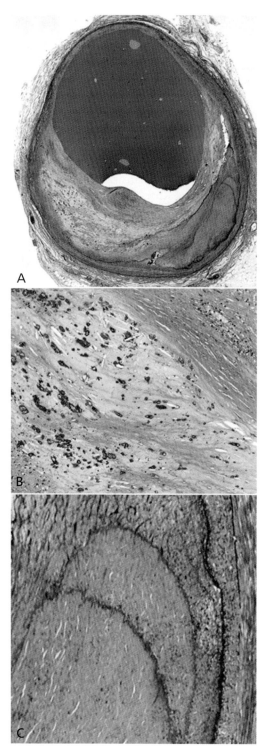

Haversian canals, bony lamella, and occasionally marrow (Figure 5.11).

The smooth muscle cell is historically considered to be the source of atherosclerotic plaque calcification, by an active process involving calcification of portions of the cell organcelles called matrix vesicles. The biology of intimal calcification within atherosclerotic regions has been recently reviewed, emphasizing the putative role for matrix vesicles (related to apoptotic bodies), bone-associated proteins, lipids, and inflammation in the formation of extracellular intimal calcifications.[1] However, the role of macrophages, which are morphologically clearly related to the deposition of irregular calcium deposits (Figures 5.5–5.9), has been relatively ignored. The role of apoptotic macrophages in calcification of necrotic cores is unclear, but may be equally as important in coronary artery calcification as in smooth muscle cell apoptosis.

Immunohistochemical studies have demonstrated the co-localization of osteopontin and other calcium binding proteins in areas of microcalcifications.[2–4] We have observed that microcalcifications begin at the base of the core, towards the internal elastic lamina (Figure 5.8B). Subsequent ruptures or superficial fissuring leading to luminal thrombosis result in layers of calcification, with the result that the heaviest concentrations of calcium are towards the internal elastic lamina (Figures 5.12–5.15). Occasionally, calcification may occur at the surface of the plaque with underlying inflammation (Figure 5.16); however, this arrangement is the

Figure 5.4 (*opposite*) Smooth muscle cell calcification: progression of punctate calcification to smooth muscle cell plates. In areas of extensive calcification, decalcification is necessary before routine histologic preparations are possible. Calcified matrix can be identified by blue-purple staining using the Movat pentachrome. A, A calcified fibroatheromatous plaque demonstrates mild luminal narrowing with positive remodeling in the area of plaque (lower portion of artery segment). B, The early core demonstrates typical punctate calcifications, presumably resulting from apoptotic macrophages seen in fibroatheroma C. The portion of the plaque closest to the internal elastic lamina shows layers of sheet-like calcification of the collagen. Such calcification appears to occur in cores that have elicited relatively little macrophage infiltrates.

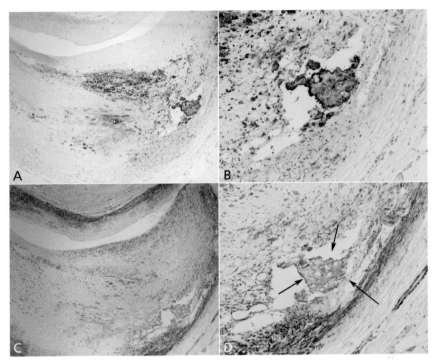

Figure 5.5 Macrophage calcification in late cores. A, A late necrotic core stained for macrophages (CD68 immunohistochemical stain). B, A higher magnification demonstrates an irregular area of calcification that is diffusely positive for macrophage antigen. C, The same core stained for smooth muscle actin. Note that there is staining for smooth muscle cells in the media and surface of the plaque towards the lumen, but the core is negative. D, A higher magnification demonstrates absence of actin staining in the calcified area (arrows).

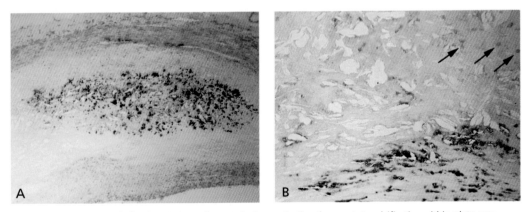

Figure 5.6 Macrophage calcification. A, A von Kossa stain demonstrating the punctate calcification within a late core. B, The macrophage-rich necrotic core (CD68 macrophage immunohistochemical stain) demonstrates macrophage staining, strongest at the periphery of the core, and blue calcium deposits barely visible as hematoxylin-stained bodies (arrows).

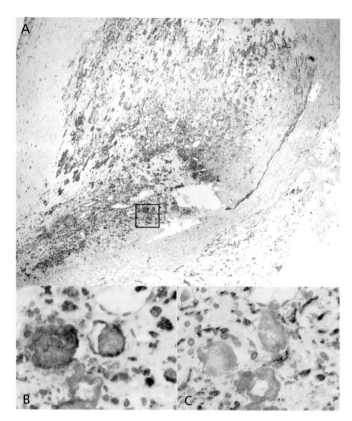

Figure 5.7 Macrophage calcification. A, A low magnification of a calcified necrotic core stained for macrophages (CD8 immunohistochemical stain) demonstrates bluish hematoxylin-stained calcium and macrophages (red-brown, alkaline phosphatase reagent). B, The area boxed in A demonstrates three calcified bodies that show variable amounts of staining for CD68 antigen. C, A smooth muscle cell stain (anti-smooth muscle actin) of the same area shows that the calcified bodies do not stain with smooth muscle actin; note spindled smooth muscle cells surrounding the bodies.

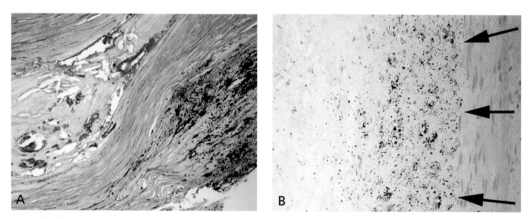

Figure 5.8 Comparison of smooth muscle cell and macrophage calcification in same plaque. A, There is a macrophage-rich necrotic core at the left, characterized by large cholesterol crystals and large calcifications. At the right, finer calcifications of a smooth muscle cell rich apoptotic core are seen (Movat pentachrome stain, calcified matrix staining dark (decalcified specimen)). B, A smooth muscle cell apoptotic core adjacent to the internal elastic lamina (arrows). The media is seen to the right of the arrows. The calcifications, stained by von Kossa stain, are predominantly adjacent to the internal elastic lamina.

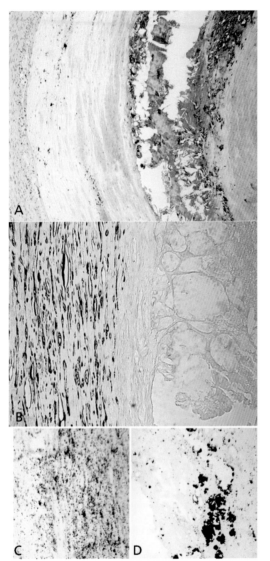

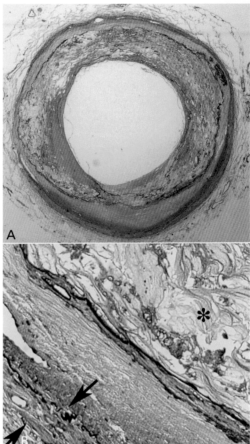

Figure 5.10 Pipestem calcification. Occasionally, a majority of the plaque area may become calcified, with little resulting luminal narrowing due to positive remodeling. A, A low magnification demonstrates circumferential calcification with patent lumen. B, A high magnification of the media shows thinned media (arrows), a narrow uncalcified area of plaque, and a calcified core (asterisk).

Figure 5.9 Comparison of smooth muscle cell and macrophage calcification in the same plaque. A, A late core is strongly positive for CD68 (macrophage marker), without staining in smooth muscle cell region at left, near the internal elastic lamina. B, Smooth muscle cells are identified by anti-alpha actin staining at left, with no staining in late core at right. The smooth muscle cell staining is characteristic of apoptotic smooth muscle cells, in that there is pronounced staining of the cell membranes with central clearing. C, A von Kossa stain in the smooth muscle cell-rich area shows typical microscopic fine calcifications of apoptotic smooth muscle cells. By contrast, the late core (D) shows blocky, larger calcifications when seen at the same magnification.

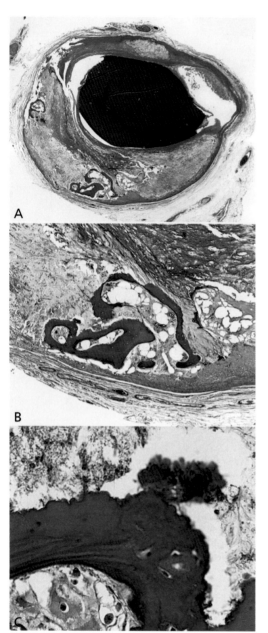

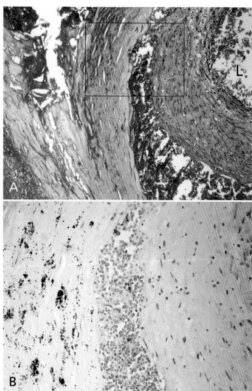

Figure 5.12 Calcium in smooth muscle cell layering of plaque after prior ruptures. A, A Movat pentachrome stain demonstrates the lumen (L), a smooth muscle cell-rich zone beneath the endothelium, an area of hemorrhage, and a deeper area rich in smooth muscle cells with underlying late core. The boxed area demonstrates two layers of smooth muscle cells separated by the hemorrhagic area. B, The boxed area at higher magnification shows that there is speckled calcium (von Kossa stain) in the older smooth muscle cell layer, indicative of ongoing apoptosis, but a lack of calcification in the superficial viable smooth muscle cells at the right of the field.

Figure 5.11 Plaque ossification. Ossification in coronary plaque. A, A low magnification image of a coronary artery section (proximal left anterior descending artery) of an obese elderly woman with hypertensive atherosclerotic heart disease. A is a low magnification of the cross-section of the artery; contrast material (black) was injected in the artery postmortem. The stable atherosclerotic plaque has a large calcified necrotic core. B, A higher magnification demonstrating ossification with osteoid and bony trabeculae. C, The highest magnification showing lacunae containing osteoblasts. Ossification is an uncommon outcome of calcified cores, early or late.

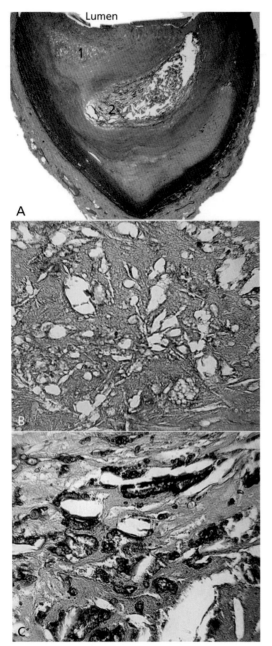

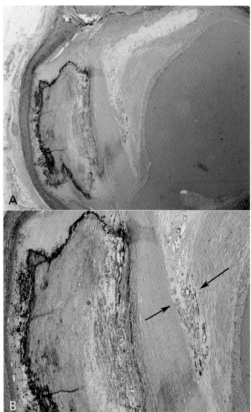

Figure 5.14 Calcium in layers of early and late cores within same plaque. A, This complex plaque demonstrates a deep area of large calcification, and superficial layering indicative of prior ruptures/fissures. B, A high magnification demonstrates formation of superficial core (arrows) with mild blocky calcification, and the deeper plate-like calcification. In general, calcification is greatest towards the internal elastic lamina, because the older portions of the plaque with established calcification occur in this area (Movat pentachrome stain).

Figure 5.13 Calcium in macrophages within layering of late cores forming after prior ruptures. A, There is a superficial core (1) with a deeper core that has ruptured remotely (2). B, The superficial core is rich in macrophages and cholesterol, and shows little if any calcification. C, The deeper macrophage core demonstrates numerous, large calcifications (Movat pentachrome stain).

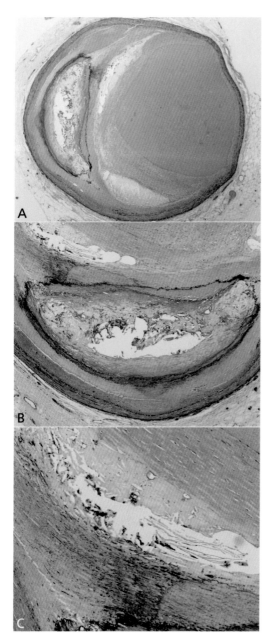

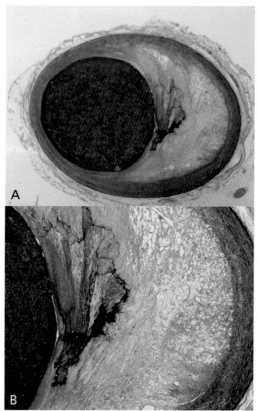

Figure 5.16 Superficial calcification. In contrast to the general rule, calcification in coronary plaques may be primarily superficial, near the lumen as in this example. A, This artery with minimal luminal compromise shows a macrophage-rich necrotic core, with superficial plate-like calcification. B, A higher magnification demonstrates the macrophage-rich necrotic core with a superficial area of calcified plate, with a superficial area suggestive of a calcified plate secondary to remote smooth muscle cell apoptosis (Movat pentachrome).

Figure 5.15 Calcium in layers of necrotic cores. A, A plaque demonstrates three necrotic cores, with one deep heavily calcified core. B, A higher magnification of the deep core reveals almost complete calcification of this core. C, The necrotic core superficial to this core demonstrates blocky macrophage calcification; in between the two cores is a layer of apoptotic smooth muscle cells with punctate fine calcifications progressing to a plate. As is typical, the degree of calcification increases towards the internal elastic lamina (Movat pentachrome stain).

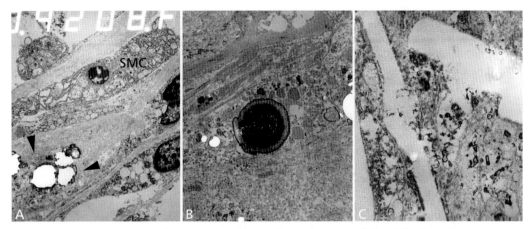

Figure 5.17 Ultrastructural images of coronary atherosclerotic plaques show extracellular calcifications adjacent to an apoptotic smooth muscle cell (SMC)(A), spherical calcification associated with degenerating smooth muscle cell organelles (B), and small calcifications surrounding cholesterol clefts in an area of macrophage degeneration (C).

exception rather than the rule. Ultrastructural study of coronary plaques demonstrates calcifications in close contact with dying smooth muscle cells, macrophages, and surrounding cholesterol clefts (Figure 5.17).

Plaque rupture, organization

The microscopic study of nondecalcified arterial segments by routine histologic methods is possible only if there is mild calcification. In these cases, usually of earlier plaques, sensitive methods such as the von Kossa stain will highlight small vesicle calcifications. In late plaques, fibrous cores and macrophage-rich cores will often demonstrate dense, plate-like calcium deposits that cannot be cut by a standard microtome. In these cases, the study of calcification is possible by evaluating calcified matrix, which can be identified in sections that have been decalcified using a weak acid solution or calcium chelating agents. We have shown an excellent correlation between morphometric measurements of decalcified calcium matrix with radiographs of ex vivo coronary arteries performed prior to decalcification.[5]

Advanced atherosclerotic plaques are characterized by thrombosis, often resulting from exposure of apoptotic cells and tissue factor-rich gruel to the vessel lumen. Although fatal and symptomatic thrombi are associated with arteries with significant cross-sectional luminal narrowing, thrombi also occur in plaques with little stenosis, and are a mechanism of plaque progression.[6] Calcification does not in itself appear to play a role in the thrombotic process, except under unusual circumstances (see below). Successive ruptures or fissures of the fibrous cap result in layering of the plaque, and the deeper layers close to the internal elastic lamina typically demonstrate more severe calcification than the surface layers (Figures 5.12–5.16). Although there is wide variation, acute ruptures are often associated with speckled calcification as assessed radiologically, whereas healed ruptures are associated with larger fragmented or diffuse calcification (Figure 5.18). The smooth muscle cell-rich proliferation that occurs soon after subclinical rupture is, as would be expected, devoid of microcalcifications, as these cells are in a proliferating phase and are not undergoing apoptosis.

We have performed quantitative analysis of calcified matrix in intermediate and later plaque stages, including fibroatheromas, acute and healed plaque ruptures, total occlusions, and plaque erosion. In contrast to rupture, plaque erosion does not expose the contents of the necrotic core to the lumen. Eroded plaques, perhaps partly as a function of their pathogenesis, do not typically occur in calcified arteries, and demonstrate far less calcified matrix than acute or healed ruptures. The degree of calcification by plaque type is illustrated in Figures 5.19 and 5.20.

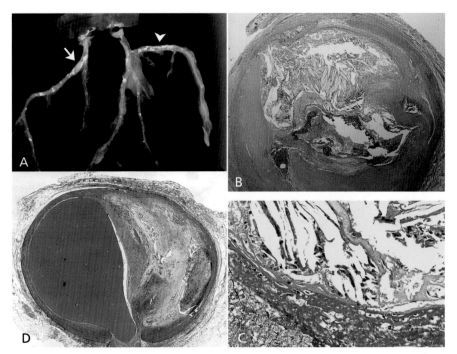

Figure 5.18 Acute and healed plaque ruptures, postmortem radiographic–pathologic correlation. In A, the coronary arterial tree of a sudden death victim has been removed and X-rayed. Subsequent histologic analysis demonstrated an acute rupture in the proximal right coronary artery (arrow) and a healed plaque rupture in the proximal left circumflex (arrowhead). There were a variety of atheromatous plaques in the left anterior descending artery and other branches. The acute rupture (arrow) is located in an area largely devoid of calcium except for barely discernible fine stippling, surrounded by larger fragments. By contrast, the healed rupture (arrowhead) demonstrates fragmented calcification. B, The corresponding histologic section of the acute rupture, with the rupture site shown at higher magnification in C. D, The histologic section of the healed rupture site, with a large area of calcification near the internal elastic lamina.

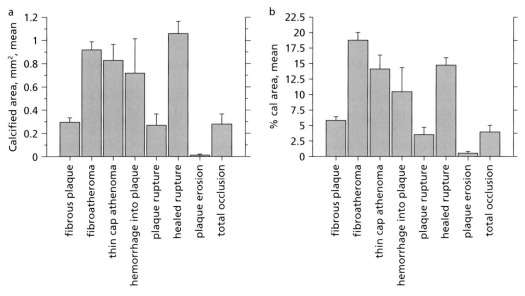

Figure 5.19 Amount of calcification by plaque morphology. Morphometric measurements were made of calcified matrix in several hundred coronary lesions classified by plaque type. a, Healed ruptures demonstrated the greatest mean area of calcification; plaque erosions demonstrate almost no calcification. b, When expressed as a percentage of the plaque area, total occlusion and plaque ruptures have relatively little calcium, and plaque erosions the least. Fibroatheroma and healed ruptures demonstrate the greatest amount of calcified matrix. (Reproduced with permission from Burke et al., Herz 2001;26:239–44.)

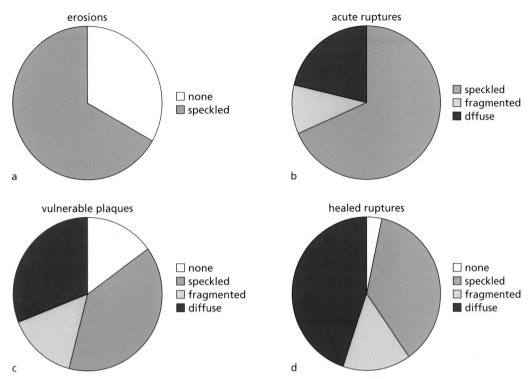

Figure 5.20 Relationship between plaque morphology and radiographic calcification. Plaque erosions (a) were exclusively present in areas with stippled or no calcification. Plaque ruptures (b) were most frequently seen in areas of speckled calcification, but were also present in blocky or diffuse calcification. Curiously, there were no ruptures in segments devoid of any calcification. Thin-capped atheromas were most frequently present in areas of speckled calcification (c), but were also seen in heavily calcified or uncalcified areas, suggesting that calcification pattern is not helpful in diagnosing these lesions. Healed ruptures are almost always seen in areas of calcification, and most frequently in diffusely calcified areas (d). (Reproduced with permission from Burke et al., Herz 2001;26:239–244.)

Systemic factors

It is clear that the initiation of calcification in the coronary atherosclerotic plaque is dependent on cell breakdown, which is a component of virtually all atherosclerotic plaques beyond the earliest stages. However, the degree of calcification from patient to patient varies significantly, and must in part be a function of factors in the circulation which may be under genetic control. Tomographically or radiographically detectable calcification is not present in all patients who die with severe coronary artery disease, but is a function of age, renal function, vitamin D levels and other aspects of bone metabolism,[7] the I/D polymorphism for angiotensin converting enzyme,[8] and diabetes.[9] Chronic renal disease increases coronary calcification as well as peripheral vascular calcification.[10,11] Genetic variations in matrix inhibitory proteins and metalloprotease 3 have been shown to play a role in the degree of atherosclerotic plaque calcification in the coronary arteries,[12,13]

and polymorphisms for tumor necrosis factor, and inflammatory cytokines, may also influence coronary artery calcification.[14] Black race is negatively correlated with coronary calcification, adjusted for other risk factors and plaque burden.[15–17] As age progresses, patients dying with severe coronary disease have increasing amounts of calcium in their plaques, with virtually 100% of patients having radiographically detectable calcification by the sixth decade. Gender appears to have an effect on the degree of plaque calcification, as women dying with severe coronary artery disease have less calcified arteries than men.[18] The reason for this variation is likely due to the protective effect of estrogen against inflammatory components of the plaque and plaque rupture, features that result in plaque calcification. The degree of calcification in women with severe coronary disease increases markedly after menopause (Figure 5.21), and approaches that of men in later years (Figure 5.22).[19]

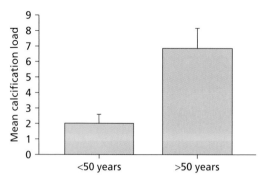

Figure 5.21 Mean calcification score in 51 women who died suddenly from severe coronary disease. The degree of coronary calcification in each segment was determined on a six-point scale and a mean calcification score was calculated for each heart. The left bar shows the mean calcification score in younger women, and the right bar, mean score in older women. The difference was significant (*P* = 0.0007, Student's *t*-test). (Reproduced from Burke et al., Am Heart J, 2001;141:S58–62.)

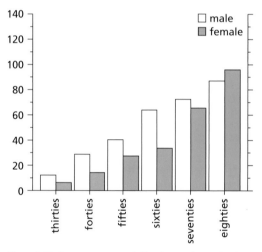

Figure 5.22 Coronary artery calcification, as determined by postmortem radiography, as a factor of age at death and gender, sudden coronary death victims. The x-axis represents the decade of age at death and the y-axis represents a calcification score determined on the basis of area of calcification of coronary arteries (not density) by morphometric scoring. All patients had lethal coronary artery disease resulting in sudden death without other cause at autopsy; cases with and without acute thrombi were included together. Note that although there is a lag in women in the degree of coronary artery calcification, the gender difference vanishes by the eighth decade. These data were derived from cases of sudden death seen in consultation at the Armed Forces Institute of Pathology during the years 1995–2003 (*n* = 413: 335 men, 78 women).

Clinical implications of coronary calcification

Screening

There have been numerous studies on screening patients for coronary artery disease using electron beam computed tomography, a sensitive indicator of coronary artery calcification. The prognostic implications of absolute and relative calcium scores have been reviewed.[20] Coronary calcification, as a marker for coronary artery plaque, is increased in patients with their first coronary event, compared to controls.[21–23] Symptomatic patients with elevated calcium scores are at greater risk for further events.[24] Although the increased benefit of coronary calcium screening in addition to conventional risk factors has not been demonstrated conclusively, some studies suggest that coronary calcification score is a marker for future coronary events independent of conventional risk factors, adding a few percentage points to the receiver operator curve concordance index.[25] Prospective studies showing a large increased risk imparted by coronary calcium independent of other risk factors have been hampered by self-referral and lack of rigorous determination of traditional risk factors.[26] There is evidence that the prediction of sudden cardiac death using the Framingham risk index and the measurement of coronary calcification are distinct methods of assessing risk for sudden cardiac death, and that neither method accurately predicts risk of coronary plaque erosion.

In general, it has been determined that although calcification is a good marker for plaque burden, absolute calcium scores do not indicate plaques that are unstable or prone to result in clinical events. With some exceptions,[27] most studies have not shown an association between serum inflammatory markers and coronary calcification.[28,29] It has been stated that calcification is a "disease marker" as opposed to a "process marker" unlike markers of inflammation.[29] These findings are corroborated by autopsy studies that demonstrate a good correlation between plaque size and morphometric analysis of calcification, but no correlation between residual lumen and calcification (Table 5.2).[20] However, if calcium scores are adjusted for gender and age, relative calcium scores may be more important in identifying patients at risk for myocardial

Table 5.2 Relationship between calcification and % luminal narrowing and residual lumen, by arterial section. (Reproduced with permission from Burke AP, et al. Herz 2001;26:239–44.)

| | Calcified area vs. % luminal narrowing (simple regression) | | | | | | Calcified area vs. residual lumen area (simple regression) | |
| | Men | | | Women | | | Men and women (combined) | |
Artery	r*	P	d.f.	r*	P	d.f.	r†	P
LM	0.20	0.20	30	0.15	0.59	14	0.14	0.58
PLAD	**0.56**	**<0.0001**	122	0.15	0.27	53	0.07	0.53
MLAD	**0.45**	**<0.0001**	91	**0.50**	**<0.0001**	66	0.10	0.29
DLAD	**0.64**	**0.0003**	27	0.31	0.11	24	0.18	0.28
LD	**0.59**	**0.001**	26	**0.75**	**0.0004**	17	0.13	0.71
PLC	0.30	0.01	78	0.25	0.07	51	0.11	0.32
MLC	0.02	0.90	35	0.31	0.29	13	0.21	0.40
LOM	**0.60**	**0.0001**	34	**0.72**	**0.01**	11	0.13	0.30
PRC	0.12	0.15	143	0.09	0.54	54	0.09	0.38
MRC	0.29	0.001	127	**0.63**	**<0.0001**	68	0.09	0.37
DRC	0.32	0.0004	116	0.36	0.06	27	0.17	0.29

* *T* values are all positive (the correlation is positive correlation between calcified area and dependent variable: % luminal narrowing in all cells).

† Correlation is negative (PLAD, MRC, DRC, LD) or positive (LM, LOM, MLAD, PLC, MLC, PRC).

Values in bold show *r* values >0.4 and a significant correlation *P* < 0.05.

Abbreviations: LM = left main; PLAD = proximal left anterior descending; MLAD = mid left anterior descending; DLAD = distal left anterior descending; LD = left diagonal; PLC = proximal left circumflex; MLC = mid left circumflex; LOM = left obtuse marginal; PRC = proximal right coronary; MRC = mid right coronary; DRC = distal right coronary; d.f. = degrees of freedom.

infarction or coronary death.[20] This would be expected, given the large effect of age on degree of calcium seen in patients dying with severe coronary disease. Because plaque calcification by computed tomographic studies is a reliable marker for subclinical coronary artery disease, it is useful for correlation between risk factors and early disease.[30,31]

Plaque instability

Biomechanical studies have calculated stress at different regions of the plaque. Mathematical models using large-strain finite element analysis have shown that increased lipids are associated with areas of weakness of the fibrous cap, but not calcification.[20] Further studies are necessary to demonstrate conclusively that calcification has

no effect on biomechanical forces resulting in plaque rupture. Clinical studies suggest that relatively mild calcification is associated with acute coronary events, whereas patients with chronic ischemia have more extensive calcification.[32] By contrast, an angiographic follow-up study has shown that calcified plaques are more likely to progress than those that are not.[33] Positive arterial remodeling has been demonstrated to be increased in coronary artery plaques with calcification[34] (Figure 5.23), and has also been demonstrated as a marker for unstable plaques.[35]

Calcified nodule

Although it is unclear if calcification predicts coronary instability, there is a form of coronary

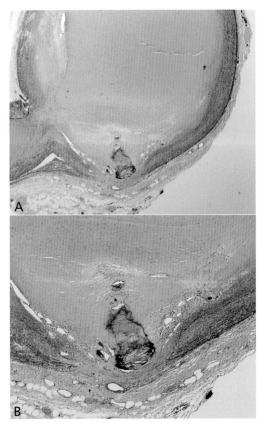

Figure 5.23 Coronary artery remodeling in calcified plaque. A, A low magnification demonstrates relatively little luminal compromise, and an area of plate-like calcification in a fibrous plaque. B, Note, at higher magnification, the destruction of media in the area of calcification, with surrounding angiogenesis (Movat pentachrome).

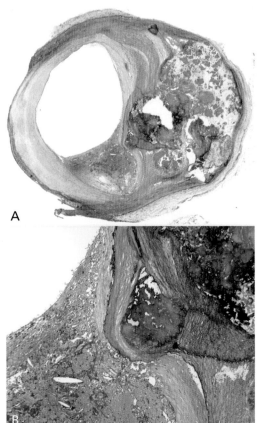

Figure 5.24 Calcified nodule. A, There is an eccentric plaque that does not result in critical stenosis; it is largely composed of calcium (Movat pentachrome stain after decalcification, calcified matrix is dark). B, A higher magnification of disrupted calcium crystals resulting in extrusion into the lumen and small luminal thrombus. (Reproduced with permission from Burke AP, et al. Herz 2001;26:239–44.)

artery calcification that may result directly in fatal thrombosis. Calcified nodules are plates of calcium in advanced plaques that have broken into fragments which erupt into the lumen, resulting in thrombosis and an intimal reaction[36] (Figure 5.24). Calcified nodules tend to occur in older men relative to ruptures or erosions. The calcium within these nodules may demonstrate an osteoclast-like reaction and osseous metaplasia. In a series of sudden death, calcified nodules resulted in only 5% of lethal coronary thrombi.[36] Nodular calcification may occur within the plaque in the absence of luminal thrombosis, and is characterized by fractured plates of calcification, often with an

inflammatory reaction (Figure 5.25). The stimulus which triggers the formation of nodular calcification is unknown, but may include the incorporation of fibrin, which is often present surrounding the calcified plates.

References

1. Proudfoot D, Shanahan CM. Biology of calcification in vascular cells: intima versus media. Herz 2001:245–51.
2. Fitzpatrick LA, Severson A, Edwards WD, Ingram RT. Diffuse calcification in human coronary arteries. Association of osteopontin with atherosclerosis. J Clin Invest 1994;94:1597–604.

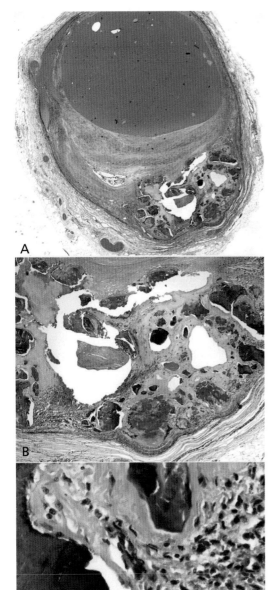

Figure 5.25 Nodular calcification, without rupture. Most cases of nodular calcification do not result in symptomatic thrombosis. A, A section of coronary artery demonstrates heavy calcification towards the internal elastic lamina. B, A higher power magnification of this area demonstrates large blocks of calcium, which appear to have broken, possibly due to shear stresses. C, The broken calcium fragments are focally surrounded by an inflammatory response.

3. Kwon HM, Hong BK, Kang TS, et al. Expression of osteopontin in calcified coronary atherosclerotic plaques. J Korean Med Sci 2000;15:485–93.

4. O'Brien ER, Garvin MR, Stewart DK, et al. Osteopontin is synthesized by macrophage, smooth muscle, and endothelial cells in primary and restenotic human coronary atherosclerotic plaques. Arterioscler Thromb 1994;14:1648–56.

5. Burke AP, Taylor A, Farb A, Malcom GT, Virmani R. Coronary calcification: insights from sudden coronary death victims. Z Kardiol 2000;89:49–53.

6. Burke AP, Kolodgie FD, Farb A, Weber DK, Malcom GT, Smialek J, Virmani R. Healed plaque ruptures and sudden coronary death: evidence that subclinical rupture has a role in plaque progression. Circulation 2001;103:934–40.

7. Watson KE, Abrolat ML, Malone LL, et al. Active serum vitamin D levels are inversely correlated with coronary calcification. Circulation 1997;96:1755–60.

8. Pfohl M, Athanasiadis A, Koch M, et al. Insertion/deletion polymorphism of the angiotensin I-converting enzyme gene is associated with coronary artery plaque calcification as assessed by intravascular ultrasound. J Am Coll Cardiol 1998;31:987–91.

9. Burke AP, Farb A, Liang Y-H, Smialek J, Virmani R. Diabetes mellitus is associated with coronary artery calcification in sudden cardiac death. J Am Coll Cardiol 1997;29:516A.

10. Schoenhagen P, Tuzcu EM. Coronary artery calcification and end-stage renal disease: vascular biology and clinical implications. Cleve Clin J Med 2002;69:S12–20.

11. Raggi P, Ali O. Phosphorus restriction and control of coronary calcification as assessed by electron beam tomography. Curr Opin Nephrol Hypertens 2002;11:391–5.

12. Herrmann SM, Whatling C, Brand E, et al. Polymorphisms of the human matrix gla protein (MGP) gene, vascular calcification, and myocardial infarction. Arterioscler Thromb Vasc Biol 2000;20:2386–93.

13. Pollanen PJ, Lehtimaki T, Ilveskoski E, et al. Coronary artery calcification is related to functional polymorphism of matrix metalloproteinase 3: the Helsinki Sudden Death Study. Atherosclerosis 2002;164:329–35.

14. Keso T, Perola M, Laippala P, et al. Polymorphisms within the tumor necrosis factor locus and prevalence of coronary artery disease in middle-aged men. Atherosclerosis 2001;154:691–7.

15. Lee TC, O'Malley PG, Feuerstein I, Taylor AJ. The prevalence and severity of coronary artery calcification on coronary artery computed tomography in black and white subjects. J Am Coll Cardiol 2003;41:39–44.

16. Newman AB, Naydeck BL, Whittle J, Sutton-Tyrrell K, Edmundowicz D, Kuller LH. Racial differences in coronary artery calcification in older adults. Arterioscler Thromb Vasc Biol 2002;22:424–30.

17. Burke AP, Farb A, Kutys R, Zieske A, Weber DK, Virmani R. Atherosclerotic coronary plaques in African Americans are less likely to calcify than coronary plaques in Caucasian Americans. Circulation 2002;106:II-481(A).

18. Burke AP, Farb A, Malcom G, Virmani R. Effect of menopause on plaque morphologic characteristics in coronary atherosclerosis. Am Heart J 2001;141:S58–62.

19. Burke AP, Weber DK, Kolodgie FD, Farb A, Taylor AJ, Virmani R. Pathophysiologie der Kalziumdeposition in Koronararterien. Herz 2001;26:239–44.

20. Raggi P. Prognostic implications of absolute and relative calcium scores. Herz 2001;26:262–9.

21. Pohle K, Ropers D, Maffert R, et al. Coronary calcifications in young patients with first, unheralded myocardial infarction: a risk factor matched analysis by electron beam tomography. Heart 2003;89:625–8.

22. Cheng YJ, Church TS, Kimball TE, et al. Comparison of coronary artery calcium detected by electron beam tomography in patients with to those without symptomatic coronary heart disease. Am J Cardiol 2003;92:498–503.

23. Vliegenthart R, Oudkerk M, Song B, van der Kuip DA, Hofman A, Witteman JC. Coronary calcification detected by electron-beam computed tomography and myocardial infarction. The Rotterdam Coronary Calcification Study. Eur Heart J 2002;23:1596–603.

24. Mohlenkamp S, Lehmann N, Schmermund A, et al. Prognostic value of extensive coronary calcium quantities in symptomatic males – a 5-year follow-up study. Eur Heart J 2003;24:845–54.

25. Shaw LJ, Raggi P, Schisterman E, Berman DS, Callister TQ. Prognostic value of cardiac risk factors and coronary artery calcium screening for all-cause mortality. Radiology 2003;17:17.

26. Kondos GT, Hoff JA, Sevrukov A, et al. Electron-beam tomography coronary artery calcium and cardiac events: a 37–month follow-up of 5635 initially asymptomatic low- to intermediate-risk adults. Circulation 2003;107:2571–6.

27. Wang TJ, Larson MG, Levy D, et al. C-reactive protein is associated with subclinical epicardial coronary calcification in men and women: the Framingham Heart Study. Circulation 2002;106:1189–91.

28. Reilly MP, Wolfe ML, Localio AR, Rader DJ. C-reactive protein and coronary artery calcification. The Study of Inherited Risk of Coronary Atherosclerosis (SIRCA). Arterioscler Thromb Vasc Biol 2003;21:21.

29. Hunt ME, O'Malley PG, Vernalis MN, Feuerstein IM, Taylor AJ. C-reactive protein is not associated with the presence or extent of calcified subclinical atherosclerosis. Am Heart J 2001;141:206–10.

30. O'Malley PG, Jones DL, Feuerstein IM, Taylor AJ. Lack of correlation between psychological factors and subclinical coronary artery disease. N Engl J Med 2000;343:1298–304.

31. Taylor AJ, Burke AP, O'Malley PG, et al. A comparison of the Framingham risk index, coronary artery calcification, and culprit plaque morphology in sudden cardiac death. Circulation 2000;101:1243–8.

32. Shemesh J, Apter S, Itzchak Y, Motro M. Coronary calcification compared in patients with acute versus in those with chronic coronary events by using dual-sector spiral CT. Radiology 2003;226:483–8.

33. Casscells W, Hassan K, Vaseghi MF, et al. Plaque blush, branch location, and calcification are angiographic predictors of progression of mild to moderate coronary stenoses. Am Heart J 2003;145:813–20.

34. Burke AP, Kolodgie FD, Farb A, Weber D, Virmani R. Morphological predictors of arterial remodeling in coronary atherosclerosis. Circulation 2002;105:297–303.

35. Von Birgelen C, Klinkhart W, Mintz GS, et al. Plaque distribution and vascular remodeling of ruptured and nonruptured coronary plaques in the same vessel: an intravascular ultrasound study in vivo. J Am Coll Cardiol 2001;37:1864–70.

36. Virmani R, Kolodgie FD, Burke AP, Farb A, Schwartz SM. Lessons from sudden coronary death: a comprehensive morphological classification scheme for atherosclerotic lesions. Arterioscler Thromb Vasc Biol 2000;20:1262–75.

CHAPTER 6

Adventitial and periadventitial fat inflammation and plaque vulnerability

Silvio Litovsky, Deborah Vela, Mohammad Madjid,
Samuel Ward Casscells & James T Willerson

Because atherosclerosis is an intimal disease of large and medium arteries, most of the literature on this subject is devoted to the intimal layer and the smooth muscle cells that reach the intima from the media. Nevertheless, the adventitia has long been known to play an important role in restenosis after vascular injury and in the natural development and progression of atherosclerosis.

The following significant findings suggest that the adventitia plays a prominent role in normal vessel physiology:

1 Occlusion of the adventitial vasa vasorum of pigs results in intimal smooth-muscle-rich proliferating lesions, suggesting that arterial hypoxia is involved in the initiation of intimal hyperplasia.[1]

2 In experimental atherosclerosis, marked proliferation of angiogenic vessels is seen early in the disease process, in the adventitia as much as in the intimal plaque.[2] In swine, adventitial angiogenesis occurs within 3 days after experimental coronary angioplasty, and regression of adventitial microvessels correlates with arterial narrowing, suggesting that the adventitial microvasculature has an important influence on arterial remodeling.[3]

3 Scott and coworkers[4] and Shi and colleagues[5] reported that, after balloon overstretch injury to porcine coronary arteries, adventitial myofibroblasts contribute to intimal hyperplasia by proliferating, by synthesizing growth factors, and by migrating to

the intima. Increased synthesis of alpha-smooth-muscle actin in the adventitia was believed to be an important factor in the remodeling process. Cell proliferation after angioplasty was higher in the adventitia than in the media.

4 Adventitial fibroblasts can produce nitric oxide (NO) and, thus, can participate in endothelium-dependent relaxation in the absence of endothelium when they are successfully transfected with recombinant endothelial NO synthase.[6]

5 In a cynomolgus monkey model of atherosclerosis, inflammatory cells remain in the adventitia after they have disappeared from the plaque and media.[7]

6 Toll-like receptor-4 (TLR4) is a pattern-recognition receptor involved in the innate immune response to various microorganisms and other exogenous and endogenous stress factors potentially involved in the pathogenesis of atherosclerosis, such as lipopolysaccharide (LPS) and heat-shock proteins. Vink and colleagues[8] studied the localization of TLR4-positive cells in atherosclerotic human coronary arteries and found these cells in the plaque and adventitia. Of interest, in the adventitia not only macrophages but also fibroblasts were positive. Exposure of these fibroblasts to lipopolysaccharides led to activation of nuclear factor-kappa B (NF-κB) and to increases in several pro-inflammatory cytokine levels.

7 Radiation appears to prevent intimal hyperplasia after balloon injury, at least in part, by inhibiting adventitial cell proliferation.[9]

8 P-selectin, known to be a potent recruiter of leukocytes, also induces adventitial inflammation and vascular shrinkage in a balloon-injury model.[10]

9 In experimental hypercholesterolemia, neovascularization of enhanced coronary vasa vasorum (predominantly through an increase of second-order vasa vasorum) has been described within the first few weeks of plaque development.[11,12] Moreover, neovascularization preceded the development of endothelial dysfunction.

10 Using immunohistochemistry and polymerase chain reaction (PCR), Vink and associates[13] demonstrated the presence of *Chlamydia pneumoniae* in the adventitia of human coronary arteries. This microorganism was found more frequently in the adventitia than in the plaque and was related to the severity of the disease.

In summary, the immunologic, angiogenic, and fibroblastic/myofibroblastic responses to vessel injury suggest that the adventitia plays a major role in vascular remodeling and intimal hyperplasia. To date, the evidence is probably stronger for restenosis after mechanical injury than for the development of natural atherosclerosis.

Adventitial inflammation

Kohchi and coworkers[14] described adventitial inflammation, often associated with nerve involvement, in the adventitia of coronary arteries of patients with angina. These authors hypothesized that their findings might be related to the vasospastic component of unstable angina. In studying nonintimal factors associated with plaque disruption, Moreno and associates[15] found that – like intimomedial interface changes, media inflammation, and atrophy and fibrosis – adventitial inflammation was more prevalent among disrupted plaques. In class III lesions (American Heart Association classification), the authors observed mild adventitial inflammation that increased with progression of the disease.

Adventitial inflammation has been implicated in unstable angina,[14] in restenosis after angioplasty,[16] and even in proliferation of neovessels in the intima.[17] The complexity and frequent organization of the inflammatory infiltrate in advanced lesions suggests the local generation of humoral immune responses[18] with more B- than T-lymphocytes, similar to responses seen in mucosa-associated lymphoid tissue. It is, therefore, likely that the immunologic reaction develops in response to antigens released during a longstanding process of tissue injury and inflammation and that the reaction is more prominent in advanced atherosclerosis.

A number of reports[14,15,19] have focused on adventitial inflammation as a marker of plaque vulnerability. Interest has been devoted not only to macrophages and lymphocytes but also to mast cells, which are present in higher numbers in culprit arteries and also (in degranulated form) in segments with plaque rupture.[19] An association between neurogenic stimulation and mast cell release of vasoactive compounds has been described, being most prominent in advanced coronary lesions.[20] Proliferation of vasa vasorum into the intima may increase plaque vulnerability to both rupture and inflammation. Higuchi and coworkers confirmed those findings and found a greater density of lymphocytes in the adventitia of the culprit plaques than in their intima.[21] These results are not surprising in light of the total cross-sectional area of the vasa vasorum in the adventitia.

It should be kept in mind that the adventitia is also the site of parasympathetic innervation of the coronary arteries. Acetylcholine released by these terminals diffuses through the media, reaching the endothelium to activate its muscarinic receptors and release NO.

An elegant review of the influence of the adventitia on vascular function was published by Gutterman in 1999.[22]

The outer layers of the coronary artery (the media and particularly the adventitia) are vulnerable to diabetes-induced redox-sensitive injury,[23] leading to increased inflammatory gene expression, adventitial release of cytokines and chemokines, homing of blood-borne inflammatory cells into affected segments of the vessel wall, cellular crosstalk, and development of intimal lesions. Intercellular adhesion molecule (ICAM) and vascular cell adhesion molecule-1 (VCAM-1) are highly expressed in adventitial vasa vasorum, becoming an important vascular port of entry for inflammatory cells.[24]

Periadventitial fat and vascular physiology

In adults, almost all blood vessels are surrounded by periadventitial fat. This is especially true of the epicardial coronary arteries, where such fat is often very abundant. Nevertheless, although interest in the outer layers of the vessel has recently increased, the literature on atherosclerosis has not focused on periadventitial fat. This omission is somewhat surprising, as periadventitial fat produces a vascular relaxing factor that most probably functions through tyrosine-kinase-dependent activation of potassium channels in vascular smooth muscle cells,[25] which is NO-independent.

Using adenoviral gene transfer, Bhardwaj and associates[26] evaluated the angiogenic responses of several members of the vascular endothelial growth factor (VEGF) family in vivo. Adenoviruses encoding for VEGF-A, VEGF-B, VEGF-C, VEGF-D, VEGF-CDNDC, and VEGF-DDNDC were transferred locally to the **periadventitial space** of the rabbit carotid arteries by means of a collar technique. Seven days after the gene transfer, maximum neovessel formation was observed in VEGF-A-, VEGF-D-, and VEGF-DDNDC-transfected arteries. Although the authors did not emphasize the fat component of the periadventitial space, it seems reasonable to assume that the periadventitial fat displayed angiogenic responses to the VEGFs.

De Meyer and colleagues[27] observed inducible NO synthase (iNOS) expression in the periadventitial granulation tissue of rabbit carotid arteries after a silicone collar was positioned around the vessel. The iNOS was produced by macrophages and T-lymphocytes.

The adipose tissue has been studied mostly in the setting of obesity, diabetes, and metabolic syndrome.[28] Remarkably, adipocytes increase in size as a result of augmented fatty acid availability, but the cellular homeostasis and secretory profile of larger adipocytes evolve toward an inflammatory state compared with those of smaller adipocytes. The adipose tissue secretes cytokines known to be produced by macrophages, such as tumor necrosis factor alfa (TNF-α) and interleukin 6 (IL-6). Although macrophages and adipocytes derive from different lineages (hematopoietic and mesenchymal), the gene expression profile of fat tissue from obese individuals resembles that of macrophages.[29,30] All these studies were performed on subcutaneous or abdominal fat. To our knowledge, it has not yet been reported whether obesity, metabolic syndrome, diabetes mellitus, or all three conditions induce these findings in periadventitial fat as well.

Macrophages take up fat in the form of cholesterol and become foam cells in atherosclerotic vessels. Because the gene expression of preadipocytes is closer to that of macrophages than to adipocytes, researchers have suggested that adipocytes and macrophages may be interconvertible.[31] Of interest for the following discussion (below), the macrophages in adipose tissue are most likely derived from bone marrow, thus blurring even further the differences between the two cell types.[29,30]

Periadventitial adipose tissue and vascular disease

C-reactive protein is a widely used systemic marker for inflammation, and elevated high-sensitive C-reactive protein (hs-CRP) is an accepted risk factor for coronary artery disease.[32,33] However, hs-CRP is also associated with obesity, insulin resistance (a key component of the metabolic syndrome), and diabetes mellitus. The adipose tissue secretes several bioactive substances (e.g. leptin, hs-CRP, TNF-α, adiponectin) that have a major impact on obesity and vascular diseases. Adiponectin opposes TNF-α and is inversely associated with hs-CRP in plasma and adipose tissue.[34] Moreover, hypoadiponectemia has been observed in obesity, diabetes, and cardiovascular disease. It is unknown whether autonomic stimulation affects periadventitial fat.[35]

The adventitial response to injury has long been considered critical to the process of constrictive vascular remodeling that leads to restenosis after vascular injury. In a porcine coronary artery model of balloon angioplasty, Okamoto and coworkers[36] observed an inflammatory response that involved the entire perivascular space and extended several millimeters away from the arterial wall. The authors hypothesized that the perivascular reaction played a key role in the recruitment and proliferation of myofibroblasts, leading to vascular remodeling and restenosis.

There is growing interest in adipose tissue as a possible source of stem cells.[37,38] Planat-Benard

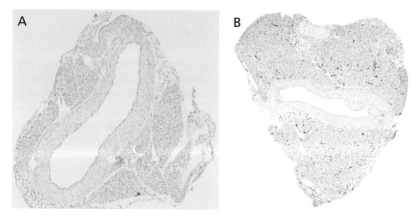

Figure 6.1 Cross-section of the thoracic aorta of a wild-type C57BL/6 mouse (A) and an apoE$^{-/-}$ mouse (B). One week before being sacrificed, the animals were injected intravenously with superparamagnetic iron oxide (1 mM/kg). Rare iron particles are seen in the periadventitial fat of the wild-type mouse. Some iron is seen in the plaque, but a much larger amount is seen in the periadventitial fat of the apoE$^{-/-}$ mouse. Note that the adventitia is extremely thin in mice ($\times$4).

and associates[39] have shown that de-differentiated human adipocytes are capable of acquiring an endothelial phenotype in vitro and inducing neovascularization in ischemic tissue.

We were able to find only a single report[40] on the possible association between the periadventitial adipose tissue and atherosclerosis. During elective coronary artery bypass grafting (CABG), the authors took samples of periadventitial fat from the right coronary arteries and compared these samples with subcutaneous fat from the same individuals with regard to expression of inflammatory cytokines. The amounts of mRNA and protein were much greater for all the inflammatory mediators in the perivascular tissue than in the subcutaneous tissue, raising the possibility that the perivascular inflammatory mediators might play a significant role in the disease process.

Superparamagnetic iron oxide and periadventitial fat

Phagocytic and microbicidal properties have been observed in the adipose tissue.[41,42] Several groups, including ours, are interested in the use of superparamagnetic iron oxide (SPIO) as a contrast agent for magnetic resonance imaging of atherosclerotic plaques. These nanoparticles are taken up by macrophages of the reticuloendothelial system and by plaque macrophages.[43] The iron localizes not

only in plaque macrophages but also in periadventitial fat. We first noticed this fact in the aortas of apoE-deficient mice. Briefly, we injected 12-month-old apoE-deficient mice and 6-month-old C57BL/6 female mice with SPIO (1 mmol/kg iron) intravenously. Six days later, the mice were killed and their aortas perfusion-fixed. The striking finding was prominent iron deposition in the periadventitial fat (Figure 6.1). Mice do not have a thick, well-defined adventitial layer, so comparison between the fat and the adventitia is not really possible. Figure 6.2 shows the stainable iron area as a function of the fat area in the periadventitial fat of apoE-deficient ($n = 22$) and wild-type C57 ($n = 11$) mice. The atherosclerotic mice had a significantly

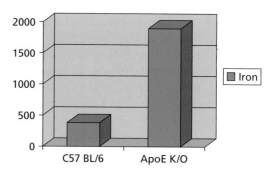

Figure 6.2 Stainable iron area as a function of the fat area in the periadventitia of wild-type C57BL/6 and atherosclerotic apoE$^{-/-}$ mice. The latter mice accumulate more iron than does the wild-type strain.

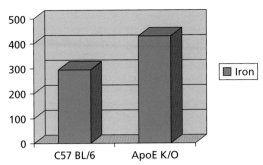

Figure 6.3 Stainable iron area as a function of the fat area in the subcutaneous fat of wild-type C57BL/6 and atherosclerotic apoE$^{-/-}$ mice. No significant difference in iron uptake is seen.

higher iron density than the wild-type mice. When the iron densities in the abdominal subcutaneous fat of apoE-deficient and C57 mice were contrasted, there was no statistical difference between the two strains (Figure 6.3). The Mac-2 stain (Figure 6.4) showed positive ovoid- and spindle-shaped cells in the fat; these cells were more numerous in the apoE

K/O mice than in the wild-type animals. Similar results were obtained with F4/80, suggesting that the positive cells were mature macrophages (Figure 6.5).

We repeated this protocol on atherosclerotic Watanabe hyperlipidemic hereditable (WHHL) rabbits and wild-type New Zealand White rabbits. In the latter animals, no iron uptake was present in the aorta. This finding was expected because no macrophages are present in the intima, and only rare iron particles occur in the periadventitial fat (Figure 6.6A). In the WHHL rabbits, however, iron was present in subendothelial macrophages (Figure 6.6B,C) and in periadventitial fat macrophages (Figure 6.6D).

The findings of Mazurek and associates[40] suggest that inflammatory cells, including macrophages, have a significant pathophysiologic effect on the periadventitial fat of coronary arteries. We compared fibroatheromas that had significant lipid cores with stable, fibrocalcific "burnt-out" plaques with regard to the presence of macrophages, as evidenced by the KP-1 monoclonal antibody. In the

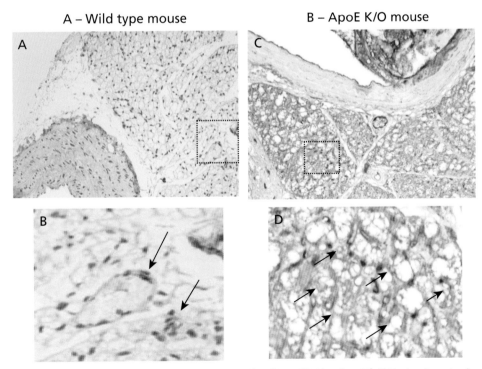

A – Wild type mouse B – ApoE K/O mouse

Figure 6.4 Macrophage (Mac2)-positive cells in periadventitial fat of C57/Bl (A,B) and apoE$^{-/-}$ (C,D) mice. A greater density of positive cells is seen in the knockout mouse (A, ×10; C, ×20; B,D, ×50).

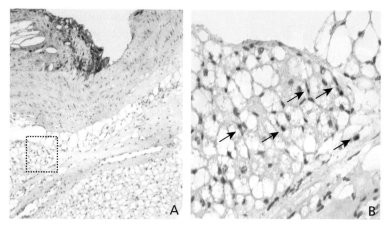

Figure 6.5 Macrophage F4/80-positive cells in apoE$^{-/-}$ mice. Positive cells are present in the periadventitial fat and also in large numbers in the atherosclerotic plaque (A, ×20; B, ×40).

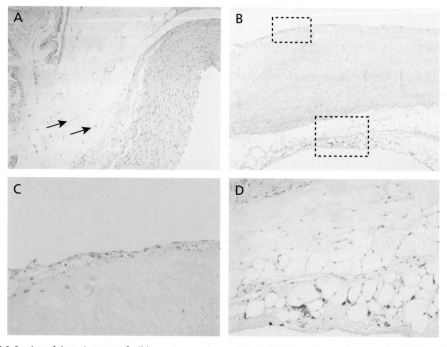

Figure 6.6 Section of thoracic aortas of wild-type New Zealand White (NZW) (A) and hypercholesterolemic Watanabe hyperlipidemic hereditable (WHHL) rabbits (B). One week before being killed, the animals were injected intravenously with superparamagnetic iron oxide (SPIO), 1 mM/kg. As with the wild-type mouse, no iron is present in the vessel layers of the New Zealand White rabbit (A), but rare amounts of iron are seen in the periadventitial fat (arrows). In the WHHL rabbit (B), intracellular iron is seen in the superficial areas of the plaque (magnified in C) and periadventitial fat (magnified in D) (A, ×10; B, ×4; C,D, ×20).

lesions with a lipid core, more macrophage infiltration was seen in the periadventitial fat (Figure 6.7). Figure 6.8A,D shows a section from a coronary artery with a fibroatheroma, including a large lipid core. In addition, a significant macrophage infiltrate was present in the adventitia and periadventitial fat. Toluidine blue and S100 stains ruled out the possibility that these cells might represent

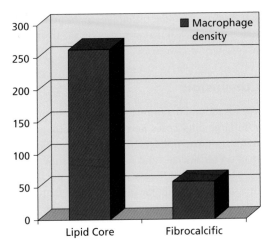

Figure 6.7 The density of macrophages in the periadventitial fat of sections with lipid cores is markedly higher than in sections with stable, fibrocalcific, "burnt-out" plaques.

mast cells or dendritic cells. The lack of clear differences between the adventitia and the immediate periadventitial fat suggests that these two structures function as a physiologic unit.

Figure 6.8B,E shows a fibrocalcific plaque with significant calcification and fibrosis but without a lipid core. Only rare macrophages are present in the periadventitial fat. Finally, two coronary artery sections from patients without atherosclerosis revealed only rare macrophages in the periadventitial fat (Figure 6.8C,F).

Our study shows that human atherosclerotic coronary arteries with large lipid cores have a significantly greater number of macrophages in their periadventitial fat than do fibrocalcific and nonatherosclerotic arteries, thus adding to the list of vulnerability variables.

Our study also suggests that the adventitia and periadventitial fat may function as a unit. The lack of a functional border between the adventitia and periadventitial fat was noted earlier by Okamoto and colleagues[36] in the setting of percutaneous transluminal coronary angioplasty (PTCA), and we believe that this finding can be extrapolated to atherosclerotic plaque.

Significant macrophage transport through the markedly expanded vasa vasorum has been seen in advanced atherosclerotic disease,[44] but no

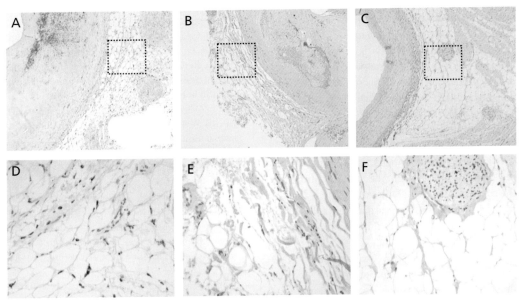

Figure 6.8 Results of CD68 immunostaining for macrophages in human coronary arteries. A, Section from a patient with a typical fibroatheroma, showing a lipid core, a large number of plaque macrophages, and a thin cap. The inset (D) shows a large number of macrophages in the periadventitial fat. B, A stable fibrocalcific plaque. The macrophage density is clearly lower in the plaque and periadventitial fat. The inset (E) shows only rare macrophages in the adventitia and periadventitial fat. C, Section of a normal coronary artery. Only a rare macrophage is seen in the adventitia and periadventitial fat. In the inset (F), hardly any macrophages are seen (A–C, ×10; D–F, ×40).

association with increased fat neovascularization has been described. Our data from mice and humans support the theory that the homing of "out-of-fat" macrophages may play a role in atherosclerosis.[29,30] All these studies suggest that, on the basis of "outside-to-inside" signaling, periadventitial fat may have a role in the development, progression, and/or complications of atherosclerosis.

Atherosclerosis is absent from the intramyocardial segments of coronary arteries, and hemodynamic factors are considered responsible for this absence.[45] Lack of periadventitial fat, however, could be an alternative explanation. Anomalous coronary arteries arising from the opposite sinus also lack atherosclerosis in the intramural aortic segments[46] and periadventitial fat in their intramural course.

Potential diagnostic and therapeutic implications

The present study suggests a potential means for imaging inflammation. The periadventitial uptake should improve MRI spatial resolution, the greatest drawback in MRI technology, and thus could represent a major advance in the noninvasive imaging of vulnerable atherosclerotic plaques.

Pericardial drug delivery is most promising because, unlike in the endovascular approach, the entire coronary tree and its surrounding fat tissue is in direct contact with the overlying pericardial fluid.

Perivascular intrapericardial delivery of NO donor has been successfully tried in experimental animals as a way of preventing restenosis after vessel injury.[47,48] It is difficult to ascertain whether the primary effect is on the periadventitial fat, the adventitia, or both. Other compounds that are being tested via intrapericardial delivery include FGF-2,[49] procainamide,[50] nitroglycerin,[51] heparin,[52] and others.

Gene therapy has been used to insert DNA encoding a number of proteins into vascular tissue.[53] Intracerebroventricular injection of an adenovirus vector with the gene for β-galactosidase has successfully transfected adventitial cells into the subarachnoid space.[54] Encoded compounds have included endothelial nitric oxide synthase,[6] superoxide dismutase,[55] and angiogenic factors.

Application of similar techniques to the pericardial space could have a major impact on the treatment of coronary artery disease.

Conclusion

We have found that human atherosclerotic arteries with large lipid cores have a significantly greater number of macrophages in their periadventitial fat than do fibrocalcific and nonatherosclerotic arteries. This may be additional evidence that the adventitia, and specifically the periadventitial fat plays a role in the atherosclerosis and its progression.

References

1. Barker SG, Tilling LC, Miller GC, et al. The adventitia and atherogenesis: removal initiates intimal proliferation in the rabbit which regresses on generation of a "neoadventitia." Atherosclerosis 1994;105:131–44.
2. Winter PM, Morawski AM, Caruthers SD, et al. Molecular imaging of angiogenesis in early-stage atherosclerosis with alpha(v)beta3-integrin-targeted nanoparticles. Circulation 2003;108:2270–4. Epub 2003 Oct 13.
3. Pels K, Labinaz M, Hoffert C, O'Brien ER. Adventitial angiogenesis early after coronary angioplasty: correlation with arterial remodeling. Arterioscler Thromb Vasc Biol 1999;19:229–38.
4. Scott NA, Cipolla GD, Ross CE, Dunn B, Martin FH, Simonet L, Wilcox JN. Identification of a potential role for the adventitia in vascular lesion formation after balloon overstretch injury of porcine coronary arteries. Circulation 1996;93:2178–87.
5. Shi Y, O'Brien JE, Fard A, Mannion JD, Wang D, Zalewski A. Adventitial myofibroblasts contribute to neointimal formation in injured porcine coronary arteries. Circulation 1996;94:1655–64.
6. Tsutsui M, Onoue H, Iida Y, Smith L, O'Brien T, Katusic ZS. Adventitia-dependent relaxations of canine basilar arteries transduced with recombinant eNOS gene. Am J Physiol 1999;276:H1846–52.
7. Padgett RC, Heistad DD, Mugge A, Armstrong ML, Piegors DJ, Lopez JA. Vascular responses to activated leukocytes after regression of atherosclerosis. Circ Res 1992;70:423–9.
8. Vink A, Schoneveld AH, van der Meer JJ, et al. In vivo evidence for a role of toll-like receptor 4 in the development of intimal lesions. Circulation 2002;106:1985–90.
9. Wilcox JN, Waksman R, King SB, Scott NA. The role of the adventitia in the arterial response to angioplasty: the effect of intravascular radiation. Int J Radiat Oncol Biol Phys 1996;36:789–96.

10. Hayashi S, Watanabe N, Nakazawa K, et al. Roles of P-selectin in inflammation, neointimal formation, and vascular remodeling in balloon-injured rat carotid arteries. Circulation 2000;102:1710–17.

11. Kwon HM, Sangiorgi G, Ritman EL, et al. Enhanced coronary vasa vasorum neovascularization in experimental hypercholesterolemia. J Clin Invest 1998;101:1551–6.

12. Herrmann J, Lerman LO, Rodriguez-Porcel M, et al. Coronary vasa vasorum neovascularization precedes epicardial endothelial dysfunction in experimental hypercholesterolemia. Cardiovasc Res 2001;51:762–6.

13. Vink A, Pasterkamp G, Poppen M, et al. The adventitia of atherosclerotic coronary arteries frequently contains *Chlamydia pneumoniae*. Atherosclerosis 2001;157:117–22.

14. Kohchi K, Takebayashi S, Hiroki T, Nobuyoshi M. Significance of adventitial inflammation of the coronary artery in patients with unstable angina: results at autopsy. Circulation 1985;71:709–16.

15. Moreno PR, Purushothaman KR, Fuster V, O'Connor WN. Intimomedial interface damage and adventitial inflammation is increased beneath disrupted atherosclerosis in the aorta: implications for plaque vulnerability. Circulation 2002;105:2504–11.

16. Li G, Chen SJ, Oparil S, Chen YF, Thompson JA. Direct in vivo evidence demonstrating neointimal migration of adventitial fibroblasts after balloon injury of rat carotid arteries. Circulation 2000;101:1362–5.

17. Kwon HM, Sangiorgi G, Ritman EL, et al. Adventitial vasa vasorum in balloon-injured coronary arteries: visualization and quantitation by a microscopic three-dimensional computed tomography technique. J Am Coll Cardiol 1998;32:2072–9.

18. Houtkamp MA, de Boer OJ, van der Loos CM, van der Wal AC, Becker AE. Adventitial infiltrates associated with advanced atherosclerotic plaques: structural organization suggests generation of local humoral immune responses. J Pathol 2001;193:263–9.

19. Laine P, Kaartinen M, Penttila A, Panula P, Paavonen T, Kovanen PT. Association between myocardial infarction and the mast cells in the adventitia of the infarct-related coronary artery. Circulation 1999;99:361–9.

20. Laine P, Naukkarinen A, Heikkila L, Penttila A, Kovanen PT. Adventitial mast cells connect with sensory nerve fibers in atherosclerotic coronary arteries. Circulation 2000;101:1665–9.

21. Higuchi ML, Gutierrez PS, Bezerra HG, et al. Comparison between adventitial and intimal inflammation of ruptured and nonruptured atherosclerotic plaques in human coronary arteries. Arq Bras Cardiol 2002;79:20–4.

22. Gutterman DD. Adventitia-dependent influences on vascular function. Am J Physiol 1999;277:H1265–72.

23. Zhang L, Zalewski A, Liu Y, et al. Diabetes-induced oxidative stress and low-grade inflammation in porcine coronary arteries. Circulation 2003;108:472–8. Epub 2003 Jul 14.

24. O'Brien KD, McDonald TO, Chait A, Allen MD, Alpers CE. Neovascular expression of E-selectin, intercellular adhesion molecule-1, and vascular cell adhesion molecule-1 in human atherosclerosis and their relation to intimal leukocyte content. Circulation 1996;93:672–82.

25. Lohn M, Dubrovska G, Lauterbach B, Luft FC, Gollasch M, Sharma AM. Periadventitial fat releases a vascular relaxing factor. Faseb J 2002;16:1057–63.

26. Bhardwaj S, Roy H, Gruchala M, et al. Angiogenic responses of vascular endothelial growth factors in periadventitial tissue. Hum Gene Ther 2003;14:1451–62.

27. De Meyer GR, Kockx MM, Cromheeke KM, Seye CI, Herman AG, Bult H. Periadventitial inducible nitric oxide synthase expression and intimal thickening. Arterioscler Thromb Vasc Biol 2000;20:1896–902.

28. Rajala MW, Scherer PE. Minireview: the adipocyte – at the crossroads of energy homeostasis, inflammation, and atherosclerosis. Endocrinology 2003;144:3765–73.

29. Xu H, Barnes GT, Yang Q, et al. Chronic inflammation in fat plays a crucial role in the development of obesity-related insulin resistance. J Clin Invest 2003;112: 1821–30.

30. Weisberg SP, McCann D, Desai M, Rosenbaum M, Leibel RL, Ferrante AW, Jr. Obesity is associated with macrophage accumulation in adipose tissue. J Clin Invest 2003;112:1796–808.

31. Charriere G, Cousin B, Arnaud E, et al. Preadipocyte conversion to macrophage. Evidence of plasticity. J Biol Chem 2003;278:9850–5. Epub 2003 Jan 7.

32. Blake GJ, Ridker PM. C-reactive protein, subclinical atherosclerosis, and risk of cardiovascular events. Arterioscler Thromb Vasc Biol 2002;22:1512–13.

33. Ridker PM. On evolutionary biology, inflammation, infection, and the causes of atherosclerosis. Circulation 2002;105:2–4.

34. Ouchi N, Kihara S, Funahashi T, et al. Reciprocal association of C-reactive protein with adiponectin in blood stream and adipose tissue. Circulation 2003;107:671–4.

35. Boden G, Hoeldtke RD. Nerves, fat, and insulin resistance. N Engl J Med 2003;349:1966–7.

36. Okamoto E, Couse T, De Leon H, et al. Perivascular inflammation after balloon angioplasty of porcine coronary arteries. Circulation 2001;104:2228–35.

37. Gaustad KG, Boquest AC, Anderson BE, Gerdes AM, Collas P. Differentiation of human adipose tissue stem cells using extracts of rat cardiomyocytes. Biochem Biophys Res Commun 2004;314:420–7.

38. Planat-Benard V, Menard C, Andre M, et al. Spontaneous cardiomyocyte differentiation from adipose tissue stroma cells. Circ Res 2004;94:223–9. Epub 2003 Dec 1.

39. Planat-Benard V, Silvestre JS, Cousin B, et al. Plasticity of human adipose lineage cells toward endothelial cells:

physiological and therapeutic perspectives. Circulation 2004;109:656–63. Epub 2004 Jan 20.

40. Mazurek T, Zhang L, Zalewski A, et al. Human epicardial adipose tissue is a source of inflammatory mediators. Circulation 2003;108:2460–6. Epub 2003 Oct 27.

41. Cousin B, Munoz O, Andre M, et al. A role for preadipocytes as macrophage-like cells. Faseb J 1999;13: 305–12.

42. Villena JA, Cousin B, Penicaud L, Casteilla L. Adipose tissues display differential phagocytic and microbicidal activities depending on their localization. Int J Obes Relat Metab Disord 2001;25:1275–80.

43. Litovsky S, Madjid M, Zarrabi A, Casscells SW, Willerson JT, Naghavi M. Superparamagnetic iron oxide-based method for quantifying recruitment of monocytes to mouse atherosclerotic lesions in vivo: enhancement by tissue necrosis factor-alpha, interleukin-1beta, and interferon-gamma. Circulation 2003;107: 1545–9.

44. Jeziorska M, McCollum C, Woolley DE. Calcification in atherosclerotic plaque of human carotid arteries: associations with mast cells and macrophages. J Pathol 1998;185:10–17.

45. Angelini P, Villason S, Chang A, Diez J. Coronary artery anomalies: a comprehensive approach. In: Normal and anomalous coronary arteries in humans. Philadelphia: Lippincott Williams & Wilkins, 1999:27–150.

46. Angelini P, Velasco JA, Ott D, Khoshnevis GR. Anomalous coronary artery arising from the opposite sinus: descriptive features and pathophysiologic mechanisms, as documented by intravascular ultrasonography. J Invasive Cardiol 2003;15:507–14.

47. Kaul S, Cercek B, Rengstrom J, et al. Polymeric-based perivascular delivery of a nitric oxide donor inhibits intimal thickening after balloon denudation arterial injury:

role of nuclear factor-kappa B. J Am Coll Cardiol 2000; 35:493–501.

48. Baek SH, Hrabie JA, Keefer LK, et al. Augmentation of intrapericardial nitric oxide level by a prolonged-release nitric oxide donor reduces luminal narrowing after porcine coronary angioplasty. Circulation 2002;105:2779–84.

49. Laham RJ, Rezaee M, Post M, Xu X, Sellke FW. Intrapericardial administration of basic fibroblast growth factor: myocardial and tissue distribution and comparison with intracoronary and intravenous administration. Catheter Cardiovasc Interv 2003;58:375–81.

50. Ujhelyi MR, Hadsall KZ, Euler DE, Mehra R. Intrapericardial therapeutics: a pharmacodynamic and pharmacokinetic comparison between pericardial and intravenous procainamide delivery. J Cardiovasc Electrophysiol 2002;13:605–11.

51. Waxman S, Moreno R, Rowe KA, Verrier RL. Persistent primary coronary dilation induced by transatrial delivery of nitroglycerin into the pericardial space: a novel approach for local cardiac drug delivery. J Am Coll Cardiol 1999;33:2073–7.

52. Edelman ER, Adams DH, Karnovsky MJ. Effect of controlled adventitial heparin delivery on smooth muscle cell proliferation following endothelial injury. Proc Natl Acad Sci USA 1990;87:3773–7.

53. Fromes Y, Salmon A, Wang X, et al. Gene delivery to the myocardium by intrapericardial injection. Gene Ther 1999;6:683–8.

54. Ooboshi H, Welsh MJ, Rios CD, Davidson BL, Heistad DD. Adenovirus-mediated gene transfer in vivo to cerebral blood vessels and perivascular tissue. Circ Res 1995;77:7–13.

55. Wang HD, Pagano PJ, Du Y, et al. Superoxide anion from the adventitia of the rat thoracic aorta inactivates nitric oxide. Circ Res 1998;82:810–18.

CHAPTER 7

Murine models of advanced atherosclerosis

Michael E Rosenfeld & Stephen M Schwartz

One hundred and fifty years after Virchow's description of the atherosclerotic plaque we have a generally accepted view of how plaques begin and how they progress to clinically significant events. This view, as shown schematically in Figure 7.1, is largely based on the concept that the initial events in lesion formation ultimately lead to an inflamed, prothrombotic lesion, encapsulated with a protective cap made up of smooth muscle cells. Loss of this protective effect leads to vascular occlusion via thrombosis and coagulation. The wide-based, modern support for an intimate tie between atherosclerosis and thrombosis is demonstrated by the renaming of the relevant council of the American Heart Association, which is now called "Council on Arteriosclerosis, Thrombosis and Vascular Biology." Overall, this conflation of disciplines is appealing, since atherosclerosis is manifest as a vascular lesion, and that lesion ultimately kills by a thrombocoagulative event. However, as we will discuss, the connection between thrombosis, coagulation, and the natural history of the lesion is often confusing because of four common assertions that are, at least in part, false. These assumptions are:

1 Risk factors for atherosclerosis are usually identified by clinical endpoints. These risk factors can be found in models of lesion initiation, i.e. fatty streak formation.

2 Thrombo-occlusion implies plaque rupture.

3 Plaque rupture is sufficient to cause thrombosis and coagulation.

4 We know the factors leading to coagulation following plaque rupture.

Lesion initiation

In 1947 Duguid developed a hypothesis, the encrustation hypothesis, positing that atherosclerotic lesions are initiated by incorporation of platelet lipids into the vessel wall following the formation of mural thrombi.[1] While platelet deposition can contribute to the lipid debris in the wall,[2] studies in the middle of the last century showed that the great

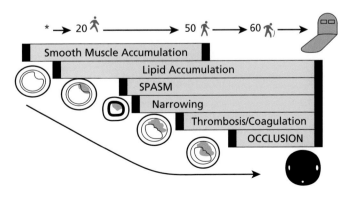

Figure 7.1 Natural history of atherosclerosis in man. This diagram shows the current consensus of how atherosclerosis begins and evolves to a clinically significant lesion. One significant difference here compared with some diagrams commonly shown is the inclusion of the intima cell mass as a pre-atherosclerotic lesion. This concept is discussed at length elsewhere.[159,160]

bulk of the lipid content of the plaque represents serum lipoproteins rather than cell membranes.[3]

Duguid's hypothesis returned with the work of Ross in the 1970s. Based on in vitro studies implicating platelet-derived products as mitogens for smooth muscle cells, Ross developed a popular hypothesis that platelet interactions with the wall could initiate atherosclerosis by contributing to accumulation of smooth muscle cells and matrix in the intima.[4] Although there is evidence that lesions begin with smooth muscle accumulation before lipid accumulates (Figure 7.2 and references 5 and 6), this hypothesis also gradually fell from favor, largely as a result of the failure of Ross or others to find evidence of widespread endothelial denudation in early lesions.[7,8] What was observed in hyperlipidemic monkeys, swine, and rabbits was focal endothelial retraction over subendothelial macrophage-derived foam cells and pointed to the increasing evidence that the earliest

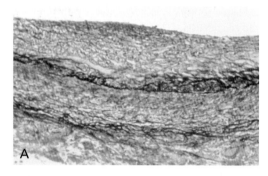

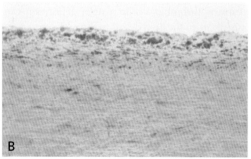

Figure 7.2 Intimal mass vs. fatty streak: two concepts of the early lesion. A, Intimal mass in the left anterior descending coronary artery of a normal 6-month-old human heart. B, Fatty streak or intimal xanthoma in the intima of a 23-year-old thoracic aorta. The intimal mass is an irreversible change that will become a lesion on all people as they age. The xanthomas may become a lesion, but may also regress.

detectable event in animal model lesions was monocytosis. This monocytosis was described first by McMillan and colleagues and then by Thomas and colleagues with early cell kinetic studies in cholesterol-fed rabbits and swine in the 1970s[9] and 1980s.[10] Emphasis on these monocyte changes has continued to increase so that the most widely accepted contemporary model for the initiation of atherosclerotic lesions is that lesions begin as a result of a focal monocytosis resulting from as yet unexplained focal accumulation of lipid and a secondary inflammatory response.[11] An alternative model, largely from our lab, is similar except that it focuses on the role of intimal smooth muscle cells as a pre-atherosclerotic lesion.[12,13] The alternative model is supported by evidence for monoclonality of the cells comprising the fibrous cap, and by evidence that the early lesion that develops at sites likely to persist into the adult human occurs as lipid deposition deep within a pre-existing intimal mass.[12] For purposes of this review, however, the models are consistent in that both models claim that lesions depend on the initiation of inflammation in response to lipid deposition, followed by accumulation of macrophages that take up lipid.

Recently, Duguid's and Ross's ideas about an initiating role for the platelet have begun to reappear in a new form as a result of studies in atherosclerotic mice. This new view, while not involving thrombus formation, hypothesizes that nonthrombotic platelet–endothelial interactions occur as an early event, perhaps even prior to the development of monocytosis itself. The literature on this subject is very confusing, perhaps because of the diversity of methods used to demonstrate platelet–endothelial interactions. The predominant opinion of morphologists, based on both transmission and scanning electron microscopy of atherosclerotic lesions in rabbits, swine, monkeys, and mice, is that any significant interaction with platelets occurs only after lesions advance to the point of widespread endothelial denudation, i.e. a very late event.[7,8,14–19]

Recently, however, Massberg et al.[20] reached a different conclusion. They used a novel in vivo intravital microscopy approach based on fluorescent-labeled platelets and found dramatic evidence of platelet deposition on the surface of carotid arteries in ApoE$^{-/-}$ mice prior to the presence of monocytosis. Furthermore, they found that treatment of these fat-fed ApoE$^{-/-}$ mice with a neutralizing antibody to Gp1b was able to dramatically reduce the incidence of atherosclerosis in this model. These authors have also shown that platelet–endothelial interactions can initiate NFκB-induced inflammatory activation of cultured endothelial cells or smooth muscle cells[21,22] and suggest, therefore, that platelet activation, presumably by some as yet unexplained effect of hyperlipemia, is a new risk factor for initiation of atherosclerosis. Two important conclusions of their work may be simply that there are a large number of transient platelet–endothelial interactions and that electron microscopy, with its need for perfusion fixation, may be misleading us about the frequency of nontransient platelet–endothelial interactions.

If this new platelet hypothesis is true, then one might expect that knockouts of molecules implicated in platelet adhesion or activation would attenuate atherosclerosis. In support of this hypothesis, Burger and Wagner found that platelet P-selectin deficiency as well as von Willebrand factor (vWF) deficiency, consistent with the Massberg's hypothesis, decreased the extent of atherosclerosis.[23,24] By contrast, Weng et al. found that a knockout of β$_3$ integrin promoted lesion formation in both the fat-fed ApoE$^{-/-}$ and the LDLR$^{-/-}$ models.[25] Weng's result, however, may be misleading since the β$_3$ integrin is important to the function of many cell types, including smooth muscle cells, endothelial cells, and, possibly, macrophages. Finally, Huo et al. may have brought together the monocyte and platelet stories. In a recent paper, they showed that injection of activated wild-type, but not P-selectin$^{-/-}$ platelets, into ApoE$^{-/-}$ mice resulted in increased monocyte entry into the vessel wall and increased lesion size.[26] Finally, platelet–endothelial interactions may promote lipid accumulation in several ways, including the recent proposal for effects of PF4, and activation of endothelial cells, promoting monocyte/macrophage entry into the vessel wall.[27]

The other component of thrombocoagulation, fibrin, may also be worth revisiting in early atherosclerosis. Westrick et al. reported an increased incidence and size of fatty lesions in ApoE$^{-/-}$ mice with a deficiency of the tissue factor pathway inhibitor (TFPI).[28] On the other hand, Xiao et al. studied fibrinogen$^{-/-}$ mice crossed with the ApoE$^{-/-}$ mouse and found no diminution of lesion formation.[29] The apparent paradox may be resolved by considering functions of tissue factor, other than its role in coagulation. Tissue factor knockout mice die in utero prior to onset of fibrinogen synthesis, implying that there is an unknown activity.[30] TFPI has an unexplained inhibitory activity toward endothelial cells.[31] Finally, while the usual emphasis in the entire coagulation pathway is on fibrin formation, the pathway generates many molecules far in excess of the need to promote fibrin formation, and several of these have intriguing activities outside of fibrin formation.[32] Thus, at least for elements of the "coagulation pathway," it is important to realize that knockouts or drugs may have effects independent of fibrin itself.

To summarize, there is reason to consider a role for platelets in early atherosclerosis, although probably not the pivotal roles proposed by Duguid or Ross. A more likely view is that the platelet can be a player in the inflammatory process whereby monocytosis occurs. In turn, especially given the dramatic claims by Massberg et al.[20] for a near complete ablation of lesions in ApoE$^{-/-}$ mice blocked in GpIb function, it may be worth considering the possibility that hyperlipemia in some way accelerates platelet–endothelial–monocyte interactions.

Role of thrombosis in progression

While Duguid's and Ross' hypotheses painted the platelet as a bad actor in plaque progression, recent thinking has raised the alternative hypothesis that the effects of platelet-released factors may be beneficial, both to keep the fibrous cap intact and to avert plaque rupture.[33,34] While Ross had suggested that PDGF was a bad actor by inducing the presence of smooth muscle cells that later became foam cells, current thinking is that growth factors, such as PDGF (platelet derived growth factor), TGF(transforming growth factor)-α, TGF-β, the heparin binding growth factors, etc. may stimulate wound repair, creating a healthy cover for the necrotic core.[33] In support of this paradigm, two groups recently showed that PDGF antagonists or deficiency in the ApoE$^{-/-}$ mouse delayed the formation of the fibrous cap.[35,36] Interestingly, these animals showed large xanthomatous lesions without the expected necrotic core, suggesting some as yet unexplained relationship between the fibrous cap and apoptosis of the plaque macrophage.

Another recent change in thinking about plaque progression and the possible role of thrombosis and coagulation is the increased interest in angiogenesis within the plaque as a factor. Plaque vasa could be important in plaque stability if, as has been suggested before, intraplaque rupture is a critical event either in further plaque rupture and/or in plaque growth.[37,38] On the other hand, abundance of plaque microvessels is associated with constrictive remodeling in human coronary arteries following angioplasty.[38] Fibrin itself has been proposed as a pro-angiogenic matrix by Dvorak and, more recently, by others.[39,40] Growth factors released by platelets have been shown to be angiogenic, including platelet-derived endothelial cell growth factor and TGF-α.[41-43] On the other hand, platelet factor 4 (PF4) appears to be anti-angiogenic. PF4, as well as proteolytic fragments of PF4, are potent anti-angiogenic molecules.[44] Until we have better models for intraplaque rupture and coagulation, we can only speculate about the role of thrombosis and coagulation in intraplaque angiogenesis, and vice versa.

Loss of lumen

The usual literature on coronary artery disease leads the public to the idea that atherosclerosis occurs because "bad" cholesterol encrusts the vessel lining, leading to constriction of the pipes much as happens when the drainpipe from your house become encrusted by household wastes. We have known that this idea is simplistic since the seminal paper by Glagov in 1987.[45] In that paper, Glagov noted that affected vessels compensate for the growth of the atherosclerotic lesion by increasing the diameter of the vessels outer boundary, the external elastic lamina (EEL), to accommodate the growth of the lesion. Figure 7.3 shows examples of two forms of atherosclerotic occlusion of the lumen due to constriction of the lumen, one in mice and one in humans. It is important to note that in neither model does lipid or foam cell mass play a significant role in vascular stenosis.

This ability to accommodate changes in wall mass is part of a fundamental, normal mechanism whereby the vessel wall simultaneously controls its wall thickness and outer diameter to maintain a physiological level of wall tension and blood flow. When wall thickness increases in a resistance artery, the resulting increased response to a constrictive response, even a normal level of vasoactivity, is an increase in vasoconstriction due to the elevated mass. In turn, this increased vasoconstriction elevates resistance and blood pressure.[46] Any increase

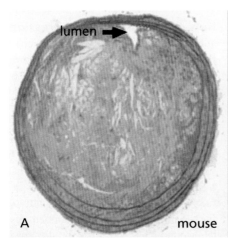 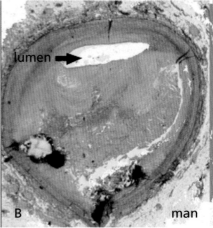

Figure 7.3 Two examples of occlusion of the lumen by atherosclerotic lesions in a mouse carotid and a human coronary artery. A, The mouse lesion is occluded secondary to rapid enlargement of the mouse lesions following intramural hemorrhage, i.e. this is ruptured plaque. This form of occlusion occurs rarely in man. Even in the ApoE[−/−] mouse we find such lesions around 40 weeks of age, and then only infrequently. More commonly, we see fibrosis, calcification, and chondroplasia with contraction of the lumen between 1 and 2 years of age. B, Loss of lumen in a human lesion showing considerable scarring. (Reproduced with permission from Rosenfeld ME, et al., Arterioscler Thromb Vasc Biol 2000;20:2587–92.)

in wall mass due to atherosclerosis or vascular injury will, therefore, be compensated for by an outward remodeling of the EEL. This is seen in animal models as well. Neointima formed in response to angioplasty in rats or rabbits results in a preservation of lumen size due to outward remodeling. The same outward remodeling is seen in atherosclerotic rabbits and mice[17,47–49] and in humans following angioplasty where, contrary to the commonly held view of many cardiologists, angioplasty with restenosis is usually due to a return of the injured vessel to its pre-injury dimensions rather than a loss of lumen due to any increase in neointima.[50,51] Studies of protease activity in aneurysms and of elastin deleted by genetic mutation suggests that this molecule may normally function as a stent, preventing collapse during development, but permitting expansion if deleted in the adult animal, e.g. by proteolysis.[52–56]

What then does ultimately lead to narrowing of an atherosclerotic vessel? Glagov's original paper suggested that there was some physical limit, and that when a vessel reaches this limit, further growth leads to loss of lumen. While this may be true, the histology of the lesions (Figure 7.3) suggests a simpler answer: that as lesions progress, multiple injuries occur that are followed by scarring; and these scars retract, constricting the lumen in what might be called pathologic inward remodeling. Consistent with this point of view, Virmani and her colleagues describe the typical narrowed vessel in man as a fibrocalcific plaque.[57] In unpublished work, we see similar scarred, constricted lesions in the murine carotid artery of ApoE mice aged up to 2 years (data not shown).

Final events

There is obviously less controversy at the other end of the natural history of atherosclerosis. Since the clinical success of thrombolytic therapies, no one can seriously doubt the importance of thrombosis and coagulation in the terminal events of this disease. Similarly, epidemiological data clearly associates alterations of platelet or coagulation function with evidence of accelerated risk of cardiovascular events.[58–67] Such correlations, however, need not address the lesion itself. For example, the risks associated with C-reactive protein, hyperfibrinogenemia, or smoking are arguably indicators of systemic conditions that increase the likelihood that an independent event in a lesion, such as plaque rupture, will lead to massive thrombosis. These systemic indicators may or may not tell us about the status of the lesion itself.

"Status of the lesion," i.e. the specific properties leading to an abrupt thrombocoagulative event, are not fully clear. Usually, these properties are combined under the term "vulnerable plaque," and attempts have been made to define both the morphological and biochemical properties of the vulnerable plaque based on autopsy data.[68] These studies have led to the assertion that the vulnerable plaque is characterized by a thin fibrous cap overlying a necrotic core[69] with extensive infiltration of macrophages at the shoulder regions. Studies based on autopsies by Henney et al.,[70] followed by more extensive mechanistic studies by Libby and others, have proposed that plaques rupture because of the release of proteases by macrophages located in the shoulder regions of the plaque.[71] Although animal data have been cited in support of this hypothesis,[72] so far all of that data is from relatively early lesions, and we lack experimental animal support for the proteolytic hypothesis. The one paradoxical exception is the recent observation from Falkenberg et al., claiming that macrophage-targeted expression of urokinase enhances xanthoma formation and does not lead to plaque rupture.[73] Consistent with this observation, it is important to note that the usual model in mice has, at best, a thin fibrous cap (Figure 7.4). Many of these lesions are composed of endothelium overlying fatty macrophage, so the use of such models to study what is and is not a "vulnerable plaque" makes little sense.[74–80] Another confusing concept in human lesions is the importance of cellularity. As shown in Figure 7.5, the typical fibrous cap of the carotid lesion may be nearly acellular. The fibrous cap in this figure resembles a tendon, and at high power, one can find extremely attenuated cells that appear to be sufficient to maintain integrity of the cap.

A possible resolution to the lack of experimental animal data may come from new methods for study of human lesions. As convincing as such postmortem data may be, it is essential to remember that advanced lesions are seen in all patients with atherosclerosis of long duration, and such lesions show similar morphology, even when the cause of

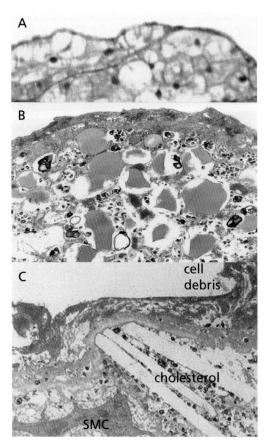

Figure 7.4 Fatty streaks as a model for plaque rupture. Although there are many papers using the mouse lesion as a model for the vulnerable plaque, most of these are based on the misapprehension that the mouse lesions, like the human lesion, has a thick cap. This does happen as the lesion develops; however, in the early lesions shown here, the covering over the lesions is very tenuous. The fatty streak shown in A may have a thin layer of endothelium, as in B, or even no endothelium, as in C. Thus, the idea that rupture occurs simply by the loss of a fibrous cap is incorrect.

death is obviously not atherosclerotic.[81,82] While this image of a vulnerable lesion as being composed of a thin fibrous cap with shoulder regions replete with macrophage-derived proteases is widely held, the critical histology is more diverse than the proponents of this hypothesis suggest.[83] For example, Farb and colleagues[84] describe a lesion without rupture seen at autopsy of young women with total occlusion of their coronary arteries. These lesions, called "erosions," have no evidence of disruption of the fibrous cap and, in some cases, not even the

presence of a necrotic core. Since it is clear from the work of Farb et al. that properties of lesions other than a thin fibrous cap and macrophages in the shoulders can contribute to thrombosis, we may need to consider whether the thin fibrous cap and macrophage-rich regions, while likely to make lesions labile, could still be independent of the actual events initiating thrombosis, even in the advanced lesions. More direct tests for the "fragile plaque as a risk factor" hypothesis may come from longitudinal MRI studies in living humans.[85] Yuan and colleagues have produced near histological images of carotid lesions and can show a very high correlation with a history of ischemic events and evidence of plaque disruption, i.e. exactly the sort of changes predicted by Libby and others. Presumably, prospective MRI studies will confirm or deny our current concept of the structure of the vulnerable plaque.

Even knowing the morphology of the vulnerable lesion, however, would still leave us with mysteries. Conventional wisdom today is that the toxic effects of lipids and proteolytic activities in the plaque (e.g. pro-thrombotic activities due to phospholipid and collagen degradation) are key to the final clinical events.[11,69,86] The commonly held concept is that plaque disruption is followed by exposure of this thrombogenic/procoagulant necrotic core. However, while debris from an advanced plaque is procoagulant,[87] it is not at all obvious why coagulation should be accelerated by rupture, since the intact plaque contains abundant procoagulant proteins.[88,89] Of course, the plaque also contains anticoagulant proteins, including TFPI, annexin V, plasminogen activators, and so on. Thus, the critical factor initiating coagulation is not simply access of plasma following rupture. Moreover, it is clear that thrombosis and coagulation can occur over a lesion even in the absence of a thrombogenic/procoagulant necrotic core. In the case of the "erosion" lesions described above, occlusive thrombi develop even though there is little or no evidence of inflammation in the vessel wall and no tissue factor in the wall.[84] Absence of tissue factor in the wall implies that coagulation and, therefore, thrombus stabilization in these lesions depends on activation of the extrinsic pathway by factors intrinsic to the blood. Indeed the thrombi in the lumen of these vessels display abundant tissue factor by

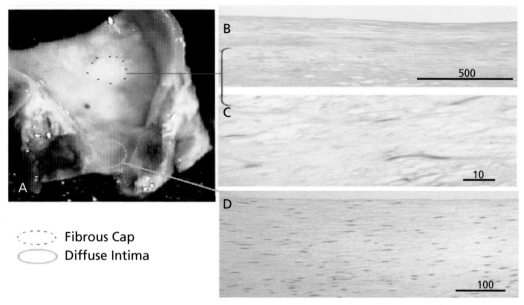

Figure 7.5 The fibrous cap can be very acellular, as in this example from human carotid arteries. A, Macrophotograph of a carotid endarterectomy specimen shows a thin white structure (dotted lines) (courtesy R. Geary). B and C, Typical histology of this structure. Note the tissue is largely acellular, but at higher power one can find extremely attenuated cells with thin nuclei and little cytoplasm. C, As a comparison this shows the adjacent nonatherosclerotic intima.

immunocytochemistry. This is paradoxical because tissue factor was traditionally believed to be absent in normal blood and to become activated only in the atherosclerotic wall where it is present in macrophages and smooth muscle cells.[90] The resolution of the paradox appears to be that there is a "stealth" form of tissue factor present in plasma as a small, high-density liposome. The mechanisms of activation of this liposome are not yet known.[91–93]

Prospects for study of advanced lesions in humans

The existing literature on advanced lesions is confusing for three reasons. First, autopsy data is our major current source of morphological information. Epidemiology of such data is notoriously difficult to evaluate, since there is no randomness in who comes to autopsy. The other sources of data (ultrasound and angiography) are largely limited to images of the lumen. Second, epidemiological studies, including most genetic studies, use clinical endpoints to define the advanced lesions. Such an approach will equate any systemic factor that increases the likelihood of death from a plaque

event with changes in the plaque itself. Thus, as we have already discussed, elevation of fibrinogen is likely not related to the plaque, but to the likelihood that if a plaque ruptures, it will eventuate in thrombotic occlusion. Third, manipulations in humans are very difficult to achieve because of ethical concerns. Thus, once we know that a drug, e.g. the statins, is of clinical value, it is difficult to design a study.

The answers to these problems in man are emerging from the use of MRI and the identification of a site that is more easily studied than the coronary arteries.[94,95] Such studies have already demonstrated profound effects of the statins on plaque morphology.[96,97] That site is the carotid artery. Unlike the coronary artery, the carotid is relatively unaffected by movement of the heart or lungs. As a result, spatial resolution is already at 250 μm.[85] While this is not the 0.2 μm of light microscopy, it approaches a histological level of detail and, combined with the use of contrast media, is adequate to recognize such features as the necrotic core, fibrous cap, intraplaque hemorrhage and, recently, again via innovative uses of contrast media, intraplaque vessels.[98–101] In a recent retrospective study, evidence of plaque rupture was very highly correlated with a clinical history of cerebral events.[102] Thus, for the first time we should be able to follow serial changes in human vessels and assay the effects of drugs, genes, and environment in a prospective fashion.

One simple step that is vital for any progress in understanding the pathology of the human lesion is the use of standardized terminology.[57] The most widely used such terminology, however, is that developed by an AHA consensus committee.[83,103,104] The good aspect of this terminology is that it includes a very large range of lesions. The bad news is twofold. The simplest issue is that in an effort to classify all lesions, the consensus committee developed an alphabetically coded set of terms that is very complex. Investigators using these codes in place of descriptive terminology may or may not be rigorous in following the original scheme. As a result one reads all too many papers where a "correlation" is drawn between some code or term defined at autopsy, e.g. "vulnerable" or "early," and some clinical parameter measured in life.

The second, and probably more difficult, problem is that the AHA scheme includes terms, e.g. "early" or "vulnerable," that are conclusions rather than descriptions. One example will suffice. The AHA terminology equates the presence of a thin fibrous cap with a lesion prone to rupture, i.e. a vulnerable plaque. This is a reasonable hypothesis, but not a proven fact. For example, studies from Virmani and her colleagues have shown that vessels can occlude by thrombosis in the absence of a thin fibrous cap, even without a necrotic core or much inflammation. Knowing that such "erosion" events can occur means that it is impossible to prove that the occlusion seen in a ruptured plaque is the result of the rupture, rather than the result of "erosion" occurring elsewhere in the vessel. Defining the mechanism of erosion is a major challenge. Furthermore, the AHA definition of "ruptured plaque" is itself problematic, since it requires the presence of a break in the plaque (a fissure) associated with thrombocoagulative occlusion. Fissures, along with evidence of scarring attributed to old fissure/ruptures, are expected features of the advanced lesion and are commonly seen in advanced lesions of people dying from other causes.[82] Moreover, in a recent MRI study, there was evidence of extensive plaque rupture, defined as hemorrhage into the plaque, and this correlated with the incidence of stroke. However, the carotid itself was patent, and histological studies of such vessels suggest that rather than a terminal event, rupture is an ongoing, repetitive process contributing to thrombotic rather than occlusive end points.[102] Clearly most of these events must have occurred without the catastrophic results implied by the equation of plaque rupture with a terminal occlusive event.

The obvious conclusion of this part of our discussion is that it is essential for human studies of plaque morphology to use an objective, nonconclusionary set of terms like the scheme introduced by our group working with Virmani (Table 7.1).[57] If the AHA scheme is to be used, the study needs to carefully explain how the criteria are applied, and the analysis must be stripped of any implications

Table 7.1 Defining features of end-stage disease. (Adapted from Virmani R, et al. Arterioscler Thromb Vasc Biol 2000;20:1262–75).[57]

Erosion	Formation of thrombo-occlusive mass without evidence of plaque rupture
Thin fibrous cap atheroma	May or may not show evidence of recent rupture, usually also shows abundant macrophages in the shoulder regions. Sometimes called the "vulnerable plaque". Lumen often not narrowed
Plaque rupture	Thrombosis and occlusion over a thin-cap atheroma, with at least one fissure connected to the thrombus and usually with evidence of scarring and fissures. Lumen often not narrowed
Fibrocalcific plaque	Scarred lesions, suggestive of multiple ruptures and healing. Usually calcified. Lumen usually narrowed
Calcified nodule	Eruptive calcification usually over fibrocalcific plaque. Mural thrombus usually nonocclusive and lumen usually narrowed

that a particular morphology has functional implications. The combination of an objective set of descriptions that can be confirmed at the MRI level, as well as the histological level,[105,106] the assumptions that the carotid can serve as a surrogate for studies of the coronaries themselves, and a more open-minded approach to drawing mechanistic conclusions should, within the next few years, allow us to know what actually happens as the human plaque progresses. Such studies in humans are essential to determine the relevance of any study in mice.

Prospects for study of advanced lesions in mice

As discussed above, Virmani and colleagues developed a simple descriptive set of terms that is easy to use and applicable to animal models, as well as to man.[57] These criteria became necessary when Williams et al. and our group tried to apply the traditional terms used in man to the lesions in mice. Both groups discovered that the carotid artery in the mouse (Figure 7.6) undergoes changes much closer to those seen in human vessels, including stenosis,[107] formation of a fibrous cap,[17] effects of estrogen,[108] and rupture.[17,109] Figures 7.7 and 7.8 illustrate the application of this terminology to typical murine lesions in the ApoE[-/-], chow-fed mouse. The animals are between 30 and 40 weeks of age.

Unfortunately, most studies in mice have equated atherosclerotic severity with the accumulation of intimal xanthomata (Figures 7.4, 7.6), the lesions called fatty streaks or early lesions in the AHA scheme. This literature vaguely equates initiation of lesions, i.e. accumulation of lipid in the wall, with the entire progress of lesions. We know this view is false. For example, addition of estrogen to male ApoE[-/-] mice totally ablates new lesion formation without having any observable effect on the progression of already existing lesions.[108] Similarly, current reviews[110] emphasize factors such as local formation of oxidation products or expression of proteases that seem intuitively more likely to affect later stages of the lesion rather than the initial events leading to monocytosis and lipid accumulation. Finally, we need to be concerned that factors likely to be involved in the late stages of human lesion progression may have quite different effects when manifest in the much thinner wall of a mouse. For example, Daugherty et al. have shown that hypertension in ApoE[-/-] mice leads to a highly localized formation of aneurysm in the abdominal aorta. This appears likely to be due to monocytosis and secretion of metalloproteinases, factors considered critical to lesion rupture in the human.[56,111]

The role of the mouse in atherosclerosis research has changed dramatically over the last decade. Mice were traditionally viewed as an atherosclerosis-resistant species. The pioneering studies of Paigen

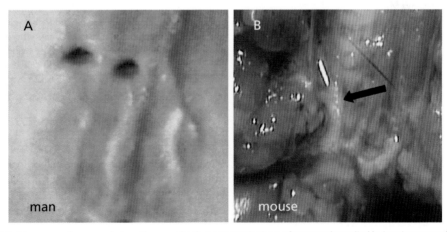

Figure 7.6 A human and a mouse lesion. These are both macroscopic views of commonly studied lesions in man and mouse. The lesion in man is a fatty streak, called an intimal xanthoma in the Virmani criteria. Histology of similar lesions in mice is shown in Figure 7.4. The mouse lesion is seen from the outside and is a very extensive "advanced" lesion of the sort shown microscopically in Figures 7.7 and 7.8.

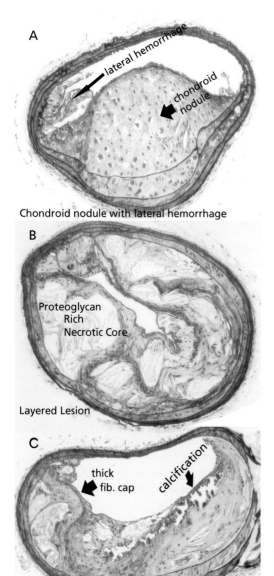

A

lateral hemorrhage

chondroid nodule

Chondroid nodule with lateral hemorrhage

B

Proteoglycan Rich Necrotic Core

Layered Lesion

C

thick fib. cap

calcification

Fibrocalcific Lesion

Figure 7.7 Three lesions in the brachiocephalic artery of ApoE$^{-/-}$ mice. A, This would be a very unusual lesion in a human. In the Virmani terminology this is a thick fibrous cap lesion without an atheroma, since there is no necrotic core. However, in places where we might expect to see a mass of macrophages, this lesion shows cells with the morphology of chondrocytes. In an unpublished work, we find type II collagen in such lesions. Type II collagen is a canonical marker for cartilage. B, This lesion, like the lesion in A, could not be described by the AHA criteria. In the Virmani classification it is a thin fibrous cap lesion. "Thin fibrous cap," however, fails to recognize that this lesion is apparently made up of several overlapping layers of necrotic lesions, each of which still has only a thin cap. Such "layered lesions" are sometimes, incorrectly used as evidenced for multiple rupture. In our data, layered lesions are seen as early as, or even earlier than, evidence of rupture. C, This lesion shows two features of an advanced human lesion, though in a somewhat different pattern then one ever sees in man. The lesion shows a thick fibrous cap and an area of calcification. Usually in man the fibrous cap would overlie the calcified lesion, although in mice it may be that the calcification is sequential to the chondroplasia shown in Figure 7.7A.

et al. first demonstrated that there were in fact strains of mice such as the C57Bl/6, that could be induced to form fatty streaks in the aortic sinus with addition of fat, cholesterol, and cholate to the diet.[112] Quantitative trait locus analysis later revealed a gene on chromosome 1 referred to as *Ath 1* that, in part, accounts for the susceptibility of C57Bl/6 mice to diet-induced atherosclerosis. However, because lesions are largely restricted to the aortic sinus and don't progress much past the fatty streak stage of lesion development (likely due to the modest

hypercholesterolemia that results from simple fat-feeding in mice), this approach has not contributed to modeling the advanced stages of the disease. With the advent of knockout and transgenic technology, however, mice again became the central focus for atherosclerosis research. Targets such as apolipo-proteins and lipoprotein receptors that regulate the clearance of lipoproteins from the circulation were chosen and led to the development of the two most widely utilized models, the apolipo-protein E and LDL receptor knockout strains.

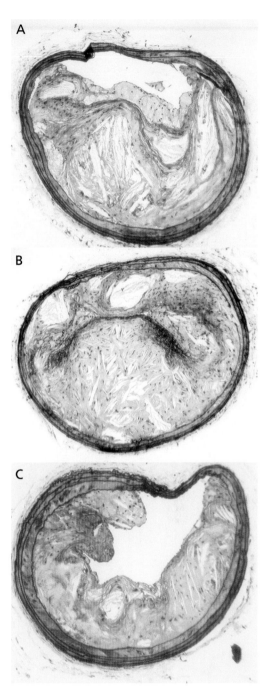

Figure 7.8 Additional lesions classified by the Virmani criteria. A, This is a superficial xanthoma overlying a thin fibrous cap xanthoma. Superficial xanthomas are a common feature of both men and mice. As noted in Figure 7.7B, these superficial lesions can form multiple layers, creating a tree rung structure. At least in the mouse, this layering is unrelated to multiple periods of rupture. Deep in this lesion is an atheroma, the cholesterol-rich, necrotic structure first called an atheroma by Virchow. The presence of the atheroma is the critical criteria for identification of a classical atherosclerotic lesion. However, as noted in the text, even a thick fibrous cap without atheromas may cause thrombocoagulative occlusion. B, This nearly occlusive lesion shows a thick fibrous cap on top and a thin cap on the bottom. Both parts of the cap overlay necrotic cores. Note that, even here, the extent of fibrous cap formation does not approach the extent seen in Figure 7.5. C, The most notable feature of this lesion is rupture through a superficial xanthoma located at the lateral surface of this plaque. Lateral xanthoma formation is typical of most murine carotid lesions in both ApoE$^{-/-}$, as shown here, and in LDL R$^{-/-}$ (not shown).

These were bred onto the C57Bl/6 background and, in the case of the ApoE-deficient strain, spontaneously and rapidly develop lesions throughout the vasculature, even without feeding of fat and cholesterol.[17,19,113]

Since the establishment of these two models, there have been a large number of reports of additional genetic or pharmacologic manipulations of both models as a means of accelerating lesion development. Table 7.2 contains a compilation of

Table 7.2 Selected reports of additional genetic or pharmacologic manipulations of both LDLR−/− and ApoE−/− models as a means of accelerating lesion development.

Model	Pro-atherogenic changes	Evidence of unstable plaque				Reference
		Rupture (intraplaque hemorrhage)	Thrombosis	Decreased collagen	Spontaneous death or MI	
Apo E−/− (chow-fed)	Increased VLDL/LDL. Develops lesions throughout the vasculature within 20 weeks and exhibits intraplaque hemorrhage in the innominate artery and other sites	Yes	No	No	No	17,19,113,140,141
Apo E−/− (fat-fed)	Radically increased VLDL. Very rapid onset of lesions. Exhibits rupture and hemorrhage within 8 weeks in the innominate artery. Evidence of associated thrombosis. Plasma cholesterol in excess of 1500 mg/dl	Yes	Yes	No	Yes	109,114,115
LDL-R−/− (fat-fed)	Increased IDL/LDL. Requires a high fat and cholesterol diet. Rate of lesion development slower than apo E−/− mice. Lesions largely fatty streaks. Evidence of intraplaque hemorrhage	Yes	No	No	No	113,142
Apo E−/− X LDL-R−/− (chow-fed)	Increased IDL/LDL/VLDL. Severe hyperlipidemia. One report of myocardial infarction	No	No	No	Yes	143,144
Apo E−/− X SRB1−/− (chow-fed)	Increased VLDL/IDL/LDL. Evidence of myocardial infarction	No	No	No	Yes	123
Apo E−/− X gulonolactone−/−	Vitamin C deficiency leads to decreased collagen synthesis and evidence of reduced plaque stability	No	No	Yes	No	78
Apo B100/100 X LDL-R−/− (chow-fed)	Increased apo B100/IDL/LDL. Severe hyperlipidemia with lipoprotein profile similar to humans. Rapid onset of lesions	No	No	No	No	145,146
Apo BEC−/− X LDL-R−/− (chow-fed)	Increased apo B100/IDL/LDL. Severe hyperlipidemia with lipoprotein profile similar to humans. Rapid onset of lesions	No	No	No	No	147
LDL-R−/− X SRB1−/−	Increased VLDL/IDL/LDL	No	No	No	No	148
Apo E3 Leiden (fat-fed)	Increased VLDL. Lesions slowly progress to advanced stages	No	No	No	No	149
Apo E*2 (arg158 − cys) (fat-fed)	Increased VLDL. Similar to apo E3 Leiden mice	No	No	No	No	150
Apo E−/− X hCETP++ (chow-fed)	Increased VLDL, decreased HDL	No	No	No	No	151
LDL-R−/− X hCETP++ (fat-fed)	Increased IDL/LDL, decreased HDL	No	No	No	No	146
LDL-R−/− X human apo CIII++ (chow or fat-fed)	Increased VLDL, IDL/LDL	No	No	No	No	152
Apo E−/− X human Apo AII++	Increased VLDL	No	No	No	No	153
LDL-R−/− X ACAT-1−/− (macrophages)	Increased free cholesterol in plaques	No	No	No	No	154
Apo E3 Leiden X p53−/− (macrophages)	Increased proliferation and cell death in plaques	No	No	No	No	155
LDL-R−/− X Leptin−/− (chow fed)	Increased VLDL/remnants. Plaque composition not yet described	No	No	No	No	156
Apo E−/− plus angiotensin II	Increased macrophage cholesterol synthesis. Not hypertensive	No	No	No	No	157
Human angiotensinogen plus rennin ++ in C57Bl/6 (fat-fed)	Hypertensive	No	No	No	No	158

many of these reports. Of particular notice have been those manipulations that radically increase plasma lipid levels and/or induce lipoprotein profiles similar to known human dyslipidemias. These have included increased expression of human ApoB-100, expression of the cholesterol ester transfer protein (CETP), which is normally not expressed in mice, and knockout of the type B1 scavenger receptor. These have produced mice with significant increases in remnant lipoproteins and LDL, reductions in HDL, and exhibit rapid onset of lesion formation.

Unfortunately, very few of these studies have focused on questions of plaque composition and stability in older animals and have largely restricted their analyses to changes in plaque size, particularly in the aortic sinus. The few exceptions have been studies we and others have conducted that have focused primarily on lesions that develop in the innominate/brachiocephalic artery (Figure 7.6B), as described above in this review.[17,74,114,115] Lesions at this site exhibit thinning of the fibrous cap and intraplaque hemorrhage. Formation of these measures of plaque stability can be radically accelerated by feeding the animals excess fat and cholesterol.[114] Calara et al. have also reported the occasional occurrence of intraplaque hemorrhage in older ApoE[−/−] and LDL-R[−/−] mice in both the aorta and aortic sinus.

A major problem with using mouse models has been the unfortunate claim that the lesions are similar to human lesions, especially to advanced lesions in humans. For example many, perhaps most, studies of murine disease have focused on the extent of atherosclerosis behind the valves or in the coronary orifices. Neither of these are significant sites of atherosclerotic vascular disease in humans. Moreover, histology at these sites can be extremely confusing because of the involvement of the valve leaflets and extension of the retrovalvular lesions to the coronary arteries, a process identified in humans as atherosclerotic valvular disease, a distinct process from coronary artery disease. In a careful study of coronary arteries in ApoE[−/−] mice, we have found no coronary artery lesions in the major arteries, other than extensions of the retrovalvular disease.[116]

The criteria offered by Virmani et al. to classify human lesions may be our best guide to suggesting how to define advanced lesions in mice.[57] The defining features of end-stage disease in her classification include those in Table 7.1.

To date the most advanced lesions seen to appear consistently by 30–40 weeks of age and, in studies from this lab of ApoE[−/−] mice, are found to progress as late as 2 years from birth. After a systematic survey, we focused on the innominate artery (Figure 7.6B), a location where late-stage lesions in mice have qualities of late-stage human lesions, such as large and central necrotic cores, calcification, proteoglycan and collagen deposition, and areas of hemorrhage.[17] These mouse models, both in our work and in the work of others,[74,108,109] have demonstrated that plaque fissures and ruptures occur consistently at this site and, more episodically, at other sites.[115]

Figures 7.7 and 7.8 shows lesions in these mice classified as closely as we can to the Virmani criteria. These murine lesions differ from the conventional view of the human lesion in three ways. The first difference between murine rupture and the conventional view of human rupture is that the rupture, while also occurring in the shoulder region,[117] seems to occur by apoptosis within the dense accumulation of foamy macrophages in the lateral xanthomas (Figure 7.8). These structures occur over the pre-existing lesions, new xanthomas, and can themselves progress to form multilayered lesions (Figure 7.7B) or to plaque rupture (Figures 7.8C, 7.9). As shown in Figure 7.9, the mechanism of rupture in the murine lesion is quite clear. The superficial xanthomas located lateral to the main lesion, "lateral xanthomas," often, and perhaps usually, interrupt the fibrous cap (Figures 7.8C, 7.9A,C, 7.10). Just as the original intimal xanthoma undergoes death to form a necrotic core, these superficial xanthomas undergo death. In Figure 7.9D1 and D2, serial sections show the result: hemorrhage entering the necrotic xanthomas penetrates all the way into the necrotic core. In extreme cases, the result may even be interplaque hemorrhage resulting in occlusion of the lumen, as in Figure 7.3A.

This rather simple mechanism of plaque rupture is distinct from plaque rupture as digestion of a collagenous matrix, as proposed first by Davies[117] and now more extensively by Libby.[71] The proteolytic hypothesis is supported by extensive autopsy studies, as discussed above. The better temporal

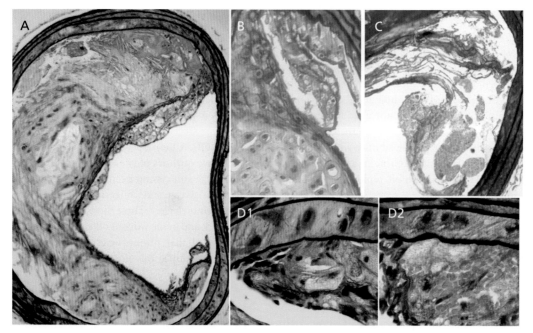

Figure 7.9 Plaque rupture begins within the lateral xanthomas. A, There is massive cell death and hemorrhage through the lateral xanthoma undergoing necrosis. B and D1, Two more of many examples we found of this form of plaque rupture. C, A picture of a thin section, stained with methylene blue and showing the dying macrophage. D2, A serial section of D1 showing what otherwise might be seen as an isolated pool of red cells, or even an intraplaque vessel. (Reproduced with permission from Rosenfeld ME et al., Arterioscler Thromb Vasc Biol 2000;20:2587–92.)

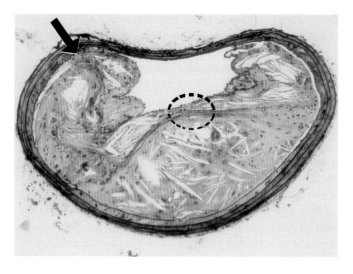

Figure 7.10 A superficial xanthoma over a thick fibrous cap lesion. Two features are worth noting. The fibrous cap is fairly thick for a mouse lesion, but obviously not as extensive as seen in human lesions. For example, even the attenuated, acellular cap in Figure 7.5 is much thicker than this. Second, the mouse cap is incomplete and is typically interrupted laterally by the lateral xanthoma (arrow) that penetrates the cap. The dotted line shows the fibrous cap.

definition of the murine model, as opposed to autopsy studies in humans, may mean that it is worth asking whether macrophage death in the shoulders is also important in man. In a recent careful morphologic study of human lesions, Kolodgie and colleagues suggested that such apop-totic or necrotic macrophages were, in fact, the major feature of rupture sites.[118] Combined with recent studies of the properties of dying cells from our lab,[119] it seems possible that cytokine release and proteolytic events are greatly enhanced by the apoptotic process itself.

The second difference between the human lesion and the mouse model is the lack of fibrin or thrombus formation at sites of rupture in murine lesions.[17,109,115] Even if we had satisfactory models for thrombosis with rupture in the mouse, the issue of thrombosis with "erosion," as discussed above, would remain. There is no model for this phenomenon in the mouse, although it is possible to produce such a model using fine forceps to squeeze the artery at lesion sites,[120] or lasers to injure the wall.[121] There is also a relevant model in dogs.[122] Part of the problem with studies in the mouse may be attributed to technology for detection of fibrin in the mouse. For example, the antibody used to see fibrin in the coronary arteries of SRB-1$^{-/-}$ X ApoE$^{-/-}$ mice by Braun et al.[123] is known not to be able to detect fibrin other than in humans.[89] Other studies have relied on histochemical stains that may not distinguish fibrin from other coagulated proteins, such as apoptotic debris.[110] Nonetheless, when Johnson and Jackson[114] fed ApoE$^{-/-}$ mice of a mixed genetic background a high fat diet supplemented with 21% beef lard (instead of the typical milk fat, which contains more n-3 fatty acids), their animals died with occluded carotid arteries. Therefore, there may be dietary changes or strain choices required to produce thrombosis in murine models.

Given the obvious importance of coagulation and thrombus in the advanced human plaque, the absence of an animal model for this step is a serious limitation of the mouse model. As noted, this limitation may already have been overcome by feeding lard and cholesterol to ApoE$^{-/-}$ mice on a mixed genetic background.[69,77] However, as this diet induces plasma cholesterol levels in excess of 1500 mg/dl in these mice, it is unclear whether there is any physiological relevance to the formation of thrombus in this model. It is well known that dietary fat and cholesterol increases thromboxane A2 production in hyperlipidemic mice[124] and accelerates thrombus formation postinjury.[125] There is also evidence that there are distinct differences in platelet function between mouse strains[126] and questions related to dietary cholesterol induced hepatotoxicity.[127]

Aside from concerns about such an extreme diet, it is difficult to evaluate postmortem the validity of the thrombosis in animals. If, however, we are to learn the specific mechanistic requirement for thrombosis in the presence of atherosclerosis, the experimental solution will combine prothrombotic mutations with atherosclerotic models. Potential mouse models of thrombosis or elevated coagulation could be promising when crossed onto the ApoE or LDL receptor deficient backgrounds. In some cases, this has already been done, and it would be interesting to look at drug and gene therapy interventions in the older, double knockout mice. These include Factor V Leiden mutation,[128] PAI-1$^{-/-}$ X ApoE$^{-/-}$[63], SRBI$^{-/-}$ X ApoE$^{-/-}$,[123] heterozygotes for protein C deficiency,[129] and antithrombin knockout mice.[130] Finally, somewhat controversial human data has implicated polymorphisms in molecules associated with platelet function with increases in coronary artery death.[59] To our knowledge, animal models for these platelet defects have not as yet been crossed with hyperlipidemic models.

The third difference between mouse and man may be the presence or absence of angiogenesis in the advanced murine lesions. Moulton and her collaborators have described CD31+ vessels within murine plaques and have attributed a proatherogenic role to these structures.[131] Although we have seen similar structures, as in Figures 7.11 and 7.12, CD31 is also able to stain macrophages,[132] suggesting that these structures may be macrophage rather than endothelial-lined channels. Moreover, in our hands, these "vessels" fail to stain with VE-cadherin antibodies and do not show permeation when the vasculature is perfused with horseradish peroxidase, a traditional marker of vascular flow.[133] (unpublished observations)

Conclusions

For the most part, studies of murine lesions of atherosclerosis have focused on the formation of fatty streaks, i.e. on accumulations of fat-filled macrophages, termed intimal xanthomas in the Virmani classification scheme. These lesions occur within the intima of the large arteries, primarily the aortic root, the lesser curvature of the outflow track, and the descending aorta. By and large, these sites are either rarely seen as sites of advanced disease in human vessels or are rarely important in late stage human disease. Thus, at best, efforts to

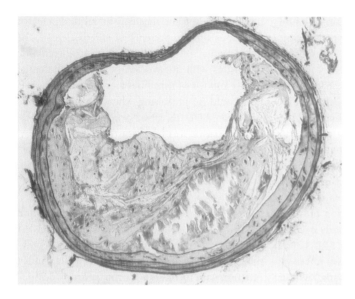

Figure 7.11 A superficial xanthoma over a thin fibrous cap lesion with pseudo-angiogenesis within the lesion. While the small structure deep in the lesions could be vessels, electron microscopy of these lesions, as well as stain with a macrophage-specific marker, shows that these channels are either unlined or lined by a thin layer of macrophage-extended cytoplasm. Moreover, as in Figure 7.9D, we have been able to use serial sections to trace blood like this to ruptures through the lateral xanthomas.

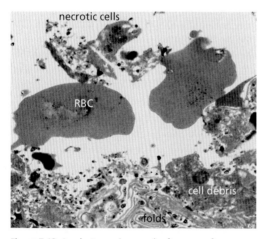

Figure 7.12 An electron micrograph of an area of intraplaque hemorrhage. Necrotic debris, red cells (RBC), and red cell debris are evident. The lower part of the image shows a typical cell found lining one of these cavities. The cells can be quite flattened, but unlike endothelial cells, typically contain phagosomes, lack Weibell–Palade bodies, lack functional complexes, lack a basement membrane, and show areas of extensive membrane folding typical of macrophage.

characterize such lesions as "typical" of "advanced" human lesions may be appropriate if similar mechanisms operate in anatomically distinct lesions in the two distinct species.[97] Whether the mechanisms involved in a slowed or accelerated formation of xanthomatous intimal masses apply to mechanisms controlling advanced lesions in man is only conjectural unless, as discussed above, the murine observations can be supported by prospective studies in human vessels using MRI.

To date, another limitation of the murine model is that coronary arteries do not show advanced disease. Reports claiming to see lesions in the coronaries need to be tempered by the likelihood that the narrow murine coronary arteries can become occluded by extensions into the coronary vessels by the typical retrovalvular atherosclerotic lesions, characteristic of the mouse, but very rare in man.

Studies in any animal model depend on reproducibility. So far in the mouse, the most reproducible site for studies of advanced lesions is the carotid artery. Even with the carotid model, there are a number of cautions to consider:

1 Rupture in the mouse carotid appears to be due to death of macrophages forming the shoulder of the plaque. These macrophages form a continuous channel between the lumen and the necrotic core. We do not know that similar structures exist in human disease.

2 The pathology of the mouse lesions seems to be primarily fatty and fibrotic. The thrombus and fibrin seen in humans are rarely, if ever, seen. The reasons for this discrepancy are not clear, and as we have described above, there may be exceptions in some mice with accelerated coagulation.

3 The mouse vessel is much smaller than any relevant human vessel. As such, hemodynamic issues believed to be relevant to the human lesion may tell us little. On the other hand, the murine carotid lesions described here do progress, do rupture, and do stenose. Thus, one can argue that the mouse carotid is a better model for human coronary artery disease than is, for example, the ascending aorta of the atherosclerotic mouse, or for that matter, the typical lesions that rarely progress to clinically significant status, as seen in rabbits, monkeys, or swine. Combined with this reproducibility, the manipulability of the mouse, especially the potential for combining mutations affecting different parts of the existing hypotheses, does offer a great opportunity for progress. Recent breakthroughs have been particularly important in identifying promoters that allow gene targeting to macrophages, smooth muscle cells, and endothelial cells in the plaque.[134–139]

Finally, an obvious point raised by the mouse studies to date is that mouse lesions, like human lesions, are highly localized. This includes not only the apparent location of xanthomas at sites predicted by shear, but the locations of advanced lesions at specific sites, or the propensity for certain sites to develop aneurysm.[56] Explaining this region-specific pathology may be the most important opportunity growing out of the mouse models.

References

1. Duguid JB. Atherogenesis of atherosclerosis. Lancet 1947;257:925–936.
2. Chandler AB, Hand RA. Phagocytized platelets: a source of lipids in human thrombi and atherosclerotic plaques. Science 1961;134:946–7.
3. Hollander W. Role of arterial lipoproteins in the formation of the fibrous plaque. Adv Exp Med Biol 1977;82:793–9.
4. Ross R, Glomset JA. Atherosclerosis and the arterial smooth muscle cell: proliferation of smooth muscle is a key event in the genesis of the lesions of atherosclerosis. Science 1973;180:1332–9.
5. Schwartz SM, Majesky MW, Murry CE. The intima: development and monoclonal responses to injury. Atherosclerosis 1995;118:S125–40.
6. Yee KO, Ikari Y, Schwartz SM. An update of the Grutzbalg hypothesis: the role of thrombosis and coagulation in atherosclerotic progression. Thromb Haemost 2001;85:207–17.
7. Davies PF, Bowyer DE. Scanning electron microscopy: arterial endothelial integrity after fixation at physiological pressure. Atherosclerosis 1975;21:463–9.
8. Faggiotto A, Ross R, Harker L. Studies of hypercholesterolemia in the non-human primate. I. Changes that lead to fatty streak formation. Arteriosclerosis 1984;4:323–40.
9. Stary HC, McMillan GC. Kinetics of cellular proliferation in experimental atherosclerosis. Radioautography with grain counts in cholesterol-fed rabbits. Arch Pathol 1970;89:173–83.
10. Kim DN, Schmee J, Lee KT, Thomas WA. Atherosclerotic lesions in the coronary arteries of hyperlipidemic swine. Part 1. Cell increases, divisions, losses and cells of origin in first 90 days on diet. Atherosclerosis 1987;64:231–42.
11. Glass CK, Witztum JL. Atherosclerosis. The road ahead. Cell 2001;104:503–516.
12. Ikari Y, McManus BM, Kenyon J, Schwartz SM. Neonatal intima formation in the human coronary artery. Arterioscler Thromb Vasc Biol 1999;19:2036–40.
13. Williams KJ, Tabas I. The response-to-retention hypothesis of early atherogenesis. Arterioscler Thromb Vasc Biol 1995;15:551–61.
14. Davies PF, Reidy MA, Goode TB, Bowyer DE. Scanning electron microscopy in the evaluation of endothelial integrity of the fatty lesion in atherosclerosis. Atherosclerosis 1976;25:125–30.
15. Goode TB, Davies PF, Reidy MA, Bowyer DE. Aortic endothelial cell morphology observed in situ by scanning electron microscopy during atherogenesis in rabbits. Atherosclerosis 1977;27:235–51.
16. Gerrity RG. The role of the monocyte in atherogenesis. I. Transition of blood-borne monocytes into foam cells in fatty lesions. Am J Pathol 1981;103:181–90.
17. Rosenfeld ME, Polinsky P, Virmani R, Kauser K, Rubanyi G, Schwartz SM. Advanced atherosclerotic lesions in the innominate artery of the ApoE knockout mouse. Arterioscler Thromb Vasc Biol 2000;20:2587–92.
18. Rosenfeld ME, Carson KG, Johnson JL, Williams H, Jackson CL, Schwartz SM. Animal models of spontaneous plaque rupture: the holy grail of experimental atherosclerosis research. Curr Atheroscler Rep 2002;4:238–42.
19. Reddick RL, Zhang SH, Maeda N. Atherosclerosis in mice lacking apo E. Evaluation of lesional development and progression. Arterioscler Thromb. 1994;14:141–7 [published erratum appears in Arterioscler Thromb 1994;14(5):839].
20. Massberg S, Brand K, Gruner S, et al. A critical role of platelet adhesion in the initiation of atherosclerotic lesion formation. J Exp Med 2002;196:887–96.

21. Gawaz M, Page S, Massberg S, et al. Transient platelet interaction induces MCP-1 production by endothelial cells via I kappa B kinase complex activation. Thromb Haemost 2002;88:307–14.

22. Massberg S, Vogt F, Dickfeld T, Brand K, Page S, Gawaz M. Activated platelets trigger an inflammatory response and enhance migration of aortic smooth muscle cells. Thromb Res 2003;110:187–94.

23. Burger PC, Wagner DD. Platelet P-selectin facilitates atherosclerotic lesion development. Blood 2003;101: 2661–6.

24. Methia N, Andre P, Denis CV, Economopoulos M, Wagner DD. Localized reduction of atherosclerosis in von Willebrand factor-deficient mice. Blood 2001;98:1424–8.

25. Weng S, Zemany L, Standley KN, et al. Beta3 integrin deficiency promotes atherosclerosis and pulmonary inflammation in high-fat-fed, hyperlipidemic mice. Proc Natl Acad Sci USA 2003;100:6730–5.

26. Huo Y, Schober A, Forlow SB, et al. Circulating activated platelets exacerbate atherosclerosis in mice deficient in apolipoprotein E. Nat Med 2003;9:61–7.

27. Gawaz M, Neumann FJ, Dickfeld T, et al. Activated platelets induce monocyte chemotactic protein-1 secretion and surface expression of intercellular adhesion molecule-1 on endothelial cells. Circulation 1998;98: 1164–71.

28. Westrick RJ, Bodary PF, Xu Z, Shen YC, Broze GJ, Eitzman DT. Deficiency of tissue factor pathway inhibitor promotes atherosclerosis and thrombosis in mice. Circulation 2001;103:3044–6.

29. Xiao Q, Danton MJ, Witte DP, Kowala MC, Valentine MT, Degen JL. Fibrinogen deficiency is compatible with the development of atherosclerosis in mice. J Clin Invest 1998;101:1184–94.

30. Parry GC, Mackman N. Mouse embryogenesis requires the tissue factor extracellular domain but not the cytoplasmic domain. J Clin Invest 2000;105:1547–54.

31. Hembrough TA, Ruiz JF, Papathanassiu AE, Green SJ, Strickland DK. Tissue factor pathway inhibitor inhibits endothelial cell proliferation via association with the very low density lipoprotein receptor. J Biol Chem 2001;276:12241–8.

32. Mann KG, Brummel K, Butenas S. What is all that thrombin for? J Thromb Haemost 2003;1:1504–14.

33. Schwartz SM, Virmani R, Rosenfeld ME. The good smooth muscle cells in atherosclerosis. Curr Atheroscler Rep 2000;2:422–9.

34. Kockx MM, Herman AG. Apoptosis in atherosclerosis: beneficial or detrimental? Cardiovasc Res 2000;45: 736–46.

35. Sano H, Sudo T, Yokode M, et al. Functional blockade of platelet-derived growth factor receptor-beta but not of receptor-alpha prevents vascular smooth muscle cell accumulation in fibrous cap lesions in apolipoprotein E-deficient mice. Circulation 2001;103:2955–60.

36. Kozaki K, Kaminski WE, Tang J, et al. Blockade of platelet-derived growth factor or its receptors transiently delays but does not prevent fibrous cap formation in ApoE null mice. Am J Pathol 2002;161: 1395–407.

37. Geiringer E. Intimal vascularization and atherosclerosis. J Pathol Bacteriol 1951;63:201–11.

38. Assiri A, Veinot JP, Woodend K, et al. Abundance of plaque microvessels is associated with constrictive remodeling in angioplastied human coronary arteries. Jpn Circ J 2001;65:429–33.

39. Dvorak HF, Harvey VS, Estrella P, Brown LF, McDonagh J, Dvorak AM. Fibrin containing gels induce angiogenesis. Implications for tumor stroma generation and wound healing. Lab Invest 1987;57: 673–86.

40. Staton CA, Brown NJ, Lewis CE. The role of fibrinogen and related fragments in tumour angiogenesis and metastasis. Expert Opin Biol Ther 2003;3:1105–20.

41. Guo P, Hu B, Gu W, et al. Platelet-derived growth factor-B enhances glioma angiogenesis by stimulating vascular endothelial growth factor expression in tumor endothelia and by promoting pericyte recruitment. Am J Pathol 2003;162:1083–93.

42. Manegold PC, Hutter J, Pahernik SA, Messmer K, Dellian M. Platelet-endothelial interaction in tumor angiogenesis and microcirculation. Blood 2003;101: 1970–6.

43. Lindahl P, Bostrom H, Karlsson L, Hellstrom M, Kalen M, Betsholtz C. Role of platelet-derived growth factors in angiogenesis and alveogenesis. Curr Top Pathol 1999;93:27–33.

44. Hagedorn M, Zilberberg L, Lozano RM, et al. A short peptide domain of platelet factor 4 blocks angiogenic key events induced by FGF-2. FASEB J 2001;15:550–2.

45. Glagov S, Weisenberg E, Zarins CK, Stankunavicius R, Kolettis GJ. Compensatory enlargement of human atherosclerotic coronary arteries. N Engl J Med 1987;316:1371–5.

46. Folkow B. Physiological aspects of primary hypertension. Physiol Rev 1982;62:347–504.

47. Stadius ML, Gown AM, Kernoff R, Schwartz SM. Does sequential balloon injury of an artery lead to a different outcome than a single injury? An experimental study of angioplasty. Coron Artery Dis 1996;7:247–55.

48. Courtman DW, Schwartz SM, Hart CE. Sequential injury of the rabbit abdominal aorta induces intramural coagulation and luminal narrowing independent of intimal mass: extrinsic pathway inhibition eliminates luminal narrowing. Circ Res 1998;82:996–1006.

49. Stadius ML, Rowan R, Fleischhauer JF, Kernoff R, Billingham M, Gown AM. Time course and cellular characteristics of the iliac artery response to acute balloon injury. An angiographic, morphometric, and immunocytochemical analysis in the cholesterol-fed New Zealand white rabbit. Arterioscler Thromb 1992;12:1267–73.

50. Mintz GS, Kovach JA, Javier SP, Ditrano CJ, Leon MB. Geometric remodeling is the predominant mechanism of late lumen loss after coronary angioplasty (abstract). Circulation 1993;88:I-654.

51. O'Brien ER, Alpers CE, Stewart DK, et al. Proliferation in primary and restenotic coronary atherectomy tissue. Implications for antiproliferative therapy. Circ Res 1993;73:223–31.

52. Milewicz DM, Urban Z, Boyd C. Genetic disorders of the elastic fiber system. Matrix Biol 2000;19:471–80.

53. Li DY, Brooke B, Davis EC, et al. Elastin is an essential determinant of arterial morphogenesis. Nature 1998; 393:276–80.

54. Curci JA, Liao S, Huffman MD, Shapiro SD, Thompson RW. Expression and localization of macrophage elastase (matrix metalloproteinase-12) in abdominal aortic aneurysms. J Clin Invest 1998;102:1900–10.

55. Krettek A, Sukhova GK, Libby P. Elastogenesis in human arterial disease: a role for macrophages in disordered elastin synthesis. Arterioscler Thromb Vasc Biol 2003;23:582–7.

56. Daugherty A, Cassis LA. Mechanisms of abdominal aortic aneurysm formation. Curr Atheroscler Rep 2002;4:222–7.

57. Virmani R, Kolodgie FD, Burke AP, Farb A, Schwartz SM. Lessons from sudden coronary death: a comprehensive morphological classification scheme for atherosclerotic lesions. Arterioscler Thromb Vasc Biol 2000;20:1262–75.

58. Atherosclerosis Thrombosis and Vascular Biology Italian Study Group. No evidence of association between prothrombotic gene polymorphisms and the development of acute myocardial infarction at a young age. Circulation 2003;107:1117–22.

59. Aleksic N, Juneja H, Folsom AR, et al. Platelet Pl(A2) allele and incidence of coronary heart disease: results from the Atherosclerosis Risk In Communities (ARIC) Study. Circulation 2000;102:1901–5.

60. Mikkelsson J, Perola M, Penttila A, Karhunen PJ. Platelet glycoprotein Ibalpha HPA-2 Met/VNTR B haplotype as a genetic predictor of myocardial infarction and sudden cardiac death. Circulation 2001;104: 876–80.

61. Rosengren A, Wilhelmsen L. Fibrinogen, coronary heart disease and mortality from all causes in smokers and nonsmokers. The study of men born in 1933. J Intern Med 1996;239:499–507.

62. Blake GJ, Schmitz C, Lindpaintner K, Ridker PM. Mutation in the promoter region of the beta-fibrinogen gene and the risk of future myocardial infarction, stroke and venous thrombosis. Eur Heart J 2001;22:2262–6.

63. Eitzman DT, Westrick RJ, Xu Z, Tyson J, Ginsburg D. Plasminogen activator inhibitor-1 deficiency protects against atherosclerosis progression in the mouse carotid artery. Blood 2000;96:4212–15.

64. Humphries SE, Ye S, Talmud P, Bara L, Wilhelmsen L, Tiret L. European Atherosclerosis Research Study: genotype at the fibrinogen locus (G-455–A beta-gene) is associated with differences in plasma fibrinogen levels in young men and women from different regions in Europe. Evidence for gender–genotype–environment interaction. Arterioscler Thromb Vasc Biol 1995;15: 96–104.

65. Kannel WB, Wolf PA, Castelli WP, D'Agostino RB. Fibrinogen and risk of cardiovascular disease. The Framingham Study. JAMA 1987;258:1183–6.

66. Quinn MJ, Topol EJ. Common variations in platelet glycoproteins: pharmacogenomic implications. Pharmacogenomics 2001;2:341–52.

67. Ridker PM, Stampfer MJ, Rifai N. Novel risk factors for systemic atherosclerosis: a comparison of C-reactive protein, fibrinogen, homocysteine, lipoprotein(a), and standard cholesterol screening as predictors of peripheral arterial disease. JAMA 2001;285:2481–5.

68. Davies MJ, Thomas AC. Plaque fissuring – the cause of acute myocardial infarction, sudden ischemic death, and crescendo angina. Br Heart J 1985;53:363–73.

69. Fuster V. Elucidation of the role of plaque instability and rupture in acute coronary events. Am J Cardiol 1996;76:24C–33C.

70. Henney AM, Wakeley PR, Davies MJ, et al. Localization of stromelysin gene expression in atherosclerotic plaques by in situ hybridization. Proc Natl Acad Sci USA 1991;88:8154–8.

71. Libby P. Inflammation in atherosclerosis. Nature 2002;420:868–74.

72. Shah PK, Galis ZS. Matrix metalloproteinase hypothesis of plaque rupture: players keep piling up but questions remain. Circulation 2001;104:1878–80.

73. Falkenberg M, Tom C, DeYoung MB, Wen S, Linnemann R, Dichek DA. Increased expression of urokinase during atherosclerotic lesion development causes arterial constriction and lumen loss, and accelerates lesion growth. Proc Natl Acad Sci USA 2002;99:10665–70.

74. Bea F, Blessing E, Bennett B, Levitz M, Wallace EP, Rosenfeld ME. Simvastatin promotes atherosclerotic plaque stability in apoE-deficient mice independently of lipid lowering. Arterioscler Thromb Vasc Biol 2002;22:1832–7.

75. Blanc J, Alves-Guerra MC, Esposito B, et al. Protective role of uncoupling protein 2 in atherosclerosis. Circulation 2003;107:388–90.

76. Gojova A, Brun V, Esposito B, et al. Specific abrogation of transforming growth factor-beta signaling in T cells alters atherosclerotic lesion size and composition in mice. Blood 2003;102:4052–8.

77. Merched AJ, Williams E, Chan L. Macrophage-specific p53 expression plays a crucial role in atherosclerosis development and plaque remodeling. Arterioscler Thromb Vasc Biol 2003;23:1608–14.

78. Nakata Y, Maeda N. Vulnerable atherosclerotic plaque morphology in apolipoprotein E-deficient mice unable to make ascorbic acid. Circulation 2002;105:1485–90.

79. Rekhter MD. How to evaluate plaque vulnerability in animal models of atherosclerosis? Cardiovasc Res 2002;54:36–41.

80. Robertson AK, Rudling M, Zhou X, Gorelik L, Flavell RA, Hansson GK. Disruption of TGF-beta signaling in T cells accelerates atherosclerosis. J Clin Invest 2003;112:1342–50.

81. Arbustini E, Grasso M, Diegoli M, et al. Coronary atherosclerotic plaques with and without thrombus in ischemic heart syndromes: a morphologic, immuno-histochemical, and biochemical study. Am J Cardiol 1991;68:36B–50B.

82. Arbustini E, Grasso M, Diegoli M, et al. Coronary thrombosis in non-cardiac death. Coron Artery Dis 1993;4:751–9.

83. Stary HC. Natural history and histological classification of atherosclerotic lesions: an update [comment]. Arterioscler Thromb Vasc Biol 2000;20:1177–8.

84. Farb A, Burke AP, Tang AL, et al. Coronary plaque erosion without rupture into a lipid core. A frequent cause of coronary thrombosis in sudden coronary death. Circulation 1996;93:1354–63.

85. Luo Y, Polissar N, Han C, et al. Accuracy and unique-ness of three in vivo measurements of atherosclerotic carotid plaque morphology with black blood MRI. Magn Reson Med 2003;50:75–82.

86. Sheth SS, Deluna A, Allayee H, Lusis AJ. Understanding atherosclerosis through mouse genetics. Curr Opin Lipidol 2002;13:181–9.

87. Badimon JJ, Lettino M, Toschi V, et al. Local inhibition of tissue factor reduces the thrombogenicity of disrupted human atherosclerotic plaques: effects of tissue factor pathway inhibitor on plaque thrombo-genicity under flow conditions. Circulation 1999;99:1780–7.

88. Smith EB. Fibrin deposition and fibrin degradation products in atherosclerotic plaques. Thromb Res 1994;75:329–35.

89. Kudryk BJ, Bini A. Monoclonal antibody designated T2G1 reacts with human fibrin beta-chain but not with the corresponding chain from mouse fibrin. Arterioscler Thromb Vasc Biol 2000;20:1848–9.

90. Wilcox JN, Smith KM, Schwartz SM, Gordon D. Localization of tissue factor in the normal vessel wall and in the atherosclerotic plaque. Proc Natl Acad Sci USA 1989;86:2839–43.

91. Taubman MB, Fallon JT, Schecter AD, et al. Tissue factor in the pathogenesis of atherosclerosis. Thromb Haemost 1997;78:200–4.

92. Schecter AD, Spirn B, Rossikhina M, et al. Release of active tissue factor by human arterial smooth muscle cells. Circ Res 2000;87:126–32.

93. Bogdanov VY, Balasubramanian V, Hathcock J, Vele O, Lieb M, Nemerson Y. Alternatively spliced human tissue factor: a circulating, soluble, thrombogenic protein. Nat Med 2003;9:458–62.

94. Fayad ZA, Fuster V. The human high-risk plaque and its detection by magnetic resonance imaging. Am J Cardiol 2001;88:42E–45E.

95. Helft G, Worthley SG, Fuster V, et al. Atherosclerotic aortic component quantification by noninvasive mag-netic resonance imaging: an in vivo study in rabbits. J Am Coll Cardiol 2001;37:1149–54.

96. Corti R, Fayad ZA, Fuster V, et al. Effects of lipid-lowering by simvastatin on human atherosclerotic lesions: a longitudinal study by high-resolution, noninvasive magnetic resonance imaging. Circulation 2001;104:249–52.

97. de Paepe A, Devereux RB, Dietz HC, Hennekam RC, Pyeritz RE. Revised diagnostic criteria for the Marfan syndrome. Am J Med Genet 1996;62:417–26.

98. Yuan C, Kerwin WS, Ferguson MS, et al. Contrast-enhanced high resolution MRI for atherosclerotic carotid artery tissue characterization. J Magn Reson Imaging 2002;15:62–7.

99. Yuan C, Mitsumori LM, Ferguson MS, et al. In vivo accuracy of multispectral magnetic resonance imaging for identifying lipid-rich necrotic cores and intraplaque hemorrhage in advanced human carotid plaques. Circulation 2001;104:2051–6.

100. Fayad ZA, Fuster V, Fallon JT, Jayasundera T, et al. Noninvasive in vivo human coronary artery lumen and wall imaging using black-blood magnetic resonance imaging. Circulation 2000;102:506–10.

101. Crispe IN. Fatal interactions: Fas-induced apoptosis of mature T cells. Immunity 1994;1:347–9.

102. Yuan C, Zhang SX, et al. Identification of fibrous cap rupture with magnetic resonance imaging is highly associated with recent transient ischemic attack or stroke. Circulation 2002;105:181–5.

103. Stary HC, Chandler AB, Dinsmore RE. A definition

of advanced types of atherosclerotic lesions and a histological classification of atherosclerosis. A report from
the Committee on Vascular Lesions of the Council
on Arteriosclerosis, American Heart Association.
Arterioscler Thromb Vasc Biol 1995;15:1512–31.

104. Stary HC, Chandler AB, Glagov S, et al. A definition of
initial, fatty streak and intermediate lesions of atherosclerosis. A report from the Committee on Vascular
Lesions of the Council on Arteriosclerosis, American
Heart Association. Circulation 1994;89:2462–78.

105. Yuan C, Zhao XQ, Hatsukami TS. Quantitative evaluation of carotid atherosclerotic plaques by magnetic
resonance imaging. Curr Atheroscler Rep 2002;4:
351–7.

106. Schwartz SM, Hatsukami TS, Yuan C. Molecular
markers, fibrous cap rupture, and the vulnerable plaque:
new experimental opportunities. Circ Res 2001;89:471–3.

107. Seo HS, Lombardi DM, Polinsky P, et al. Peripheral
vascular stenosis in apolipoprotein E-deficient mice.
Potential roles of lipid deposition, medial atrophy,
and adventitial inflammation. Arterioscler Thromb
Vasc Biol 1997;17:3593–601.

108. Rosenfeld ME, Kauser K, Martin-McNulty B, Polinsky
P, Schwartz SM, Rubanyi GM. Estrogen inhibits the
initiation of fatty streaks throughout the vasculature
but does not inhibit intra-plaque hemorrhage and the
progression of established lesions in apolipoprotein E
deficient mice. Atherosclerosis 2002;164:251–9.

109. Williams H, Johnson JL, Carson KG, Jackson CL.
Characteristics of intact and ruptured atherosclerotic
plaques in brachiocephalic arteries of apolipoprotein
E knockout mice. Arterioscler Thromb Vasc Biol
2002;22:788–92.

110. Li AC, Glass CK. The macrophage foam cell as a target
for therapeutic intervention. Nat Med 2002;8:1235–42.

111. Sukhova GK, Schonbeck U, Rabkin E, et al. Evidence
for increased collagenolysis by interstitial collagenases-
1 and -3 in vulnerable human atheromatous plaques.
Circulation 1999;99:2503–9.

112. Paigen B. Genetics of responsiveness to high-fat and
high-cholesterol diets in the mouse. Am J Clin Nutr
1995;62:458S–62S.

113. Nakashima Y, Plump AS, Raines EW, Breslow JL, Ross
R. ApoE-deficient mice develop lesions of all phases of
atherosclerosis throughout the arterial tree. Arterioscler
Thromb 1994;14:133–40.

114. Johnson JL, Jackson CL. Atherosclerotic plaque rupture
in the apolipoprotein E knockout mouse. Atherosclerosis 2001;154:399–406.

115. Calara F, Silvestre M, Casanada F, Yuan N, Napoli C,
Palinski W. Spontaneous plaque rupture and secondary
thrombosis in apolipoprotein E-deficient and LDL
receptor-deficient mice. J Pathol 2001;195:257–63.

116. Hu W, Polinsky P, Rosenfeld ME, Schwartz S.M.
Atherosclerotic lesions in the common coronary arteries of ApoE knockout mice. Cardiorosc Pathol 2005;
14:120–25.

117. Davies MJ. Stability and instability: two faces of coronary atherosclerosis. The Paul Dudley White Lecture
1995. Circulation 1996;94:2013–20.

118. Kolodgie FD, Narula J, Burke AP, et al. Localization of
apoptotic macrophages at the site of plaque rupture in
sudden coronary death. Am J Pathol 2000;157:1259–68.

119. Park DR, Thomsen AR, Frevert CW, et al. Fas (CD95)
induces proinflammatory cytokine responses by human
monocytes and monocyte-derived macrophages. J
Immunol 2003;170:6209–16.

120. Reddick RL, Zhang SH, Maeda N. Aortic atherosclerotic plaque injury in apolipoprotein E deficient mice.
Atherosclerosis 1998;140:297–305.

121. Bodary PF, Westrick RJ, Wickenheiser KJ, Shen Y,
Eitzman DT. Effect of leptin on arterial thrombosis
following vascular injury in mice. JAMA 2002;287:
1706–9.

122. Anderson HV, McNatt J, Clubb FJ, et al. Platelet
inhibition reduces cyclic flow variations and neointimal proliferation in normal and hypercholesterolemic-
atherosclerotic canine coronary arteries. Circulation
2001;104:2331–7.

123. Braun A, Trigatti BL, Post MJ, et al. Loss of SR-BI
expression leads to the early onset of occlusive
atherosclerotic coronary artery disease, spontaneous
myocardial infarctions, severe cardiac dysfunction,
and premature death in apolipoprotein E-deficient
mice. Circ Res 2002;90:270–6.

124. Cyrus T, Pratico D, Zhao L, et al. Absence of 12/15-
lipoxygenase expression decreases lipid peroxidation
and atherogenesis in apolipoprotein e-deficient mice.
Circulation 2001;103:2277–82.

125. Eitzman DT, Westrick RJ, Xu Z, Tyson J, Ginsburg D.
Hyperlipidemia promotes thrombosis after injury to
atherosclerotic vessels in apolipoprotein E-deficient
mice. Arterioscler Thromb Vasc Biol 2000;20:1831–
4.

126. Paigen B, Holmes PA, Novak EK, Swank RT.
Analysis of atherosclerosis susceptibility in mice with
genetic defects in platelet function. Arteriosclerosis
1990;10:648–52.

127. Sugano M, Hori K, Wada M. Hepatotoxicity and
plasma cholesterol esterification by rats. Arch Biochem
Biophys 1969;129:588–96.

128. Cui J, Eitzman DT, Westrick RJ, et al. Spontaneous
thrombosis in mice carrying the factor V Leiden mutation. Blood 2000;96:4222–6.

129. Levi M, Dorffler-Melly J, Reitsma P, et al. Aggravation
of endotoxin-induced disseminated intravascular

coagulation and cytokine activation in heterozygous protein-C-deficient mice. Blood 2003;101:4823–7.

130. Kojima T. Targeted gene disruption of natural anticoagulant proteins in mice. Int J Hematol 2002;76 (suppl 2):36–9.

131. Moulton KS, Vakili K, Zurakowski D, et al. Inhibition of plaque neovascularization reduces macrophage accumulation and progression of advanced atherosclerosis. Proc Natl Acad Sci USA 2003;100:4736–41.

132. Newman PJ, Berndt MC, Gorski J, et al. PECAM-1 (CD31) cloning and relation to adhesion molecules of the immunoglobulin gene superfamily. Science 1990;247:1219.

133. Kelly SM, MacDougall ED, Pabón-Peña LM, Rosenfeld ME, Schwartz SM. Absence of small vessels in advanced lesions in the innominate arteries of hyperlipidemic mice. Unpublished observations.

134. Horvai A, Palinski W, Wu H, Moulton KS, Kalla K, Glass CK. Scavenger receptor A gene regulatory elements target gene expression to macrophages and to foam cells of atherosclerotic lesions. Proc Natl Acad Sci USA 1995;92:5391–5.

135. Greaves DR, Quinn CM, Seldin MF, Gordon S. Functional comparison of the murine macrosialin and human CD68 promoters in macrophage and non-macrophage cell lines. Genomics 1998;54:165–8.

136. Clarke S, Greaves DR, Chung LP, Tree P, Gordon S. The human lysozyme promoter directs reporter gene expression to activated myelomonocytic cells in transgenic mice. Proc Natl Acad Sci USA 1996;93:1434–8.

137. Moessler H, Mericskay M, Li Z, Nagl S, Paulin D, Small JV. The SM 22 promoter directs tissue-specific expression in arterial but not in venous or visceral smooth muscle cells in transgenic mice. Development 1996;122:2415–25.

138. Hoggatt AM, Simon GM, Herring BP. Cell-specific regulatory modules control expression of genes in vascular and visceral smooth muscle tissues. Circ Res 2002;91:1151–9.

139. Cowan PJ, Shinkel TA, Fisicaro N, et al. Targeting gene expression to endothelium in transgenic animals: a comparison of the human ICAM-2, PECAM-1 and endoglin promoters. Xenotransplantation 2003;10:223–31.

140. Plump AS, Smith JD, Hayek T, Aalto-Setälä K, Walsh A, Verstuyft JG, Rubin EM, Breslow JL. Severe hypercholesterolemia and atherosclerosis in apolipoprotein E-deficient mice created by homologous recombination in ES cells. *Cell* 1992 October 16;71(2):343–53.

141. Zhang SH, Reddick RL, Piedrahita JA, Maeda N. Spontaneous hypercholesterolemia and arterial lesions in mice lacking apolipoprotein E. Science 1992; 16;258(5081):468–71.

142. Ishibashi S, Goldstein JL, Brown MS, Herz J, Burns DK. Massive xanthomatosis and atherosclerosis in cholesterol-fed low density lipoprotein receptor-negative mice. J Clin Invest 1994;93:1885–93.

143. Tokuno S, Hinokiyama K, Tokuno K, Lowbeer C, Hansson LO, Valen G. Spontaneous ischemic events in the brain and heart adapt the hearts of severely atherosclerotic mice to ischemia. Arterioscler Throm Vasc Biol 2002;22:995–1001.

144. Bonthu S, Heistad DD, Chappell DA, Lamping KG, Faraci FM. Atherosclerosis, vascular remodeling, and impairment of endothelium-dependent relaxation in genetically altered hyperlipidemic mice. Arterioscler Throm Vasc Biol 1997;17:2333–40.

145. Sanan DA, Newland DL, Tao R, et al. Low density lipoprotein receptor-negative mice expressing human apolipoprotein B-100 develop complex atherosclerotic lesions on a chow diet: no accentuation by apolipoprotein(a). Proc Natl Acad Sci USA 1998;95(8):4544–9.

146. Veniant MM, Withycombe S, Young SG. Lipoprotein size and atherosclerosis susceptibility in Apoe(-/-) and Ldlr(-/-) mice. Arterioscler Throm Vasc Biol 2001;21: 1567–70.

147. Powell-Braxton L, Véniant M, Latvala RD, et al. A mouse model of human familial hypercholesterolemia: markedly elevated low density lipoprotein cholesterol levels and severe atherosclerosis on a low-fat chow diet [see comments]. Nat Med 1998;4:934–8.

148. Covey SD, Krieger M, Wang W, Penman M, Trigatti BL. Scavenger receptor class B type I-mediated protection against atherosclerosis in LDL receptor-negative mice involves its expression in bone marrow-derived cells. Arterioscler Throm Vasc Biol 2003;23:1589–94.

149. Lutgens E, de Muinck ED, Heeneman S, Daemen MJ. Compensatory enlargement and stenosis develop in apoe(-/-) and apoe*3-leiden transgenic mice. Arterioscler Thromb Vasc Biol 2001;21:1359–65.

150. van Vlijmen BJ, van Dijk KW, van't Hof HB, et al. In the absence of endogenous mouse apolipoprotein E, apolipoprotein E*2(Arg-158 → Cys) transgenic mice develop more severe hyperlipoproteinemia than apolipoprotein E*3-Leiden transgenic mice. J Biol Chem 1996;271:30595–602.

151. Plump AS, Masucci-Magoulas L, Bruce C, Bisgaier CL, Breslow JL, Tall AR. Increased atherosclerosis in ApoE and LDL receptor gene knock-out mice as a result of human cholesteryl ester transfer protein transgene expression. Arterioscler Thromb Vasc Biol 1999;19: 1105–10.

152. Masucci-Magoulas L, Goldberg IJ, Bisgaier CL, Serajuddin H, Francone OL, Breslow JL, Tall AR. A

mouse model with features of familial combined hyper-lipidemia. Science 1997;275(5298):391–4.

153. Escola-Gil JC, Julve J, Marzal-Casacuberta A, Ordonez-LLanos J, Gonzalez-Sastre F, Blanco-Vaca F. Expression of human apolipoprotein A-II in apolipoprotein E-deficient mice induces features of familial combined hyperlipidemia. J Lipid Res 2000;41:1328–38.

154. Fazio S, Major AS, Swift LL, Gleaves LA, Accad M, Linton MF, Farese RV, Jr. Increased atherosclerosis in LDL receptor-null mice lacking ACAT1 in macrophages. J Clin Invest 2001;107:163–71.

155. van Vlijmen BJ, Gerritsen G, Franken AL, et al. Macrophage p53 deficiency leads to enhanced atherosclerosis in APOE*3-Leiden transgenic mice. Circ Res 2001;88:780–6.

156. Hasty AH, Shimano H, Osuga J, et al. Severe hyper-cholesterolemia, hypertriglyceridemia, and atheroscle-rosis in mice lacking both leptin and the low density lipoprotein receptor. J Biol Chem 2001;276:37402–8.

157. Keidar S, Attias J, Heinrich R, Coleman R, Aviram M. Angiotensin II atherogenicity in apolipoprotein E deficient mice is associated with increased cellular cholesterol biosynthesis. Atherosclerosis 1999;146:249–57.

158. Sugiyama F, Haraoka S, Watanabe T, et al. Acceleration of atherosclerotic lesions in transgenic mice with hypertension by the activated renin-angiotensin system. Lab Invest 1997;76:835–42.

159. Schwartz SM, Majesky MW, Murry CE. The intima: development and monoclonal responses to injury. Atherosclerosis 1995;118(suppl):S125–40.

160. Yee KO, Ikari Y, Schwartz SM. An update of the Grutzbalg hypothesis: the role of thrombosis and coagulation in atherosclerotic progression. Thromb Haemost 2001;85:207–17.

PART 3

Triggers for plaque rupture

CHAPTER 8

Physical and mechanical stress

Luis E Rohde & Richard T Lee

Plaques that are predisposed to disruption frequently share specific morphological, mechanical and biochemical properties, and early determination of these characteristics may provide a broad temporal window to implement preventive therapeutic strategies. With the anticipated success of drug-eluting stents, the prospects for prevention of acute ischemic events have never been as promising. In this chapter we will introduce basic concepts and terms of solid mechanics to provide the common-ground understanding for a more detailed discussion of the complex biomechanical interactions that take place during atherosclerotic plaque initiation, progression, and rupture.

Basics of vascular mechanics

Fracture or rupture is a probability distribution determined by the nature of imposed stresses and the strength of a particular material. Strength is a property that results from the structure of the material, which includes the distribution, orientation, and interconnection of its constituents. To be sure that a structure will be mechanically stable when confronted with different forces we must consider the behavior of materials under distinct conditions. Understanding basic concepts of solid mechanics,[1,2] such as stress, strain, and their relationship, is essential to comprehend the intricate biomechanical interactions that take place in atherosclerotic lesions. Table 8.1 summarizes important concepts in vascular mechanics.

Stress, strain, and the stress–strain relationship

Stress and strain are interrelated concepts that are frequently confused. **Stress** is defined as the force acting on a surface, while **strain** is the resulting deformation caused by a stress. For these reasons stress is expressed in units of force divided by the area of the surface, and strain is usually expressed as a fraction or a percentage of the change in length. Forces can be applied in several directions on a specific surface: "normal" stresses represent perpendicular forces, while "shear" or "tangential" stresses are parallel to the surface. Endothelial cells, for example, are subjected to both normal (in the radial direction) and shear stresses, because forces from the blood flow and blood pressure are in different directions. Stresses and strain may also be characterized as compressive, when the structure is compressed, or tensile, when the structure is stretched. Within an artery or plaque, there are compressive normal stresses but also tensile stresses in the other dimensions.

Laplace's relation, also known as Lame's equation, tells us that the tensile wall stress is proportional to the pressure and the radius of the vessel and inversely related to the thickness of its wall or $\sigma = Pr/h$ (where σ is the tensile wall stress, P is the pressure, r is the radius, and h is the thickness of the vessel). This relation holds true when the wall of the cylinder is thin relative to the diameter of the vessel. In abdominal aortic aneurysms, for example, greater diameters and increases in arterial blood pressure

Table 8.1 Definitions of important terms in vascular mechanics.

Stress	Force acting on a surface, per unit of area. Stress is directional: normal/radial, tangential/shear or circumferential
Strain	Deformation resulting from a force, usually expressed as a fraction or a percentage of the change in length
Stiffness	General term describing resistance to deformation
Compliance	Change in volume per change in pressure
Elastic modulus	Fundamental material property that describes the relation between stress and strain
Linear behavior	Occurs when the stress–strain relations are constant over the range of stresses
Nonlinear elasticity	Occurs when increments in strain are changed for each increment in stress; common in biological materials
Isotropy	Property that describes materials in which the direction of stresses does not alter the stress–strain relation
Anisotropy	Property that describes materials in which the direction of stresses interfere with the stress–strain relation; common in biological materials
Viscoelasticity	Time-dependence of stress–strain responses

are important factors that contribute to the probability of rupture, as they are major determinants of wall stress. Although understanding stresses within heterogeneous structures such as the atherosclerotic lesion is much more challenging, these three basic components – diameter, pressure, and thickness – will always be pivotal determinants of stress. Thin fibrous caps in complex atherosclerotic plaques and thin myocardial walls after acute infarctions, for example, are well-known features of mechanical vulnerability and propensity to rupture.

It is common – and useful – to focus on the dominant force in a given configuration, but we must realize that stresses on the vessel and vascular cells cannot be reduced to a single number. Forces may be applied in multiple directions, and one type of stress can lead to other types of stress, leading to interactions throughout the vessel and even within a single cell.

The amount of deformation that occurs after applying a stress to a material will depend on its intrinsic mechanical properties. The relationship between force and deformation (stress–strain relationship) of a particular material is a central characterization of its mechanical behavior. The **elastic modulus** (or **Young's modulus**) represents this ratio: $E = $ stress/strain. Stiff materials (such as steel, bone tissue, or a thick fibrous cap) will respond to large increases in stress with minute deformations.

When the elastic modulus is constant over the range of stresses imposed on a material, the stress–strain behavior is called **linear elastic**. As most biological materials are composed of different layers of tissue with distinct mechanical properties, we usually do not observe linear elastic behavior in tissues. In fact, increments in strain often decrease for each increment of stress, so that the material actually becomes stiffer when exposed to higher levels of stress, a property called **nonlinear elasticity**. In addition, most biological materials have three-dimensional asymmetry that leads to different stress–strain relationships according to the vector of the forces; this important property is called **anisotropy**. The highly anisotropic nature of the vessel makes its biomechanical characterization much more difficult, particularly in the diseased state. Another important factor that must be considered in order to understand the stress–strain relationships is that they are time-dependent. A perfectly elastic material will immediately assume its unstressed shape after stress is removed. **Viscoelastic** materials, however, will gradually reassume their previous shape over time, a phenomenon called creep. In summary, most biological structures behave as nonlinear elastic materials that are highly anistropic with viscoelastic properties. Although researchers use sophisticated modern engineering techniques to incorporate most of these factors in stress analysis, there is a useful tendency to oversimplify the mechanics of the normal vessel and the atherosclerotic lesion to allow clinically-useful approximations.

Vascular mechanics of the normal vessel

The basic principles discussed above are instrumental to understanding the specific role of components of the normal vessel in maintaining vascular integrity. The structural integrity of the arterial wall results primarily from layers of smooth muscle cells, collagen and elastin, which are the main components of the tunica media. Elastin is a highly extensible fiber that can be stretched to many times its initial length without rupturing, although it can fracture at relatively low levels of stress.[3] Elastin behaves very much like a linear elastic material, hence its name. Although elastin is an important contributor to the pulsatile behavior of the vessel, it is much less important in determining its overall strength, since elastin fibers are easily broken. Collagen fibers, by contrast, have much higher fracture stresses when compared to elastin fibers; collagen fibers can withstand stresses orders of magnitude greater than levels that fracture elastin fibers.[4,5] Elastin fibers dominate the mechanical behavior of the artery at low stresses and strains, while at higher levels, elastin fibers stretch to their limit, and collagen fibers are sequentially recruited so that the vessel becomes stiffer and more resistant to rupture.[6]

Vascular biomechanical behavior may be studied in both active and passive states. In the absence of smooth muscle tone, most arteries demonstrate stress relaxation under constant extension and creep under constant loads, indicating viscoelastic behavior.[7] The active behavior of normal arteries has been evaluated by pressure–diameter and axial force–length tests on cylindrical segments, demonstrating that the active response is similar for various arteries, is length dependent, and peaks at a particular circumferential stretch.[8,9]

Vascular mechanics of the diseased vessel

Several studies have evaluated mechanical properties of the atherosclerotic vessel by comparing diseased arteries and nondiseased control vessels. One basic approach to study vascular mechanics is to evaluate the entire diseased vessel, using tension applied in one direction. Although this line of investigation is conceptually limited because it does not consider the distinct mechanical properties of different components of the atherosclerotic plaque, initial findings were consistent in demonstrating that the atherosclerotic vessel wall is stiffer, displaying limited distensibility when compared to the nondiseased wall. The atheroma, however, is a complex three-dimensional structure of many cell types and matrix components with great spatial and cellular heterogeneity. We then must consider separately the predominant components of a typical atherosclerotic lesion to understand its fundamental mechanical behavior.

The plaque cap

Description of plaque cap mechanical properties has been a focus of attention from biomechanical investigations. Pivotal studies, notably from Lendon, Born, Richardson, and Davies, revealed the nonlinear behavior of plaque caps and the influence of cellular content on the mechanical behavior of atherosclerotic lesions.[10,11] These investigators evaluated plaque caps from ulcerated and nonulcerated human aortas and demonstrated important interactions of structural, physical and biological features, such as vessel stiffness, stress, and collagen content.[10] Ex vivo studies also suggested that propensity to rupture depends on these characteristics. Human coronary artery plaque caps subjected to uniaxial tensile tests demonstrated less elongation than normal intima for a given level of stress and a sudden rise in stress with trivial increases in elongation, demonstrating the distinctive nonlinear behavior of atherosclerotic lesions. Also, when intact aortic strips were subjected to mechanical testing, plaque caps that developed intimal tearing had significantly fewer macrophages than lesions without fissures, suggesting that macrophage density, a cellular surrogate of the inflammatory burden, decreases plaque cap strength.[11]

Data from our laboratory extended these findings, demonstrating the role of fibrous cap composition in determining physical forces and propensity to rupture.[12] First, we evaluated if plaque cap histology – cellular, hypocellular, or calcific – would change the stress–strain relationship after dynamic and static uniaxial compression tests in aortic atherosclerotic lesions. We found that stiffness is two- to five-fold higher in calcific lesions when compared to hypocellular and cellular caps and that the viscoelastic component is prominent in plaque caps with cellular dominance. Subsequently, we demonstrated that the tangential modulus increased progressively with the percent strain, providing direct evidence of the nonlinear tensile behavior of plaque caps.[13] Taken together our findings indicate that the stress–strain behavior of plaque caps is also composition dependent, anisotropic, and nonlinear.

The lipid core

One common approach to study the mechanical properties of atherosclerotic lesions is to evaluate how plaques behave after in vivo or ex vivo angioplasty. High and prolonged pressure compression after transluminal coronary angioplasty causes a significantly greater reduction in plaque thickness in lipoid lesions when compared to fibrotic plaques.[14] Using reconstituted plaque lipid pools we evaluated whether lipid composition of the plaque core could affect the biomechanical balance within the atheroma. A significant positive association was observed between dynamic shear moduli and the concentration of cholesterol monohydrate in each specimen, indicating that lipid pool stiffness itself may be variable.[15] However, irrespective of specific lipid content, the lipid pool is so soft that it bears little stress.

Calcified plaques

Arterial calcification is a common feature of atherosclerosis, and imaging techniques such as electron-beam computerized tomography can accurately identify calcified plaques. Identification of vascular calcification may be important for several reasons. First, calcifications may impact vascular interventions, where calcium deposits may accentuate the dissection that generally accompanies successful procedures.[16] Second, there is compelling evidence from observational data that coronary artery calcification is associated with a worse cardiovascular prognosis. Calcification is probably a marker of overall extent of disease, rather than a primary promoter of plaque instability. Most lesions that rupture are in fact not heavily calcified.[17] To test the hypotheses that calcification impacts biomechanical stresses in human atherosclerosis, we studied 20 human coronary lesions with a structural analysis approach called finite element analysis (see below for further description). In this analysis, maximal stress was not associated with calcification, but it was markedly dependent on the degree of lipid deposition. We also explored an alternative approach to evaluate the contribution of calcium to plaque stress by computationally replacing calcified sections with fibrous tissue. This analysis is illustrated in Figure 8.1 and demonstrates that the "no calcium" solution leads to insignificant changes in plaque stress.[18]

Residual stress

Another important concept that is relevant to understand vascular mechanics is residual stress. Residual stress is the inherent force that exists in a body in the absence of externally applied forces. This intrinsic configuration represents the original stress-free state to which the material will return following any reversible process. Pivotal work from Fung and Vaishnav determined the role of residual stress in determining arteries' biomechanical behavior along the vascular tree.[19,20] They observed, for example, that intact unloaded artery rings open up at different angles in response to longitudinal cuts, representing distinct levels of residual stress.[21,22] Using a similar methodology, Hong et al. elegantly demonstrated that vascular biomechanical properties are altered in early atherogenesis even before subtle structural changes have occurred. These investigators evaluated hypercholesterolemic and normal rabbits that underwent angiography, intravascular ultrasound evaluation, and ex vivo aortic residual strain measurements. Residual strain was significantly increased in hypercholesterolemic rabbits, although angiography was completely normal in both groups of animals and intravascular ultrasound analysis showed only minor atherosclerotic plaques (<10% of cross-sectional area).[23] Interestingly, changes in residual strain were inversely correlated with the aortic cholesterol content in all segments of the aorta.

Finite element analysis

One striking finding from postmortem studies in the early 1980s was that severe coronary stenosis is a

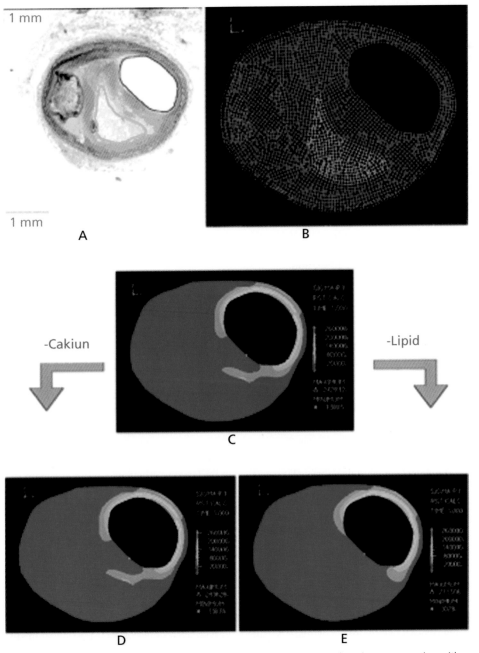

Figure 8.1 Example of an atherosclerotic lesion and finite element analysis. A, Original specimen cross-section, with purple lines designating regions of calcification, bold green line designating the lipid pool, blue lines indicating lumen, and fine green lines indicating arterial media. B, Finite element mesh corresponding to this section. C, A stress map of an unaltered lesion. D, A lesion with replacement of calcification by fibrous plaque. E, A lesion with replacement of lipid by fibrous plaque. (From Huang H, et al. Circulation 2001;103:1051–6.)

relatively uncommon anatomic presentation in most patients suffering acute coronary events. Biomechanical analysis based on the finite element method helped to unravel this apparent paradox, providing insight into important features of the vulnerable lesion. Finite element analysis is a widely used engineering technique employed to study complex three-dimensional structures. By subdividing a complex geometrical structure into much smaller sections and by assigning specific mechanical properties for each element, the distribution of stresses within the original structure can be more easily estimated (Figure 8.1). Finite element analysis is particularly amenable to the study of different constituents of atherosclerotic plaques, because one can individualize the impact of structural and morphological features – such as luminal area reduction, fibrous cap thickness, and the lipid pool – on stress estimation.

Using the finite element method, Richardson et al. published a landmark study that greatly influenced our contemporary knowledge of the vulnerable lesion and propensity to rupture.[24] These investigators suggested that plaque fissures were due to high circumferential tensile stress concentrated at the edges of the fibrous cap near the border of normal intima, particularly in lesions with large lipid pools. Subsequently, data from our laboratory indicated that maximal circumferential stress is significantly higher in culprit plaques responsible for acute and fatal coronary events when compared to stable control lesions. Interestingly, the location of plaque rupture was not always the area of greatest stress in an individual lesion.[25] This initially unexpected finding suggests that other factors, possibly mediated by biological processes or structural features, may determine which high stress regions actually evolve to rupture. Furthermore, using finite element analysis, we demonstrated that increasing stenosis severity solely by incrementing the fibrous cap thickness actually induced a five-fold decrease in maximum circumferential stress.[26] Conversely, when fibrous cap thickness falls below a critical threshold (approximately 200 μm), stress increases dramatically, achieving levels that have been shown to induce fracture human atherosclerotic tissue. Figure 8.2 illustrates the effect of plaque cap thickness on maximum circumferential stress normalized to luminal pressure. Thus, analysis of

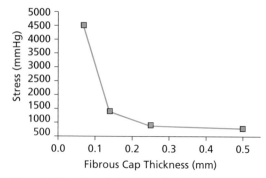

Figure 8.2 The effect of plaque cap thickness on maximum circumferential stress normalized to luminal pressure. When fibrous cap thickness falls below 0.2 mm, circumferential stress increases exponentially, reaching levels shown to be necessary to fracture human atherosclerotic tissue. (From Loree HM, et al. Circ Res 1992;71:850–8.)

plaque structures have helped explain confusing clinical observations – that very severe stenoses tend to progress to occlusion without rupture, and that moderate stenoses with thin fibrous caps as most unstable.

Imaging, mechanical behavior, and atherosclerosis

Because current data indicate that the degree that the lumen is narrowed is not a dominant factor in determining stress in the fibrous cap, it is easy to understand why angiography is a poor tool for determining plaque stability. Current clinical tools are unable to precisely measure the thickness of the atherosclerotic plaque layers in vivo, particularly in the submillimeter range necessary to characterize unstable lesions, but great improvement has been made in the last few years. Several new noninvasive and invasive imaging tools have received great attention as potentially useful and safe methods to evaluate atherosclerotic lesions in vivo. Advances in these techniques make it possible at the present time to identify some constituents of the human atherosclerotic plaque. For example, coronary plaque composition can be predicted with reasonable accuracy through real-time intravascular ultrasound radiofrequency analysis.[27] We have demonstrated that ex vivo ultrasound-based plaque cap classification has a good agreement with histology analysis.[28] Biomechanical parameters, such as static compressive stiffness, were also shown to correlate with intravascular ultrasound plaque classifications, suggesting that intravascular imaging could be eventually applied to identify specific lesions predisposed to instability. In fact, structural analysis based on intravascular ultrasound imaging before in vitro balloon angioplasty predicts most locations of plaque fracture.[29] Similarly, high-spatial-resolution magnetic resonance imaging is capable of visualizing fibrous cap thickness and rupture[30] and identifying lipid-rich cores and intraplaque hemorrhage in human carotid plaques before endarterectomy.[31]

Pathology and biomechanical[10,24,26,32] studies are remarkably consistent in demonstrating that thin plaque caps are a central element of vulnerability. Data from these studies indicate that plaque rupture is more likely to occur when plaque cap thickness falls below 100 µm. Although most imaging techniques at the present lack this resolution, we are on the verge of clinically identifying the vulnerable lesion, particularly in vascular locations that are easily evaluated by noninvasive imaging methods, such as the neck extracranial arteries.

Mechanical forces and plaque biology

It is becoming apparent that atherosclerotic plaque fatigue and rupture depend on the interplay of plaque architecture and composition, its mechanical properties, and extracellular matrix biology. Mechanical forces act in combination with biological processes within the atheroma, particularly extracellular matrix degradation, and influence plaque vulnerability and propensity to rupture. Several lines of evidence in fact support this hypothesis. First, it has been known for over 20 years that mechanical deformation regulates extracellular matrix synthesis by vascular smooth muscle cells in vivo.[33] Second, fluid shear stresses control several endothelial molecular responses. For example, shear stress selectively upregulates intercellular adhesion molecule 1 expression in cultured human endothelial cells.[34] Third, we have demonstrated that regions of high circumferential stress in the shoulder area of atherosclerotic plaques are the same regions where matrix metalloproteinase 1 (MMP-1) – a proteolytic enzyme that initiates fibrillar collagen degradation – is expressed.[35] Finally, recent studies demonstrate that very small mechanical strains can modulate cellular signaling.

For example, mechanical deformation of monocytes/macrophages induces MMP-1 and MMP-3 expression,[36] and biaxial strains of human vascular smooth muscle cells interact with growth factor regulation of MMP-1.[37] Taken together these findings clearly demonstrate an exquisite sensitivity of the cell to mechanical stimuli.

The signaling pathways responsible for mechanotransduction are just now beginning to be characterized and possibly multiple pathways may participate in the processes in converting physical stimuli into biochemical products. These pathways may involve stretch-activated ion channels, paracrine growth factors, G proteins, MAP kinases, integrins, tyrosine kinases, and phospholipid metabolism.[38,39]

Conclusions

There is a general understanding that the phenomenon of plaque fracture is an acute local event with catastrophic consequences. A growing body of evidence, however, suggests that atherosclerotic lesions frequently fracture without causing symptoms.[40,41] This may, in fact, be an important mechanism for plaque growth. In addition, several recent studies support the concept that acute coronary events are not sporadic and unpredictable episodes due to instability of one isolated coronary lesion, but in fact they are the "tip of a vulnerable iceberg" of widespread instability.[42,43] The specific locations of rupture will depend on structural, physical and biological factors that interact to create regions of vulnerability. It is clear that mechanical forces and biological processes are not separate factors in this process, but intricately associated as the cells of the atherosclerotic lesion struggle to maintain stability. Our challenge in the near future will be to detect the "vulnerable vascular environment" with enough time to implement specific therapies aimed to improve the structural integrity of the vulnerable atherosclerotic lesion and avoid acute vascular events.

References

1. Lee RT, Kamm RD. Vascular mechanics for the cardiologists. J Am Coll Cardiol 1994;23:1289–5.

2. Rohde LE, Lee RT. Mechanical stress and strain and the vulnerable atherosclerotic lesion. In: Valentin Fuster, ed. The vulnerable atherosclerotic plaque: understanding, identification and modification. Armonk, New York: Futura Publishing, 1999:305–16.

3. Mukherjee DP, Kagan HM Jordan RE, Franzblau C. Effects of hydrophobic elastin ligans on the stress–strain properties of elastin fibers. Connect Tissue Res 1976;4:177.

4. Kato YP, Christiansen DL, Hahn RA, Shien JJ, Golstein JD, Silver FH. Mechanical properties of collagen fibers: a comparison of reconstituted and rat tail tendon fibers. Biomaterials 1989;10:38–42.

5. Kato YP, Silver FH. Formation of continuous collagen fibers: evaluation of biocompatibility and mechanical properties. Biomaterials 1990;11:169–75.

6. Roach MR, Burton AC. The reason for the shape of the distensibility curve of arteries. Can J Biochem. Physiol 1957;35:681–90.

7. Humphrey JD. Mechanics of arterial wall: reviews and directions. Crit Rev Biomed Eng 1995;23(1–2):1–162.

8. Dobrin PB. Biaxial anisotropy of dog carotid artery: estimation of circumferential elastic modulus. J Biomech 1986;19:351–8.

9. Cox RH. Comparison of carotid artery mechanics in rat, rabbit and dog. Am J Physiol 1978;234:H280–8.

10. Lendon CL, Briggs AD, Born GVR, Burleigh MC, Davies MJ. Mechanical testing of the connective tissue in the search for determinants of atherosclerotic plaque cap rupture. Biochem Soc Trans 1988;16:1032–3.

11. Lendon CL, Davies MJ. Born GVR, Richardson PD. Atherosclerotic plaque caps are locally weakened when macrophages density is increased. Atherosclerosis 1991; 87:87–90.

12. Lee RT, Grodzinsky AJ, Franf EH, Kamm RD, Schoen FJ. Structure dependent dynamic mechanical behavior of fibrous caps from human atherosclerotic plaque. Circulation 1991;83:1764–70.

13. Loree HM, Grodzinsky AJ, Park SY, Gibson LJ, Lee RT. Static circumferential modulus of human atherosclerotic tissue. J Biomechanics 1994;27:195–204.

14. Kaltenbach M, Beyer J, Waltr S, Klepzig H, Schmidts L. Prolonged application of pressure in transluminal coronary angioplasty. Catheterization Cardiovasc Diagn 1984;10:213–19.

15. Loree HM, Tobias BJ, Gibson LJ, Kamm RD, Small DM, Lee RT. Mechanical properties of model atherosclerotic lesion lipid pools. Arterioscler Thromb 1994;14:230–4.

16. Fitzgerald PJ, Ports TA, Yock PG. Contribution of localized calcium deposits to dissection after angioplasty: an observational study using intravascular ultrasound. Circulation 1992;86:64–70.

17. Moriuchi M, Saito S, Takaiwa Y, et al. Assessment of plaque rupture by intravascular ultrasound. Heart Vessels 1997;12:178–81.

18. Huang H, Virmani R, Younis H, Burke AP, Kamm RD, Lee RT. The impact of calcification on the biomechanical stability of atherosclerotic plaques. Circulation 2001; 103:1051–6.

19. Chuong CJ, Fung YC. On residual stress in arteries. ASME J Biomech Engr 1986;108:189–92.

20. Vaishnav RN, Vossoughi J. Residual stress and strain in aortic segments. J Biomech 1987;20:235–9.

21. Han HC, Fung YC. Species dependence of the zero-stress state of aorta: pigs versus rat. ASME J Biomech Engr 1991;113:446–51.

22. Fung YC, Liu SQ. Changes in zero-stress state of rat pulmonary arteries in hypoxic hypertension. J Appl. Physiol 1991;70:2455–70.

23. Hong MK, Vossoughi J, Mintz GS, et al. Altered compliance and residual strain precede angiographically detectable early atherosclerosis in low-density lipoprotein receptor deficiency. Arterioscler Thromb Vasc Biol 1997;17:2209–17.

24. Richardson PD, Davies MJ, Born GVR. Influence of plaque configuration and stress distribution on fissuring of coronary atherosclerotic plaques. Lancet. 1989; 2:941–4.

25. Cheng GC, Loree HM, Kamm RD, Fishbein MC, Lee RT. Distribution of circumferential mechanical stress in ruptured and stable atherosclerotic lesions: a structural analysis with histopathological correlation. Circulation. 1993;87:1179–87.

26. Loree HM, Kamm RD, Stringfellow RG, Lee RT. Effects of fibrous cap thickness on peak circumferential stress in model atherosclerotic vessels. Circ Res 1992;71:850–8.

27. Nair A, Kuban BD, Tuzcu M, Schoenhagen P, Nissen SE, Vince DG. Coronary plaque classification with intravascular ultrasound radiofrequency data analysis. Circulation 2002;106:2200–6.

28. Lee TR, Richardson G, Loree HM, et al. Prediction of mechanical properties of human atherosclerotic tissue by high-frequency intravascular ultrasound imaging. Arterioscler Thromb 1992;12:1–5.

29. Lee RT, Lorree HM, Cheng GC, Lieberman EH, Jaramillo N, Schoen FJ. Computational structural analysis based on intravascular ultrasound imaging before in vitro angioplasty: prediction of plaque fracture location. J Am Coll Cardiol 1993;21:777–82.

30. Hatsukami TS, Ross R, Polissar NL, Yuan C. Visualization of fibrous cap thickness and rupture in human atherosclerotic carotid plaque in vivo with high-resolution magnetic resonance imaging. Circulation 2000;102:959–64.

31. Yuan C, Mitsumori LM, Ferguson MS, et al. In vivo assuracy of multispectral magnetic resonance imaging for identifying lipid-rich necrotic cores and intraplaque hemorrhage in advanced human carotid plaques. Circulation 2001;104:2051–6.

32. Virmani R, Burke AP, Kolodgie FD, Farb A. Vulnerable plaque: the pathology of unstable coronary lesions. J Interv Cardiol. 2002;15:439–46.

33. Leung DY, Glagov S, Mathews MB. Cyclic stretching stimulates synthesis of matrix components by arterial smooth muscle cells in vitro. Science 1976;191:475–7.

34. Hagel T, Resnick N, Atkinson WJ, Dewey CF Jr, Gimbrone MA Jr. Shear stress selectively upregulates intercellular adhesion molecule-1 expression in cultured human vascular endothelial cells. J Clin Invest 1994;94: 885–91.

35. Lee RT, Schoen FJ, Loree HM, Lark MW, Libby P. Circumferential stress and matrix metalloproteinase 1 in human coronary atherosclerosis. Implications for plaque rupture. Arterioscler Thromb Vasc Biol. 1996;16: 1070–3.

36. Yang J-H, Lee RT. Small mechanical deformations induce immediate-early gene expression and augment matrix metalloproteinase expression by human monocyte/macrophages. Circulation 1998;98:I47.

37. Yang J-H, Briggs WH, Libby P, Lee RT. Small mechanical strains selectively suppress matrix metalloproteinase-1 expression by human vascular smooth muscle cells. J Biol Chem 1998;273:6550–5.

38. Banes AJ, Tauzaki M, Yamamoto J, et al. Mechanoreception at the cellular level: the detection, interpretation, and diversity of responses to mechanical signals. Biochem Cell Biol 1995;73:349–65.

39. Lee RT, Huang H. Mechanotransduction and arterial smooth muscle cells: new insights into hypertension and atherosclerosis. Ann Med 2000;32:233–5.

40. Rioufol G, Finet G, Ginon I, et al. Multiple atherosclerotic plaque rupture in acute coronary syndrome: a three-vessel intravascular ultrasound study. Circulation 2002;106:804–8.

41. Spagnoli LG, Bonanno E, Mauriello A, et al. Multicentric inflammation in epicardial coronary arteries of patients dying of acute myocardial infarction. J Am Coll Cardiol 2002;40:1579–88.

42. Goldstein JA, Demetriou D, Grines CL, Pica M, Shoukfen M, O'Neill WW. Multiple complex coronary plaques in patients with acute myocardial infarction. N Engl J Med 2000;343:343:915–22.

43. Buffon A, Biasucci LM, Liuzzo G, D'onofrio G, Crea F, Maseri A. Widespread coronary inflammation in unstable angina. N Engl J Med 2002;347:5–12.

CHAPTER 9

Inflammation and matrix metalloproteinases

Zorina S Galis & Susan M Lessner

The story of inflammatory cell and matrix metalloproteinase contributions to plaque destabilization is somewhat reminiscent of a classic murder mystery, in which a motley assortment of characters – each with both the motives and the opportunities for creating mayhem – is gathered together at the scene of the crime (Figure 9.1). Several potential weapons are scattered about the grounds, and a few red herrings are likely thrown in for good measure. Now it is up to the distinguished investigator (and her audience) to sift through a wealth of clues to identify the guilty party or parties and to establish a case which will hold up in court.

A cast of highly suspicious characters – inflammatory cells in atherosclerosis

Inflammatory cells are commonly found within human atheroma, particularly in culprit lesions. The concept of atherosclerosis as a chronic inflammatory disease has become well established over the past 10–15 years.[1] Several types of inflammatory cells are implicated in the pathogenesis of the human disease from its earliest stages. Genetically engineered mouse models lacking various components of the immune system or deficient in specific inflammatory mediators have proven particularly useful in efforts to dissect out the specific roles of the various players.

Monocytes/macrophages

Observations from experimental models and autopsy findings in young human subjects suggest that monocyte adhesion to the endothelial surface and transmigration into the intima are among the earliest events in the development of atherosclerotic lesions.[2–4] Specific endothelial adhesion molecules, including vascular cell adhesion molecule (VCAM)-1 and intracellular adhesion molecule (ICAM)-1, and chemokines such as monocyte chemotactic protein (MCP)-1, mediate monocyte recruitment into the arterial wall.[5–9] The molecular mechanisms underlying monocyte adhesion and chemotaxis are regulated both by systemic factors, including hypercholesterolemia,[6,10] and by site-specific factors, such as local hemodynamics.[7] Strategies to block monocyte recruitment to the endothelial wall, including deletion of genes for MCP-1 or its receptor CCR-2, effectively reduce early lesion formation in mouse models of atherosclerosis.[11–13] Similarly, mice deficient in macrophage colony-stimulating factor (M-CSF), a cytokine important for maturation and differentiation of monocytic cells, show a dramatic reduction in the development of atherosclerotic lesions, indicating a primary role for monocytes in lesion initiation and growth.[14]

After crossing the endothelial barrier and migrating into the arterial intima, monocytes accumulate lipid and differentiate into macrophage-derived foam cells, the distinctive cell type of the early fatty streak lesion. Within the vascular wall, macrophage foam cells function in a number of ways to promote further growth and destabilization of the plaque: secretion of cytokines and chemokines,[15] generation of reactive oxygen species,[16] presentation of immune activation markers to lymphocytes, such as HLA-DR, a human major histocompatibility complex[17,18] or macrophage scavenger receptor,[19]

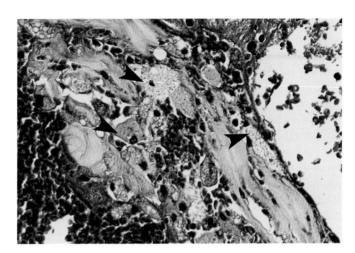

Figure 9.1 Murder most foul. Rupture of an atherosclerotic plaque having a thin fibrous cap and heavy infiltration of inflammatory cells (arrowheads) leads to intramural thrombosis. Not a pretty picture, but autopsy studies suggest that many ruptured plaques do heal without producing acute coronary events.

production of matrix-degrading proteases,[20] and release of inflammatory debris into the plaque core following necrosis or apoptosis.[21]

T-lymphocytes

Various lines of evidence, reviewed in several recent papers,[22,23] point to a role for both humoral and cell-mediated immunity in the development and progression of the atherosclerotic plaque. T-lymphocytes are seen in atherosclerotic plaques at nearly all stages of development, where they may account for up to 20% of the total nucleated cells.[24–26] Most T-lymphocytes within atherosclerotic lesions belong to the CD4+ Th1 T-cell subtype. T-lymphocytes within atherosclerotic lesions represent a polyclonal population, suggesting that limited expansion in response to antigen stimulation occurs in the plaque.[27] In support of this view, Paulsson and coworkers have shown using spectratyping of T-cell receptor (TCR) mRNA that oligoclonal expansion of T-lymphocytes takes place within aortic lesions in the apoE knockout mouse model of atherosclerosis.[28] Antigens suggested as possible mediators of T-cell activation within the atherosclerotic plaque include oxidized low density lipoprotein (LDL), heat shock proteins, and microbial proteins.[29–31] Activated, CD4+ T-lymphocytes expressing CD40 ligand have been demonstrated immunohistochemically in human lesions.[32] T-lymphocytes contribute to plaque vulnerability by producing proinflammatory cytokines, including interferon gamma (IFN-γ) and tumor necrosis factor alfa (TNF-α).[33] Direct evidence for a pro-atherogenic role for T-lymphocytes has emerged from studies in an immunodeficient apoE knockout mouse model of atherosclerosis.[34] Adoptive transfer of CD4+ T-cells in these animals, which normally lack functional T-lymphocytes, resulted in increased lesion development.

B-lymphocytes

B-lymphocytes have been detected by immunohistochemistry in advanced human atherosclerotic lesions and in animal models of atherosclerosis,[35,36] but their precise role is not known. Some researchers suggest that B-cell-mediated adaptive immunity may play an atheroprotective role, in contrast to the proatherogenic role of monocytes and T-lymphocytes.[37] Evidence for an atheroprotective role for B-lymphocytes has emerged from studies in which B-cells from mice having established lesions were adoptively transferred to younger, congenic animals, resulting in reduced lesion development in the recipients.[38] In immunodeficient apoE knockout mouse models of atherosclerosis, lesions develop in the absence of both T- and B-lymphocytes but remain smaller than in immunocompetent apoE knockout mice.[34,39] While inferences drawn from an animal model may not be directly applicable to human disease, these studies suggest that B- and T-lymphocytes play a secondary role to monocytes in atherogenesis.

Mast cells

Mast cells, although relatively uncommon compared to the other types of inflammatory cells involved in atherosclerosis, have the potential to play a critical role in destabilization of the atherosclerotic lesion. Mast cells are characterized by an abundance of cytoplasmic granules. While allergen binding to IgE is the classic mediator of mast cell degranulation, other stimuli more likely to occur in the context of the vulnerable plaque can also provoke this phenomenon. These include soluble factors secreted by activated T-cells or macrophages[40,41] and collagen-derived peptides.[42] In the process of degranulation, the granule contents, including heparin, inflammatory mediators such as histamine, and neutral proteases such as tryptase and chymase, are released into the surrounding medium. Activated mast cells often occur in the vulnerable shoulder regions of mature plaques.[43] Furthermore, mast cell infiltrates were identified in regions of plaque rupture or erosion in association with myocardial infarction,[44] and it is thought that their neutral proteases may serve to trigger activation of macrophage-released matrix metalloproteinases.[45]

A choice of lethal weapons – introduction to matrix metalloproteinases

Matrix metalloproteinases (MMPs) constitute a large class of related, zinc-dependent endopeptidases sharing several features of structural homology and common mechanisms of activation. These enzymes are among the most useful tools in the cellular arsenal for degradation of the extracellular matrix, but when not kept under tight control they also have the potential to cause destructive mischief.

Subclasses and substrate specificities

MMPs can be divided into several subfamilies, based either on structural similarities or on substrate specificities. For example, the MT-MMPs are distinguished from other members of the class by the fact that they are tethered to the cell membrane by means of a transmembrane domain or a glyco-phosphatidylinositol (GPI) anchor. On the other hand, other MMPs, such as the gelatinases MMP-2 and MMP-9, are grouped together primarily on the basis of similar substrate preferences. Both the gelatinases preferentially degrade short collagen molecules, such as the type IV and V collagens of the basement membrane.

Regulation of MMP activity – overview

As befits molecules which have a high potential for destruction of tissue, MMP activity is tightly regulated at a number of levels. At the transcriptional level, the levels of messenger RNA transcribed by cells from MMP genes are regulated both by soluble factors such as cytokines and by mechanical forces that act on the cells. Furthermore, most MMPs, with the exception of the membrane-type MMPs, are secreted by cells as inactive zymogens. Activation requires the exposure of the catalytic site, thereby allowing substrate binding and degradation. This can be achieved following molecular conformational changes of latent MMPs and/or by cleavage of their prodomain, which shields the catalytic active site. Activated MMPs catalyze their own autolysis, resulting in the eventual loss of enzymatic activity. Thus, their lifetime in tissue as catalytically active molecules is intrinsically self-limited.

In addition, MMP activity in vivo is controlled by specific, native inhibitors, known as tissue inhibitors of metalloproteinases (TIMPs). The TIMPs are relatively nonspecific in terms of their interactions with individual MMPs.[46] TIMP-1 binds to the active forms of most vascular MMPs.[47,48] MMP-2 is inhibited selectively by TIMP-2 but not by TIMP-1.[49] TIMPs are expressed constitutively by smooth muscle cells and endothelial cells in the vascular wall. Current evidence obtained from pathological investigations of human atherosclerotic specimens as well as experimental studies suggests that an imbalance between MMPs and their respective natural inhibitors is associated with active destruction of matrix in pathological conditions.

Factors which regulate vascular MMP expression

The microenvironment of the atherosclerotic plaque contains an abundance of potential stimuli capable of inducing MMP production in one or more populations of vascular cells, as depicted schematically in Figure 9.2. Macrophages and other inflammatory cells within the plaque are the source of many of these stimuli, although activated

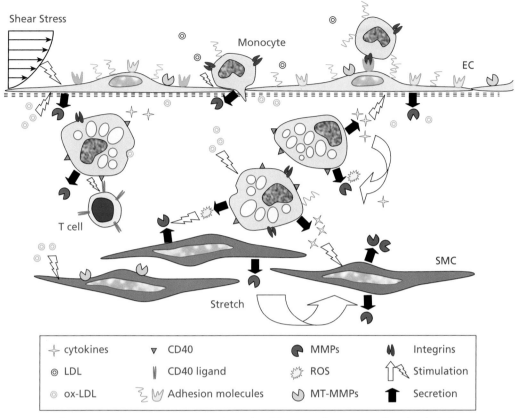

Figure 9.2 Inflammatory cells are prime suspects in plaque destabilization. Inflammatory cells within the intima secrete their own MMPs as well as stimulatory factors such as cytokines which can upregulate MMP expression in endothelial cells (ECs) and smooth muscle cells (SMCs). In addition, leukocytes within the plaque release reactive oxygen species which can activate MMP zymogens. Contact-dependent interactions between inflammatory cells and other cells within the plaque, mediated either through adhesion molecule–integrin binding or through CD40 binding to its ligand, can also stimulate production of MMPs. Finally, mechanical forces acting on the vessel wall modulate MMP expression.

vascular cells can also contribute. In vitro studies have provided much of the evidence to implicate these factors in stimulation of MMP activity, but in many cases their relative importance to MMP expression in human lesions remains unknown.

Cytokines and other inflammatory mediators

An important route by which inflammatory cells influence plaque stability is through secretion of cytokines which, among their many effects, can regulate the expression of MMPs by other vascular cells. Interleukin 1alfa (IL-1α) and TNF-α, two cytokines expressed by activated inflammatory cells in human lesions, stimulate smooth muscle cells and/or endothelial cells to produce a wide range of MMPs, including MMP-1, MMP-3, MMP-8, MMP-9, and MT1-MMP.[50–52] Figure 9.3 demonstrates that IL-1

is among the pro-inflammatory cytokines which colocalize with areas of macrophage infiltration in human atheroma, leading to possible upregulation of MMP secretion by the surrounding cells. Cytokine stimulation of MMP production may also occur through an indirect pathway involving generation of downstream inflammatory mediators such as eicosanoids. For example, the pro-inflammatory cytokine IL-1β can upregulate monocyte expression of enzymes essential to the synthesis of prostaglandin E_2, a major eicosanoid product of macrophages.[17] Prostaglandin E_2, in turn, strongly stimulates production of MMP-2 and MMP-9 by human monocytes.[53] Thus, cytokine secretion by inflammatory cells may lead to elevated MMP levels in the vulnerable plaque through both paracrine and autocrine routes.

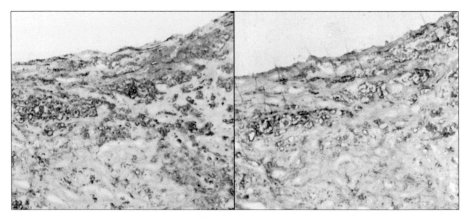

Figure 9.3 Bad company? Macrophages frequently infiltrate the vulnerable shoulder regions of human atherosclerotic lesions and secrete cytokines which can stimulate matrix metalloproteinase production by surrounding vascular cells. Immunohistochemical detection of human macrophages (left panel) and interleukin 1 (right panel). (Serial sections of human endarterectomy specimen; immunoperoxidase staining with DAB detection (brown color) counterstained with hematoxylin.)

Oxidized lipoproteins

Oxidation of lipoproteins sequestered in the microenvironment of the atherosclerotic plaque has important consequences for plaque progression and destabilization, which include promoting the ongoing recruitment of inflammatory cells.[54] In addition to its role in monocyte recruitment and foam cell formation, oxidized low density lipoprotein (LDL) stimulates production of several MMPs by cultured human endothelial cells and monocyte/macrophages.[55,56] Oxidized lipoproteins also modulate the cell surface expression of membrane-type metalloproteinases, potentially important for their ability to initiate a proteolytic cascade by activating other MMPs. In vitro exposure of human vascular smooth muscle cells (VSMCs) to oxidized LDL results in increased production of both mRNA and protein for MT1-MMP.[57] In cultured human macrophages, oxidized LDL stimulates increased production of mRNA and protein for MT3-MMP in a time- and dose-dependent manner.[58]

Mechanical forces

A correlation thought to be highly relevant for the development of atherosclerotic lesions and pathological vascular remodeling in general is related to the complex mechanical environment which characterizes arteries compared to other blood vessels. The entire arterial wall, and thus all the cell types within the wall, are normally exposed to longitudinal stretching as well as circumferential tensile stresses resulting from the pulsating high fluid (blood) pressure. In addition, blood flow exerts tangential shear forces upon the inner endothelial lining. Disease processes, such as hypertension or atherosclerotic lesion growth, or medical interventions, such as balloon angioplasty or intravascular stenting, induce additional changes in the mechanical environment of the arterial wall. In either case, changes in the mechanical forces acting on the vascular wall have the potential to alter the stability of atherosclerotic plaques by modulating the expression of matrix-degrading metalloproteinases.

Experimental models are necessary in order to confirm relations suggested by circumstantial evidence from human pathological specimens. We and others have used an in vivo mouse model in which carotid artery remodeling is induced by cessation of blood flow produced by ligation,[59] and found a time-dependent increase in both MMP-9 and MMP-2.[60] In larger animal models, arterial injury induced by balloon angioplasty provides a practical means to trigger vascular remodeling, precipitated by changes in both shear stress and wall stress. In a pig angioplasty model, ballooned iliac arteries in animals treated with the nonspecific MMP inhibitor batimastat remodeled so as to normalize shear stress, but not wall stress, in contrast to ballooned arteries in control animals, in which both shear stress and wall stress were normalized.[61] The complexity of these and other in vivo models complicates the task of drawing a direct inference between changes in mechanical forces and MMP regulation. Ex vivo studies using porcine carotid arteries maintained in an organ culture system, in which transmural pressure and shear stress could be independently controlled, demonstrated increased production of MMP-2 and MMP-9 in response to elevated pressure over a 24- to 48-hour time course.[62] In this system, changes in shear stress had no effect on gelatinase production. In these experiments, increases in MMP-2 and MMP-9 protein expression quantified by SDS–PAGE zymography correlated with enhanced gelatinolytic activity in tissue specimens as measured by in situ zymography, along with increased degradation of elastic lamellae.[62] In vitro studies of the response of human vascular smooth muscle cells to mechanical stretch corroborated these results by demonstrating that stationary uniaxial strain significantly increases both mRNA and protein levels of MMP-2 and MMP-9, while extended periods of cyclical strain at a physiologically relevant frequency of 1 Hz result in decreased secretion of MMP-2.[63] Furthermore, Yang and coworkers showed that in vitro mechanical deformation also activated monocyte-macrophages, inducing selective augmentation of MMPs, immediate early genes, and M-CSF receptors.[64] These observations may help to explain why MMP activity is generally elevated in the rupture-prone shoulder regions of plaques, since these areas also experience the highest levels of tensile stress.[65] In addition, these areas are characterized by complex patterns of shear stress,[66] which in vitro induces the expression of MMP-9 by endothelial cells.[67]

Cell–cell interactions

Direct cell–cell interactions involving several types of receptor–ligand pairs result in increased MMP production. Both monocytes and T-lymphocytes display contact-dependent regulation of MMP secretion. Several studies have implicated interactions between leukocyte integrins and adhesion receptors on endothelial cells in modulating gelatinase expression and secretion. Binding to VCAM-1, an adhesion molecule expressed by activated endothelial cells, stimulated increased expression of MMP-2 by T-lymphocytes.[68] In addition, Aoudjit and coworkers have reported that T-lymphocytes upregulate their production of MMP-9, as well as its inhibitor TIMP-1, upon binding to endothelial cells via ICAM-1.[69] Human monocytic cells also increased secretion of MMP-9 after binding to human endothelial cells, but the molecular mechanism responsible for this effect has not been established.[70] Interaction of CD40, a cell-surface receptor, with its ligand CD154 (previously known as CD40L) upregulates expression of MMP-1, MMP-3, MMP-8, and MMP-9 in monocytes/macrophages.[52,71,72] In addition, CD40-mediated signaling promotes MMP expression by vascular smooth muscle cells.[73]

Guilt by association – inflammatory cells, MMPs, and plaque vulnerability

Analysis of human lesions has revealed a correlation between inflammatory cell infiltration and plaque vulnerability to rupture and/or erosion.[18,74–77] Recent research has pointed to several possible routes by which inflammatory cells, with their arsenal of matrix-degrading enzymes, can promote destabilization of atherosclerotic plaques. The most important of these routes includes formation of an acellular necrotic core, direct degradation of the fibrous cap, outward remodeling of the vessel wall, and facilitation of intraplaque angiogenesis.

The lipid-rich core which is the classic hallmark of atheroma varies greatly in size among individual lesions. This core typically consists of extracellular lipids, including both free cholesterol and cholesterol esters, and cell debris. Studies of autopsy material obtained from patients with atherosclerosis have demonstrated a correlation between the size of the atheromatous core and the frequency of plaque rupture, with plaques having a lipid core occupying 40% or more of the cross-sectional area at greatest risk.[78] Longitudinal studies of lesion development in animal models suggest that the lipid core originates via apoptosis or necrosis of macrophage foam cells, with the consequent release of free lipids into the extracellular space. Apoptosis of inflammatory cells frequently occurs in human lesions as well.[21]

Thinning or loss of the fibrous cap has been correlated with plaque rupture in human autopsy specimens.[79,80] Proposed mechanisms for thinning of the fibrous cap include degradation of collagen I, the main structural protein of the cap, and loss of smooth muscle cells by apoptosis or necrosis. These mechanisms are closely intertwined, since collagen degradation becomes problematic only when collagen synthesis is reduced to the point where there is a net loss of extracellular matrix, a situation likely to occur following loss of smooth muscle cells. Furthermore, inflammatory cell infiltration and thinning of the fibrous cap often occur together in pathological specimens of culprit lesions, suggesting the possibility of a causal connection. Macrophage foam cells obtained from rabbit fatty streak lesions constitutively produce a range of MMPs in vitro, including MMP-1, MMP-3, and MMP-9,[20] indicating that foam cells have the potential to promote collagen degradation. Furthermore, in vitro studies have shown that human monocyte/macrophages cultured in the presence of atherosclerotic vessel segments can induce collagen breakdown in the fibrous caps of these lesions.[81] Clinical studies correlating the composition of atherectomy specimens to symptomatic evidence of plaque vulnerability such as unstable angina or myocardial infarction have shown that vulnerable lesions tend to have a larger component of inflammatory cells and a lower collagen content than do stable lesions.[75] Similarly, in a rabbit model of plaque rupture, hypercholesterolemic animals developed macrophage-rich plaques which had lower collagen content and decreased mechanical strength compared to lesions in normocholesterolemic controls.[82] Furthermore, enzymatically cleaved type I collagen occurs in association with macrophages expressing the interstitial collagenases MMP-1 and MMP-13 in human atheromatous lesions.[83] In the apoE knockout mouse model of atherosclerosis, deficiency in MMP-3 was associated with development of lesions containing fewer macrophages and more fibrillar collagen, suggesting that decreased expression of MMP-3 correlates with histological features which characterize stable plaques.[84] In addition, MMPs may potentially contribute to the death of vascular cells, which are anchorage dependent cells, by severing their contacts with the surrounding matrix. This specific type of cell death through the removal of potential integrin adhesion sites is known as "anoikis," from the Greek term suggesting "homelessness."[85]

Outward or compensatory remodeling, defined as an enduring increase in diameter of an adult blood vessel, frequently occurs in the context of atherosclerotic lesion development. In fact, examination of human coronary vessels by intravascular ultrasound (IVUS) has demonstrated that even relatively large atherosclerotic plaques may produce no stenosis detectable by angiography, owing to compensatory enlargement of the affected artery.[86] Although compensatory remodeling may confer some benefit in terms of maintaining normal lumen size despite plaque growth, this process has also been related to plaque vulnerability.[87] Outward remodeling necessitates coordinated matrix degradation and synthesis to maintain the normal cross-sectional structure of the vessel wall as its overall diameter expands. MMP activity has been implicated in matrix reorganization in several animal models of compensatory remodeling, both in response to flow loading[88] and in response to arterial lesion growth.[60,89,80] Of note, compensatory enlargement of arteries in experimental models correlated with the size of atherosclerotic lesions having a high macrophage foam cell content, but not with the size of lesions arising mainly from intimal smooth muscle cell hyperplasia.[89]

Atherosclerotic lesions, somewhat like tumors, need to develop their own blood supply as they expand in size, to compensate for decreased oxygen and nutrient transport from the vessel lumen. Some authors have referred to the network of new capillaries within a growing plaque as the "vasa plaquorum," by analogy to the vasa vasorum of the adventitia. Vulnerable plaques frequently show evidence of intraplaque angiogenesis, sometimes associated with hemorrhage of the microvessels.[91–93] In human autopsy studies, Burke and colleagues found that both acute plaque rupture and intraplaque hemorrhage were more frequent in men who had died during exertion than in those who died while at rest, but the authors did not demonstrate a direct causal association.[94] Inflammatory cells contribute to the growth of the vasa plaquorum by production of reactive oxygen species (ROS) such as hydrogen peroxide and superoxide anion, which can stimulate angiogenesis even in the absence of hypoxia.[95,96] Both vascular smooth muscle cells and macrophages respond to hydrogen peroxide exposure by secreting vascular endothelial

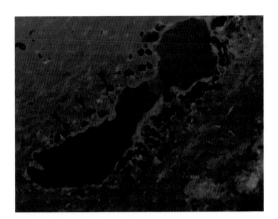

Figure 9.4 Red herring or red alert? In situ zymography reveals MMP activity around the periphery of microvessels within an atherosclerotic plaque. Mounting evidence suggests that intraplaque angiogenesis may destabilize lesions. In this example, dark areas (arrowheads) indicate regions where MMPs have degraded the fluorescently-labeled gelatin (red) which overlays the tissue specimen.

growth factor (VEGF), a potent mediator of angiogenesis.[97,98] MMPs contribute to plaque angiogenesis by at least two distinct mechanisms. They can release the active forms of several angiogenic cytokines, including VEGF, from membrane-bound or matrix-bound precursors, thus increasing their bioavailability and promoting angiogenic signaling in target cells.[99,100] In addition, the growth of angiogenic vessels requires invasion of the extracellular matrix, likely through the degrading action of MMPs. As shown in Figure 9.4, MMP activity was detected in intraplaque capillaries[101] and was correlated with intraplaque hemorrhage.[102] MMPs produced by inflammatory cells may contribute to the opening of channels through ischemic tissue, thereby facilitating capillary growth.[103]

Abdominal aortic aneurysm as a special case of arterial vulnerability

The etiology of abdominal aortic aneurysm (AAA) remains incompletely understood, but several pathological features of this condition suggest that it represents an extreme endpoint of vascular remodeling associated with atherosclerotic disease. AAA typically occurs in the context of pre-existing intimal atherosclerosis. Inflammatory cell infiltration of the media and medial elastin breakdown, two of the hallmarks of AAA, occur to a lesser extent in nonaneurysmal atherosclerotic arteries.

In mouse models of atherosclerosis, such as the apoE knockout mouse, microaneurysms characterized by focal breakdown of the elastic laminae commonly appear in association with advanced lesions.[104,105] However, the evidence available to date is insufficient to prove that microaneurysms in these models share a common mechanism of origin with human aortic aneurysms.

The scene of the crime – histological evidence for MMP involvement in atherosclerosis

MMP messenger RNA (mRNA) is present in atherosclerotic lesions

The mRNA of several MMPs, required as a template for their production by cells, was detected in human atherosclerotic plaques by means of in situ hybridization.[106–108] In situ hybridization has also revealed the presence of mRNA for elastolytic MMPs in specimens of AAA.[107,109] In vitro studies of the major cell types found in human atheroma, including smooth muscle cells, endothelial cells, and monocyte/macrophages, have yielded a substantial body of knowledge regarding factors which regulate expression of MMP mRNA. Nevertheless, expression of mRNA in itself points only to the potential for enzyme production and activation, and thus cannot provide information on the proximate causes of plaque destabilization. For this reason, our discussion will focus primarily on evidence for MMP proteins and enzymatic activity in the human atherosclerotic lesion.

Immunohistochemistry demonstrates that several classes of MMPs and their inhibitors are present in atherosclerotic lesions

Expression of a wide variety of MMPs in specimens of atherosclerotic human arteries was demonstrated using immunohistochemical methods, as summarized in Table 9.1. Thus, the MMPs implicated in human disease include molecules having substrate specificity for virtually every component of vascular ECM, including interstitial collagen, basement membrane collagens, elastin, fibronectin, laminin, and proteoglycans. Here we have a case where the means at hand are more than sufficient to dispatch the victim, but the challenge

Table 9.1 Summary of matrix metalloproteinase (MMP) involvement in human atherosclerosis and aneurysm development as demonstrated by immunohistochemical methods. (Several alternative names for each MMP are listed.)

MMP	Cell type	Location	Stimulus	Reference
MMP-1 Interstitial collagenase, collagenase 1	SMC	In vitro	TNF-α and IL-1	51
	Macrophage foam cell and SMC	Overexpression at shoulder region of carotid plaque	TNF-α and IL-1	101, 122
	SMC, endothelial cells	Carotid plaque		102
	Macrophage	In vitro		81
	Macrophage	Carotid plaque		83
	Endothelial cell	Umbilical vein, aorta	Ox-LDL	55
	Macrophage	Carotid artery	Mast cell degranulation	45
MMP-2 72-kDa gelatinase, gelatinase A	SMC	In vitro		51
	Macrophage foam cell, SMC	Throughout normal carotid artery		101, 149
		Atherosclerotic coronary artery with expansive remodeling		111
	Macrophage	In vitro		81
		Serum level in acute coronary syndrome		150
	SMC	Abdominal aortic aneurysm		116
	SMC	Abdominal aortic aneurysm		151
		Cerebral artery aneurysm		152
	SMC	In vitro	Thrombin	128
MMP-3 Stromelysin 1	SMC	In vitro	TNF-α and IL-1	51
	Macrophage foam cell, SMC	Overexpression at shoulder region of carotid plaque	? TNF-α and IL-1	101, 149
	Macrophage	Carotid artery	Mast cell degranulation	45
MMP-7 Matrilysin	Macrophage foam cell	Carotid plaque		153
MMP-8 Neutrophil collagenase	Macrophage, EC, SMC	Carotid plaque and in vitro	TNF-α, IL-1β, CD40L	52
MMP-9 92-kDa gelatinase, gelatinase B	SMC	In vitro	TNF-α and IL-1	51
	Macrophage foam cell, SMC	Overexpression at shoulder region of carotid plaque	TNF-α and IL-1	101, 149
	Macrophage, SMC	Coronary atherectomy specimens in the setting of unstable angina		154
		Unstable carotid plaques		155
	Macrophage	In vitro	Adhesion to collagen I	156
	Macrophage	In vitro	Ox-LDL	56
	Macrophage	In vitro	TNF-α, IL-1β	157
	Peripheral blood monocyte	In vitro	Ox-LDL	158
		Plasma level in acute coronary syndrome		150
	SMC	Abdominal aortic aneurysm		116
	Macrophages	Abdominal aortic aneurysm		117

Table 9.1 (Cont'd)

MMP	Cell type	Location	Stimulus	Reference
MMP-12	Macrophages	In vitro		159
Metalloelastase	Macrophages	Abdominal aortic aneurysm		109
MMP-13 Interstitial collagenase, Collagenase 3	Macrophages, endothelial cells, SMC	Carotid plaques and in vitro	TNF-α and IL-1β	83
MMP-14 Membrane	Macrophages, SMC	Coronary plaques	TNF-α, IL-1 β, ox-LDL	57
type 1-MMP	Endothelial cell	In vitro	TNF-α, IL-1α, IL-1β, ox-LDL	50
		Cerebral artery aneurysm		152
MMP-16 Membrane type 3-MMP	Macrophages, SMC	Coronary plaques Macrophages in vitro	TNF-α, M-CSF, ox-LDL	58

IL 'interleukin; LDL = low density lipoprotein; M-CSF = macrophage-colony stimulating factor; ox-LDL = oxidized low density lipoprotein; SMC = smooth muscle cell; TNF = tumor necrosis factor.

lies in determining which – if any – were actually responsible for rupture of the plaque.

Interstitial collagenases

The role of the interstitial collagenases, which include MMP-1 (collagenase-1), MMP-8 (neutrophil collagenase), and MMP-13, may be critically important to the stability of the atherosclerotic plaque, since these enzymes have the ability to degrade fibrillar collagen I, the major structural component of the fibrous cap. While these interstitial collagenases were not detectable in the normal arterial wall, all three were identified by immunohistochemistry within human atherosclerotic lesions.[52,83,101] MMP-1 protein was localized particularly in the vulnerable shoulder region where the lesion merges with the adjacent, uninvolved vessel wall, within the fibrous cap, and at the base of the lipid core.[101] All cell types in the atheroma, including smooth muscle cells, macrophage foam cells, endothelial cells, and infiltrating leukocytes, expressed MMP-1, suggesting their activation. MMP-8, originally described as a neutrophil-derived collagenase, also colocalizes with most of the major cell types (endothelial cells, smooth muscle cells,

and macrophages) in human atheroma.[52,110] Furthermore, immunostaining for MMP-1, MMP-8, and MMP-13 coincided with positive staining for cleaved collagen fragments but not for intact collagen I,[52,83] suggesting that matrix degradation actively takes place in regions of collagenase accumulation.

Gelatinases

Immunohistochemical methods have demonstrated the presence of both the gelatinases, MMP-2 and MMP-9, in specimens of atherosclerotic human arteries.[110,111] MMP-2 is also expressed constitutively by both smooth muscle cells and endothelial cells in vitro and in nondiseased human arteries, where it may play a role in normal turnover of cell basement membranes.[112] The gelatinases may affect plaque stability through at least two distinct routes. The ability of gelatinases to degrade basement membrane components such as collagen IV raises the possibility that these MMPs participate in atherosclerotic plaque erosion, characterized by frank loss of endothelium overlying the atheroma. Plaque erosion, like plaque rupture, is frequently associated with thrombus formation and its acute consequences.[113] Besides their ability to degrade short collagens, the gelatinases also possess elastolytic activity. Evidence from animal studies suggests that gelatinase activity is important in vascular remodeling in response to changes in blood flow and other stimuli, including mechanical injury produced by surgical intervention in a variety of experimental models.[60,88,114] In human atherosclerotic specimens, MMP-2 activity is higher in expansively remodeled segments than in constrictively remodeled segments of coronary arteries.[111] MMP-9, in particular, has been implicated in the destruction of elastic lamellae, which characterizes aneurysmal dilatation of advanced atherosclerosis.[115–117]

Elastases

Elastin, a major structural protein responsible for the elastic properties of the arterial wall, resists degradation by most proteases in its mature, insoluble form and has a very low turnover rate in normal, adult tissues. However, several MMPs have the unusual capacity to degrade mature elastin, including the gelatinases MMP-2 and MMP-9, macrophage metalloelastase (MMP-12), and matrilysin (MMP-7).[118–120] Since all of these elastolytic MMPs have been detected by immunohistochemistry in human atheroma (Table 9.1), the challenge lies in determining which ones are actually responsible for elastin degradation in this pathological condition. Elastases may also play a

significant role in the pathogenesis of AAA. Both mRNA and protein levels of MMP-12 are elevated in tissue specimens of AAA relative to normal arteries.[109] Immunoreactive MMP-12 has been detected in association with infiltrating macrophages in the degenerating media of human AAA specimens, where it also appears to be bound to residual elastin fragments.[109] As mentioned in the previous section, increased levels of MMP-9 are also present in human aneurysm specimens.[115–117]

Other MMPs

In specimens of human atherosclerotic plaques, areas of macrophage infiltration and plaque shoulder regions displayed increased expression of stromelysin (MMP-3), which is absent in normal human arteries.[101] Both smooth muscle cell- and macrophage-derived foam cells stained positively for MMP-3.

TIMPs – every MMP has its alibi

The task of relating MMP protein localization to areas at risk for matrix degradation is complicated by the ubiquitous presence of the endogenous metalloproteinase inhibitors, or TIMPs. Immunoreactive TIMP-1 and TIMP-2 are present throughout the vessel wall in both normal and atherosclerotic human arteries.[101] TIMP-3 occurs in human lesions as well.[121] As shown in Figure 9.5, TIMP

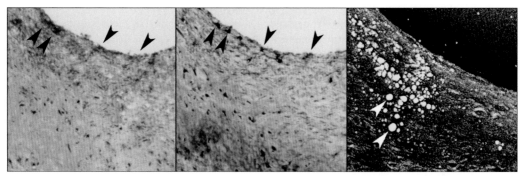

Figure 9.5 Caught in the act! Under normal circumstances, MMP activity in the vascular wall is kept in check by the presence of endogenous inhibitors, the TIMPs. Immunohistochemistry demonstrates that TIMPs frequently colocalize with MMPs in the atherosclerotic vessel as well (black arrowheads), but it cannot tell us whether their presence is sufficient to counteract increased MMP levels. Immunoperoxidase staining for MMP-1 (left panel) and TIMP-1 (center panel) in serial sections of human arterectomy specimen with diaminobenzidine detection (brown areas). In situ zymography (right panel) clearly demonstrates regions where the balance has tipped in favor of active matrix degradation, revealed by areas of substrate lysis in the plaque shoulder (round white regions at arrowheads). Since the substrate in this instance is a gelatin-based film emulsion, the guilty party is likely to be a gelatinase – but is it MMP-2 or MMP-9?

immunoreactivity frequently colocalizes with MMP immunoreactivity in atherosclerotic lesions, confounding the issue of whether MMPs present within the plaque are free to cause trouble or effectively kept in check by locally produced inhibitors. Immunohistochemical staining does not provide quantitative information on the actual concentration ratio of MMPs to TIMPs in a given specimen; therefore, this approach cannot tell us whether the balance of power is shifted in favor of inhibition or activation of matrix degradation. Direct evidence of MMP activity must come from alternative approaches, such in situ zymography,[122] a method that reveals enzymatic activity within the tissue, which will be described below.

Studies in genetically deficient mouse models of atherosclerosis have provided some evidence for the role of TIMPs in vivo during lesion development. Although the added deficiency in TIMP-1 did seem to affect aortic lesion development or composition of lesions per se in the apoE knockout mouse model,[105] these atherosclerotic lesions developed more aortic medial ruptures (or pseudo-microaneurysms), suggesting that TIMP-1 may limit medial elastin degradation in the context of atherosclerosis.

In situ zymography provides convincing evidence of MMP activity in atherosclerotic lesions

While immunohistochemistry provides an abundance of specific information regarding localization and expression of potentially destructive metalloproteases in the vulnerable plaque, the availability of an enzyme does not necessarily translate into enzymatic activity and consequently does not imply matrix degradation. The multiple mechanisms by which MMP activity is tightly regulated, such as inhibition by TIMPs, ensure that extracellular matrix (ECM) degradation does not occur in normal vessels or at best is limited in scope. Alternative methods, such as fluorescent substrate assays and in situ zymography, are required to differentiate enzyme activity from total protein levels.

Specifically designed substrates, tailored to mimic the preferred amino acid recognition sequence of the substrate for individual MMPs, are useful in assaying enzyme activity in tissue homogenates and in samples of culture media or body fluids.

Enzymatic cleavage of such substrates, which are quenched unless digested, by the specialized MMP releases a bound fluorophore into the medium, resulting in an increase in fluorescence intensity proportional to the enzyme activity. Since these fluorescently labeled substrates are small, readily diffusible molecules, they are not useful for spatial localization of enzymatic activity in intact tissue specimens.

The technique of in situ zymography[122] has provided the most convincing evidence to date of localized MMP enzymatic activity in vulnerable regions of human atherosclerotic plaques.[45,101] Currently there are several variations of this technique, but all of them involve direct contact between the unfixed tissue specimen and a thin film containing an appropriate substrate such as gelatin or casein. Degradation of the substrate by metalloproteinases in the sample produces zones of lysis which, depending on the substrates employed, appear as areas which are either brighter or darker than the surrounding tissue. Quenched substrates which become fluorescent only when degraded yield bright areas in zones of enzymatic activity, while other types of labeled substrates produce dark zones when the label is lost through enzymatic degradation. Figure 9.5 demonstrates the localization of gelatinolytic activity in the shoulder region of a human lesion using in situ zymography. While very valuable in confirming the presence of localized enzymatic activity, the choice of substrates currently available for in situ zymography does allow the distinction between MMPs with similar substrate affinities.

Who fired the fatal shot? Mechanisms of MMP activation in the environment of atherosclerotic lesions

As described in the preceding section, immunohistochemical methods demonstrate that a wide range of ECM-degrading MMPs are present in human atherosclerotic lesions, and in situ zymography tells us that at least some of these enzymes are actively degrading the matrix. As mentioned earlier, MMPs exert this biological function only after the activation of secreted MMP zymogens. Thus, in terms of preventing the consequences of plaque destabilization, an effective strategy would be to determine and prevent activation of MMPs within the plaque. Much of the data regarding potential mechanisms of MMP activation has been derived either from in vitro studies or from animal models of disease. There is a notable shortage of direct evidence for mechanisms of activation in vivo in human disease, although immunohistochemical methods have suggested several potential players in human plaque specimens.

MT-MMPs

The MT-MMPs, which unlike most MMPs are expressed on the cell surface in the mature, active form rather than as inactive zymogens, have the capacity to activate other MMPs.[123,124] The best-studied example involves activation of pro-MMP-2 by MT1-MMP, which appears to occur through formation of a ternary cell-surface complex with TIMP-2.[125] Pericellular activation of MMP zymogens by MT-MMPs provides a mechanism by which MMP activity can be precisely localized and controlled, which may be particularly important in vectorial processes such as cell migration. Two members of the MT-MMP subfamily, MT1-MMP and MT3-MMP, have been detected by immunohistochemistry in specimens of atherosclerotic human vessels as well as in normal human arteries.[50,58] MT1-MMP, together with its potential substrate MMP-2, colocalized with smooth muscle cells (SMCs) and macrophages in human coronary atherosclerotic lesions.[50]

Plasmin

Immunohistochemical studies have demonstrated increased levels of fibrinolytic activators, including urokinase-type plasminogen activator (u-PA) and tissue-type plasminogen activator (t-PA), in human atherosclerotic plaques, suggesting that plasmin-mediated proteolysis may play a role in lesion development.[126] Expression of u-PA is particularly strong in plaque macrophages at the intimal–medial boundary.[126] Evidence for plasmin-mediated activation of MMPs comes both from in vitro experiments and from in vivo studies in genetically engineered mice having deficiencies in the fibrinolytic system.[104,127] ApoE knockout mice deficient in u-PA (but not those deficient in t-PA) were protected from medial elastin

degradation and aneurysmal dilatation of the vessel wall.[104] Since plasmin itself does not degrade elastin or collagen, the protective effect of plasmin deficiency was attributed to a reduced activation of matrix-degrading MMPs. In vitro, macrophages from wild-type or t-PA-deficient mice, but not those from u-PA-deficient mice, can activate the zymogens of MMP-3, MMP-9, MMP-12, and MMP-13 in a plasminogen-dependent manner.[104]

Thrombin

In atherosclerotic plaques which have been compromised either by rupture of the fibrous cap or by intraplaque hemorrhage, MMPs produced by vascular cells are likely to come into contact with thrombin. In vitro studies have shown that thrombin, in contrast to plasmin and several other proteases, can activate pro-MMP-2 in a cell-independent manner.[128] Thrombin-mediated activation of MMP-2 may provide a mechanism by which intraplaque hemorrhage could contribute to plaque destabilization and rupture.

Other proteases

As mentioned earlier, mast cells produce the neutral proteases tryptase and chymase, which are released from the cells in the process of degranulation. In vitro, mast cell proteases have the ability to activate the zymogens of MMP-1 and MMP-3.[129] Johnson and colleagues showed that mast cells in human atherectomy specimens colocalized with immunoreactive MMP-1 and MMP-3 proteins. Furthermore, ex vivo treatment of these specimens with a pharmacological agent that induces mast cell degranulation resulted in a 1.5-fold increase in total MMP activity measured using a fluorogenic substrate, which could be partially blocked by treatment with tryptase or chymase inhibitors.[45]

Reactive oxygen species (ROS)

Interestingly, due to their chemical properties, ROS provide a protease-independent mechanism for activation of MMPs. ROS are generated within the environment of atheroma,[130] and while the relative contributions of ROS generated by resident inflammatory cells or by activated vascular cells remain to be determined, lesions with a high

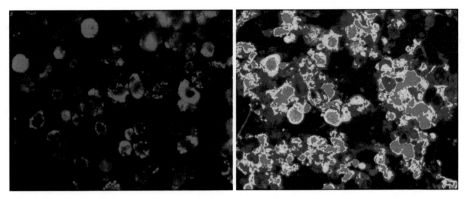

Figure 9.6 Armed and dangerous. Macrophages in the atherosclerotic plaque accumulate lipids and develop into foam cells (left panel, Nile Red staining of macrophage foam cells from experimental rabbit atheroma). These macrophage-derived foam cells constitutively express a range of MMPs, together with the reactive oxygen species capable of activating them. The localized production of both MMPs and their activators puts macrophage-rich areas of an atherosclerotic plaque at particular risk. (Right panel: confocal microscopy of macrophage foam cells stained with dihydroethidium to demonstrate production of hydrogen peroxide, shown in red in this pseudocolored image).

inflammatory content are more likely to be under increased oxidative stress. Inflammatory cells can produce a full spectrum of ROS, including hydrogen peroxide and superoxide anion. Macrophage-derived foam cells isolated from rabbit atheroma continue to generate superoxide, nitric oxide, and hydrogen peroxide in culture without exogenous stimulation[16] (Figure 9.6). In vitro studies have demonstrated that certain ROS can activate MMP zymogens at physiologically relevant concentrations. At concentrations below 10 μmol, hydrogen peroxide activated the latent form of MMP-2, but nitric oxide had no effect.[16] However, peroxynitrite ion, a reaction product of nitric oxide and superoxide anion, also demonstrated the ability to activate pro-MMP-2 in vitro. Generation of ROS provides a route by which inflammatory cells may autoactivate their own MMP zymogens as well as those secreted by surrounding cells. Treatment of explanted lesions of rabbit atheroma with the antioxidant N-acetyl-cysteine (NAC) abolished gelatinase enzymatic activity and, surprisingly, reduced MMP-9 protein expression as well.[131] Deficiencies in ROS production were shown to inhibit the development of lesions in mouse models of atherosclerosis. ApoE knockout mice deficient in the p47 subunit of the NADPH oxidase, an enzymatic source of superoxide anion, displayed reduced lesion formation compared to control apoE knockout mice.[132]

Crime prevention – does inhibition of MMPs offer a means to stabilize the vulnerable plaque?

Given the evidence that MMPs are major players in destabilization of the vulnerable atherosclerotic plaque, we now must ask whether the corollary also holds true – will inhibition of MMPs provide a route to reduce plaque vulnerability and its potentially devastating clinical consequences? Two major obstacles stand in the way of finding an answer to this question: first, the absence of good animal models of plaque rupture and aneurysm formation; and second, the lack of specific pharmacological inhibitors targeting individual MMPs. Despite these obstacles, the evidence which has begun to accumulate suggests that MMP inhibition may have beneficial results in some situations.

Animal models which accurately reflect the natural history and clinical consequences of human plaque rupture or erosion remain virtually nonexistent, despite strenuous efforts to develop them.[133] Therefore, studies on the effects of MMP deficiency or inhibition in animal models of atherosclerosis have to date focused primarily on alterations in lesion size, morphology, or composition which might be indicative of plaque "stabilization," such as decreased inflammatory cell infiltration or increased collagen content. Treatment with the currently available broad-spectrum MMP inhibitors has had mixed results in animal models of atherosclerosis.[134–136] For instance, the MMP inhibitor marimastat inhibited constrictive arterial remodeling in favor of both neutral and expansive remodeling in an experimental pig model of balloon angioplasty.[135] Marimastat was also found to inhibit neointimal thickening in cultured human saphenous veins in a concentration-dependent manner.[136] By contrast, the broad-spectrum MMP inhibitor CGS 27023A had no effect on the extent of aortic atherosclerosis in the LDL receptor knockout mouse model, and it delayed but did not prevent intimal lesion development in a rat model of carotid injury.[134] The specific inhibition of MMP-9 through targeted genetic deficiency in murine models was found to suppress development of experimental abdominal aortic aneurysms,[137] reduce intimal hyperplasia, and diminish constrictive remodeling of carotid arteries.[90]

Recent research has shown that some common pharmacological treatments for cardiovascular disease, while not directly aimed at inhibition of MMPs, may produce clinical benefits partially through this mechanism. Antioxidant therapy, while not conclusively proven as a treatment for atherosclerosis in large-scale clinical trials, most likely due to use of inappropriate antioxidants, dosage, or patient selection,[138–141] has the potential to reduce MMP activity in the vascular wall by scavenging of ROS. Lipid lowering therapy may improve plaque stability by a number of mechanisms, including reduction in MMP activity. In a rabbit model of atherosclerosis, Aikawa and colleagues found that 8–16 months of dietary lipid lowering altered the composition of established plaques, resulting in diminished macrophage content, increased aortic collagen, and decreased levels of immunoreactive MMP-1 in comparison to lesions of animals which remained on a high-fat diet.[142] Dietary lipid lowering also reduced matrix-degrading proteolytic activity attributable to MMP-2, MMP-3, and MMP-9 in aortic specimens. Treatment of hypercholesterolemic rabbits with avasimibe, an acyl-CoA:cholesterol O-acyltransferase (ACAT) inhibitor, similarly decreased monocyte-macrophage content and reduced the macrophage-to-lesion ratio, which correlated with a decrease in the activity of MMP-9 and to a lesser extent of MMP-1 and MMP-3.[143]

Statins, a class of hydroxymethyl-glutaryl coenzyme A (HMG-CoA) inhibitors frequently prescribed to lower plasma cholesterol, demonstrate a range of beneficial effects not directly related to lipid lowering.[144,145] Pleiotropic effects of statins observed in vitro include inhibition of MMP expression and/or secretion.[146,147] Most interestingly, patients treated with a statin for 3 months prior to carotid endarterectomy demonstrated reduced levels of immunoreactive MMP-2 in the specimen recovered during surgery, together with increased levels of immunoreactive TIMP-1 and greater collagen content.[148]

Conclusion

All the evidence available from examination of pathological specimens of normal and atherosclerotic arteries, experimental atherosclerotic lesions, and in vitro experiments with vascular and inflammatory cells points to the contribution of MMPs, particularly of macrophage-derived MMPs, in the progression and complications of atherosclerotic plaques. However, the lack of live witnesses does not allow us to convict macrophages and their MMPs beyond any reasonable doubt, and thus leaves us no choice but to continue to investigate this case while the suspects are still at large.

Acknowledgments

ZSG is the recipient of an American Heart Association Established Investigator Award 0040087N. SML is supported by a National Research Service Postdoctoral Award 1 F32 HL68449. Research in Dr Galis' laboratory was partially funded through grants from the National Institutes of Health Heart and Lung Blood Institute RO1 64689 and RO1 71061. We thank Dr Renu Virmani of the Armed Forces Institute of Pathology for providing the photomicrograph shown in Figure 9.1.

References

1. Ross R. Atherosclerosis – an inflammatory disease. N Engl J Med 1999;340:115–26.
2. Gerrity RG. The role of the monocyte in atherogenesis: I. Transition of blood-borne monocytes into foam cells in fatty lesions. Am J Pathol 1981;103:181–90.

3. Faggiotto A, Ross R, Harker L. Studies of hypercholesterolemia in the nonhuman primate. I. Changes that lead to fatty streak formation. Arteriosclerosis 1984;4: 323–40.

4. Stary HC. Changes in components and structure of atherosclerotic lesions developing from childhood to middle age in coronary arteries. Basic Res Cardiol 1994;89:17–32.

5. Yla-Herttuala S, Lipton BA, Rosenfeld ME, et al. Expression of monocyte chemoattractant protein 1 in macrophage-rich areas of human and rabbit atherosclerotic lesions. Proc Natl Acad Sci USA 1991;88: 5252–6.

6. Li H, Cybulsky MI, Gimbrone Jr, MA, Libby P. An atherogenic diet rapidly induces VCAM-1, a cytokine regulatable mononuclear leukocyte adhesion molecule, in rabbit endothelium. Arterioscler Thromb 1993;3: 197–204.

7. Walpola PL, Gotlieb AI, Cybulsky MI, Langille BL. Expression of ICAM-1 and VCAM-1 and monocyte adherence in arteries exposed to altered shear stress. Arterioscler Thromb Vasc Biol 1995;15:2–10.

8. Cybulsky MI, Lichtman AH, Hajra L, Iiyama K. Leukocyte adhesion molecules in atherogenesis. Clin Chim Acta 1999;286:207–18.

9. Patel SS, Thiagarajan R, Willerson JT, Yeh ET. Inhibition of alpha4 integrin and ICAM-1 markedly attenuate macrophage homing to atherosclerotic plaques in ApoE-deficient mice. Circulation 1998;97:75–81.

10. Cybulsky MI, Gimbrone Jr MA. Endothelial expression of a mononuclear leukocyte adhesion molecule during atherogenesis. Science 1991;251:788–91.

11. Gu L, Okada Y, Clinton SK, Gerard C, Sukhova GK, Libby P, Rollins BJ. Absence of monocyte chemoattractant protein-1 reduces atherosclerosis in low density lipoprotein receptor-deficient mice. Mol Cell 1998;2:275–81.

12. Guo J, Van Eck M, Twisk J, Maeda N, Benson GM, Groot PH, Van Berkel TJ. Transplantation of monocyte CC-chemokine receptor 2-deficient bone marrow into ApoE3–Leiden mice inhibits atherogenesis. Arterioscler Thromb Vasc Biol 2003;23:447–53.

13. Boring L, Gosling J, Cleary M, Charo IF. Decreased lesion formation in CCR2-/- mice reveals a role for chemokines in the initiation of atherosclerosis. Nature 1998;394:894–7.

14. Smith JD, Trogan E, Ginsberg M, Grigaux C, Tian J, Miyata M. Decreased atherosclerosis in mice deficient in both macrophage colony-stimulating factor (op) and apolipoprotein E. Proc Natl Acad Sci USA 1995; 92:8264–8.

15. Barath P, Fishbein MC, Cao J, Berenson J, Helfant RH, Forrester JS. Detection and localization of tumor necrosis factor in human atheroma. Am J Cardiol 1990;65:297–302.

16. Rajagopalan S, Meng XP, Ramasamy S, Harrison DG, Galis ZS. Reactive oxygen species produced by macrophage-derived foam cells regulate the activity of vascular matrix metalloproteinases in vitro. Implications for atherosclerotic plaque stability. J Clin Invest 1996;98:2572–9.

17. Cipollone F, Prontera C, Pini B, et al. Overexpression of functionally coupled cyclooxygenase-2 and prostaglandin E synthase in symptomatic atherosclerotic plaques as a basis of prostaglandin E(2)-dependent plaque instability. Circulation 2001;104:921–7.

18. van der Wal AC, Becker AE, van der Loos CM, Das PK. Site of intimal rupture or erosion of thrombosed coronary atherosclerotic plaques is characterized by an inflammatory process irrespective of the dominant plaque morphology. Circulation 1994;89:36–44.

19. Geng YJ, Holm J, Nygren S, Bruzelius M, Stemme S, Hansson GK. Expression of the macrophage scavenger receptor in atheroma. Relationship to immune activation and the T-cell cytokine interferon-gamma. Arterioscler Thromb Vasc Biol 1995;15:1995–2002.

20. Galis ZS, Sukhova GK, Kranzhöfer R, Clark S, Libby P. Macrophage foam cells from experimental atheroma constitutively produce matrix-degrading proteinases. Proc Natl Acad Sci USA 1995;92:402–6.

21. Bjorkerud S, Bjorkerud B. Apoptosis is abundant in human atherosclerotic lesions, especially in inflammatory cells (macrophages and T-cells), may contribute to the accumulation of gruel and plaque instability. Am J Pathol 1996;149:367–80.

22. Hansson GK. Cell-mediated immunity in atherosclerosis. Curr Opin Lipidol 1997;8:301–11.

23. Hansson GK, Libby P, Schonbeck U, Yan ZQ. Innate and adaptive immunity in the pathogenesis of atherosclerosis. Circ Res 2002;91:281–91.

24. Hansson GK, Jonasson L, Lojsthed B, Stemme S, Kocher O, Gabbiani G. Localization of T-lymphocytes and macrophages in fibrous and complicated human atherosclerotic plaques. Atherosclerosis 1988;72: 135–41.

25. Emeson EE, Robertson AL Jr. T-lymphocytes in aortic and coronary intimas. Their potential role in atherogenesis. Am J Pathol 1988;130:369–76.

26. Xu QB, Oberhuber G, Gruschwitz M, Wick G. Immunology of atherosclerosis: cellular composition and major histocompatibility complex class II antigen expression in aortic intima, fatty streaks, atherosclerotic plaques in young and aged human specimens. Clin Immunol Immunopathol 1990;56:344–59.

27. Stemme S, Rymo L, Hansson GK. Polyclonal origin of T-lymphocytes in human atherosclerotic plaques. Lab Invest 1991;65:654–60.

28. Paulsson G, Zhou X, Tornquist E, Hansson GK. Oligoclonal T-cell expansions in atherosclerotic lesions of apolipoprotein E-deficient mice. Arterioscler Thromb Vasc Biol 2000;20:10–17.

29. Kuo CC, Gown AM, Benditt EP, Grayston JT. Detection of *Chlamydia pneumoniae* in aortic lesions of atherosclerosis by immunocytochemical stain. Arterioscler Thromb 1993;13:1501–4.

30. Xu Q, Willeit J, Marosi M, et al. Association of serum antibodies to heat-shock protein 65 with carotid atherosclerosis. Lancet 1993;341:255–9.

31. Yla-Herttuala S, Palinski W, Butler SW, Picard S, Steinberg D, Witztum JL. Rabbit and human athero-sclerotic lesions contain IgG that recognizes epitopes of oxidized LDL. Arterioscler Thromb 1994;14:32–40.

32. Mach F, Schonbeck U, Sukhova GK, Bourcier T, Bonnefoy JY, Pober JS, Libby P. Functional CD40 ligand is expressed on human vascular endothelial cells, smooth muscle cells, macrophages: implications for CD40–CD40 ligand signaling in atherosclerosis. Proc Natl Acad Sci USA 1997;94:1931–6.

33. Hansson GK. Immune mechanisms in atherosclerosis. Arterioscler Thromb Vasc Biol 2001;21:1876–90.

34. Zhou X, Nicoletti A, Elhage R, Hansson GK. Trans-fer of CD4(+) T-cells aggravates atherosclerosis in immunodeficient apolipoprotein E knockout mice. Circulation 2000;102:2919–22.

35. Parums DV, Chadwick DR, Mitchinson MJ. The local-isation of immunoglobulin in chronic periaortitis. Atherosclerosis 1986;61:117–23.

36. Zhou X, Hansson GK. Detection of B-cells and proinflammatory cytokines in atherosclerotic plaques of hypercholesterolaemic apolipoprotein E knockout mice. Scand J Immunol 1999;50:25–30.

37. Hansson GK. The B-cell: a good guy in vascular disease? Arterioscler Thromb Vasc Biol 2002;22:523–4.

38. Caligiuri G, Nicoletti A, Poirier B, Hansson GK. Protective immunity against atherosclerosis carried by B-cells of hypercholesterolemic mice. J Clin Invest 2002;109:745–53.

39. Dansky HM, Charlton SA, Harper MM, Smith JD. T and B-lymphocytes play a minor role in atherosclerotic plaque formation in the apolipoprotein E-deficient mouse. Proc Natl Acad Sci USA 1997;94:4642–6.

40. Liu MC, Proud D, Lichtenstein LM, et al. Human lung macrophage-derived histamine-releasing activity is due to IgE-dependent factors. J Immunol 1986;136:2588–95.

41. Sedgwick JD, Holt PG, Turner KJ. Production of a histamine-releasing lymphokine by antigen- or mitogen-stimulated human peripheral T-cells. Clin Exp Immunol 1981;45:409–18.

42. Wize J, Wojtecka-Lukasik E, Maslinski S. Collagen-derived peptides release mast cell histamine. Agents Actions 1986;18:262–5.

43. Kaartinen M, Penttila A, Kovanen PT. Accumulation of activated mast cells in the shoulder region of human coronary atheroma, the predilection site of atherom-atous rupture. Circulation 1994;90:1669–78.

44. Kovanen PT, Kaartinen M, Paavonen T. Infiltrates of activated mast cells at the site of coronary atherom-atous erosion or rupture in myocardial infarction. Circulation 1995;92:1084–8.

45. Johnson JL, Jackson CL, Angelini GD, George SJ. Activation of matrix-degrading metalloproteinases by mast cell proteases in atherosclerotic plaques. Arterioscler Thromb Vasc Biol 1998;18:1707–15.

46. Vu TH, Werb Z. Gelatinase B: structure, regulation, function. In Parks WC, Mecham RP, eds. Matrix metalloproteinases. San Diego: Academic Press, 1998:115–49.

47. Gomis-Ruth FX, Maskos K, Betz M, et al. Mechanism of inhibition of the human matrix metalloproteinase stromelysin-1 by TIMP-1. Nature 1997;389:77–81.

48. Brew K, Dinakarpandian D, Nagase H. Tissue inhibitors of metalloproteinases: evolution, structure and func-tion. Biochim Biophys Acta 2000;1477:267–83.

49. Stetler-Stevenson WG, Krutzsch HC, Liotta LA. Tissue inhibitor of metalloproteinase (TIMP-2). A new mem-ber of the metalloproteinase inhibitor family. J Biol Chem 1989;264:17374–8.

50. Rajavashisth TB, Liao JK, Galis ZS, et al. Inflammatory cytokines and oxidized low density lipoproteins increase endothelial cell expression of membrane type 1-matrix metalloproteinase. J Biol Chem 1999;274:11924–9.

51. Galis ZS, Muszynski M, Sukhova GK, et al. Cytokine-stimulated human vascular smooth muscle cells syn-thesize a complement of enzymes required for extracellular matrix digestion. Circ Res 1994;75:181–9.

52. Herman MP, Sukhova GK, Libby P, et al. Expression of neutrophil collagenase (matrix metalloproteinase-8) in human atheroma: a novel collagenolytic pathway suggested by transcriptional profiling. Circulation 2001;104:1899–904.

53. Corcoran ML, Stetler-Stevenson WG, DeWitt DL, Wahl LM. Effect of cholera toxin and pertussis toxin on prostaglandin H synthase-2, prostaglandin E2, matrix metalloproteinase production by human monocytes. Arch Biochem Biophys 1994;310:481–8.

54. Berliner JA, Heinecke JW. The role of oxidized lipo-proteins in atherogenesis. Free Radical Biol Med 1996;20:707–27.

55. Huang Y, Mironova M, Lopes-Virella MF. Oxidized LDL stimulates matrix metalloproteinase-1 expression in human vascular endothelial cells. Arterioscler Thromb Vasc Biol 1999;19:2640–7.

56. Xu XP, Meisel SR, Ong JM, et al. Oxidized low-density lipoprotein regulates matrix metalloproteinase-9 and its tissue inhibitor in human monocyte-derived macrophages. Circulation 1999;99:993–8.

57. Rajavashisth TB, Xu X-P, Jovinge S, et al. Membrane type 1 matrix metalloproteinase expression in human atherosclerotic plaques: evidence for activation by proinflammatory mediators. Circulation 1999;99: 3103–9.

58. Uzui H, Harpf A, Liu M, et al. Increased expression of membrane type 3-matrix metalloproteinase in human atherosclerotic plaque: role of activated macrophages and inflammatory cytokines. Circulation 2002;106: 3024–30.

59. Kumar A, Lindner V. Remodeling with neointima formation in the mouse carotid artery after cessation of blood flow. Arterioscler Thromb Vasc Biol 1997;17: 2238–44.

60. Godin D, Ivan E, Johnson C, Magid R, Galis ZS. Remodeling of carotid artery is associated with increased expression of matrix metalloproteinases in mouse blood flow cessation model. Circulation 2000;102:2861–6.

61. Wentzel JJ, Kloet J, Hyiswara I, et al. Shear-stress and wall-stress regulation of vascular remodeling after balloon angioplasty: effect of matrix metalloproteinase inhibition. Circulation 2001;104:91–6.

62. Chesler N, Ku D, Galis ZS. Transmural pressure induces matrix-degrading activity in porcine arteries ex vivo. Am J Physiol 1999;277:H2002–9.

63. Asanuma K, Magid R, Johnson C, Nerem RM, Galis ZS. Uniaxial strain upregulates matrix-degrading enzymes produced by human vascular smooth muscle cells. Am J Physiol Heart Circ Physiol 2003;284:H1778–84.

64. Yang JH, Sakamoto H, Xu EC, Lee RT. Biomechanical regulation of human monocyte/macrophage molecular function. Am J Pathol 2000;156:1797–804.

65. Lee RT, Schoen FJ, Loree HM, Lark MW, Libby P. Circumferential stress and matrix metalloproteinase 1 in human coronary atherosclerosis. Implications for plaque rupture. Arterioscler Thromb Vasc Biol 1996; 16:1070–3.

66. Davies PF. Spatial hemodynamics, the endothelium, focal atherogenesis: a cell cycle link? [letter; comment]. Circ Res 2000;86:114–16.

67. Magid R, Murphy TJ, Galis ZS. Expression of matrix metalloproteinase-9 in endothelial cells is differentially regulated by shear stress: role of c-Myc. J Biol Chem 2003; [on-line ahead of print].

68. Romanic AM, Madri JA. The induction of 72-kD gelatinase in T-cells upon adhesion to endothelial cells is VCAM-1 dependent. J Cell Biol 1994;125:1165–78.

69. Aoudjit F, Potworowski EF, St-Pierre Y. Bi-directional induction of matrix metalloproteinase-9 and tissue inhibitor of matrix metalloproteinase-1 during T lymphoma/endothelial cell contact: implication of ICAM-1. J Immunol 1998;160:2967–73.

70. Amorino GP, Hoover RL. Interactions of monocytic cells with human endothelial cells stimulate monocytic metalloproteinase production. Am J Pathol 1998;152: 199–207.

71. Mach F, Schonbeck U, Bonnefoy JY, Pober JS, Libby P. Activation of monocyte/macrophage functions related to acute atheroma complication by ligation of CD40: induction of collagenase, stromelysin, tissue factor. Circulation 1997;96:396–9.

72. Malik N, Greenfield BW, Wahl AF, Kiener PA. Activation of human monocytes through CD40 induces matrix metalloproteinases. J Immunol 1996;156: 3952–60.

73. Schonbeck U, Mach F, Sukhova GK, Murphy C, Bonnefoy JY, Fabunmi RP, Libby P. Regulation of matrix metalloproteinase expression in human vascular smooth muscle cells by T-lymphocytes: a role for CD40 signaling in plaque rupture? Circ Res 1997;81: 448–54.

74. Lendon CL, Davies MJ, Born GV, Richardson PD. Atherosclerotic plaque caps are locally weakened when macrophages density is increased. Atherosclerosis 1991;87:87–90.

75. Moreno P, Falk E, Palacios I, Newell J, Fuster V, Fallon J. Macrophage infiltration in acute coronary syndromes. Implications for plaque rupture. Circulation 1994;90:775–8.

76. Boyle JJ. Association of coronary plaque rupture and atherosclerotic inflammation. J Pathol 1997;181: 93–9.

77. Buja LM, Willerson JT. Role of inflammation in coronary plaque disruption. Circulation 1994;89:503–5.

78. Davies MJ, Richardson PD, Woolf N, Katz DR, Mann J. Risk of thrombosis in human atherosclerotic plaques: role of extracellular lipid, macrophage, smooth muscle cell content. Br Heart J 1993;69:377–81.

79. Burke A, Farb A, Malcom G, Liang YH, Smialek J, Virmani R. Coronary risk factors and plaque morphology in men with coronary disease who died suddenly. N Engl J Med 1997;336:1276–82.

80. Virmani R, Kolodgie FD, Burke AP, Farb A, Schwartz SM. Lessons from sudden coronary death: a comprehensive morphological classification scheme for atherosclerotic lesions. Arterioscl Thromb Vasc Biol 2000;20:1262–75.

81. Shah PK, Falk E, Badimon JJ, et al. Human monocyte-derived macrophages induce collagen breakdown in fibrous caps of atherosclerotic plaques. Potential role of matrix-degrading metalloproteinases and implications for plaque rupture. Circulation 1995;92:1565–9.

82. Rekhter MD, Hicks GW, Brammer DW, et al. Hypercholesterolemia causes mechanical weakening of rabbit atheroma: local collagen loss as a prerequisite of plaque rupture. Circ Res 2000;86:101–8.

83. Sukhova GK, Schonbeck U, Rabkin E, Schoen FJ, Poole AR, Billinghurst RC, Libby P. Evidence for increased collagenolysis by interstitial collagenases-1 and -3 in vulnerable human atheromatous plaques. Circulation 1999;99:2503–9.

84. Silence J, Lupu F, Collen D, Lijnen HR. Persistence of atherosclerotic plaque but reduced aneurysm formation in mice with stromelysin-1 (MMP-3) gene inactivation. Arterioscler Thromb Vasc Biol 2001;21:1440–5.

85. Frisch SM, Ruoslahti E. Integrins and anoikis. Curr Opin Cell Biol 1997;9:701–6.

86. Schoenhagen P, Ziada KM, Vince DG, Nissen SE, Tuzcu EM. Arterial remodeling and coronary artery disease: the concept of "dilated" versus "obstructive" coronary atherosclerosis. J Am Coll Cardiol 2001;38: 297–306.

87. Schoenhagen P, Ziada KM, Kapadia SR, Crowe TD, Nissen SE, Tuzcu EM. Extent and direction of arterial remodeling in stable versus unstable coronary syndromes: an intravascular ultrasound study. Circulation 2000;101:598–603.

88. Tronc F, Mallat Z, Lehoux S, Wassef M, Esposito B, Tedgui A. Role of matrix metalloproteinases in blood flow-induced arterial enlargement: interaction with NO. Arterioscler Thromb Vasc Biol 2000;20:E120–6.

89. Ivan E, Khatri JJ, Johnson C, et al. Expansive arterial remodeling is associated with increased neointimal macrophage foam cell content: the murine model of macrophage-rich carotid artery lesions. Circulation 2002;105:2686–91.

90. Galis ZS, Johnson C, Godin D, Magid R, Shipley JM, Senior RM, Ivan E. Targeted disruption of the matrix metalloproteinase-9 gene impairs smooth muscle cell migration and geometrical arterial remodeling. Circ Res 2002;91:852–9.

91. Barger AC, Beeuwkes R, 3rd. Rupture of coronary vasa vasorum as a trigger of acute myocardial infarction. Am J Cardiol 1990;66:41G–43G.

92. Tenaglia AN, Peters KG, Sketch MH Jr, Annex BH. Neovascularization in atherectomy specimens from patients with unstable angina: implications for pathogenesis of unstable angina. Am Heart J 1998;135:10–14.

93. Kockx MM, Cromheeke KM, Knaapen MW, Bosmans JM, De Meyer GR, Herman AG, Bult H. Phagocytosis and macrophage activation associated with hemorrhagic microvessels in human atherosclerosis. Arterioscler Thromb Vasc Biol 2003;23:440–6.

94. Burke AP, Farb A, Malcom GT, Liang Y, Smialek JE, Virmani R. Plaque rupture and sudden death related to exertion in men with coronary artery disease. JAMA 1999;281:921–6.

95. Haddad JJ, Land SC. A non-hypoxic, ROS-sensitive pathway mediates TNF-alpha-dependent regulation of HIF-1alpha. FEBS Lett 2001;505:269–74.

96. Richard DE, Berra E, Pouyssegur J. Nonhypoxic pathway mediates the induction of hypoxia-inducible factor 1alpha in vascular smooth muscle cells. J Biol Chem 2000;275:26765–71.

97. Cho M, Hunt TK, Hussain MZ. Hydrogen peroxide stimulates macrophage vascular endothelial growth factor release. Am J Physiol Heart Circ Physiol 2001;280:H2357–63.

98. Ruef J, Hu ZY, Yin LY, et al. Induction of vascular endothelial growth factor in balloon-injured baboon arteries. A novel role for reactive oxygen species in atherosclerosis. Circ Res 1997;81:24–33.

99. Bergers G, Brekken R, McMahon G, et al. Matrix metalloproteinase-9 triggers the angiogenic switch during carcinogenesis. Nature Cell Biology 2000;2:737–44.

100. Vu TH, Werb Z. Matrix metalloproteinases: effectors of development and normal physiology. Genes Dev 2000;14:2123–33.

101. Galis ZS, Sukhova GK, Lark MW, Libby P. Increased expression of matrix metalloproteinases and matrix degrading activity in vulnerable regions of human atherosclerotic plaques. J Clin Invest 1994;94:2493–503.

102. Nikkari ST, O'Brien KD, Ferguson M, Hatsukami T, Welgus HG, Alpers CE, Clowes AW. Interstitial collagenase (MMP-1) expression in human carotid atherosclerosis. Circulation 1995;92:1393–8.

103. Moldovan NI, Goldschmidt-Clermont PJ, Parker-Thornburg J, Shapiro SD, Kolattukudy PE. Contribution of monocytes/macrophages to compensatory neovascularization: the drilling of metalloelastase-positive tunnels in ischemic myocardium. Circ Res 2000;87:378–84.

104. Carmeliet P, Moons L, Lijnen R, et al. Urokinase-generated plasmin activates matrix metalloproteinases during aneurysm formation. Nature Genetics 1997;17: 439–44.

105. Lemaitre V, Soloway PD, D'Armiento J. Increased medial degradation with pseudo-aneurysm formation in apolipoprotein E-knockout mice deficient in tissue inhibitor of metalloproteinases-1. Circulation 2003;107: 333–8.

106. McMillan WD, Patterson BK, Keen RR, Pearce WH. In situ localization and quantification of seventy-

two-kilodalton type IV collagenase in aneurysmal, occlusive, normal aorta. J Vasc Surg 1995;22:295–305.

107. McMillan WD, Patterson BK, Keen RR, Shively VP, Cipollone M, Pearce WH. In situ localization and quantification of mRNA for 92-kD type IV collagenase and its inhibitor in aneurysmal, occlusive, normal aorta. Arterioscler Thromb Vasc Biol 1995;15:1139–44.

108. Henney AM, Wakeley PR, Davies MJ, Foster K, Hembry R, Murphy G, Humphries S. Localization of stromelysin gene expression in atherosclerotic plaques by in situ hybridization. Proc Natl Acad Sci USA 1991;88:8154–8.

109. Curci JA, Liao S, Huffman MD, Shapiro SD, Thompson RW. Expression and localization of macrophage elastase (matrix metalloproteinase-12) in abdominal aortic aneurysms. J Clin Invest 1998;102:1900–10.

110. Hasty KA, Pourmotabbed TF, Goldberg GI, Thompson JP, Spinella DG, Stevens RM, Mainardi CL. Human neutrophil collagenase. A distinct gene product with homology to other matrix metalloproteinases. J Biol Chem 1990;265:11421–4.

111. Pasterkamp G, Schoneveld AH, Hijnen DJ, de Kleijn DP, Teepen H, van der Wal AC, Borst C. Atherosclerotic arterial remodeling and the localization of macrophages and matrix metalloproteases 1, 2 and 9 in the human coronary artery. Atherosclerosis 2000;150:245–53.

112. Yu AE, Murphy AN, Stetler-Stevenson WG. 72-kDa gelatinase (Gelatinase A): structure, activation regulation, substrate specificity. In Parks WC, Mecham RP, eds. Matrix metalloproteinases. San Diego: Academic Press, 1998:85–113.

113. Farb A, Burke AP, Tang AL, Liang TY, Mannan P, Smialek J, Virmani R. Coronary plaque erosion without rupture into a lipid core. A frequent cause of coronary thrombosis in sudden coronary death. Circulation 1996;93:1354–63.

114. Zempo N, Kenagy RD, Au YPT, Bendeck M, Clowes MM, Reidy MA, Clowes AW. Matrix metalloproteinases of vascular wall cells are increased in balloon-injured rat carotid artery. J Vasc Surg 1994;20:209–17.

115. Freestone T, Turner RJ, Coady A, Higman DJ, Greenhalgh RM, Powell JT. Inflammation and matrix metalloproteinases in the enlarging abdominal aortic aneurysm. Arterioscler Thromb Vasc Biol 1995;15:1145–51.

116. Patel MI, Melrose J, Ghosh P, Appleberg M. Increased synthesis of matrix metalloproteinases by aortic smooth muscle cells is implicated in the etiopathogenesis of abdominal aortic aneurysms. J Vasc Surg 1996;24:82–92.

117. Thompson RW, Holmes DR, Mertens RA, et al. Production and localization of 92–kilodalton gelatinase in abdominal aortic aneurysms. An elastolytic metalloproteinase expressed by aneurysm-infiltrating macrophages. J Clin Invest 1995;96:318–26.

118. Senior RM, Griffin GL, Fliszar CJ, Shapiro SD, Goldberg GI, Welgus HG. Human 92- and 72-kilodalton type IV collagenases are elastases. J Biol Chem 1991;266:7870–5.

119. Shapiro SD, Kobayashi DK, Ley TJ. Cloning and characterization of a unique elastolytic metalloproteinase produced by human alveolar macrophages. J Biol Chem 1993;268:23824–9.

120. Woessner JF Jr. Quantification of matrix metalloproteinases in tissue samples. Methods Enzymol 1995;248:510–28.

121. Fabunmi RP, Sukhova GK, Sugiyama S, Libby P. Expression of tissue inhibitor of metalloproteinases-3 in human atheroma and regulation in lesion-associated cells: a potential protective mechanism in plaque stability. Circ Res 1998;83:270–8.

122. Galis Z, Sukhova G, Libby P. Microscopic localization of active proteases by in situ zymography: detection of matrix metalloproteinase activity in vascular tissue. FASEB J 1995;9:974–80.

123. d'Ortho MP, Will H, Atkinson S, et al. Membrane-type matrix metalloproteinases 1 and 2 exhibit broad-spectrum proteolytic capacities comparable to many matrix metalloproteinases. Eur J Biochem 1997;250:751–7.

124. Strongin AY, Collier I, Bannikov G, Marmer BL, Grant GA, Goldberg GI. Mechanism of cell surface activation of 72-kDa type IV collagenase. Isolation of the activated form of the membrane metalloprotease. J Biol Chem 1995;270:5331–8.

125. Knauper V, Murphy G. Membrane-type matrix metalloproteinases and cell surface-associated activation cascades for matrix metalloproteinases. In: Parks WC, Mecham RP, eds. Matrix metalloproteinases. San Diego: Academic Press, 1998:199–218.

126. Lupu F, Heim DA, Bachmann F, Hurni M, Kakkar VV, Kruithof EK. Plasminogen activator expression in human atherosclerotic lesions. Arterioscler Thromb Vasc Biol 1995;15:1444–55.

127. Carmeliet P, Collen D. Development and disease in proteinase-deficient mice: role of the plasminogen, matrix metalloproteinase and coagulation system. Thrombosis Res 1998;91:255–85.

128. Galis ZS, Kranzhöfer R, Fenton II J, Libby P. Thrombin promotes actvation of matrix metalloproteinase-2 (MMP-2) produced by cultured smooth muscle cells. Arterioscler Thromb Vasc Biol 1997;17:483–89.

129. Lees M, Taylor DJ, Woolley DE. Mast cell proteinases activate precursor forms of collagenase and stromelysin, but not of gelatinases A and B. Eur J Biochem 1994;223:171–7.

130. Sorescu D, Weiss D, Lassegue B, et al. Superoxide production and expression of nox family proteins in human atherosclerosis. Circulation 2002;105:1429–35.

131. Galis ZS, Asanuma K, Godin D, Meng X. *N*-acetyl-cysteine decreases the matrix-degrading capacity of macrophage-derived foam cells: new target for antioxidant therapy? Circulation 1998;97:2445–53.

132. Barry-Lane PA, Patterson C, van der Merwe M, Hu Z, Holland SM, Yeh ET, Runge MS. p47phox is required for atherosclerotic lesion progression in ApoE(-/-) mice. J Clin Invest 2001;108:1513–22.

133. Cullen P, Baetta R, Bellosta S, et al. Rupture of the atherosclerotic plaque: does a good animal model exist? Arterioscler Thromb Vasc Biol 2003;23:535–42.

134. Prescott MF, Sawyer WK, Von Linden-Reed J, Jeune M, Chou M, Caplan SL, Jeng AY. Effect of matrix metalloproteinase inhibition on progression of atherosclerosis and aneurysm in LDL receptor-deficient mice overexpressing MMP-3, MMP-12, MMP-13 and on restenosis in rats after balloon injury. Ann NY Acad Sci 1999;878: 179–90.

135. Sierevogel MJ, Pasterkamp G, Velema E, et al. Oral matrix metalloproteinase inhibition and arterial remodeling after balloon dilation: an intravascular ultrasound study in the pig. Circulation 2001;103: 302–7.

136. Porter KE, Loftus IM, Peterson M, Bell PR, London NJ, Thompson MM. Marimastat inhibits neointimal thickening in a model of human vein graft stenosis. Br J Surg 1998;85:1373–7.

137. Pyo R, Lee JK, Shipley JM, et al. Targeted gene disruption of matrix metalloproteinase-9 (gelatinase B) suppresses development of experimental abdominal aortic aneurysms. J Clin Invest 2000;105:1641–9.

138. Jialal I, Devaraj S. Antioxidants and atherosclerosis: don't throw out the baby with the bath water. Circulation 2003;107:926–8.

139. Meagher E, Rader DJ. Antioxidant therapy and atherosclerosis: animal and human studies. Trends Cardiovasc Med 2001;11:162–5.

140. Heinecke JW. Is the emperor wearing clothes? Clinical trials of vitamin E and the LDL oxidation hypothesis. Arterioscler Thromb Vasc Biol 2001;21:1261–4.

141. Parthasarathy S, Khan-Merchant N, Penumetcha M, Khan BV, Santanam N. Did the antioxidant trials fail to validate the oxidation hypothesis? Curr Atheroscler Rep 2001;3:392–8.

142. Aikawa M, Rabkin E, Okada Y, et al. Lipid lowering by diet reduces matrix metalloproteinase activity and increases collagen content of rabbit atheroma: a potential mechanism of lesion stabilization. Circulation 1998;97:2433–44.

143. Bocan TM, Krause BR, Rosebury WS, et al. The ACAT inhibitor avasimibe reduces macrophages and matrix metalloproteinase expression in atherosclerotic lesions of hypercholesterolemic rabbits. Arterioscler Thromb Vasc Biol 2000;20:70–9.

144. Palinski W, Napoli C. Unraveling pleiotropic effects of statins on plaque rupture. Arterioscler Thromb Vasc Biol 2002;22:1745–50.

145. Takemoto M, Liao JK. Pleiotropic effects of 3-hydroxy-3-methylglutaryl coenzyme a reductase inhibitors. Arterioscler Thromb Vasc Biol 2001;21:1712–19.

146. Luan Z, Chase AJ, Newby AC. Statins inhibit secretion of metalloproteinases-1, -2, -3, -9 from vascular smooth muscle cells and macrophages. Arterioscler Thromb Vasc Biol 2003;23:769–75.

147. Bellosta S, Via D, Canavesi M, Pfister P, Fumagalli R, Paoletti R, Bernini F. HMG-CoA reductase inhibitors reduce MMP-9 secretion by macrophages. Arterioscler Thromb Vasc Biol 1998;18:1671–8.

148. Crisby M, Nordin-Fredriksson G, Shah PK, Yano J, Zhu J, Nilsson J. Pravastatin treatment increases collagen content and decreases lipid content, inflammation, metalloproteinases, cell death in human carotid plaques: implications for plaque stabilization. Circulation 2001;103:926–33.

149. Galis ZS, Muszynski M, Sukhova GK, Simon-Morrissey E, Libby P. Enhanced expression of vascular matrix metalloproteinases induced in vitro by cytokines and in regions of human atherosclerotic lesions. Ann NY Acad Sci 1995;748:501–7.

150. Kai H, Ikeda H, Yasukawa H, et al. Peripheral blood levels of matrix metalloproteases-2 and -9 are elevated in patients with acute coronary syndromes. J Am Coll Cardiol 1998;32:368–72.

151. Goodall S, Crowther M, Hemingway DM, Bell PR, Thompson MM. Ubiquitous elevation of matrix metalloproteinase-2 expression in the vasculature of patients with abdominal aneurysms. Circulation 2001;104:304–9.

152. Bruno G, Todor R, Lewis I, Chyatte D. Vascular extracellular matrix remodeling in cerebral aneurysms. J Neurosurg 1998;89:431–40.

153. Halpert I, Sires UI, Roby JD, et al. Matrilysin is expressed by lipid-laden macrophages at sites of potential rupture in atherosclerotic lesions and localizes to areas of versican deposition, a proteoglycan substrate for the enzyme. Proc Natl Acad Sci USA 1996;93: 9748–53.

154. Brown DL, Hibbs MS, Kearney M, Loushin C, Isner JM. Identification of 92–kD gelatinase in human coronary

atherosclerotic lesions. Association of active enzyme synthesis with unstable angina. Circulation 1995;91: 2125–31.

155. Loftus IM, Naylor AR, Goodall S, Crowther M, Jones L, Bell PR, Thompson MM. Increased matrix metallo-proteinase-9 activity in unstable carotid plaques. A potential role in acute plaque disruption. Stroke 2000;31:40–7.

156. Wesley RB, 2nd, Meng X, Godin D, Galis ZS. Extracellular matrix modulates macrophage functions characteristic to atheroma: collagen type I enhances acquisition of resident macrophage traits by human peripheral blood monocytes in vitro. Arterioscl Thromb Vasc Biol 1998;18:432–40.

157. Saren P, Welgus HG, Kovanen PT. TNF-alpha and IL-1beta selectively induce expression of 92-kDa gelatinase by human macrophages. J Immunol 1996; 157:4159–65.

158. Ganne F, Vasse M, Beaudeux JL, et al. Cerivastatin, an inhibitor of HMG-CoA reductase, inhibits urokinase/urokinase-receptor expression and MMP-9 secretion by peripheral blood monocytes – a possible protective mechanism against atherothrombosis. Thromb Haemost 2000;84:680–8.

159. Gronski TJ Jr, Martin RL, Kobayashi DK, et al. Hydrolysis of a broad spectrum of extracellular matrix proteins by human macrophage elastase. J Biol Chem 1997;272:12189–94.

CHAPTER 10

Apoptosis in atherosclerosis

Mark M Kockx, Wim Martinet & Michiel Knaapen

Regions of cell death in atherosclerotic plaques are very common and are known as necrotic cores. The extension of these regions was considered to be a passive phenomenon and a consequence of plaque progression. Cell death in atherosclerosis has already been suggested by Virchow, the father of cellular pathology, in 1858. Virchow stated that atherosclerotic plaques form by cells that replicate and then die. He called this stage fibro-fatty degeneration.[1] Imai and Thomas studied diet-induced cerebral atherosclerosis in swine some 25 years ago[2] and examined the induced atherosclerotic lesions extensively by transmission electron microscopy. They found SMC death in the plaques and described this type of death as necrosis although their description of the nuclear and cytoplasmic changes fulfilled the criteria of apoptotic cell death. Kerr, Wyllie, and Currie introduced the term "apoptosis" to distinguish a special form of cell death different from necrosis.[3] When a cell receives a signal to die an apoptotic death, it goes through a series of morphological changes detectable by light microscopy, starting from shrinkage of the cell membrane, to condensation of nuclear chromatin, cellular fragmentation, and engulfment of the apoptotic bodies by neighboring cells. Although the term apoptosis was introduced only 25 years ago, the typical morphology of apoptosis has already been described by embryologists at the beginning of the 20th century. Embryologists recognized it as a mechanism to counterbalance the excess of cellular proliferation during the development of organs and limbs.[4] More recently, apoptosis has also been implicated in the development of arteries. Cho et al. have studied apoptosis during arterial wall development[5] and Slomp et al. focused on apoptosis and the changes

that occur in the ductus arteriosus.[6] Apoptosis, however, is not limited to cell elimination during vascular development. In recent years, apoptosis has been implicated in atherosclerosis.[7–21] Theoretically, it would be ideal to induce regression of restenotic lesions and primary atherosclerotic plaques by the induction of apoptosis.[22,23] However, apoptosis could also have negative effects on the stability of atherosclerotic plaques and may be a trigger for plaque rupture.

Apoptosis: the extrinsic versus the intrinsic pathway and the execution phase

Apoptosis is a form of programmed cell death required for the development and the homeostasis of a multicellular organism, for immune regulation, and elimination of infected and damaged cells. The family of cysteine-dependent aspartate-specific proteases, also known as caspases, have been identified as a crucial cascade system that is activated during apoptosis.[24] Nevertheless, it becomes more and more evident that the caspase-dependent pathway is not necessary to kill cells.[25] During apoptosis caspases could be activated by both the **extrinsic** and the **intrinsic** pathway (Figure 10.1).

The extrinsic pathway of apoptosis

The extrinsic pathway starts at the cell membrane when a death receptor such as Fas or TNF-R1 (tumour necrosis factor receptor 1) is activated by ligand binding. This pathway will stimulate the initiator caspases, which in turn could activate the executioner caspases. The death receptors contain a homologous cytoplasmic sequence termed the death

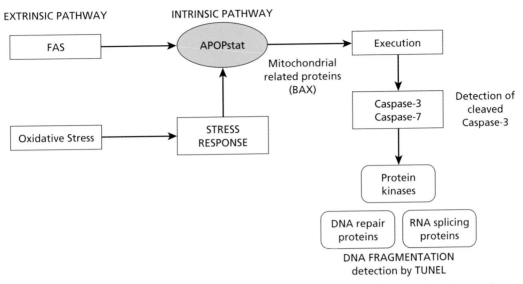

Figure 10.1 Relationship between the extrinsic and the intrinsic pathways of apoptotic cell death. Both pathways activate the downstream caspases which result in cleavage of caspase-3 and ultimately in DNA fragmentation that can be detected by the TUNEL assay.

domain[26] enabling the protein to engage the apoptotic machinery. The best characterized and most important death receptors are Fas (also called CD95 or Apo1), TNF-R1 (also called p55 or CD120a),[27,28] and TRAIL2 (also called Apo2, TRICK, or KILLER).[29–31] The death domains have a propensity to associate with one another leading to clustering of the receptors. An adapter molecule FADD (Fas-associated death domain) binds through its own death domain to the clustered receptor death domains.[32] FADD also contains a domain that binds to an analogous domain repeated in tandem within the zymogen of procaspase-8 (also called FLICE). The complex formed by procaspase-8 and adaptors like FADD is called the death-induced signaling complex or DISC.[33] Upon recruitment by FADD, caspase-8 oligomerization drives its activation through self-cleavage[34] and activates downstream caspases such as caspase-3 (directly) or caspase-9 (via the mitochondrial pathway).

The intrinsic pathway of apoptosis

In contrast to the extrinsic pathway, the intrinsic pathway does not require receptor activation and can be triggered by different apoptotic stimuli such as DNA damaging agents, oxidative damage, toxic agents, and growth factor withdrawal. Recent data suggest that this pathway is important to understand cell death in atherosclerosis via the induction of oxidative DNA damage. An important step of the intrinsic pathway is the mitochondrial membrane permeabilization.

Indeed, it has been demonstrated that mitochondria play a central role in this cytoplamic decision between life and death and thus in the apoptotic effector phase.[35,36] Generally, death signals converge to the mitochondria where cell death is mediated through members of the Bcl-2 protein family that encode only the Bcl-2 homology domain 3 or BH3 domain such as Bid and Bad. The activation of caspase-8 by the complex of FADD/Fas and procaspase-8 could induce cleavage of Bid into truncated Bid (tBid), which then translocates from the cytoplasm to the mitochondria thereby triggering cytochrome c release.[37,38] Moreover, tBid interacts directly with Bax and translocates Bax to the mitochondria where its conformation will be changed into the active form.[39] The activated form of Bax induces outer membrane permeabilization of the mitochondria, resulting in a release of the apoptogenic proteins cytochrome c,[9,40,41] apoptosis inducing factor (AIF),[42,43] and procaspase-9.[44]

Importantly, Bax could also directly induce cytochrome c release indicating that caspases do not participate specifically in the release of cytochrome c.[45,46] The exact mechanism of rupture of the outer membrane to release cytochrome c and other mitochondrial proteins is still under investigation. However, several theories exist such as: (i) the closure of the voltage-dependent anion channel (VDAC) and impairment of ATP-APD exchange;[47] (ii) binding of Bax to the adenine-nucleotide translocator (ANT);[48] (iii) channel formation by Bax;[49,50] (iv) association of Bax with VDAC;[51] and (v) formation of lipid–protein complexes after Bax insertion.[52]

Recently, it became more evident that the decision between life and death depends on the regulation of the mitochondrial permeability transition (MPT). In this concept, the caspases and Bcl-2 protein family play a very important role in regulating the homeostasis of the mitochondria.[53] Bcl-2 can prevent the MPT-mediated mitochondrial depolarization in intact cells and isolated mitochondria.[36,54] Also the Bcl-2 homolog Bcl-X_L prevents MPT-induced reactive oxygen species, the ceramide complex or death receptors.[43,55,56] By contrast, Bax provokes loss of the mitochondrial membrane potential ($\Delta\Psi_m$), matrix swelling, and cytochrome c release,[57,58] and could trigger MPT opening through binding to the adenosine-nucleotide translocator (ANT).[48] Taken together, these data suggest a regulatory role for the Bcl-2 family and emphasize the functional importance of the MPT in the decision between life and death. Moreover, the MPT could also decide on the verdict between necrosis and apoptosis when ATP depletion occurs induced by oxidative stress, pH-dependent ischemia/reperfusion injury, and Ca^{2+}.[39,59] It is also of note that antiapoptotic proteins can act downstream of cytochrome c release and might interact with Apaf-1 preventing it from activating caspase-9.[60,61]

Activation of the executioner caspases and DNA degradation phase

Initiation of active caspase-8 by death receptors at the DISC (extrinsic pathway) directly leads to the activation of downstream procaspases.[33] On the other hand, when DISC formation is strongly reduced active caspase-8 could induce the mitochondrial pathway resulting in the release of cytochrome c

in the cytosol. Cytosolic cytochrome c, Apaf-1, procaspase-9, and dATP will form a complex, also called the apoptosome, leading to activation of caspase-9.[61] Active caspase-9 will activate downstream procaspases. The downstream procaspases are also called the executioner procaspases because activation of these caspases will lead to characteristics of apoptosis such as chromatin condensation and DNA fragmentation. The chromatin condensation factor activated by the caspase cascade is caspase activated DNase (CAD/DFF40).[62,63] In nonapoptotic cells, CAD is localized in the cytoplasm where it is bound to its inhibitor (ICAD/DFF45). ICAD needs to be cleaved by caspase-3 to be released from CAD, after which it translocates to the nucleus. CAD uses its DNase activity to cleave chromatin at internucleosomal regions generating DNA fragments of approximately 180 basepairs. Moreover, CAD activity is controlled by the Cl^- efflux-dependent process[64] which occurs during the execution phase of apoptosis.[65] Another DNA fragmentation factor is the acidic cation-independent L-DNase II. L-DNaseII is derived from an ubiquitous serpin, the leukocyte elastase inhibitor (LEI), by acidic-dependent post-translational modification.[66] LEI is activated by the loss of its elastase-inhibiting activity and translocates to the nucleus where it induces chromatin condensation and DNA fragmentation. Also a caspase-independent peripheral chromatin condensation factor, namely apoptosis inducing factor (AIF), has been identified. AIF is a flavoprotein that is normally confined to the mitochondrial intermembrane space.[42,67] During apoptosis, AIF is translocated to the nucleus, where it causes chromatin condensation in the periphery of the nucleus. In addition to caspase-dependent chromatin condensation and DNA fragmentation, several proteins are activated or inactivated by caspases during apoptosis. Nuclear structural proteins such as lamin A, lamin B, and nuclear mitotic apparatus protein (NuMA) are inactivated by caspases.[68,69] This causes the disassembly of the nuclear matrix, which is required for chromatin condensation and nuclear shrinkage. Also DNA repair enzymes such as poly(ADP-ribose) polymerase (PARP), DNA-dependent protein kinase (DNA-PK), and hsRAD51 are inactivated.[70–72] Furthermore, the 70-kDa component of the U1 small ribonucleoprotein is inactivated by caspases resulting in an inhibition of RNA splicing.[73] The overall effect of the inactivation or cleavage of these proteins and enzymes is that the rate of protein synthesis as well as DNA repair is rapidly down-regulated during apoptosis. The end stage of the execution phase of apoptotic cell death induced by either the extrinsic or the intrinsic pathway is the oligonucleosomal DNA fragmentation.

Apoptosis in atherosclerotic plaques: quantitative aspects?

The detection of DNA fragmentation by the use of the terminal deoxynucleotidyl transferase end labeling (TUNEL) technique or in situ nick translation has become a standard technique for the detection of apoptosis in tissue sections. Different studies have used this technique to demonstrate that cells can die in atherosclerotic plaques through apoptosis. However, a large variation in the percentage of TUNEL-positive nuclei has been found, ranging from less than 2%[13,14,17] up to 30%.[10–12,20] The TUNEL technique labels the execution phase of apoptosis which takes in cell cultures less than 6 hours. Some of the reported values would indicate that plaques are in an imminent state of collapse which is certainly not the case, as remarked by Andrew Newby.[21] This suggests that the TUNEL technique is not without pitfalls. In accordance with Hegyi[74] we reported that the technique is very sensitive and needs a careful titration of proteolytic pretreatment and Tdt concentration, otherwise a high fraction of nonapoptotic nuclei will be labeled. In a recent study, a molecular explanation for this phenomenon was found.[75] Besides apoptotic nuclei, nonapoptotic nuclei that show signs of active gene transcription are labeled by the TUNEL technique. These cells are still active and transcribe genes that are related or completely unrelated to the apoptotic cell death pathway. In a true apoptotic cell, the nuclear DNA is cleaved in oligonucleosomal sized fragments and molecular processes such as RNA transcription and splicing are abolished. Moreover, even in the early execution phase of apoptosis caspase-3 cleaves the 70-kDa protein component of splicing factor U1 snRNP.[73] The loss of RNA splicing can be considered as an early step in the execution phase of apoptosis. Therefore, it is evident that TUNEL-positive nuclei with signs of high RNA synthesis and splicing activity are clearly not in the execution phase of apoptosis. These findings were recently confirmed by Kanoh et al. These authors found that TUNEL-labeled cardiomyocytes are not undergoing apoptosis but show signs of RNA and DNA synthesis/repair.[76] The fact that the TUNEL technique labels nuclei with high RNA synthetic activity is not surprising, since in the past several groups have employed a modification of the DNA in situ nick translation method to allow the in situ detection of active gene transcription.[77,78] Therefore, the TUNEL technique, although a useful technique to detect the execution phase of apoptosis, should always be combined with additional techniques such as markers for transcription and morphologic criteria. Using these stringent conditions, we and others have still found convincing evidence that cells can die within atherosclerotic plaques through apoptosis. The level of apoptotic cell death is also strongly related to the stage of development of the atherosclerotic plaque.[18,79,80] Therefore, a large variability can be expected when atherosclerotic plaques of different stages are compared. In general, adaptive intimal thickening and fatty streaks show very little apoptosis, whereas advanced atherosclerotic plaques show foci of apoptosis. Most of these foci are associated with regions of macrophage infiltration.[18,80] Kolodgie showed extensive macrophage apoptosis predominantly at the rupture site of the plaque.[81] Isner et al. found evidence for apoptotic cell death in primary atherosclerotic lesions and restenotic lesions.[14] Apoptotic cell death was positively linked to cell replication. Restenotic lesions showing high replication rates also demonstrated more apoptotic nuclei. In an in vitro study, Bennett et al. demonstrated that proliferating SMCs show more apoptotic cell death than nonproliferating SMCs.[82] A similar result was found by Bochaton-Piallat in the intimal thickening of rat aorta after endothelial denudation.[83] Bauriedel et al., however, found that human restenotic intimal thickenings showed less apoptotic cell death than primary advanced atherosclerotic plaques. A major difference could be the presence of replicating foam cells of macrophage origin in advanced human atherosclerotic plaques.[18,80] In a study of vein graft atherosclerosis which is considered a form of accelerated human atherosclerosis, a consistent association was found between foam cell accumulation and SMC death in the fibrous cap.[16] Recently, Boyle et al. found evidence that macrophages could induce SMC death in culture.[84] In the next paragraphs we will discuss apoptosis of plaque SMCs, macrophages, and endothelial cells of primary atherosclerotic plaques. It will become clear that the significance and the mechanisms of apoptosis in each of these cell types show similarities but also many differences.

Apoptosis of smooth muscle cells in primary atherosclerotic plaques: a possible role in the thinning of the fibrous cap

Atherosclerotic plaques are complex structures that consist of SMCs, macrophages, lymphocytes, microvessels, and different collagen types. The plaques often contain a central necrotic core that is separated from the vascular lumen by a fibrous cap. The fibrous cap is composed of SMCs and interstitial collagen fibers. Plaque rupture occurs when the mechanical stress in the fibrous cap exceeds a critical level. Factors increasing mechanical stress are thinning of the fibrous cap, a large lipid-rich necrotic core, a relatively small stenosis, and the fluidity of the lipid pool.[85–88] In addition, a number of biological factors may weaken the fibrous cap (Figure 10.2). These include infiltration of macrophages and T-lymphocytes at the shoulder region of the cap and a loss of SMCs.[89] The macrophages can promote local expression and/or activation of matrix metalloproteinases, which decrease the strength of the cap by degrading interstitial collagen fibers.[90,91] Furthermore, loss of the SMCs will decrease the biosynthesis of interstitial collagen fibers. We have demonstrated that SMCs can disappear in the plaque via apoptosis.[18] The consequence of SMC apoptosis depends on the stage and the location of SMC death in the plaque. SMC apoptosis will lead to a loss of the cells that are responsible for the synthesis of the interstitial collagen fibers.[92] Collagen synthesis in vitro is strongly associated with cell replication. Indeed, it was demonstrated in primary cultures of adult rat and rabbit aortic SMCs that the transition into a

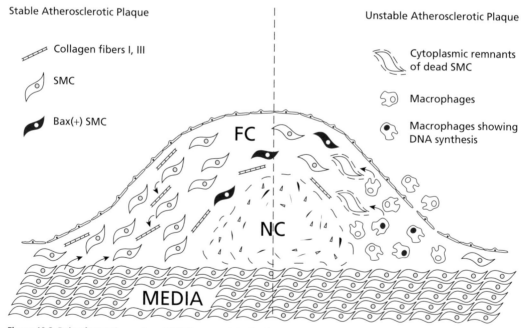

Figure 10.2 Role of smooth muscle cell (SMC) apoptosis in the destabilization of atherosclerotic plaques. A stable atherosclerotic plaque contains a small necrotic core (NC) that is separated from the lumen by a thick fibrous cap. The fibrous cap (FC) is mainly composed of smooth muscle cells and collagen fibers. The SMCs are the cellular source of type I and III collagen fibers that are responsible for the tensile strength of the fibrous cap. Plaque destabilization occurs when macrophages accumulate in the fibrous cap and SMCs undergo apoptosis

synthetic phenotype was accompanied by an increase in collagen secretion.[93] However, the situation in atherosclerosis is clearly different. Rekhter et al.[94] demonstrated that although proliferation and type I collagen expression could occur in the same cell, this is a rare event and that the majority of collagen-producing cells do not show proliferative activity. There are also arguments that SMCs in human and experimental atherosclerotic plaques show very low values of cell replication.[18] This indicates that a slight increase in the levels of SMC apoptosis in the plaque will rapidly lead to a drastic decrease of the smooth muscle content which in turn will have a major influence on the collagen type I synthesis and plaque stability.

Do smooth muscle cells of atherosclerotic plaques show an increased susceptibility for undergoing apoptosis? Microarray studies, simulation in cell culture studies

Smooth muscle cells derived from atherosclerotic plaques but not from the media die when brought into culture.[9] This phenomenon is not completely understood but we previously demonstrated that the pro-apoptotic factor Bax is strongly increased in SMCs of human atherosclerotic plaques.[18] In a recent study, we applied cDNA expression arrays to analyze transcript levels of 205 genes which are associated with apoptotic cell death in human atherosclerotic plaques (Figure 10.3). We found 17 apoptosis-related genes including two housekeeping genes with a two- to five-fold difference in expression level between carotid endarterectomy specimens and nonatherosclerotic mammary arteries (Table 10.1). Interestingly, this systematic approach confirmed Bax upregulation. Moreover, other pro-apoptotic factors were upregulated in the plaque which might suggest that plaque SMCs are more susceptible for undergoing cell death. One of the most remarkable changes related to apoptosis in human atherosclerotic plaques was the overexpression of DAP kinase both at the mRNA and protein level.[95] DAP kinase is a pro-apoptotic calmodulin-regulated serine/threonine kinase that carries interesting modules such as a C-terminal death domain.[96] The death-promoting effects of DAP kinase depend on its catalytic activity, its correct intracellular localiza-

Table 10.1 Differentially expressed apoptosis-related genes in atherosclerotic plaques of carotid endarterectomy specimens versus nonatherosclerotic mammary arteries.

Accession number	Definition	Total fold change
Upregulated		
X76104	Death-associated protein kinase (DAP kinase)	4.97
M11886	HLA class I histocompatibility antigen C-4 alpha subunit (HLAC)	3.62
M32315, M55994	Tumor necrosis factor receptor 2 precursor	3.47
U13699, M87507, X65019	Caspase-1 precursor	3.41
L22474	Apoptosis regulator BAX	2.97
L29511, M96995	Growth factor receptor-bound protein 2 (GRB2) isoform	2.88
U90313	Glutathione-S-transferase homolog	2.77
X01677	Liver glyceraldehyde 3-phosphate dehydrogenase (GAPDH)	2.38
M15796, J04718	Proliferating cyclic nuclear antigen (PCNA)	2.03
Downregulated		
J04111	c-jun proto-oncogene	5.26
M29039	jun-B	5.00
U10564, U09579, L25610	wee 1 Hu CDK tyrosine 15-kinase (CDKN1A)	5.00
M60974	Growth arrest and DNA damage-inducible protein (GADD45)	3.45
M29645	Insulin-like growth factor II (IGF2)	2.56
M74816	Clusterin precursor (CLU)	2.27
X04434, M24599	Insulin-like growth factor I receptor (IGF1R)	2.17
L13698	Growth-arrest-specific protein 1 (GAS1)	2.13

Mammary artery

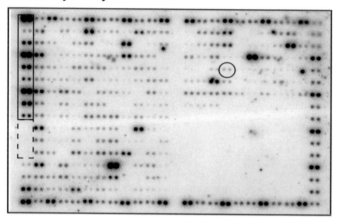

Carotid endarterectomy specimen

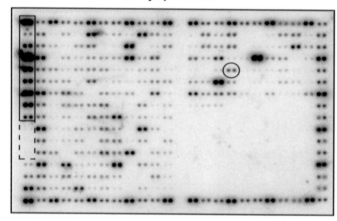

Figure 10.3 Comparative analysis of cDNA generated from nonatherosclerotic mammary arteries and carotid endarterectomy specimens by cDNA expression array hybridization. The cDNA expression array contains 205 apoptosis-related genes, nine housekeeping genes (box, full line) and three negative control cDNAs (box, dashed line). See www.atlas.clontech.com to view the array layout and complete list of genes. Genomic DNA is spotted at the right side, top and bottom of array. Differential expression of DAP kinase mRNA is marked by circles.

tion to actin microfilaments, and the presence of the death domain.[97–99] According to recent evidence, DAP kinase mRNA increases prior to cell death induced by interferon alfa (IFN-α)[97] or transient ischemia.[100] DAP kinase was overexpressed predominantly in lipid-laden SMCs of human plaques (Figure 10.4). Moreover, DAP kinase expression was stimulated in cultured aortic SMCs when cells were exposed to aggregated LDL or C_6-ceramide (Figure 10.5). As the ceramide content of aggregated LDL in atherosclerotic lesions is 10- to 50-fold higher than that of nonaggregated plasma LDL,[101] ceramide could be a potential trigger for DAP kinase expression both in vivo and in vitro. The difference between foam cells of macrophage or SMC origin in respect of DAP kinase expression is presently unclear. However,

recent reports suggest that plaque macrophages develop several anti-apoptotic mechanisms, some of which are mediated by uptake of oxidized low density lipopolysaccharide (oxLDL) or aggregated low density lipopolysaccharide (agLDL). From this point of view, it is reasonable to assume that the absence of DAP kinase upregulation in macrophages from human plaques contributes to the long-term protection against cell death. Interestingly, our cell culture data demonstrate simultaneous upregulation of DAP kinase and Bax in lipid-laden SMCs. DAP kinase and Bax mRNA in cultured SMCs treated with agLDL were upregulated to the same extent (approximately threefold). The expression of Bax and DAP kinase is regulated by lipid accumulation which could explain the in vivo expression of Bax in the different stages of

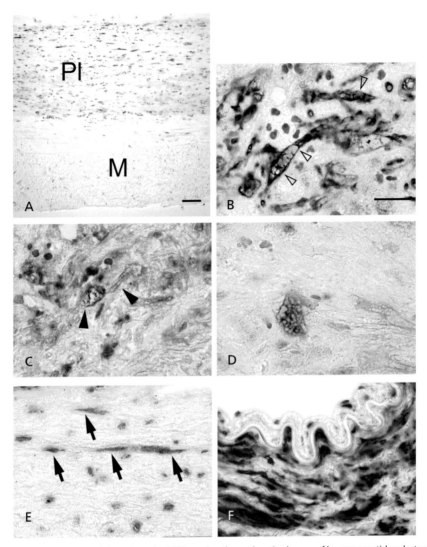

Figure 10.4 Immunohistochemical detection of DAP kinase in atherosclerotic plaques of human carotid endarterectomy specimens. A, Low-power photomicrograph of endarterectomy specimen showing DAP kinase expression in the plaque (Pl) but not in the media (M). B, Double immunohistochemical staining for DAP kinase (brown) and α-SMC actin (blue) in the plaque. Open arrowheads show that DAP kinase is expressed in lipid-laden SMCs. C, Double immunohistochemical staining for DAP kinase (brown) and CD68 (blue) in the plaque. Only SMCs (CD68–) show DAP kinase expression (arrowheads). D, DAP kinase immunolabeling (blue) combined with TUNEL (brown) in the plaque. DAP kinase positive cells were TUNEL negative. E, Double immunohistochemical staining for DAP kinase (blue) and Bax (brown, arrows) in the plaque. F, Double immunohistochemical staining for DAP kinase (brown) and α-SMC actin (blue) in mammary arteries. SMCs are DAP kinase negative. Scale bar = 100 μm (panel A) or 20 μm (panel B–F).

atherosclerotic plaques. SMCs that were present in the different stages showed striking differences regarding their expression of the pro-apoptotic protein Bax. We could distinguish three types of SMC based on their Bax expression and morphology.

The first type of SMCs was mainly present in the normal media and the adaptive intimal thickening. These SMCs showed no Bax expression and were also negative for caspase-3. From an ultrastructural point of view, these SMCs showed the classical aspects of a contractile phenotype (numerous microfilaments but without lipid vacuoles). The second type

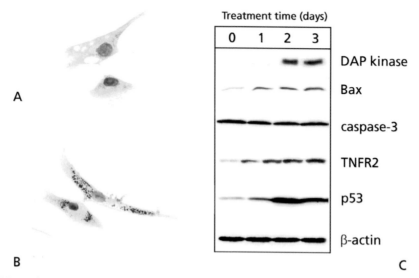

Figure 10.5 Bax and DAP kinase expression in smooth muscle cell culture treated with ag-LDL. A, Untreated smooth muscle cells. B, Smooth muscle incubated with ag-LDL. C, Western Blots of the different proteins at 0 h, 1, 2, and 3 days after incubation with ag-LDL.

includes lipid-laden SMCs. These SMCs showed a strong Bax expression and could be found already in early atherosclerotic plaques like fatty streaks (fibroxanthomata). However, the execution phase of apoptosis as detected by the TUNEL technique was very rare in these early plaques. What could be the underlying cause of Bax expression in lipid laden SMCs? One possibility is that Bax can be upregulated via a p53-dependent pathway. Indeed, it was demonstrated that p53 is a direct transcriptional activator of the human Bax gene.[102] Moreover, p53 is overexpressed but not mutated in atherosclerotic plaques.[103] The reason for the p53 upregulation is not clear but increased oxidative stress and DNA damage has to be considered. Current evidence suggests that DNA damage is sensed by kinases such as DNA-dependent protein kinase (DNA-PK) leading to the phosphorylation and activation of p53.[104] Therefore, it is intriguing to speculate that SMCs show an upregulation of Bax via a p53-dependent mechanism as a response to increased oxidative DNA damage in the plaques.[18] Bax is also upregulated in SMCs of experimental atherosclerotic plaques.[105] This upregulation could be reversed after a period of lipid lowering and indicates that the susceptibility of SMCs in plaques can possibly be reversed by lipid lowering.

The third type of SMC includes SMCs that were composed of completely disintegrated cytoplasmic fragments. The SMC origin could still be demonstrated because these cytoplasmic fragments were enclosed by cages of thickened basal laminae (Figure 10.6). Russel Ross called these cells pancake-like SMCs.[106] This particular form of SMC cell death was already described by Stehbens as granulovesicular degeneration of the SMC.[107] Recent work by our group revealed that this form of cell death has numerous characteristics that point to apoptotic cell death.[18] Indeed, the cytoplasmic fragments of the type 3 SMC showed a very high expression of Bax and caspase-3. Furthermore, it was possible to detect DNA fragmentation with the TUNEL technique in some SMCs of this type. Interestingly, this type of SMCs was completely similar to that found in unstable plaques of saphenous vein grafts adjacent to foam cells of macrophage origin.[16] This suggests that SMCs in plaques can be killed by factors derived from the macrophages (foam cell derived killing factors) as demonstrated by Boyle et al.[84] Cytokines from induced macrophages and T-lymphocytes can induce apoptosis of human and rat vascular SMCs in culture and can sensitize SMCs to Fas-mediated apoptosis via upregulation of cell surface Fas.[108] Human SMCs express Fas

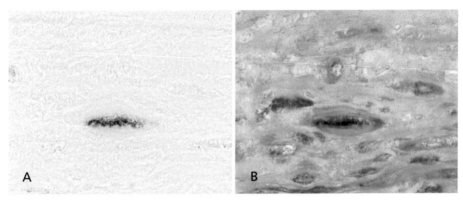

Figure 10.6 Apoptotic smooth muscle cell in the fibrous cap of an advanced atherosclerotic plaque. A TUNEL positive cell is demonstrated (A). B, The same TUNEL-stained section that was additionally stained with a PAS stain to show basal laminae. The TUNEL positive cell is surrounded by a cage of PAS-positive thickened basal laminae, which indicates their smooth muscle cell origin. These pancake smooth muscle cells are typical for the fibrous cap region of atherosclerotic plaques.

whereas T-lymphocytes, macrophages, endothelial cells, and SMCs express Fas ligand so that Fas/Fas ligand-mediated apoptosis of SMCs may occur at sites with high levels of inflammation.[109] Dong et al. found that in transplant coronary arteriopathy nearly all vascular cells show Fas expression whereas the typical atherosclerotic plaque and normal controls contain low levels of Fas.[110] This finding supports the hypothesis that the significance and the molecular mechanisms of apoptosis in different coronary pathologies (primary atherosclerosis, vein graft atherosclerosis, restenosis, and transplant arteriopathies) can be different.[111]

Conclusion

Apoptosis of SMCs will lead to a loss of collagen type I which could lead to unstable plaques that are prone to rupture. Moreover, apoptotic SMCs in the plaques are often not scavenged and could be the main source of calcifying matrix vesicles.[16,18] These matrix vesicles could lead to plaque calcification. Apoptotic SMCs can also increase the plaque thrombogenicity.[112] Indeed, plaque SMCs undergoing apoptosis have the same potency to generate thrombin as platelets. This is due to the fact that apoptotic cells expose phosphatidylserine on the surface early in the process.[112] In the presence of factors V and VII, exposed phosphatidylserine can then act as a substrate for thrombin generation. Apoptosis of SMCs in primary atherosclerotic plaques could be detrimental for plaque stability and increase the risk for thrombosis.

Apoptosis of macrophages: expansion of the necrotic core, decreased scavenging, survival in the plaque

Apoptosis of macrophages is mainly found in cellular macrophage-rich regions that also show signs of DNA synthesis. This was demonstrated with Ki-67, PCNA, and BrdU incorporation. Mitotic figures are rarely found in these regions. This finding could indicate that DNA synthesis in these cells points to DNA repair. Recently, we have found that the macrophages contain inducible nitric oxide synthase, nitrotyrosine, and oxidized lipids.[113] This point to high levels of oxidative stress and peroxynitrite. The high levels of DNA synthesis/repair could be a response to oxidative DNA damage. In early studies, it was noted that NO targets naked DNA[114,115] and induces oxidative damage in activated macrophages. Both deamination (abasic site formation) and oxidative modifications have been described in DNA as a consequence of NO damage.[116] In extension of these observations, it is widely accepted that NO-damaged DNA elicits DNA repair mechanisms in mammalian cells. In this concept, NO-induced apoptotic cell death can be considered as a mechanism that is used by the cell if DNA repair mechanisms fail.

Detection of DNA damage in human atherosclerotic plaques

Alkaline single cell gel electrophoresis revealed that the number of DNA strand breaks was significantly higher in cells of the carotid endarterectomy specimens as compared with cells derived from mammary arteries.[117] Most cells in the plaque (>90%) contained DNA strand breaks with varying outcome (Figure 10.7). However, only a minority of cells (1–2%) showed TUNEL reactivity. Cells containing a massive amount of DNA strand breaks were localized predominantly in regions of the plaque that contained large amounts of oxidized lipid deposits. In mammary arteries and peripheral blood monocytes, DNA strand breaks were scarce or completely absent.

Expression of DNA repair enzymes

Several proteins involved in DNA repair were upregulated in plaques of carotid endarterectomy specimens as compared with nonatherosclerotic vessels. Western blots revealed an increased expression of p53, p53 phosphorylated at Ser15 and Ser392, DNA-PK, endonuclease Ref-1 and PARP-1, but a constitutive expression of DNA polymerase β, the N-glycosylases hOgg1 and hNTH1 and 8-oxoGTPase (MTH1). Western blots were confirmed by immunohistochemistry. Strong nuclear immunoreactivity for Ref-1 and DNA-PK was present

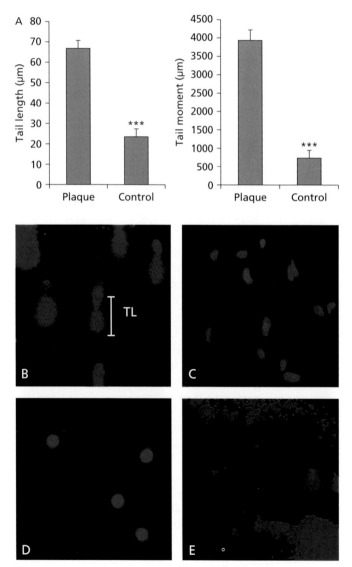

Figure 10.7 Detection of DNA strand breaks in individual cells of nonatherosclerotic mammary arteries versus plaque cells from carotid endarterectomy specimens. A, Freshly isolated mammary arteries (control, n = 8) and carotid endarterectomy specimens (plaque, n = 13) were gently pressed against an agarose-coated microscope slide. Cells which adhered to the slide were immediately covered with a second layer of low melting point agarose and analyzed using the alkaline comet assay. Slides contained both macrophages and smooth muscle cells in a ratio similar to the one found in tissue sections. Tail length (TL) as well as tail moment (TM = tail length × %DNA in tail) increased significantly in all atheromas studied. B,C, Digitized comet images of cells isolated from atherosclerotic plaques of the carotid artery (B) versus mammary arteries (C). D, Comet image of peripheral blood monocytes. E, Digitized image of a comet slide containing plaque cells with an extensive amount of DNA strand breaks surrounded by autofluorescent lipid deposits (blue). The results are expressed as mean ± SEM. ***$P < 0.001$ vs. carotid endarterectomy specimens.

in the entire plaque, both in macrophages and SMCs. The carotid artery endothelium and endothelial cells from microvessels were negative for Ref-1 and DNA-PK or showed occasional staining. SMCs from the media adjacent to the plaque and from mammary arteries hardly stained. In contrast with Ref-1 and DNA-PK immunolabeling, only a subpopulation of cells in the plaque stained for p53, phospho-p53, or PARP-1. Upregulation of p53 and PARP-1 occurred predominantly in the macrophage population of the plaque, but was undetectable in the adjacent media and mammary arteries. Overexpression of DNA repair enzymes was associated with elevated levels of PCNA. Immunoreactivity for Ref-1 and DNA-PK did not differ in intimal xanthomata from thin fibrous cap atheromas. However, overexpression of PARP-1, p53, and PCNA was found predominantly in macrophages around the necrotic core of thin fibrous cap atheromata.

DNA damage/repair and its relationship with cell death in the plaque

Two repair mechanisms have been studied in this context: (i) the p53/p21 and NO-induced DNA repair and apoptosis; (ii) the PARP pathway.

p53/p21 and NO-induced DNA repair and apoptosis

The tumor suppressor gene p53 has been recognized as a master guardian of the genome and a member of the DNA damage–response pathway.[118] Therefore, NO-induced DNA damage may upregulate p53, which in turn will arrest the cell cycle in G1 via p21 (WAF1/ Cip 1), an inhibitor of cyclin-dependent kinases. Ihling et al. demonstrated expression of p53 and p21 in human atherosclerotic plaques.[119] Induction of apoptosis via p53/p21 is less well understood but can be activated both by transactivation and transactivation-independent pathways. Recent evidence indicates that the Bcl-2 protein family can be involved. It was demonstrated that the pro-apoptotic protein Bax is upregulated in close association with NO.[120] The promotor site of the Bax gene contains a p53 binding domain.[121] Therefore, p53 could act as a sensor for DNA damage which may lead to a cell cycle arrest and DNA repair or to upregulation of pro-

apoptotic factors and increased susceptibility of apoptosis (Figure 10.8). A recent in vivo study in apoE knockout mice demonstrated that p53 is essential for the cell cycle control (G1 arrest) but not for the induction of apoptotic cell death in atherosclerosis.[122] It was demonstrated that the increased plaque size in apoE$^{-/-}$ p53$^{-/-}$ mice compared to apoE$^{-/-}$ mice was mainly a consequence of increased cell replication of the macrophages in the plaques. The accelerated proliferation rate in the plaques of these apoE$^{-/-}$ p53$^{-/-}$ mice may be mediated at least partly by the loss of the p53-dependent G1 checkpoint control and the ongoing apoptotic cell death points to p53-independent apoptosis pathways in atherosclerosis.

PARP and NO-induced DNA repair and apoptosis

DNA damage will induce attachment of poly(ADP-ribose) polymerase (PARP) to the strand breaks and extensive synthesis of short-lived polymers by the bound polymerase.[123,124] Although PARP has no direct role in DNA excision repair, the enzyme binds tightly to the DNA strand breaks and repair can be suppressed if PARP synthesis is prevented.[124] Massive PARP activation following extensive DNA damage upon exposure to peroxynitrite leads to depletion of NAD$^+$, the ADP ribose donor.[125] In an effort to resynthesize NAD$^+$, ATP becomes depleted which ultimately leads to cell death due to energy deprivation. Moreover, inhibition of mitochondrial respiration (thereby affecting ATP synthesis) via destruction of Fe-S clusters has been noted.[126] Initially, it was stated that it is unlikely that energy depletion due to PARP activation is a general pathway of this NO-mediated apoptotic cell death, since apoptotic cell death is an energy-requiring process and PARP is cleaved by caspases in the early execution phase of apoptotic cell death. However, recent findings indicate that caspases, a family of cysteine proteases that execute the cell death program, can be inactivated by a nitrosylation step.[127–129] This was demonstrated for endothelial cells[130,131] but more recently it was also demonstrated that it could be a feature of NOS-expressing cells.[128] This could indicate that NOS-expressing cells, like macrophages in atherosclerotic plaques, do not cleave PARP and other DNA repair proteins since their caspases are

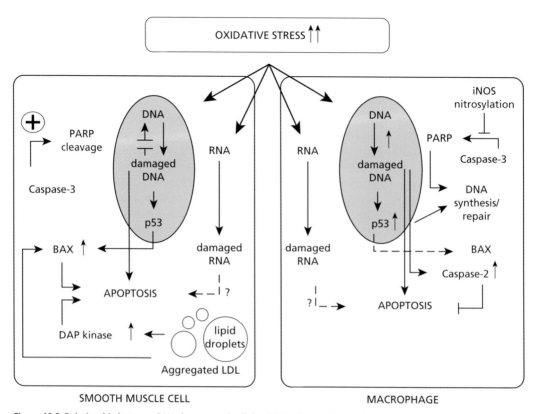

Figure 10.8 Relationship between DNA damage and cell death in both smooth muscle cells and macrophages.

inactivated. Therefore, the macrophages continously repair their DNA damage. This could be an explanation for the presence of the high levels of DNA synthesis in macrophages in human and experimental atherosclerotic plaques. Moreover, it was demonstrated that NOS-expressing cells can denitrosylate and reactivate their caspases when their Fas apoptotic pathway is activated.[128] If the nitrosylation/denitrosylation hypothesis can be demonstrated in vivo in atherosclerotic plaques new pharmacological tools can be developed to modulate apoptosis in the plaques.

Apoptosis of macrophages in atherosclerotic plaques: beneficial or detrimental?

As already explained in the previous paragraph, macrophages are responsible for collagen breakdown in the plaque. Loss of macrophages will lead to less metalloproteinase activity and to decreased collagen breakdown. This may lead to plaque stab-

ilization and a decreased risk for plaque rupture. However, the situation is not that simple. In normal development, apoptosis is followed by engulfment of the apoptotic bodies by neighboring cells. A loss of macrophages will lead to a decrease in scavenging of apoptotic bodies. Accumulation of apoptotic bodies could lead to complement and thrombin activation. This will be discussed in the next paragraph.

Scavenging of apoptotic bodies in atherosclerotic plaques

Recognition and uptake of dying cells is an important component of the apoptotic process, preventing the release of toxic intracellular contents and the formation of an inflammatory infiltrate. The finding that apoptosis can be demonstrated in atherosclerotic plaques might reflect a failure of the uptake mechanism, which could contribute to the progressive accumulation of inflammatory cells in the lesions. The mechanism by which apoptotic cells are recognized and phagocytized are incompletely understood and appear to vary according to the cell type.

Which cells and factors are involved in the uptake of apoptotic bodies in the plaque?

Although most of the apoptotic bodies are phagocytized by macrophages, it is possible that the SMCs can also ingest apoptotic bodies. For macrophages, it was demonstrated that the scavenger receptors are involved in the recognition and uptake of apoptotic bodies.[132,133] Besides their high affinity for acetylated and oxidized LDL,[134] it was demonstrated that the scavenger receptor might recognize any damaged cell by virtue of its oxidized cell membranes, which might contain domains analogues to those found in oxLDL.[134,135] In a global sense, scavenger receptors might represent a means of removing oxidatively damaged components which could otherwise injure surrounding tissues.[136] There is evidence that oxidative damage is a component of the apoptotic program.[137] Krieger et al.[138] have reviewed the structure and binding properties of macrophage scavenger receptors. In addition to oxLDL and acLDL, the receptors bind polyribonucleotides, polysaccharides, and anionic phospholipids such as phosphatidylserine. This is important because apoptotic cells expose phosphatidylserine on the external leaflet of their plasma membrane. Phosphatidylserine, which is normally sequestered in the internal leaflet of the plasma membrane, may be recognized by the macrophages via the scavenger receptors. Apoptotic bodies are cleared before damage to the plasma membrane is evident so that a stable fibrous plaque will form with a low thrombogenicity. However, if apoptotic SMCs or macrophages are not engulfed, a necrotic core with high thrombogenicity will form. This indicates that scavenging of apoptotic bodies in atherosclerotic plaques could determine whether a plaque will be stable or unstable.[136]

Lack of scavenging of apoptotic bodies in atherosclerotic plaques could also be important for the futher influx of mononuclear cells in the plaque. This is suggested by the finding that during tissue remodeling in embryonic development regions with excessive apoptosis show upregulation of the endothelial monocyte-activating polypeptide II (EMAP-II). Mature EMAP-II can attract mono- and polymorpho-nuclear cells to the site of inflammation and can induce tissue factor in endothelial cells.[139,140] This is another argument that excessive apoptosis could transform the stable plaque in an unstable plaque with high thrombogenicity.

Decreased scavenging activity of the macrophages in plaques?

Macrophages that have phagocytized erythrocytes become deficient for their phagocytosis activity.[141] This is relevant for understanding the signifcance of apoptosis in atherosclerosis since macrophages in advanced human atherosclerotic plaques show signs of platelet and erythrophagocytosis.[113] This could indicate that macrophages in advanced human atherosclerotic plaques become deficient for the scavenging of apoptotic bodies. Accordingly, apoptotic bodies in these regions are not adequately removed leading to the accumulation of necrotic debris in some regions of the plaque. This is exactly what is seen in some regions of atherosclerotic plaques. The formation of the necrotic core could be the result of both an increased apoptosis and a lack of scavenging by the remaining cells.

Apoptosis and thrombin activation/tissue factor activity

Induction of apoptosis in endothelial cells is associated with increased expression of phosphatidylserine and loss of anticoagulant membrane components.[142] Moreover, apoptotic cells show increased tissue factor activity.[143] These findings indicate that increased apoptosis in the plaque could be responsible for the increased pro-coagulant status. It was indeed demonstrated that tissue factor is mainly localized in the necrotic core of advanced atherosclerotic plaques.[144] Interestingly, Mallat et al[145] have found that most of the extracellular tissue factor expression is located around apoptotic cells in the necrotic core of human atherosclerotic plaques. This suggests that tissue factor may be shed from apoptotic cells via apoptotic microparticles. It was also demonstrated that high levels of shed membrane particles of monocytic and lymphocytic origin are produced in atherosclerotic plaques that are associated with increased tissue factor activity. Therefore, increased apoptosis in the plaque could lead to an increased level of thrombogenicity and a higher risk for plaque complications (Figure 10.9).

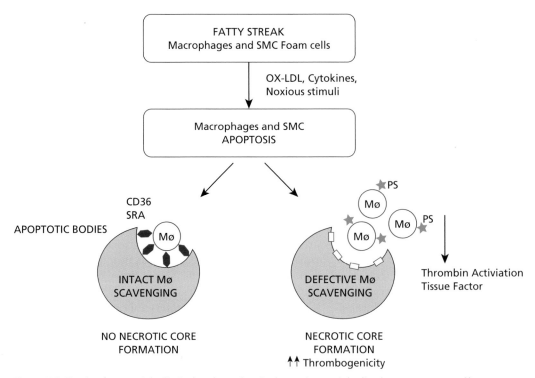

Figure 10.9 Uptake of apoptotic bodies in the atherosclerotic plaque. Apoptotic bodies that are not removed by phagocytosis can accumulate and expand the necrotic core. Unremoved apoptotic bodies increase the thrombogenicity of the plaque.

Apoptosis of endothelial cells in atherosclerotic plaques: a role in plaque erosion?

Injury of the vascular endothelium is a critical event in the pathogenesis of atherosclerosis. Importantly, endothelial cells in lesion-prone regions are characterized by increased turnover rates, suggesting a mechanistic link beween turnover of endothelial cells and the susceptibiliy of atherosclerotic plaque development. The enhanced turnover is most likely due to increased apoptosis.[146] Interestingly, traditional risk factors for atherosclerosis such as high glucose concentrations,[121] oxidized LDL,[147] increased oxidative stress, and angiotensin II stimulate apoptosis of endothelial cells.[148,149] It is also of note that endothelial cells in the normal arterial wall protect themselves against apoptosis by two NO-dependent mechanisms. The low levels of NO that are formed by the low output isoform ecNOS protect against apoptosis via cyclic GMP-dependent and cyclic GMP-independent mechanisms. Activation of cyclic GMP-dependent protein kinases is associated with protection against apoptosis.[150] Another possible mechanism is S-nitrosylation of caspases, enzymes involved in the executive steps of apoptotic cell death. All caspases contain an essential cysteine within their active center which is potentially susceptible to S-nitrosylation. Recently, it has indeed been demonstrated that nitric oxide can nitrosylate the caspases interleukin-β-converting enzyme and cystein protease protein 32,[130,131] thereby affording protection against TNF-α-induced apoptotic cell death. Endothelial cells exposed to shear stress increase their NO production which could protect the endothelial cells against different apoptotic stimuli via a cGMP-independent mechanism. This indicates that in the normal arterial wall NO is protective for different cell types. In atherosclerotic plaques, the situation is fundamentally different since the high output isoform iNOS is expressed in an environment with high levels of oxidative stress.[151–153]

Effects of lipid lowering on apoptosis in atherosclerotic plaques

It was previously demonstrated that the thickness of atherosclerotic plaques induced by feeding rabbits a cholesterol supplement did not decrease after a period of cholesterol withdrawal. However, most of the macrophages disappear from the plaques after a period of cholesterol withdrawal and the plaques are transformed in fibrous plaques. These changes were also associated with a strong decrease in metalloproteinase activity.[154] It is not clear whether the macrophages after this aggresive lipid lowering disappear from the plaques by increased apoptosis or by decreased cell replication and/or accumulation. This information is important for understanding the effects of aggressive lipid lowering since induction of excessive apoptosis could increase the thrombogenicity of the plaques as discussed in the previous paragraphs. In a recent study, we could demonstrate that apoptotic cell death[105] and DNA damage/repair[155] showed a steady decline after lipid lowering. Moreover, the pro-apoptotic protein Bax, which is upregulated in both human and experimental atherosclerotic plaques, strongly decreased after lipid lowering. These changes indicate that apoptosis (and also the susceptibility of cells in the plaque to undergo apoptosis) did not increase after lipid lowering but show a steady decline. Furthermore, it was demonstrated that the changes in cell composition of the plaques were mainly a consequence of a strong decrease in DNA synthesis of the macrophages. DNA synthesis of SMCs did not decrease after lipid lowering. SMCs remained present and lost their lipid accumulation whereas macrophages almost completely disappeared from the plaques. Interestingly, atherosclerotic plaques of the animals that remained on the cholesterol-rich diet for 52 weeks showed the same characteristics as the plaques at 26 weeks of cholesterol supplementation, which excludes age-associated changes in the plaques. Taken together, lipid lowering does not decrease the thickness of atherosclerotic plaques but increases the fibrous components without increasing the thrombogenicity.

Summary

Apoptosis of endothelial cells and SMCs is detrimental for plaque stability. Apoptosis of macrophages could be beneficial for plaque stability. Recent data, however, indicate that nonscavenged apoptotic macrophages remain in the plaque as shed microparticles which could be a potent source for tissue factor. Therefore, it is not clear whether induction of macrophage apoptosis would be beneficial for plaque stability. Lipid lowering does not induce an increase of macrophage apoptosis but a decreased macrophage accumulation in the plaque. More studies are necessary to find out whether selective induction of macrophage apoptosis could lead to the same result on plaque stability. This information is essential for understanding the effects of new apoptosis modifying drugs on plaque stability.

Acknowledgments

This work was supported by a grant of the Flemish Fund for Scientific Research (FWO). M. Kockx is holder of a fund for fundamental clinical research of the Flemish Fund for Scientific Research (FWO).

References

1. Virchow R. Die Cellularpathologie: Sechzehnte verlesung, 14 april 1858. Hildesheim OG, ed. 1966:317–329.
2. Imai H, Thomas WA. Cerebral atherosclerosis in swine: role of necrosis in progression of diet-induced lesions from proliferative to atheromatous stage. Exp Mol Pathol 1968;8:330–57.
3. Kerr JF, Wyllie AH, Currie AR. Apoptosis: a basic biological phenomenon with wide-ranging implications in tissue kinetics. Br J Cancer 1972;26:239–57.
4. Saunders JW, Jr. Death in embryonic systems. Science 1966;154:604–12.
5. Cho A, Courtman DW, Langille BL. Apoptosis (programmed cell death) in arteries of the neonatal lamb. Circ Res 1995;76:168–75.
6. Slomp J, Gittenberger-de Groot AC, Glukhova MA, Conny VM, Kockx MM, Schwartz SM, Koteliansky VE. Differentiation, dedifferentiation, apoptosis of smooth

muscle cells during the development of the human ductus arteriosus. Arterioscler Thromb Vasc Biol 1997;17:1003–9.

7. Bauriedel G, Schluckebier S, Hutter R, Welsch U, Kandolf R, Luderitz B, Prescott MF. Apoptosis in restenosis versus stable-angina atherosclerosis: implications for the pathogenesis of restenosis. Arterioscler Thromb Vasc Biol 1998;18:1132–9.

8. Bennett MR. Apoptosis of vascular smooth muscle cells in vascular remodelling and atherosclerotic plaque rupture. Cardiovasc Res 1999;41:361–8.

9. Bennett MR, Evan GI, Schwartz SM. Apoptosis of human vascular smooth muscle cells derived from normal vessels and coronary atherosclerotic plaques. J Clin Invest 1995;95:2266–74.

10. Björkerud S, Bjorkerud B: Apoptosis is abundant in human atherosclerotic lesions, especially in inflammatory cells (macrophages and T cells), and may contribute to the accumulation of gruel and plaque instability. Am J Pathol 1996;149:367–80.

11. Geng YJ, Libby P. Evidence for apoptosis in advanced human atheroma. Colocalization with interleukin-1β-converting enzyme. Am J Pathol 1995;147:251–66.

12. Han DK, Haudenschild CC, Hong MK, Tinkle BT, Leon MB, Liau G. Evidence for apoptosis in human atherogenesis and in a rat vascular injury model. Am J Pathol 1995;147:267–77.

13. Hegyi L, Skepper JN, Cary NR, Mitchinson MJ. Foam cell apoptosis and the development of the lipid core of human atherosclerosis. J Pathol 1996;180: 423–9.

14. Isner JM, Kearney M, Bortman S, Passeri J. Apoptosis in human atherosclerosis and restenosis. Circulation 1995;91:2703–11.

15. Kockx MM. Apoptosis in the atherosclerotic plaque: quantitative and qualitative aspects. Arterioscler Thromb Vasc Biol 1998;18:1519–22.

16. Kockx MM, De Meyer GR, Bortier H, et al. Luminal foam cell accumulation is associated with smooth muscle cell death in the intimal thickening of human saphenous vein grafts. Circulation 1996;94:1255–62.

17. Kockx MM, De Meyer GR, Muhring J, Bult H, Bultinck J, Herman AG. Distribution of cell replication and apoptosis in atherosclerotic plaques of cholesterol-fed rabbits. Atherosclerosis 1996;120:115–24.

18. Kockx MM, De Meyer GR, Muhring J, Jacob W, Bult H, Herman AG. Apoptosis and related proteins in different stages of human atherosclerotic plaques. Circulation 1998;97:2307–15.

19. Kockx MM, Herman AG. Apoptosis in atherogenesis: implications for plaque destabilization. Eur Heart J 1998;19(suppl G):G23–8.

20. Mallat Z, Ohan J, Leseche G, Tedgui A. Colocalization of CPP-32 with apoptotic cells in human atherosclerotic plaques. Circulation 1997;96:424–8.

21. Newby AC, George SJ. Proliferation, migration, matrix turnover, death of smooth muscle cells in native coronary and vein graft atherosclerosis. Curr Opin Cardiol 1996;11:574–82.

22. Pollman MJ, Hall JL, Mann MJ, Zhang L, Gibbons GH. Inhibition of neointimal cell bcl-x expression induces apoptosis and regression of vascular disease. Nat Med 1998;4:222–7.

23. Wang BY, Ho HK, Lin PS, et al. Regression of atherosclerosis: role of nitric oxide and apoptosis. Circulation 1999;99:1236–41.

24. Samali A, Zhivotovsky B, Jones D, Nagata S, Orrenius S. Apoptosis: cell death defined by caspase activation [letter]. Cell Death Differ 1999;6:495–6.

25. Fiers W, Beyaert R, Declercq W, Vandenabeele P. More than one way to die: apoptosis, necrosis and reactive oxygen damage. Oncogene 1999;18:7719–30.

26. Tartaglia LA, Ayres TM, Wong GH, Goeddel DV. A novel domain within the 55 kd TNF receptor signals cell death. Cell 1993;74:845–53.

27. Gruss HJ and Dower SK. The TNF ligand superfamily and its relevance for human diseases. Cytokines Mol Ther 1995;1:75–105.

28. Gruss HJ, Dower SK. Tumor necrosis factor ligand superfamily: involvement in the pathology of malignant lymphomas. Blood 1995;85:3378–404.

29. Screaton GR, Mongkolsapaya J, Xu XN, Cowper AE, McMichael AJ, Bell JI. TRICK2, a new alternatively spliced receptor that transduces the cytotoxic signal from TRAIL. Curr Biol 1997;7:693–6.

30. Walczak H, Degli-Esposti MA, Johnson RS, et al. TRAIL-R2: a novel apoptosis-mediating receptor for TRAIL. EMBO J 1997;16:5386–97.

31. Wu GS, Burns TF, Zhan Y, Alnemri ES, el Deiry WS. Molecular cloning and functional analysis of the mouse homologue of the KILLER/DR5 tumor necrosis factor-related apoptosis-inducing ligand (TRAIL) death receptor. Cancer Res 1999;59:2770–5.

32. Chinnaiyan AM, O'Rourke K, Tewari M, Dixit VM. FADD, a novel death domain-containing protein, interacts with the death domain of Fas and initiates apoptosis. Cell 1995;81:505–12.

33. Kischkel FC, Hellbardt S, Behrmann I, Germer M, Pawlita M, Krammer PH, Peter ME. Cytotoxicity-dependent APO-1 (Fas/CD95)-associated proteins form a death-inducing signaling complex (DISC) with the receptor. EMBO J 1995;14:5579–88.

34. Muzio M, Stockwell BR, Stennicke HR, Salvesen GS, Dixit VM. An induced proximity model for caspase-8 activation. J Biol Chem 1998;273:2926–30.

35. Green DR, Reed JC. Mitochondria and apoptosis. Science 1998;281:1309–12.

36. Kroemer G. Mitochondrial control of apoptosis: an overview. Biochem Soc Symp 1999;66:1–15.

37. Desagher S, Osen-Sand A, Nichols A, et al. Bid-induced conformational change of Bax is responsible for mitochondrial cytochrome c release during apoptosis. J Cell Biol 1999;144:891–901.

38. Eskes R, Desagher S, Antonsson B, Martinou JC. Bid induces the oligomerization and insertion of Bax into the outer mitochondrial membrane. Mol Cell Biol 2000;20:929–35.

39. Crompton M. Bax, Bid and the permeabilization of the mitochondrial outer membrane in apoptosis. Curr Opin Cell Biol 2000;12:414–19.

40. Kluck RM, Bossy-Wetzel E, Green DR, Newmeyer DD. The release of cytochrome c from mitochondria: a primary site for Bcl-2 regulation of apoptosis [see comments]. Science 1997;275:1132–6.

41. Martinou I, Desagher S, Eskes R, Antonsson B, Fakan S, Martinou JC. The release of cytochrome c from mitochondria during apoptosis of NGF-deprived sympathetic neurons is a reversible event. J Cell Biol 1999;144:883–9.

42. Susin SA, Lorenzo HK, Zamzami N, et al. Molecular characterization of mitochondrial apoptosis-inducing factor [see comments]. Nature 1999;397:441–6.

43. Susin SA, Zamzami N, Castedo M, et al. Bcl-2 inhibits the mitochondrial release of an apoptogenic protease. J Exp Med 1996;184:1331–41.

44. Krajewski S, Krajewska M, Ellerby LM, et al. Release of caspase-9 from mitochondria during neuronal apoptosis and cerebral ischemia. Proc Natl Acad Sci USA 1999;96:5752–7.

45. Jürgensmeier JM, Xie ZH, Deveraux QL, Ellerby LM, Bredesen DE, Reed JC. Bax directly induces release of cytochrome c from isolated mitochondria. Proc Natl Acad Sci USA 1998;95:4997–5002.

46. Rosse T, Olivier R, Monney L, et al. Bcl-2 prolongs cell survival after Bax-induced release of cytochrome c [see comments]. Nature 1998;391:496–9.

47. Vander Heiden MG, Chandel NS, Schumacker PT, Thompson CB. Bcl-xL prevents cell death following growth factor withdrawal by facilitating mitochondrial ATP/ADP exchange. Mol Cell 1999;3:159–67.

48. Marzo I, Brenner C, Zamzami N, et al. Bax and adenine nucleotide translocator cooperate in the mitochondrial control of apoptosis. Science 1998;281:2027–31.

49. Antonsson B, Conti F, Ciavatta A, et al. Inhibition of Bax channel-forming activity by Bcl-2. Science 1997;277:370–2.

50. Antonsson B, Montessuit S, Lauper S, Eskes R, Martinou JC. Bax oligomerization is required for channel-forming activity in liposomes and to trigger cytochrome c release from mitochondria. Biochem J 2000;345(Pt 2):271–8.

51. Shimizu S, Narita M, Tsujimoto Y. Bcl-2 family proteins regulate the release of apoptogenic cytochrome c by the mitochondrial channel VDAC [see comments]. Nature 1999;399:483–7.

52. Basanez G, Nechushtan A, Drozhinin O, et al. Bax, but not Bcl-xL, decreases the lifetime of planar phospholipid bilayer membranes at subnanomolar concentrations. Proc Natl Acad Sci USA 1999;96:5492–7.

53. Marzo I, Brenner C, Zamzami N, et al. The permeability transition pore complex: a target for apoptosis regulation by caspases and bcl-2–related proteins. J Exp Med 1998;187:1261–71.

54. Shimizu S, Eguchi Y, Kamiike W, et al. Bcl-2 prevents apoptotic mitochondrial dysfunction by regulating proton flux. Proc Natl Acad Sci USA 1998;95:1455–9.

55. Decaudin D, Geley S, Hirsch T, et al. Bcl-2 and Bcl-XL antagonize the mitochondrial dysfunction preceding nuclear apoptosis induced by chemotherapeutic agents. Cancer Res 1997;57:62–7.

56. Zamzami N, Susin SA, Marchetti P, Hirsch T, Gomez-Monterrey I, Castedo M, Kroemer G. Mitochondrial control of nuclear apoptosis [see comments]. J Exp Med 1996;183:1533–44.

57. Pastorino JG, Chen ST, Tafani M, Snyder JW, Farber JL. The overexpression of Bax produces cell death upon induction of the mitochondrial permeability transition. J Biol Chem 1998;273:7770–5.

58. Pastorino JG, Tafani M, Rothman RJ, Marcinkeviciute A, Hoek JB, Farber JL, Marcinkeviciute A. Functional consequences of the sustained or transient activation by Bax of the mitochondrial permeability transition pore. J Biol Chem 1999;274:31734–9.

59. Lemasters JJ, Nieminen AL, Qian T, et al. The mitochondrial permeability transition in cell death: a common mechanism in necrosis, apoptosis and autophagy. Biochim Biophys Acta 1998;1366:177–96.

60. Hu Y, Benedict MA, Wu D, Inohara N, Nunez G. Bcl-XL interacts with Apaf-1 and inhibits Apaf-1-dependent caspase-9 activation. Proc Natl Acad Sci USA 1998;95:4386–91.

61. Pan G, O'Rourke K, Dixit VM. Caspase-9, Bcl-XL. Apaf-1 form a ternary complex. J Biol Chem 1998;273:5841–5.

62. Enari M, Sakahira H, Yokoyama H, Okawa K, Iwamatsu A, Nagata S. A caspase-activated DNase that degrades DNA during apoptosis, its inhibitor ICAD. Nature 1998;391:43–50.

63. Liu X, Li P, Widlak P, Zou H, Luo X, Garrard WT, Wang X. The 40-kDa subunit of DNA fragmentation factor induces DNA fragmentation and chromatin

condensation during apoptosis. Proc Natl Acad Sci USA 1998;95:8461–6.

64. Rasola A, Farahi-Far D, Hofman P, Rossi B. Lack of internucleosomal DNA fragmentation is related to Cl(⁻) efflux impairment in hematopoietic cell apoptosis. FASEB J 1999;13:1711–23.

65. Buja LM, Eigenbrodt ML, Eigenbrodt EH. Apoptosis and necrosis. Basic types and mechanisms of cell death. Arch Pathol Lab Med 1993;117:1208–14.

66. Torriglia A, Perani P, Brossas JY, Chaudun E, Treton J, Courtois Y, Counis MF. L-DNase II, a molecule that links proteases and endonucleases in apoptosis, derives from the ubiquitous serpin leukocyte elastase inhibitor. Mol Cell Biol 1998;18:3612–19.

67. Daugas E, Susin SA, Zamzami N, et al. Mitochondrio-nuclear translocation of AIF in apoptosis and necrosis. FASEB J 2000;14:729–39.

68. Casiano CA, Tan EM. Antinuclear autoantibodies: probes for defining proteolytic events associated with apoptosis. Mol Biol Rep 1996;23:211–16.

69. Duband-Goulet I, Courvalin JC, Buendia B. LBR, a chromatin and lamin binding protein from the inner nuclear membrane is proteolyzed at late stages of apoptosis. J Cell Sci 1998;111(Pt 10):1441–51.

70. Han Z, Malik N, Carter T, Reeves WH, Wyche JH, Hendrickson EA. DNA-dependent protein kinase is a target for a CPP32-like apoptotic protease. J Biol Chem 1996;271:25035–40.

71. Song Q, Lees-Miller SP, Kumar S, et al. DNA-dependent protein kinase catalytic subunit: a target for an ICE-like protease in apoptosis. EMBO J 1996;15:3238–46.

72. Tewari M, Quan LT, O'Rourke K, et al. Yama/CPP32 beta, a mammalian homolog of CED-3, is a CrmA-inhibitable protease that cleaves the death substrate poly(ADP-ribose) polymerase. Cell 1995;81:801–9.

73. Casciola-Rosen LA, Miller DK, Anhalt GJ, Rosen A. Specific cleavage of the 70-kDa protein component of the U1 small nuclear ribonucleoprotein is a characteristic biochemical feature of apoptotic cell death. J Biol Chem 1994;269:30757–60.

74. Hegyi L, Hardwick SJ, Mitchinson MJ, Skepper JN. The presence of apoptotic cells in human atherosclerotic lesions. Am J Pathol 1997;150:371–3.

75. Kockx MM, Muhring J, Knaapen MW, De Meyer GR. RNA synthesis and splicing interferes with DNA in situ end labeling techniques used to detect apoptosis. Am J Pathol 1998;152:885–8.

76. Kanoh M, Takemura G, Misao J, et al. Significance of myocytes with positive DNA in situ nick end-labeling (TUNEL) in hearts with dilated cardiomyopathy: not apoptosis but DNA repair. Circulation 1999;99:2757–64.

77. Adolph S, Hameister H. In situ nick translation of metaphase chromosomes with biotin-labeled d-UTP. Hum Genet 1985;69:117–21.

78. Murer-Orlando ML, Peterson AC. In situ nick translation of human and mouse chromosomes detected with a biotinylated nucleotide. Exp Cell Res 1985;157:322–34.

79. Lutgens E, Daemen M, Kockx M, et al. Atherosclerosis in APOE*3-Leiden transgenic mice:from proliferative to atheromatous stage. Circulation 1999;99:276–83.

80. Lutgens E, de Muinck ED, Kitslaar PJ, Tordoir JH, Wellens HJ, Daemen MJ. Biphasic pattern of cell turnover characterizes the progression from fatty streaks to ruptured human atherosclerotic plaques. Cardiovasc Res 1999;41:473–9.

81. Kolodgie FD, Narula J, Burke AP, et al. Localization of apoptotic macrophages at the site of plaque rupture in sudden coronary death. Am J Pathol 2000;157:1259–68.

82. Bennett MR, Evan GI, Newby AC. Deregulated expression of the c-myc oncogene abolishes inhibition of proliferation of rat vascular smooth muscle cells by serum reduction, interferon-gamma, heparin, cyclic nucleotide analogues and induces apoptosis. Circ Res 1994;74:525–36.

83. Bochaton-Piallat ML, Gabbiani F, Redard M, Desmouliere A, Gabbiani G. Apoptosis participates in cellularity regulation during rat aortic intimal thickening. Am J Pathol 1995;146:1059–64.

84. Boyle JJ, Bowyer DE, Proudfoot D, Weisberg PL, Bennet MR. Human monocyte/macrophages induce human vascular smooth muscle cell apoptosis in culture. Circulation 1998;98:598.

85. Arroyo LH, Lee RT. Mechanisms of plaque rupture: mechanical and biologic interactions. Cardiovasc Res 1999;41:369–75.

86. Davies MJ. Stability and instability: two faces of coronary atherosclerosis. The Paul Dudley White Lecture 1995. Circulation 1996;94:2013–20.

87. Libby P. Molecular bases of acute coronary syndromes. Circulation 1993;91:2844–50.

88. Libby P, Geng YJ, Aikawa M, et al. Macrophages and atherosclerotic plaque stability. Curr Opin Lipidol 1996;7:330–5.

89. van der Wal AC, Becker AE. Atherosclerotic plaque rupture – pathologic basis of plaque stability and instability. Cardiovasc Res 1999;41:334–44.

90. Galis ZS, Sukhova GK, Lark MW, Libby P. Increased expression of matrix metalloproteinases and matrix degrading activity in vulnerable regions of human atherosclerotic plaques. J Clin Invest 1994;94:2493–503.

91. Newby AC, Zaltsman AB. Fibrous cap formation or destruction – the critical importance of vascular

smooth muscle cell proliferation, migration and matrix formation. Cardiovasc Res 1999;41:345–60.

92. Rekhter MD. Collagen synthesis in atherosclerosis: too much and not enough. Cardiovasc Res 1999;41:376–84.

93. Ang AH, Tachas G, Campbell JH, Bateman JF, Campbell GR. Collagen synthesis by cultured rabbit aortic smooth-muscle cells. Alteration with phenotype. Biochem J 1990;265:461–9.

94. Rekhter MD, Gordon D. Cell proliferation and collagen synthesis are two independent events in human atherosclerotic plaques. J Vasc Res 1994;31:280–6.

95. Martinet W, Schrijvers DM, De Meyer GR, Thielemans J, Knaapen MW, Herman AG, Kockx MM. Gene expression profiling of apoptosis-related genes in human atherosclerosis: upregulation of death-associated protein kinase. Arterioscler Thromb Vasc Biol 2002;22:2023–9.

96. Deiss LP, Feinstein E, Berissi H, Cohen O, Kimchi A. Identification of a novel serine/threonine kinase and a novel 15-kD protein as potential mediators of the gamma interferon-induced cell death. Genes Dev 1995;9:15–30.

97. Cohen O, Feinstein E, Kimchi A. DAP-kinase is a Ca^{2+}/calmodulin-dependent, cytoskeletal-associated protein kinase, with cell death-inducing functions that depend on its catalytic activity. EMBO J 1997;16:998–1008.

98. Cohen O, Inbal B, Kissil JL, et al. DAP-kinase participates in TNF-α and Fas-induced apoptosis and its function requires the death domain. J Cell Biol 1999;146:141–8.

99. Raveh T, Berissi H, Eisenstein M, Spivak T, Kimchi A. A functional genetic screen identifies regions at the C-terminal tail and death-domain of death-associated protein kinase that are critical for its proapoptotic activity. Proc Natl Acad Sci USA 2000;97:1572–7.

100. Yamamoto M, Takahashi H, Nakamura T, et al. Developmental changes in distribution of death-associated protein kinase mRNAs. J Neurosci Res 1999;58:674–83.

101. Schissel SL, Tweedie-Hardman J, Rapp JH, Graham G, Williams KJ, Tabas I. Rabbit aorta and human atherosclerotic lesions hydrolyze the sphingomyelin of retained low-density lipoprotein. Proposed role for arterial-wall sphingomyelinase in subendothelial retention and aggregation of atherogenic lipoproteins. J Clin Invest 1996;98:1455–64.

102. Miyashita T, Reed JC. Tumor suppressor p53 is a direct transcriptional activator of the human bax gene. Cell 1995;80:293–9.

103. Iacopetta B, Wysocki S, Norman P, House A. The p53 tumour suppressor gene is overexpressed but not mutated in human atherosclerotic tissue. Int J Oncol 1995;7:399–402.

104. Woo RA, McLure KG, Lees-Miller SP, Rancourt DE, Lee PW. DNA-dependent protein kinase acts upstream of p53 in response to DNA damage. Nature 1998;394:700–4.

105. Kockx MM, De Meyer GR, Buyssens N, Knaapen MW, Bult H, Herman AG. Cell composition, replication, apoptosis in atherosclerotic plaques after 6 months of cholesterol withdrawal. Circ Res 1998;83:378–87.

106. Ross R, Wight TN, Strandness E, Thiele B. Human atherosclerosis. I. Cell constitution and characteristics of advanced lesions of the superficial femoral artery. Am J Pathol 1984;114:79–93.

107. Stehbens WE. Cerebral atherosclerosis. Intimal proliferation and atherosclerosis in the cerebral arteries. Arch Pathol 1975;99:582–91.

108. Geng YJ, Henderson LE, Levesque EB, Muszynski M, Libby P. Fas is expressed in human atherosclerotic intima and promotes apoptosis of cytokine-primed human vascular smooth muscle cells. Arterioscler Thromb Vasc Biol 1997;17:2200–8.

109. Cai W, Devaux B, Schaper W, Schaper J. The role of Fas/APO 1 and apoptosis in the development of human atherosclerotic lesions. Atherosclerosis 1997;131:177–86.

110. Dong C, Wilson JE, Winters GL, McManus BM. Human transplant coronary artery disease: pathological evidence for Fas-mediated apoptotic cytotoxicity in allograft arteriopathy. Lab Invest 1996;74:921–31.

111. Best PJ, Hasdai D, Sangiorgi G, Schwartz RS, Holmes DR, Jr., Simari RD, Lerman A. Apoptosis. Basic concepts and implications in coronary artery disease. Arterioscler Thromb Vasc Biol 1999;19:14–22.

112. Flynn PD, Byrne CD, Baglin TP, Weissberg PL, Bennett MR. Thrombin generation by apoptotic vascular smooth muscle cells. Blood 1997;89:4378–84.

113. Cromheeke KM, Kockx MM, De Meyer GR, et al. Inducible nitric oxide synthase colocalizes with signs of lipid oxidation/peroxidation in human atherosclerotic plaques. Cardiovasc Res 1999;43:744–54.

114. Nguyen T, Brunson D, Crespi CL, Penman BW, Wishnok JS, Tannenbaum SR. DNA damage and mutation in human cells exposed to nitric oxide in vitro. Proc Natl Acad Sci USA 1992;89:3030–4.

115. Wink DA, Kasprzak KS, Maragos CM, et al. DNA deaminating ability and genotoxicity of nitric oxide and its progenitors. Science 1991;254:1001–3.

116. deRojas-Walker T, Tamir S, Ji H, Wishnok JS, Tannenbaum SR. Nitric oxide induces oxidative damage in addition to deamination in macrophage DNA. Chem Res Toxicol 1995;8:473–7.

117. Martinet W, Knaapen MW, De Meyer GR, Herman AG, Kockx MM. Elevated levels of oxidative DNA damage and DNA repair enzymes in human atherosclerotic plaques. Circulation 2002;106:927–32.

118. White E. Tumour biology. p53, guardian of Rb. Nature 1994;371:21–2.
119. Ihling C, Menzel G, Wellens E, Monting JS, Schaefer HE, Zeiher AM. Topographical association between the cyclin-dependent kinases inhibitor P21, p53 accumulation, cellular proliferation in human atherosclerotic tissue. Arterioscler Thromb Vasc Biol 1997;17:2218–24.
120. Messmer UK, Reed UK, Brune B. Bcl-2 protects macrophages from nitric oxide-induced apoptosis. J Biol Chem 1996;271:20192–7.
121. Du XL, Sui GZ, Stockklauser-Farber K, et al. Introduction of apoptosis by high proinsulin and glucose in cultured human umbilical vein endothelial cells is mediated by reactive oxygen species. Diabetologia 1998;41:249–56.
122. Guevara NV, Kim HS, Antonova EI, Chan L. The absence of p53 accelerates atherosclerosis by increasing cell proliferation in vivo. Nat Med 1999;5:335–9.
123. Althaus FR, Richter C. ADP ribosylation of proteins – enzymology and biological significance. Mol Biol Biochem Biophys 1998;37:1–125.
124. de Murcia G, Menissier dM. Poly(ADP-ribose) polymerase: a molecular nick-sensor. Trends Biochem Sci 1994;19:172–6.
125. Szabo C, Zingarelli B, O'Connor M, Salzman AL. DNA strand breakage, activation of poly (ADP-ribose) synthetase, cellular energy depletion are involved in the cytotoxicity of macrophages and smooth muscle cells exposed to peroxynitrite. Proc Natl Acad Sci USA 1996;93:1753–8.
126. Henry Y, Lepoivre M, Drapier JC, Ducrocq C, Boucher JL, Guissani A. EPR characterization of molecular targets for NO in mammalian cells and organelles. FASEB J 1993;7:1124–34.
127. Kim YM, Talanian RV, Billiar TR. Nitric oxide inhibits apoptosis by preventing increases in caspase-3-like activity via two distinct mechanisms. J Biol Chem 1997;272:31138–48.
128. Mannick JB, Hausladen A, Liu L, et al. Fas-induced caspase denitrosylation. Science 1999;284:651–4.
129. Melino G, Bernassola F, Knight RA, Corasaniti MT, Nistico G, Finazzi-Agro A. S-nitrosylation regulates apoptosis. Nature 1997;388:432–3.
130. Dimmeler S, Haendeler J, Nehls M, Zeiher AM. Suppression of apoptosis by nitric oxide via inhibition of interleukin-1beta-converting enzyme (ICE)-like and cysteine protease protein (CPP)-32-like proteases. J Exp Med 1997;185:601–7.
131. Dimmeler S, Haendeler J, Sause A, Zeiher AM. Nitric oxide inhibits APO-1/Fas-mediated cell death. Cell Growth Differ 1998;9:415–22.
132. Platt N, da Silva RP, Gordon S. Recognizing death: the phagocytosis of apoptotic cells. Trends Cell Biol 1998;8:365–72.
133. Savill J. Recognition and phagocytosis of cells undergoing apoptosis. Br Med Bull 1997;53:491–508.
134. Sambrano GR, Parthasarathy S, Steinberg D. Recognition of oxidatively damaged erythrocytes by a macrophage receptor with specificity for oxidized low density lipoprotein. Proc Natl Acad Sci USA 1994;91:3265–9.
135. Sambrano GR, Steinberg D. Recognition of oxidatively damaged and apoptotic cells by an oxidized low density lipoprotein receptor on mouse peritoneal macrophages: role of membrane phosphatidylserine. Proc Natl Acad Sci USA 1995;92:1396–400.
136. Steinberg D, Lewis A. Conner Memorial Lecture. Oxidative modification of LDL and atherogenesis. Circulation 1997;95:1062–71.
137. Buttke TM, Sandstrom PA. Oxidative stress as a mediator of apoptosis. Immunol Today 1994;15:7–10.
138. Krieger M. The other side of scavenger receptors: pattern recognition for host defense. Curr Opin Lipidol 1997;8:275–80.
139. Kao J, Houck K, Fan Y, et al. Characterization of a novel tumor-derived cytokine. Endothelial-monocyte activating polypeptide II. J Biol Chem 1994;269:25106–19.
140. Knies UE, Behrensdorf HA, Mitchell CA, Deutsch U, Risau W, Drexler HC, Clauss M. Regulation of endothelial monocyte-activating polypeptide II release by apoptosis. Proc Natl Acad Sci USA 1998;95:12322–7.
141. Loegering DJ, Raley MJ, Reho TA, Eaton JW. Macrophage dysfunction following the phagocytosis of IgG-coated erythrocytes: production of lipid peroxidation products. J Leukoc Biol 1996;59:357–62.
142. Bombeli T, Karsan A, Tait JF, Harlan JM. Apoptotic vascular endothelial cells become procoagulant. Blood 1997;89:2429–42.
143. Greeno EW, Bach RR, Moldow CF. Apoptosis is associated with increased cell surface tissue factor procoagulant activity. Lab Invest 1996;75:281–9.
144. Toschi V, Gallo R, Lettino M, et al. Tissue factor modulates the thrombogenicity of human atherosclerotic plaques. Circulation 1997;95:594–9.
145. Mallat Z, Hugel B, Ohan J, Leseche G, Freyssinet JM, Tedgui A. Shed membrane microparticles with procoagulant potential in human atherosclerotic plaques: a role for apoptosis in plaque thrombogenicity. Circulation 1999;99:348–53.
146. Dimmeler S, Hermann C, Zeiher AM. Apoptosis of endothelial cells. Contribution to the pathophysio0logy of atherosclerosis? Eur Cytokine Netw 1998;9:697–8.

147. Dimmeler S, Haendeler J, Galle J, Zeiher AM. Oxidized low-density lipoprotein induces apoptosis of human endothelial cells by activation of CPP32-like proteases. A mechanistic clue to the 'response to injury' hypothesis. Circulation 1997;95:1760–3.

148. Dimmeler S, Rippmann V, Weiland U, Haendeler J, Zeiher AM. Angiotensin II induces apoptosis of human endothelial cells. Protective effect of nitric oxide. Circ Res 1997;81:970–6.

149. Lizard G, Lemaire S, Monier S, Gueldry S, Neel D, Gambert P. Induction of apoptosis and of interleukin-1beta secretion by 7beta-hydroxycholesterol and 7-ketocholesterol: partial inhibition by Bcl-2 over-expression. FEBS Lett 1997;419:276–80.

150. Polte T, Oberle S, Schroder H. Nitric oxide protects endothelial cells from tumor necrosis factor-alpha-mediated cytotoxicity: possible involvement of cyclic GMP. FEBS Lett 1997;409:46–8.

151. Buttery LD, Springall DR, Chester AH, et al. Inducible nitric oxide synthase is present within human athero-sclerotic lesions and promotes the formation and activity of peroxynitrite. Lab Invest 1996;75:77–85.

152. Esaki T, Hayashi T, Muto E, Yamada K, Kuzuya M, Iguchi A. Expression of inducible nitric oxide synthase in T lymphocytes and macrophages of cholesterol-fed rabbits. Atherosclerosis 1997;128:39–46.

153. Wilcox JN, Subramanian RR, Sundell CL, Tracey WR, Pollock JS, Harrison DG, Marsden PA. Expression of multiple isoforms of nitric oxide synthase in normal and atherosclerotic vessels. Arterioscler Thromb Vasc Biol 1997;17:2479–88.

154. Aikawa M, Rabkin E, Okada Y, et al. Lipid lowering by diet reduces matrix metalloproteinase activity and increases collagen content of rabbit atheroma: a potential mechanism of lesion stabilization. Circulation 1998;97:2433–44.

155. Martinet W, Knaapen MW, De Meyer GR, Herman AG, Kockx MM. Oxidative DNA damage and repair in experimental atherosclerosis are reversed by dietary lipid lowering. Circ Res 2001;88:733–9.

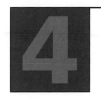

PART 4

Diagnosis

CHAPTER 11

Emerging biomarkers of instability

Sotirios Tsimikas

Specific criteria have been recently proposed to assess the relevance of plasma biomarkers in clinical care.[1] For a biomarker to have clinical utility, it should provide independent diagnostic or prognostic information, account for a significant proportion of the disease being evaluated, be accurate and reliable, provide good sensitivity, specificity and predictive value, and be available for widespread application.

Oxidative biomarkers

Oxidized low density lipoprotein

Oxidation of lipoproteins, and in particular low density lipoprotein (LDL), has been implicated as a major factor in the initiation and progression of atherosclerosis.[2] The process of lipid peroxidation involves the ability of various agents to abstract a hydrogen atom (H^+) from a methylene (carbon–carbon double bond, $C = C$) carbon. Unsaturated lipids (having one or more methylene moieties) are particularly susceptible to peroxidation in proportion to their number of methylene groups. Over the last 25 years, research from many laboratories has elucidated multiple mechanisms through which oxidized LDL (oxLDL) is atherogenic and has shown that oxidation of LDL is necessary, if not obligatory, in atherogenesis (reviewed in refs 3–5). Oxidation of LDL in the subendothelial space of the vessel wall leads to an inflammatory cascade that activates many atherogenic pathways, including the unregulated uptake of oxLDL by scavenger receptors on monocyte-derived macrophages leading to foam cell formation. Accumulation of foam cells leads to fatty streak formation, consisting primarily of cholesterol ester-laden cells, mostly derived from circulating monocytes (but also from modified smooth muscle cells) that have penetrated through the endothelial layer. Foam cell necrosis and/or apoptosis and continued accumulation of oxidized lipids in the extracellular space eventually lead to atheroma formation. The complex interplay of oxidized lipids, inflammatory processes, endothelial dysfunction, and platelet activation and thrombosis ultimately leads to plaque progression and/or disruption giving rise to clinical events. Immune mechanisms and inflammatory cells play a central role throughout all these events, resulting in atherosclerotic lesions having many features of a chronic inflammatory disease.[6]

The importance of oxLDL in the pathogenesis of atherosclerosis was initially appreciated when it was noted that oxLDL was rapidly taken up by macrophages compared to normal LDL, leading to an accelerated rate of foam cell formation. In addition, oxLDL was noted to be cytotoxic to cells and pro-inflammatory.[4] Napoli, Palinski and colleagues[7,8] have established that fatty streaks even appear during human fetal life. In fact, they documented that oxLDL was present in aortas of fetuses whose mothers were hypercholesterolemic during gestation even prior to monocyte entry into the vessel wall, suggesting that LDL oxidation is involved a priori in the recruitment of monocytes. Additionally, they showed that maternal hypercholesterolemia is an important factor in the progression of atherosclerosis of children[8] and demonstrated in animal models that altered gene expression mediates subsequent atherogenesis. Treatment of murine maternal hypercholesterolemia

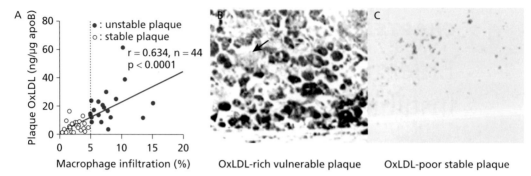

Figure 11.1 A, The presence of oxLDL compared to the extent of macrophage infiltration in stable or unstable carotid plaques (based on pathological criteria), obtained at carotid endarterectomy. B and C, Immunostaining for oxLDL in vulnerable (B) and stable (C) carotid plaques. (Reprinted from Nishi K, et al. Arterioscler Thromb Vasc Biol 2002;22:1649–54,[16] with permission from the American Heart Association.)

with antioxidants or cholestyramine reduces progression of atherosclerosis in progeny.[9,10]

Oxidized LDL is present within atherosclerotic lesions of animal models and humans.[11–14] For example, plaque specimens from human carotid and coronary arteries are significantly enriched in oxLDL[11,13] In particular, unstable plaques appear to be preferentially enriched in oxLDL (Figure 11.1),[15,16] and oxLDL in plasma has been shown to be associated with acute coronary syndromes[15,17,18] and endothelial dysfunction.[19,20] In animals, oxLDL within plaques is preferentially depleted in response to regression/antioxidant diets[21–23] and in humans oxLDL becomes depleted following treatment with statins.[24]

The association of oxidized phospholipids (oxPL) with inflammatory disorders, such as atherosclerosis and infection, is becoming more established. For example, oxPL are present on oxLDL, pneumococcal cell membranes, and apoptotic blebs.[25] oxPL are pro-inflammatory and various mechanism have evolved to bind and potentially neutralize them, such as natural monoclonal IgM autoantibodies (i.e. antibody E06)[26,27] and C-reactive protein.[25] Supporting data shows that immunization of LDLR$^{-/-}$ mice with pneumococcal vaccine results in increased titers of oxLDL-specific IgM autoantibodies and protection against atherosclerosis.[28] Several human studies have also noted an inverse association between IgM autoantibodies to oxLDL and various manifestations of cardiovascular disease.[17,29–31]

Work from our laboratory suggests that oxLDL may be imaged in the vessel wall using radiolabeled oxidation-specific antibodies, such as the murine monoclonal antibody (MAb) MDA2 and the human MAb Fab IK-17 (Figure 11.2).[12,21,32] The uptake of such antibodies is proportional to overall plaque burden, measured either by atherosclerosis surface area or aortic weight, which may allow quantitation of oxLDL in lipid-rich, "vulnerable" plaques as well as allow detection of global plaque burden.[33,34] Interestingly, regression of atherosclerosis results in significantly reduced oxLDL content in the vessel wall resulting in a proportional decrease in antibody uptake that can be quantified and detected (Figure 11.3).[21,23] If this method can be translated to human imaging, potential applications may include measurement of global oxLDL burden, measuring plaque vulnerability, assessing the efficacy of novel treatments, and screening high risk individuals.[33,34]

Although the concept of oxLDL was first described in 1979, most experimental data has been generated from in vitro studies and only in the last 10 years has it been possible to directly measure circulating oxLDL in plasma, as well as immune complexes and autoantibodies to oxLDL (Figure 11.4). This has led to a rapidly accelerating pace of new reports on the relationship of circulating oxLDL and various cardiovascular pathological processes.

oxLDL nomenclature

oxLDL is not one homogeneous entity, but may

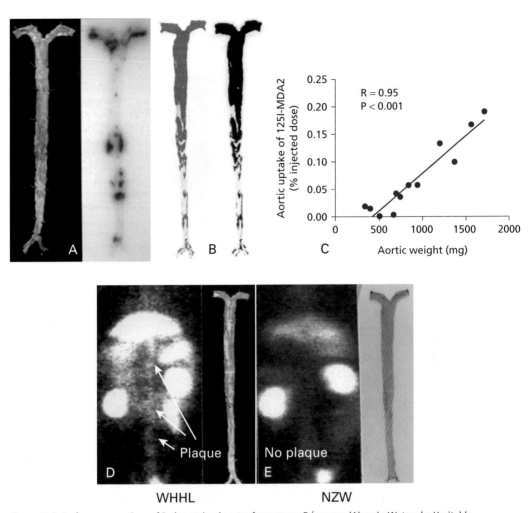

Figure 11.2 En-face preparations of Sudan-stained aortas from an apoE$^{-/-}$ mouse (A) and a Watanabe Heritable Hyperlipidemic rabbit (WHHL) (B) injected with ^{125}I-MDA2, respectively. Red color (left panels in A and B) signifies the presence of neutral lipid within the atherosclerotic plaque stained with Sudan IV and black color (right panels in A and B) in the corresponding autoradiograph signifies the presence of accumulated ^{125}I-MDA2 reflecting the presence of oxLDL. C, The relationship of ^{125}I-MDA2 uptake and plaque burden as measured by aortic weight. D and E, In vivo imaging of atherosclerotic WHHL (D) and nonatherosclerotic New Zealand White (E) rabbits with ^{99m}Tc-MDA2. (Reprinted from Tsimikas S, et al. J Nucl Cardiol 1999;6:41–53,[12] with permission from the American Society of Nuclear Cardiology.)

potentially represent tens, even hundreds, of different chemical and immunogenic modifications of both the lipid (polyunsaturated fatty acids on cholesterol esters and phospholipids) and protein moieties (apolipoprotein B-100). Because many oxLDL epitopes have not been well characterized, confusion with terminology has been created in the literature as most investigators have been using the term "oxLDL" in a generic sense for many different types of oxLDL. With the development of specific oxLDL assays based on monoclonal antibodies, the opportunity now exists to specifically describe different types of oxLDL. For this reason, we have suggested that investigators use the antibody used in their assay next to oxLDL (i.e. oxLDL-E06[35–37]) to minimize confusion in the literature. In this chapter, this type of terminology will be used to describe various oxLDL assays.

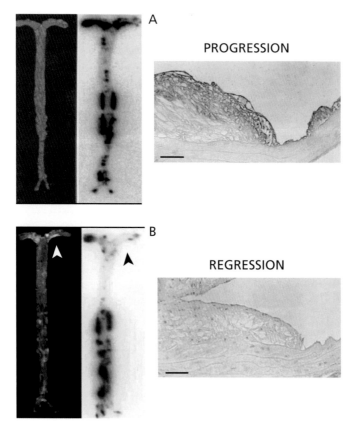

A

PROGRESSION

B

REGRESSION

Figure 11.3 En-face preparations of Sudan-stained aortas (left) and corresponding autoradiographs (right) from LDLR$^{-/-}$ mice injected with ^{125}I-MDA2. A, Aorta from a mouse fed a high fat/cholesterol diet (Progression) showing concordance of lipid staining (left panel) and ^{125}I-MDA2 uptake (right panel). Corresponding immunohistochemical staining with guinea pig antiserum MAL2 shows extensive oxLDL staining (red) within the atherosclerotic lesions. B, Aorta from a mouse after being switched to a normal mouse chow diet (Regression) for 6 months showing diminished or absent ^{125}I-MDA2 uptake (arrowheads) in some areas of lipid staining, signifying the removal of oxLDL before complete plaque regression has occurred. Corresponding immunohistochemical staining shows preferential depletion of oxLDL, even though cholesterol crystals are still present within the lesion. Scale bar = 100 μm. (Reprinted from Tsimikas S, et al. Arterioscler Thromb Vasc Biol 2000;20:689–97,[21] with permission from the American Heart Association.)

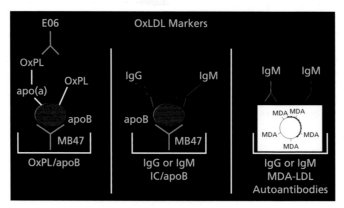

Figure 11.4 Schematic representation of one method of performing oxLDL assays. A, Direct measure of oxLDL termed oxLDL-E06. This technique captures apolipoprotein B-100 (apoB-100) from plasma and determines the presence of oxidized phospholipids (oxPL) on apoB-100 (oxPL/apoB). The antibody E06 detects oxPL present on both apoB-100 and apolipoprotein (a) [apo(a)]. B, Measurement of apoB-immune complexes (IC) by capturing apoB-100 and detecting the presence of human autoantibodies on apoB-100 (IC/apoB). C, Measurement of autoantibodies to MDA-LDL. Autoantibodies to other epitopes of oxLDL may be measured by plating the appropriate antigen on the bottom of the microtiter plate (i.e. copper oxidized LDL). (Reprinted from Tsimikas S, et al. Circulation 2004;110:1406–12,[36] with permission from the American Heart Association.)

Plasma oxLDL assays

Three major oxLDL plasma enzyme-linked immu-noabsorbent (ELISA) assays have been developed based on murine MAbs DLH3, 4E6, and E06 that bind various types of oxLDL. Itabe et al.[38] immunized mice with homogenates of human atherosclerotic plaques and cloned out IgM MAb DLH3 which binds oxidized phosphatidylcholine (the exact structure(s) have not been fully delineated) on LDL. DLH3 does not need apoB for recognition, suggesting that it detects a modified oxPL moiety. A sandwich ELISA has been developed with this anti-body by plating DLH3 on the bottom of the a microtiter plate, adding isolated LDL, and using a polyclonal anti-apoB antibody to detecting the captured apoB (oxLDL-DLH3).[39] A reference oxLDL is used to generate a standard curve and the assay results are presented as units/ml, where 1 unit equals the absorbance of 250 ng of the reference oxLDL. Potential limitations of this assay include the fact that the reference oxLDL may not be the same from batch to batch and possibly the potential need to isolate LDL from each patient by centrifugal ultracentrifugation which may limit widespread applicability.[35]

Holvoet et al. have described several murine MAbs for measuring malondialdehyde (MDA)-LDL and copper-oxLDL.[18,40,41] Recently, MAb 4E6 has been developed into a commercial assay (Mercodia, Inc, Uppsala, Sweden). 4E6 binds to a derivatized apoB moiety when at least 60 lysine groups have been modified, but the specific epitope it binds to has not been characterized as it binds to both oxLDL and MDA-LDL.[42,43] This assay can be run as a sandwich assay similar to the DLH3 assay. A limitation of this assay is the high correlation between plasma LDL and oxLDL-4E6 ($r = 0.65-0.70$ in several studies),[44–48] suggesting cross-reactivity with normal LDL epitopes. Alternatively, it is pos-sible that there is a constant relationship of LDL concentration and generation of oxLDL, although this is less likely, particularly since LDL is cleared over days to weeks whereas oxLDL is cleared in hours (reviewed in ref. 35). More recently, this assay has been modified as a competition assay by plating a reference oxLDL, then adding the plasma sample together with MAb 4E6. However, the strong association with LDL is still present.[45]

Our laboratory has used the natural murine MAb E06 to develop an in vitro assay of oxLDL, termed oxLDL-E06 (Figure 11.4). oxLDL-E06 is a measure of the content of oxPL per apoB-100 par-ticle as detected by MAb E06, which specifically binds to the phosphorylcholine head group of oxidized but not native phospholipids (reviewed in Tsimikas[17,49] and references therein). This assay is performed by capturing a constant, saturating amount of each patient's plasma apoB-100 on a microtiter plate with antibody MB-47, which spe-cifically binds to human apoB-100. Because each plate binds an equal and minute fraction of each patient's apoB-100, it is by definition independ-ent of LDL-cholesterol levels.[17,36,49] Biotinylated E06 is then added to detect the presence of oxPL on LDL that were captured on the plate, e.g. to yield oxPL/apoB. This methodology allows for two complementary but unique sets of measurements: (i) it quantitates the number of oxPL epitopes per apoB-100 particle [oxPL/apoB], and (ii) when oxPL/apoB is multiplied by (independently mea-sured) plasma apoB-100 levels, one derives total apoB-oxPL levels present on all apoB-100 particles. This assay is currently read out in relative light units per 100 milliseconds (RLU).

Circulating oxLDL studies

Preclinical atherosclerosis

Elevated circulating oxLDL levels have been associ-ated with increased carotid intima-media thickness in several studies in patients without overt cardio-vascular disease, such as in asymptomatic subjects with relatives with familial hypercholesterolemia, asymptomatic middle aged males, and even in children.[47,48,50–52] Interestingly, several studies have also shown an inverse correlation between oxLDL levels and HDL, consistent with HDL's antioxid-ative properties potentially emanating from its enrichment in several antioxidant enzymes such as platelet activating factor acetylhydrolase, para-oxonase and lecithin cholesterol acyl transferase.[3] Increased oxLDL levels have been recently associ-ated with the metabolic syndrome and small dense LDL.[44,45,53]

Endothelial dysfunction

oxPL are known to be highly inflammatory and induce vasoconstriction,[54] therefore it is possible that removal of such oxPL contributes to rapid improvement in endothelial function. This concept is supported by several studies showing improvement in coronary[55] and brachial endothelial function[19] with LDL apheresis or lovastatin treatment.[20] For example, in a study assessing the effects of LDL apheresis on acetylcholine-induced brachial artery vasodilatation, Tamai et al.[19] have shown improvement within 4 hours of the end of LDL apheresis. Interestingly, the best correlate of improvement was reduced plasma oxLDL-DLH3 levels. In a similar study, LDL apheresis significantly decreased (by 61%) plasma MDA-LDL.[56] In a human coronary regression study with lovastatin, Penny et al.[20] have shown that oxLDL-E06 was the best correlate of acetylcholine-induced coronary vasodilatation. Matsumoto et al.[57] have recently shown in patients with normal coronary arteries that oxLDL-DLH3 independently predicts coronary vasomotor tone, both in the epicardial segments and in the microcirculation, measured by Doppler wire in the left anterior descending artery. Kugiyama et al.[58] have also shown a strong correlation between elevated oxLDL-DLH3 levels and vasospastic angina as confirmed by intracoronary acetylcholine infusion.

Stable coronary artery disease

Several groups have demonstrated an association with oxLDL, measured by antibodies 4E6 and DLH3, and coronary artery disease (CAD).[42,45,53,59] Toshima et al. have shown that plasma oxLDL levels were elevated in patients with CAD compared to normal controls and that the receiver operating curves showed that the area under the curve was higher for oxLDL than for total cholesterol, apoB, HDL, and triglyceride levels.[59] Similarly, Holvoet et al. also showed that oxLDL levels were higher in patients with CAD[42] or CAD-risk equivalent and the metabolic syndrome[44,45] and that the oxLDL levels provided additive information above and beyond well accepted cardiovascular risk factors. In this study and others, oxLDL-4E6 correlated with both hypercholesterolemia and CRP.[45]

Acute coronary syndromes

Holvoet et al. initially showed that MDA-LDL levels were significantly higher in patients presenting with chest pain, and in conjunction with troponin levels a high predictive value was obtained for diagnosing

acute myocardial infarction (MI).[18] Ehara and colleagues[15] showed that circulating oxLDL-DLH3 levels, measured on isolated LDL rather than plasma, reflected the presence of immunochemically detected oxLDL in coronary atherectomy specimens, and to some extent, appeared to differentiate the severity of the underlying clinical presentation (Figure 11.5).[15] We extended these observations by showing that a specific temporal pattern occurs in oxLDL-E06 levels following acute coronary syndrome (ACS) where significant increases in oxLDL-E06 were noted at hospital discharge (54% increase above baseline levels) and at 1 month (36%) and subsequently declined near basal levels by 7 months. oxLDL-E06 correlated extremely well with Lp(a) in the entire cohort of patients ($r = 0.91$, $P < 0.0001$) and strongly paralleled the acute rise in lipoprotein (a) [Lp(a)] in the MI group, suggesting that toxic oxPL are preferentially bound to and are transported by Lp(a).[17,60]

These studies in total suggest that elevated circulating oxLDL levels at the time of presentation and at follow-up strongly reflect the presence of ACS. It also emphasizes that in a setting of plaque disruption and MI these values will be elevated reflecting an acute phase response and cannot be used to ascertain baseline values.

Percutaneous coronary intervention

Only one study to date has evaluated the role of oxLDL in percutaneous coronary intervention (PCI). oxLDL-E06 and Lp(a) were measured in 141 patients with stable angina pectoris undergoing PCI with serial venous blood samples drawn pre-PCI, post-PCI, and at 6 and 24 hours, 3 days, 1 week, and 1, 3 and 6 months. oxLDL-E06 and Lp(a) levels significantly increased immediately post-PCI by 36% ($P < 0.0001$) and 64% ($P < 0.0001$), respectively, and returned to baseline by 6 hours (Figure 11.6).[49] In vitro immunoprecipitation of Lp(a) from selected plasma samples showed that almost all of the oxPL detected by E06 was bound to Lp(a) at all timepoints, except in the post-PCI sample, suggesting independent release and subsequent re-association of oxPL with Lp(a) by 6 hours. A strong correlation was noted between oxLDL-E06 and Lp(a). oxLDL autoantibody titers decreased initially and apoB-immune complex levels increased acutely in a classical anamnestic immunization pattern. These data

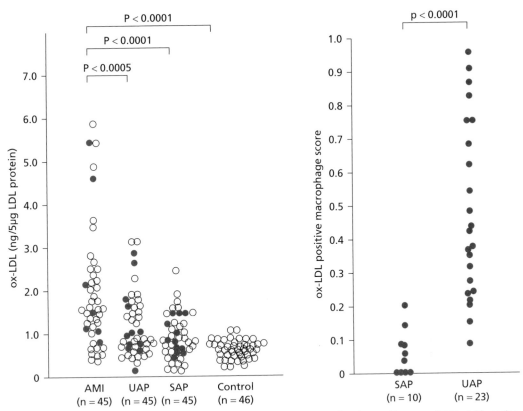

Figure 11.5 Measurement of oxLDL-DLH3 in patients presenting with acute MI (AMI), unstable angina (UAP), stable angina (SAP), and in controls. Specimens immunostained for oxLDL retrieved during atherectomy reveal a higher percentage of immunopositive macrophages in UAP. (Reprinted from Ehara S, et al. Circulation 2001;103:1955–60,[15] with permission from the American Heart Association.)

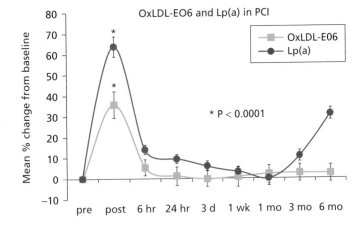

Figure 11.6 Mean percent change from pre-PCI levels in oxLDL-E06 and Lp(a) levels following PCI. *P < 0.001 compared to other timepoints. (Reprinted from Tsimikas S, et al. Circulation 2004;109:3164–70,[49] with permission from the American Heart Association.)

suggest that oxPL that are released or generated during PCI are transferred to Lp(a) suggesting that Lp(a) may contribute acutely to a protective innate immune response. These findings suggest that release and/or generation of oxLDL during PCI may have detrimental effects on coronary blood flow and thrombosis and provides impetus for further studies in this area.

Response to lipid-lowering therapies

Data on the changes in oxLDL in response to therapeutic modalities, particularly statins, is relatively sparse. In the MIRACL study, oxLDL-E06 and Lp(a) levels were measured in 2341 patients at baseline and after 16 weeks' treatment with atorvastatin 80 mg/day or placebo. Compared to baseline values, levels of total apoB-oxPL on all apoB particles were significantly reduced (−29.4%) in the atorvastatin group.[36] However, despite a smaller pool of apoB, the content of oxPL in the remaining individual apoB particles (oxPL/apoB) was increased and associated with increased Lp(a) levels, which we have recently shown bind such oxPL.[17,49,60] Additional unpublished data from our laboratory in murine, rabbit and cynomolgus monkey experiments show that following regression of established atherosclerosis by dietary-induced lipid lowering, there are similar increases in oxPL/apoB plasma levels in conjunction with marked depletion of oxPL epitopes from the vessel wall detected by immunostaining with antibody E06. Thus, in association with lesion regression, there was a clear net efflux of oxPL from the vessel wall at a time when the oxPL/apoB ratio in plasma was increased. This suggests the hypothesis that mobilization of oxPL, binding to Lp(a), and ultimate clearance represents a novel mechanism contributing to rapid plaque stabilization induced by atorvastatin. De Caterina et al. have also shown that simvastatin reduces plasma oxLDL-4E6 levels in patients treated for hypercholesterolemia, and interestingly no further effect of vitamin E was noted.[61]

Two studies with LDL apheresis have shown that oxLDL-DLH3 and MDA-LDL levels are significantly and acutely reduced by apheresis.[19,56]

oxLDL in risk prediction

The majority of studies measuring oxLDL in plasma have focused on its ability to provide diagnostic information. Only recently have prognostic studies been performed.

Shimada et al.[62] followed 238 patients for a mean of 52 months and showed that baseline levels of oxLDL-DLH3 were significantly higher in patients with subsequent development of cardiac death, nonfatal MI, and unstable angina. Unfortunately, follow-up levels were not measured to ascertain the true effect of the oxLDL measures. Recently, baseline elevated oxLDL-DLH3 levels have been shown to predict mortality in patients with congestive heart failure.[63]

Other clinical scenarios

oxLDL-DLH3 has also been shown to be elevated in acute stroke and in Alzheimer's disease,[64,65] and oxLDL-4E6 to provide both diagnostic and prognostic information in transplant-associated atherosclerosis.[43,66]

In summary, the pace of discovery in the field of measuring plasma oxLDL levels is rapidly accelerating. It is now well established that oxLDL is associated with and plays a causal role in many pathophysiological processes associated with human atherogenesis and acute coronary syndromes. In the near future, further data will be required to determine its ability to provide independent diagnostic and prognostic information above and beyond traditional and other emerging risk factors before it can be incorporated into clinical decision making.

Isoprostanes

Isoprostanes are free-radical catalyzed isomers of cyclooxygenase-derived enzymatic products. They are derived in vivo from nonenzymatic peroxidation of polyunsaturated fatty acids (PUFA), primarily arachidonic acid.[67] Arachidonic acid and other PUFA are present in cholesteryl esters and phospholipids, which are major components of lipoprotein particles and cell membranes. Isoprostanes are released by a phospholipase activity and circulate in plasma or are excreted in urine. Theoretically, up to 64 different compounds may be generated from arachidonic acid (Figure 11.7). F2 isoprostanes have been best studied in atherosclerotic disease due to their stability as end-products of lipoprotein metabolism, specificity of the mechanism of formation, and their ability to be measured with high sensitivity and specificity with gas chromatography/mass spectrometry. Interestingly, F2 isoprostanes are not only found in inflammatory disorders but also in normal biological fluids and tissues, suggesting that lipid peroxidation occurs at a basal level under normal physiological conditions. Thus, measurement of isoprostanes does not necessarily reflect LDL oxidation.

In animal models, elevated levels of F2 isoprostanes have been associated with hypercholesterolemia

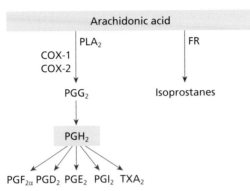

Figure 11.7 Overview of the formation of isoprostanes from arachidonic acid. Abbreviations: COX = cyclooxygenase; FR = free radicals; PLA$_2$ = phospholipase A$_2$; PGF$_{2\alpha}$ = prostaglandin F$_{2\alpha}$; PGD$_2$ = prostaglandin D$_2$; PGE$_2$ = prostaglandin E$_2$; PGG$_2$ = prostaglandin G$_2$; PGI$_2$ = prostaglandin I$_2$; TXA$_2$ = thromboxane. (Reprinted from Pratico D, et al. Trends Endocrinol Metab 2001;12:243–7,[203] with permission from Elsevier.)

and atherosclerosis and reduced levels are noted mediated by overexpression of apolipoprotein E or treatment with vitamin E concomitant with reductions in atherosclerosis.[68–71] In humans, elevated F2 isoprostanes levels are associated with hypercholesterolemia,[61,72,73] diabetes mellitus,[74,75] smoking,[76,77] renovascular hypertension,[78] and hyperhomocysteinemia.[79,80] Increased levels of isoprostanes have been detected within carotid atherosclerotic plaques and colocalize with foam cells immunocytochemically[81,82] and are correlated with unstable carotid plaques.[83] Urinary F2 isoprostane levels are strongly correlated with plasma LDL-cholesterol levels and LDL-associated isoprostanes[72,73] and have been reported to be reduced following treatment with statins, although additional studies are needed to confirm this finding.[61] Interestingly, unlike mouse models, 800 IU of vitamin E does not affect urinary isoprostane levels in humans,[61] although the doses in the mice studies were substantially higher (2000 IU/kg vs. ~10 IU/kg in humans).[69] In addition, isoprostanes are elevated in unstable angina[84] and in the coronary sinus and urine of patients undergoing PCI or thrombolysis and reperfusion during acute MI.[85–87]

Despite the promising animal and clinical data, no prognostic information is yet available. In addition, the relative sophistication required for isoprostane assays in specialized laboratories in an efficient and cost-effective manner inhibits widespread use.[88] Although ELISA kits are now available, they are limited by reduced specificity in the presence of biological fluids, such as plasma.[89] Thus, additional refinements will be required prior to widespread implementation in the clinical arena.

Cellular-derived oxidative markers

In the presence of a pro-atherogenic milieu, blood-derived monocytes enter the vessel wall after being attracted by endothelial adhesion molecules and differentiate into macrophages. Macrophages, via their possession of several scavenger receptors, take up oxLDL in an unregulated fashion and transform into foam cells. Activated macrophages and foam cells are highly pro-inflammatory and can activate T-lymphocytes, secrete cytokines and matrix-degrading metalloproteinases to destabilize lesions. Macrophage foam cells are often found in the shoulder regions of atherosclerotic plaques where the plaque is growing in an elliptical and circumferential fashion in the vessel lumen and vessel wall.[4,90] In patients with acute coronary syndromes, evidence of monocyte and neutrophil infiltration is noted in fissured and thrombosed plaques.[91,92] Many of the oxidative pathways mediated by monocyte/macrophage products, such as nitration, chlorination or tyrosyl modification, are not affected by α-tocopheral.[93–95]

Myeloperoxidase

Myeloperoxidase (MPO) is a heme peroxidase that is present in primary granules of neutrophils (5% of protein), monocytes (1%), and macrophages and is released during leukocyte activation. MPO catalyzes the production of hypochlorous acid from hydrogen peroxide and chloride anion, which are present at physiological concentrations, as follows:

$$H_2O_2 + Cl^- + H^+ \rightarrow HOCl + H_2O$$

Hypochlorous acid is a potent, metal ion-independent chlorinating oxidant that can diffuse locally to form free radicals. It is also a potent antimicrobial agent and is part of the innate immune response. Hypochlorous acid can induce lipid peroxidation, including on LDL, rendering formation of oxLDL that is a substrate for scavenger receptors.[96] In fact, oxidation products from

MPO are found on LDL isolated from atherosclerotic lesions.[94,96] Daugherty et al.[97] first showed that MPO was present in lipid-rich areas of human atherosclerotic plaques, which has been confirmed by several other groups.[91,98,99] Subsequently, Hazen and colleagues have shown that MPO can result in consumption of nitric oxide, leading to nitric-oxide derived oxidants in vitro[100–102] and in vivo.[103]

MPO deficiency is a common genetic trait with a frequency of 1 out of 2000–4000 Caucasians. MPO-deficient macrophages of humans display impaired bactericidal activity, but no major recurrent infections seem to be present in humans. Interestingly, genetic polymorphisms resulting in MPO deficiency or diminished activity are associated with lower cardiovascular risk.[104–107] However, MPO knockout mice develop more, rather than less, atherosclerosis, suggesting a disconnect between murine and human disease.[94,108]

Recent data suggests that MPO may play a mechanistic role in plaque vulnerability.[109] Libby and colleagues initially showed that MPO macrophage expression and HOCl were highly co-localized in culprit lesions of patients dying of sudden death. More recently, they showed that HOCl induced endothelial cell death by both necrosis and apoptosis at the endothelial intimal junctions, suggesting a potential mechanism between endothelial erosion and sudden death[110] (Figure 11.8).

Recent data has shown that MPO correlates with endothelial function[111] and angiographic CAD.[112] Recent studies in patients have shown that plasma levels of MPO provide diagnostic and prognostic information. In a case control study of patients with angiographically significant CAD, Zhang et al.[112] showed that blood and leukocyte MPO levels had an odds ratio of 11.9 and 20.4, respectively, for the presence of CAD in the highest vs. lowest quartiles. In a follow-up study, Brennan et al.[113] obtained MPO levels in the emergency room in 604 patients presenting with chest pain but no initial evidence of MI and showed that MPO levels predicted the subsequent in-hospital presence of elevated biomarkers of MI, independent of other markers of inflammation, such as C-reactive protein. In addition, they showed that MPO levels were strong predictors of death, MI, and revascularization at 6 month follow-up. Baldus et al.[114] studied 1090 patients with ACS derived from the CAPTURE study and showed that MPO levels were strong independent predictors of increased risk for subsequent cardiovascular events at 6-months. Interestingly, atorvastatin has been shown to reduce levels of MPO-derived oxidants, such as chlorotyrosine, suggesting specific antioxidant properties.[115]

These data suggest that MPO provides independent information on diagnosis and prognosis of patients with chest pain and may be used as an adjunct to traditional risk factors and other inflammatory markers.

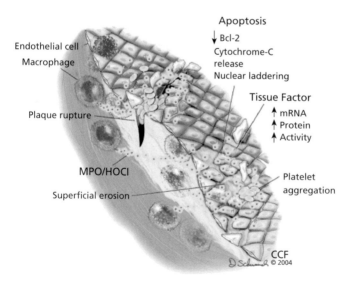

Figure 11.8 The role of myeloperoxidase to plaque vulnerability. (Reprinted from Hazen SL. Arterioscler Thromb Vasc Biol 2004;24:1143–6,[96] with permission from the American Heart Association.)

Antioxidant enzymes

Most mammalian cells synthesize several antioxidant enzymes, the principal of which is glutathione peroxidase. Glutathione peroxidase-1 detoxifies hydrogen peroxide to water, lipid peroxides to their respective alcohols, and peroxynitrite to nitrous acid. In mouse studies, reduced levels of glutathione peroxidase-1 is associated with inhibition of pro-atherogenic monocyte 5-lipoxygenase, increased cell-mediated LDL oxidation, reduced bioavailability of nitric oxide, endothelial dysfunction, and increased atherosclerosis.[116–119] A recent study in patients has shown that patients with CAD with the lowest levels of erythrocyte glutathione peroxidase-1 had a worse prognosis at an average follow-up of 1 year compared to those in the highest quartile (event rate 20.5% vs. 7.0%, respectively).[120] Interestingly, superoxide dismutase, an antioxidant enzyme that converts superoxide anion to hydrogen peroxide, and selenium levels, were not predictive of cardiovascular outcomes. More clinical research is needed before these antioxidant enzymes can be fully evaluated as biomarkers.

Lipoprotein biomarkers

Lipoprotein (a)

Lp(a) is a heavily glucosylated lipoprotein of unknown physiological function composed of apolipoprotein (a) that is covalently attached to an LDL particle via binding through a single disulfide bond on apolipoprotein B-100 (Figure 11.9). Apolipoprotein (a) is composed of kringles IV and V and an inactive protease domain that has very high homology to plasminogen (75–98%).[121] Thus, it has been hypothesized to mediate pro-thrombotic effects, although these have been demonstrated only in vitro.[122–124] Unlike plasminogen, apolipoprotein (a) does not contain kringles I–III. Kringle IV is composed of 10 subtypes, of which kringle IV-type 2 repeats are very polymorphous and may exist in 2–43 copies. Several kringle IV segments have been documented to have specific functions, such as mediating binding to apoB-100, fibrinogen, foam cells, and extracellular matrix.[122–124] Lp(a) concentrations within the vessel wall have been noted in some cases to be even higher than apoB-100.[125–127]

Lp(a) is transmitted in an autosomal dominant fashion and values range widely from essentially no measurable levels in some subjects to levels over 250 mg/dl.[121] Plasma Lp(a) levels seem to be largely determined at the transcription level of apolipoprotein (a) by its rate of synthesis in hepatocytes, rather than its rate of clearance, with smaller isoforms being secreted much faster than larger isoforms and therefore resulting in higher plasma concentrations. The number of kringle IV-type 2 repeats is moderately inversely related to plasma levels of Lp(a).[128]

Increased plasma levels of Lp(a) independently predict the presence of angiographic[129] and clinical CAD, as shown in a recent meta-analysis,[130] particularly in patients with elevated LDL cholesterol levels.[131] In general, this increased risk appears to be particularly true in high risk,[132] as opposed to low risk, populations[133] but young patients with elevated Lp(a) levels seem particularly at risk.[134,135]

Despite these potential associations between Lp(a) and cardiovascular disease, the underlying mechanisms of Lp(a) contributing to the pathogenesis of atherosclerosis are not well understood. In a series of basic[60] and clinical studies,[17,36,49] we have recently shown that Lp(a) strongly binds oxPL, as measured by antibody E06 (oxLDL-E06), which suggests both a physiological function for Lp(a) and potential explanations on its contribution to atherogenesis. For example, we have shown that Lp(a) rises acutely in a similar fashion to oxLDL-E06 following ACS[17] and immediately following PCI.[49] Additionally, we have shown in 504 patients undergoing coronary angiography that both Lp(a) and oxLDL-E06 predict the presence and extent of CAD (i.e. one-, two- and three-vessel CAD) to a similar extent and that their predictive ability for obstructive CAD are highly interdependent.[37] Interesting insights into the role of Lp(a) were recently derived from the MIRACL study[136] where we showed that high dose atorvastatin increased Lp(a) levels ~10% from baseline. Interestingly, this potential statin effect on Lp(a) has been previously noted during the treatment of hypercholesterolemia with other statins.[137–141] In association with this increase in Lp(a) was ~10% increase oxPL/apoB at the new steady state following atorvastatin treatment, despite a markedly reduced total oxPL associated with apoB-100 particles (Total apoB-oxPL).[36] We documented in other studies that these oxPL are present in both the lipid

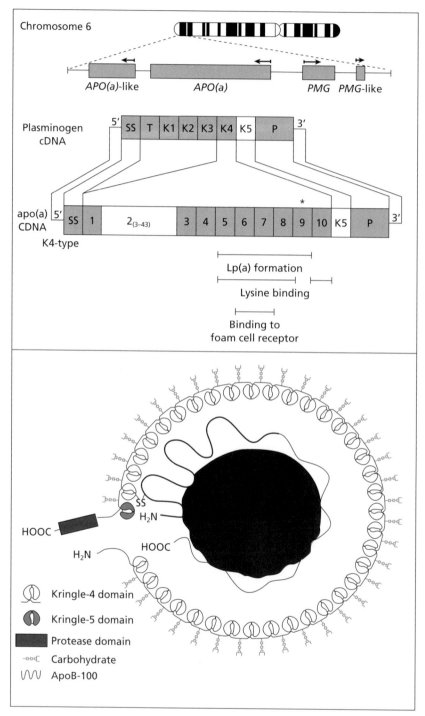

Figure 11.9 Genetic structure of apolipoprotein (a) (top panel) and structure of lipoprotein (a) (bottom panel). (Top panel reprinted from Hobbs HH, White AL. Curr Opin Lipidol 1999;10:225–36,[123] with permission.)

phase of Lp(a) and are also covalently bound to lysine residues on isolated fragments of kringle V of apolipoprotein (a) which can bind up to 2 moles of such oxPL.[17,36,49,60] These kringle V fragments have been shown to induce inflammatory responses by upregulating interleukin 8 formation from cultured human macrophages.[60,142] In all these four studies, a very strong correlation was noted between plasma levels of oxLDL-E06 and Lp(a) ($r = \sim 0.85$).

We have recently postulated that the atherogenicity of Lp(a) may be explained, in part, through its binding and transport of oxPL and that a potential physiological role of Lp(a) may be to bind and detoxify pro-inflammatory oxPL.[17,49,121,123,124] Evolutionarily, Lp(a), which is only present in humans and certain primates (hedgehogs also have an Lp(a)-like molecule derived independently through divergent evolution), may have evolved to provide protection against various oxidative stressors. For example, Lp(a) has been shown to be involved in wound healing[143] and in possibly preventing angiogenesis in tumor models.[144] Similarly, oxPL are generated in a variety of settings such as in atherosclerosis, pneumococcal infections, and apoptosis, all of which would require housekeeping clearance functions for vascular health. In that regard, Lp(a) may act similarly to C-reactive protein which has also been shown to bind pro-inflammatory oxPL.[25] Also consistent with this is that several studies have shown that Lp(a) acts as an acute phase reactant in patients with ACS.[17,49,145] Lp(a) is also known to be highly enriched in PAF-acetyl hydrolase (sevenfold higher than LDL),[146] an enzyme that potentially could detoxify such oxPL by cleaving off the oxidized fatty acid at the sn-2 position of the oxPL. However, in a milieu of elevated Lp(a) levels within a setting of chronically increased oxidative stress, such as hypercholesterolemia and other cardiovascular risk factors, Lp(a) may be pro-atherogenic, perhaps in part from its ability to bind such pro-inflammatory oxPL and deliver them to the vessel wall.[125,127]

Thus, the physiological role of Lp(a) and its mechanisms of atherogenesis are now just starting to be re-discovered. Lp(a) seems to be a viable biomarker in younger patients with multiple risk factors, especially a family history of coronary artery disease. Because it is transmitted in an autosomal dominant fashion, screening of siblings and close family members may also be warranted. Because the excess cardiovascular risk of Lp(a) seems to abate with lowering LDL cholesterol levels[131] or with aging, it seems appropriate that when patients with elevated Lp(a) levels are discovered the primary objective would be to treat the LDL (or low HDL) cholesterol aggressively with a statin, perhaps in conjunction with niacin, which is the only drug that reliably lowers Lp(a). In addition, these are the types of patients in whom early detection and treatment would derive the greatest benefit, as Lp(a) levels, except in acute phase response states, remain relatively constant throughout life and therefore these patients are exposed to the cardiovascular risk of Lp(a) starting at birth.[52] This may be similar to the risk of low HDL, which also tends to be genetically determined, but is in distinction to elevated LDL cholesterol, where, except for patients with familial hypercholesterolemia, LDL-C levels are quite low at birth ($\sim 40 - 50$ mg/dl) and gradually rise in middle age, and then tend to decrease again as patients become older.

With the recent identification of a novel potential role of Lp(a) in binding inflammatory oxPL, a new approach in studying the normal physiological role of Lp(a) and its contribution and effects on inflammation and atherogenesis can begin anew. Future studies on the atherogenicity of Lp(a) and its pathophysiological role will allow us to fine tune its usefulness as a biomarker and develop activators or inhibitors to its varied functions to prevent or treat cardiovascular disease.

LDL particle heterogeneity (small dense LDL)

The metabolic syndrome is characterized by insulin resistance, hypertension, obesity, low plasma HDL and elevated triglyceride-rich remnants and intermediate density lipoproteins. Multiple distinct subclasses of lipoprotein particles have been identified based on particle buoyant density, size, charge, and lipid and apoprotein content.[147] At least seven subclasses of LDL particles have been described based on differing densities in the range of 1.019–1.060 mg/dl and on several techniques including density gradient gel electrophoresis, ultracentrifugation, chromatographic and NMR spectroscopy techniques.[148–151] Based on these studies, two distinct LDL subclass phenotypes have been described, pattern A and pattern B. Pattern A represents larger, more buoyant LDL and pattern B small dense LDL. Small, dense LDL particles are generated in patients with the metabolic syndrome when excess triglycerides on VLDL are exchanged for cholesterol esters from LDL by cholesterol ester transfer protein (CETP), producing triglyceride-rich LDL, which then undergoes lipolysis by hepatic lipase to produce smaller and denser LDL particles (Figure 11.10). It is currently believed that different VLDL precursors lead to different pathways for small dense LDL production during remodeling of these lipoproteins in the vasculature (reviewed in Berneis and Krauss[147]). Pattern B is present in 30–35% of adult males. Genetic deter-

minants explaining 35–45% of variability have also been discovered to explain some of these findings suggesting that there are multiple genes involved, such as apo A-I, C-III, A-IV, CETP, and manganese-superoxide dismutase, in determining LDL particle size.[152] In addition, dietary fat and particularly increased carbohydrate intake can induce small dense LDL phenotype.[153,154] Small dense LDL is thought be particularly pro-atherogenic compared to more buoyant LDL because it is more amenable to oxidative modification, is easily transported to the subendothelial space, and trapped by proteoglycans.[155–159] Recent studies have also shown increased circulating oxLDL levels in patients with metabolic syndrome.[44,46] Similar events occur on HDL, resulting in a small dense HDL that is more easily

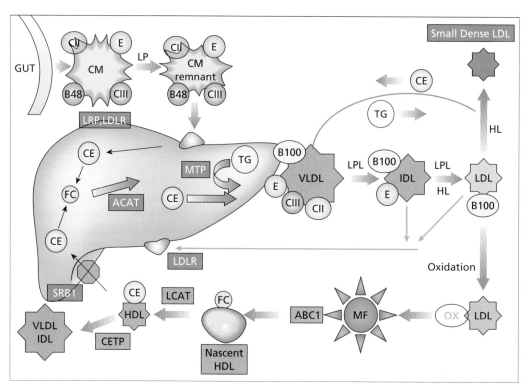

Figure 11.10 Overview of lipoprotein metabolism and generation of small dense LDL. CE = cholesterol ester; FC = free cholesterol; TG = triglycerides; LPL = lipoprotein lipase; HL = hepatic lipase; oxLDL = oxidized LDL; MΦ = macrophage; LDLR = low density lipoprotein receptor; LRP = LDL receptor-related protein receptor; CM = chylomicron; B100, B48, CII, CIII, E = polipoproteins B100, B48, CII, CIII, E, respectively; MTP = microsomal transfer protein; ACAT = acyl coenzyme A:cholesterol acyltransferase; VLDL = very low density lipoprotein receptor; IDL = intermediate density lipoprotein receptor; HDL = high density lipoprotein receptor; ABCA1 = adenosine triphosphate binding cassette transporters; LCAT = lecithin:cholesterol acyl transferase; CETP = cholesterol ester transfer protein; SRB1 = scavenger receptor B1. Other abbreviations as in text. (Reprinted from Tsimikas S, et al. In: Chien KR, ed. Molecular basis of cardiovascular disease. A companion to Braunwald's Heart Disease. Philadelphia: WB Saunders, 2004,[4] with permission.)

catabolized by the kidney resulting in lower HDL plasma levels.[160]

Case control studies of MI and angiographic CAD have shown that small dense LDL is associated with approximately threefold increased risk of CAD.[161–168] Several angiographic studies have also shown increased progression in patients with small dense LDL particles.[169–174] However, most of these studies were not able to demonstrate an independent relationship due to the strong relationship of small dense LDL to triglyceride levels.

The response to therapeutic interventions is also interesting. In the SCRIP trials, cholestyramine and niacin resulted in reduced progression of angiographic CAD, but only in those patients with predominantly small dense LDL (present in 40% of the cohort).[175] In the Helsinki Heart Trial, the major benefit of gemfibrozil occurred in those with triglyceride levels >204 mg/dl.[176] In the Familial Atherosclerosis Treatment Study (FATS) trial, treatment with colestipol/lovastatin and colestipol/niacin significantly decreased hepatic lipase activity with a concomitant conversion of small dense LDL to buoyant LDL, which was the strongest predictor of angiographic regression.[177]

Despite these findings, the independent prognostic value of small dense LDL has not been determined and no studies exist to point out the relationship between small dense LDL and vessel wall pathology.

Lipoprotein-associated phospholipase A$_2$ (Lp-PLA$_2$)

Many pathways and enzymes are involved in the remodeling and metabolism of apolipoproteins as they circulate through the blood vessels and tissues.[4] Cholesterol acyl transferases add fatty acids to cholesterol molecules during chylomicron, VLDL and HDL production. Neutral lipases, such as endothelial and hepatic lipases, cleave triglycerides on circulating lipoproteins. CETP, phospholipid transfer protein, and hepatic lipase are involved in HDL metabolism. An important set of enzymes called phospholipases are involved in phospholipid metabolism, which are major components of all lipoproteins and cell membranes. A family of phospholipases exist which cleave specific sites of phospholipids. Secretory phospholipase A2 hydrolyzes the sn2 ester bond between glycerol and

the fatty acid (generally arachidonic acid) of phospholipids creating smaller and denser lipoproteins. Lipoprotein-associated PLA2 (Lp-PLA2 – which is identical to platelet-activating factor acetylhydrolase), on the other hand, is the product of another gene and functions instead to hydrolyze oxidized phospholipids (i.e. oxidized sn2 side chains present on phospholipids) on oxLDL to yield a free oxidized fatty acid and lysophosphatidylcholine (Figure 11.11).[178,179]

Lp-PLA2 is released by inflammatory cells including monocyte-macrophages, T-cells, and mast cells.[180] Lp-PLA2 is secreted into the plasma and seems to have high affinity for particular lipoproteins, particularly Lp(a), where is found in up to seven times higher content than LDL.[4,146] However, in most patients, due to variable levels of Lp(a) and the fact that Lp(a) levels are skewed toward lower levels, the majority (~80%) of Lp-PLA2 is present on LDL but some is also present of HDL. In addition, it has been demonstrated that LDL(–), a modified subfraction of LDL present in plasma, has a fivefold higher PAF-AH (Lp-PLA2) activity and induces the release of interleukin 8 and monocyte chemotactic protein 1 from cultured endothelial cells than normal LDL in both normolipemic and familial hypercholesterolemic subjects.[181]

There is currently debate as to the potential physiological role of Lp-PLA2. When it hydrolyzes oxPL, it creates two biologically and pro-atherogenic particles from one.[182] It is not been determined if this is protective or potentially proatherogenic.[179] By contrast, it has been recently documented that the phospholipase activity of HDL is entirely due to Lp-PLA2, rather than paraoxonase, a property that would suggest anti-atherogenic and anti-inflammatory properties of HDL.[183,184]

Preliminary in vitro studies have suggested that an inhibitor of Lp-PLA2, SB-244323, does not prevent the rate of LDL oxidation, but results in decreased oxidation byproducts leading to less biological activity and decreased extent of atherosclerosis.[178] Adenovirus-mediated overexpression of PAF-AH in mice resulted in an ~100-fold increase in plasma PAF-AH activity which was present in all lipoprotein fractions and conferred more resistance against oxidative stress and was associated with lower autoantibody levels against oxLDL in plasma.[185] In apoE$^{-/-}$ mice, overexpression of

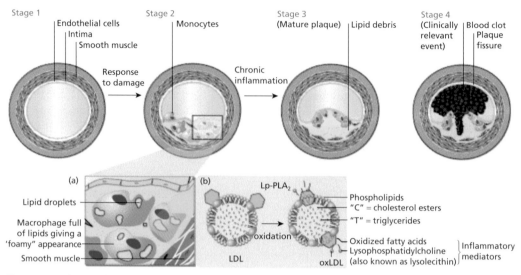

Figure 11.11 The role of Lp-PLA2 in the breakdown of oxidized products. Oxidation of polyunsaturated fatty acids at the sn-2 position of phospholipids present on LDL results in generation of short chain oxidized fatty acids. Lp-Pla2 removes this oxidized fatty acid generating a free oxidized fatty acid and lysophosphatidylcholine, both of which are inflammatory mediators. (Reprinted from Macphee CH. Current Opinion in Pharmacology 2001;1:121–5,[179] with permission from Elsevier.)

Lp-PLA2, which exclusively attaches to HDL in this model, resulted in a significant reduction in aortic wall thickness.[186] Intravenous administration of an adenovirus directing liver-specific expression of human PAF-AH in apoE[−/−] mice resulted in a 3.5-fold increase in plasma PAF-AH activity and significantly reduced oxidized lipoproteins, macrophages, and smooth muscle cells in the arterial wall, reduction in neointimal area and atherosclerotic in male mice.[187] These data suggest a beneficial effect of Lp-PLA2. However, further studies are needed to understand the role of this enzyme in reducing biologically active products and its role in atherogenesis.

In humans, Lp-PLA2 is present within atherosclerotic plaques and co-localizes with macrophages.[188] Interestingly, in Japanese populations, an inherited deficiency of Lp-PLA2 resulting from valine to phenylalanine substitution (G994 → T) and present as a heterozygous trait in 27% of the population, appears to confer increased risk of myocardial infarction, stroke, and peripheral arterial disease.[189–192]

Recently, an antibody-based ELISA has been developed to measure Lp-PLA2 levels in plasma.[193]

This assay appears to show a high correlation between plasma mass and activity of Lp-PLA2. In a nested case-control study from the West of Scotland Coronary Prevention Study, Lp-PLA2 levels were found to be an independent risk factor for death, MI, and revascularization.[194] More recently, in the MONICA (MONItoring of trends and determinants in CArdiovascular disease) study, Lp-PLA2 levels were found to predict future coronary events in hypercholesterolemic middle-aged males who were followed for 14 years.[195] However, in the Women's Health Study[196] and in the ARIC Study,[197] Lp-PLA2 was not an independent predictor of cardiac events, and in particular this seemed to be confounded by a high correlation with LDL cholesterol levels. This has been further confirmed by several studies showing similar decreases in Lp-PLA2 as LDL-C levels with several other lipid lowering agents.[198–202]

Further research is needed to dissect out the independent role of Lp-PLA2, particularly in regard to the high correlation with LDL. In the future, it appears that specific inhibitors will be tested to assess the impact of Lp-PLA2 inhibition on atherosclerosis and clinical events.

References

1. Manolio T. Novel risk markers and clinical practice. N Engl J Med 2003;349:1587–9.

2. Steinberg D. Atherogenesis in perspective: hypercholesterolemia and inflammation as partners in crime. Nat Med 2002;8:1211–17.

3. Navab M, Ananthramaiah GM, Reddy ST, et al. Thematic review series: The pathogenesis of atherosclerosis: The oxidation hypothesis of atherogenesis: the role of oxidized phospholipids and HDL. J Lipid Res 2004;45:993–1007.

4. Tsimikas S, Mooser V. Molecular biology of lipoproteins. Molecular basis of cardiovascular disease. A companion to Braunwald's Heart Disease. In: Chien KR, ed. Philadelphia: WB Saunders, 2004: pp365–384.

5. Chisolm GM, Steinberg D. The oxidative modification hypothesis of atherogenesis: an overview. Free Radic Biol Med. 2000;28:1815–26.

6. Libby P. Inflammation in atherosclerosis. Nature 2002;420:868–74.

7. Napoli C, D'Armiento FP, Mancini FP, et al. Fatty streak formation occurs in human fetal aortas and is greatly enhanced by maternal hypercholesterolemia. Intimal accumulation of low density lipoprotein and its oxidation precede monocyte recruitment into early atherosclerotic lesions. J Clin Invest 1997;100:2680–90.

8. Napoli C, Glass CK, Witztum JL, et al. Influence of maternal hypercholesterolaemia during pregnancy on progression of early atherosclerotic lesions in childhood: Fate of Early Lesions in Children (FELIC) study. Lancet 1999;354:1234–41.

9. Napoli C, Witztum JL, Calara F, et al. Maternal hypercholesterolemia enhances atherogenesis in normocholesterolemic rabbits, which is inhibited by antioxidant or lipid-lowering intervention during pregnancy: an experimental model of atherogenic mechanisms in human fetuses. Circ Res 2000;87:946–52.

10. Napoli C, de Nigris F, Welch JS, et al. Maternal hypercholesterolemia during pregnancy promotes early atherogenesis in LDL receptor-deficient mice and alters aortic gene expression determined by microarray. Circulation 2002;105:1360–7.

11. Palinski W, Rosenfeld ME, Ylä-Herttuala S, et al. Low density lipoprotein undergoes oxidative modification in vivo. Proc Natl Acad Sci USA 1989;86:1372–6.

12. Tsimikas S, Palinski W, Halpern SE, et al. Radiolabeled MDA2, an oxidation-specific, monoclonal antibody, identifies native atherosclerotic lesions in vivo. J Nucl Cardiol 1999;6:41–53.

13. Ylä-Herttuala S, Palinski W, Rosenfeld ME, et al. Evidence for the presence of oxidatively modified low density lipoprotein in atherosclerotic lesions of rabbit and man. J Clin Invest 1989;84:1086–95.

14. Witztum JL, Steinberg D. The oxidative modification hypothesis of atherosclerosis: does it hold for humans? Trends Cardiovasc Med 2001;11:93–102.

15. Ehara S, Ueda M, Naruko T, et al. Elevated levels of oxidized low density lipoprotein show a positive relationship with the severity of acute coronary syndromes. Circulation 2001;103:1955–60.

16. Nishi K, Itabe H, Uno M, et al. Oxidized LDL in carotid plaques and plasma associates with plaque instability. Arterioscler Thromb Vasc Biol 2002;22:1649–54.

17. Tsimikas S, Bergmark C, Beyer RW, et al. Temporal increases in plasma markers of oxidized low-density lipoprotein strongly reflect the presence of acute coronary syndromes. J Am Coll Cardiol 2003;41:360–70.

18. Holvoet P, Collen D, van de Werf F. Malondialdehyde-modified LDL as a marker of acute coronary syndromes. JAMA 1999;281:1718–21.

19. Tamai O, Matsuoka H, Itabe H, et al. Single LDL apheresis improves endothelium-dependent vasodilatation in hypercholesterolemic humans. Circulation 1997;95:76–82.

20. Penny WF, Ben Yehuda O, Kuroe K, et al. Improvement of coronary artery endothelial dysfunction with lipid-lowering therapy: heterogeneity of segmental response and correlation with plasma-oxidized low density lipoprotein. J Am Coll Cardiol 2001;37:766–74.

21. Tsimikas S, Shortal BP, Witztum JL, et al. In vivo uptake of radiolabeled MDA2, an oxidation-specific monoclonal antibody, provides an accurate measure of atherosclerotic lesions rich in oxidized LDL and is highly sensitive to their regression. Arterioscler Thromb Vasc Biol 2000;20:689–97.

22. Tsimikas S, Palinski W, Witztum JL. Circulating autoantibodies to oxidized LDL correlate with arterial accumulation and depletion of oxidized LDL in LDL receptor-deficient mice. Arterioscler Thromb Vasc Biol 2001;21:95–100.

23. Aikawa M, Sugiyama S, Hill CC, et al. Lipid lowering reduces oxidative stress and endothelial cell activation in rabbit atheroma. Circulation 2002;106:1390–6.

24. Crisby M, Nordin-Fredriksson G, Shah PK, et al. Pravastatin treatment increases collagen content and decreases lipid content, inflammation, metalloproteinases, and cell death in human carotid plaques: implications for plaque stabilization. Circulation 2001;103:926–33.

25. Chang MK, Binder CJ, Torzewski M, et al. C-reactive protein binds to both oxidized LDL and apoptotic cells through recognition of a common ligand: phosphorylcholine of oxidized phospholipids. Proc Natl Acad Sci USA 2002;99:13043–8.

26. Hörkkö S, Bird DA, Miller E, et al. Monoclonal autoantibodies specific for oxidized phospholipids or oxidized phospholipid-protein adducts inhibit macrophage uptake of oxidized low-density lipoproteins. J Clin Invest 1999;103:117–28.

27. Chang MK, Bergmark C, Laurila A, et al. Monoclonal antibodies against oxidized low-density lipoprotein bind to apoptotic cells and inhibit their phagocytosis by elicited macrophages: evidence that oxidation-specific epitopes mediate macrophage recognition. Proc Natl Acad Sci USA 1999;96:6353–8.

28. Binder CJ, Horkko S, Dewan A, et al. Pneumococcal vaccination decreases atherosclerotic lesion formation: molecular mimicry between *Streptococcus pneumoniae* and oxidized LDL. Nat Med 2003;9:736–43.

29. Wu R, de Faire U, Lemne C, et al. Autoantibodies to oxLDL are decreased in individuals with borderline hypertension. Hypertension 1999;33:53–9.

30. Hulthe J, Bokemark L, Fagerberg B. Antibodies to oxidized LDL in relation to intima-media thickness in carotid and femoral arteries in 58-year-old subjectively clinically healthy men. Arterioscler Thromb Vasc Biol 2001;21:101–7.

31. Karvonen J, Paivansalo M, Kesaniemi YA, et al. Immunoglobulin M type of autoantibodies to oxidized low-density lipoprotein has an inverse relation to carotid artery atherosclerosis. Circulation 2003;108:2107–12.

32. Shaw PX, Hörkkö S, Tsimikas S, et al. Human-derived antioxidized LDL autoantibody blocks uptake of oxidized LDL by macrophages and localizes to atherosclerotic lesions in vivo. Arterioscler Thromb Vasc Biol 2001;21:1333–9.

33. Tsimikas S, Shaw PX. Non-invasive imaging of vulnerable plaques by molecular targeting of oxidized LDL with tagged oxidation-specific antibodies. J Cell Biochem 2002;39:138–46.

34. Tsimikas S. Noninvasive imaging of oxidized low-density lipoprotein in atherosclerotic plaques with tagged oxidation-specific antibodies. Am J Cardiol 2002;90:L22–7.

35. Tsimikas S, Witztum JL. Measuring circulating oxidized low-density lipoprotein to evaluate coronary risk. Circulation 2001;103:1930–2.

36. Tsimikas S, Witztum JL, Miller ER, et al. High-dose atorvastatin reduces total plasma levels of oxidized phospholipids and immune complexes present on apolipoprotein B-100 in patients with acute coronary syndromes in the MIRACL trial. Circulation 2004;110:1406–12.

37. Tsimikas S, Brilakis E, Miller ER, et al. Oxidized phospholipids, Lp(a) lipoprotein, and coronary artery disease. N Engl J Med 2005;353:46–57.

38. Itabe H, Takeshima E, Iwasaki H, et al. A monoclonal antibody against oxidized lipoprotein recognizes foam cells in atherosclerotic lesions. Complex formation of oxidized phosphatidylcholines and polypeptides. J Biol Chem 1994;269:15274–9.

39. Itabe H, Yamamoto H, Imanaka T, et al. Sensitive detection of oxidatively modified low density lipoprotein using a monoclonal antibody. J Lipid Res 1996;37:45–53.

40. Holvoet P, Perez G, Zhao Z, et al. Malondialdehyde-modified low density lipoproteins in patients with atherosclerotic disease. J Clin Invest 1995;95:2611–19.

41. Holvoet P, Vanhaecke J, Janssens S, et al. Oxidized LDL and malondialdehyde-modified LDL in patients with acute coronary syndromes and stable coronary artery disease. Circulation 1998;98:1487–94.

42. Holvoet P, Mertens A, Verhamme P, et al. Circulating oxidized LDL is a useful marker for identifying patients with coronary artery disease. Arterioscler Thromb Vasc Biol 2001;21:844–8.

43. Holvoet P, Stassen JM, Van Cleemput J, et al. Oxidized low density lipoproteins in patients with transplant-associated coronary artery disease. Arterioscler Thromb Vasc Biol 1998;18:100–7.

44. Holvoet P, Kritchevsky SB, Tracy RP, et al. The metabolic syndrome, circulating oxidized LDL, and risk of myocardial infarction in well-functioning elderly people in the health, aging, and body composition cohort. Diabetes. 2004;53:1068–73.

45. Holvoet P, Harris TB, Tracy RP, et al. Association of high coronary heart disease risk status with circulating oxidized LDL in the well-functioning elderly: findings from the health, aging, and body composition study. Arterioscler Thromb Vasc Biol 2003;23:1444–8.

46. Sigurdardottir V, Fagerberg B, Hulthe J. Circulating oxidized low-density lipoprotein (LDL) is associated with risk factors of the metabolic syndrome and LDL size in clinically healthy 58-year-old men (AIR study). J Intern Med. 2002;252:440–7.

47. Hulthe J, Fagerberg B. Circulating oxidized LDL is associated with subclinical atherosclerosis development and inflammatory cytokines (AIR Study). Arterioscler Thromb Vasc Biol 2002;22:1162–7.

48. Liu ML, Ylitalo K, Salonen R, et al. Circulating oxidized low-density lipoprotein and its association with carotid intima-media thickness in asymptomatic members of familial combined hyperlipidemia families. Arterioscler Thromb Vasc Biol 2004;24:1492–7.

49. Tsimikas S, Lau HK, Han KR, et al. Percutaneous coronary intervention results in acute increases in oxidized phospholipids and lipoprotein(a): short-term and long-term immunologic responses to oxidized low-density lipoprotein. Circulation 2004;109:3164–70.

50. Zhang B, Bai H, Liu R, et al. Serum high-density lipoprotein-cholesterol levels modify the association between plasma levels of oxidatively modified low-density lipoprotein and coronary artery disease in men. Metabolism. 2004;53:423–9.

51. Jarvisalo MJ, Lehtimaki T, Raitakari OT. Determinants of arterial nitrate-mediated dilatation in children: role of oxidized low-density lipoprotein, endothelial function, and carotid intima-media thickness. Circulation 2004;109:2885–9.

52. Tsimikas S, Witztum JL. Shifting the diagnosis and treatment of atherosclerosis to children and young adults: a new paradigm for the 21st century. J Am Coll Cardiol 2002;40:2122–4.

53. Tanaga K, Bujo H, Inoue M, et al. Increased circulating malondialdehyde-modified LDL levels in patients with coronary artery diseases and their association with peak sizes of LDL particles. Arterioscler Thromb Vasc Biol 2002;22:662–6.

54. Berliner JA, Subbanagounder G, Leitinger N, et al. Evidence for a role of phospholipid oxidation products in atherogenesis. Trends Cardiovasc Med 2001;11: 142–7.

55. Mellwig KP, Baller D, Gleichmann U, et al. Improvement of coronary vasodilatation capacity through single LDL apheresis. Atherosclerosis 1998;139:173–8.

56. Kobayashi J, Katsube S, Shimoda M, et al. Single LDL apheresis improves serum remnant-like particle-cholesterol, C-reactive protein, and malondialdehyde-modified-low-density lipoprotein concentrations in Japanese hypercholesterolemic subjects. Clin Chim Acta 2002;321:107–12.

57. Matsumoto T, Takashima H, Ohira N, et al. Plasma level of oxidized low-density lipoprotein is an independent determinant of coronary macrovasomotor and microvasomotor responses induced by bradykinin. J Am Coll Cardiol 2004;44:451–7.

58. Kugiyama K, Sugiyama S, Soejima H, et al. Increase in plasma levels of oxidized low-density lipoproteins in patients with coronary spastic angina. Atherosclerosis 2001;154:463–7.

59. Toshima S, Hasegawa A, Kurabayashi M, et al. Circulating oxidized low density lipoprotein levels: a biochemical risk marker for coronary heart disease. Arterioscler Thromb Vasc Biol 2000;20:2243–7.

60. Edelstein C, Pfaffinger D, Hinman J, et al. Lysine-phosphatidylcholine adducts in Kringle V impart unique immunological and potential pro-inflammatory properties to human apolipoprotein(a). J Biol Chem 2003;278:51841–7.

61. De Caterina R, Cipollone F, Filardo FP, et al. Low-density lipoprotein level reduction by the 3-hydroxy-3-methylglutaryl coenzyme-A inhibitor simvastatin is accompanied by a related reduction of F2-isoprostane formation in hypercholesterolemic subjects: no further effect of vitamin E. Circulation 2002;106:2543–9.

62. Shimada K, Mokuno H, Matsunaga E, et al. Circulating oxidized low-density lipoprotein is an independent predictor for cardiac event in patients with coronary artery disease. Atherosclerosis 2004;174:343–7.

63. Tsutsui T, Tsutamoto T, Wada A, et al. Plasma oxidized low-density lipoprotein as a prognostic predictor in patients with chronic congestive heart failure. J Am Coll Cardiol 2002;39:957–62.

64. Uno M, Kitazato KT, Nishi K, et al. Raised plasma oxidised LDL in acute cerebral infarction. J Neurol Neurosurg Psychiatry 2003;74:312–16.

65. Dei R, Takeda A, Niwa H, et al. Lipid peroxidation and advanced glycation end products in the brain in normal aging and in Alzheimer's disease. Acta Neuropathol (Berl) 2002;104:113–22.

66. Holvoet P, Van Cleemput J, Collen D, et al. Oxidized low density lipoprotein is a prognostic marker of transplant-associated coronary artery disease. Arterioscler Thromb Vasc Biol 2000;20:698–702.

67. Pratico D, Rokach J, Lawson J, et al. F2-isoprostanes as indices of lipid peroxidation in inflammatory diseases. Chem Physics Lipids 2004;128:165–71.

68. Pratico D. Lipid peroxidation in mouse models of atherosclerosis. Trends Cardiovasc Med 2001;11: 112–16.

69. Praticó D, Tangirala RK, Rader DJ, et al. Vitamin E suppresses isoprostane generation in vivo and reduces atherosclerosis in ApoE-deficient mice. Nat Med 1998;4:1189–92.

70. Tangirala RK, Pratico D, FitzGerald GA, et al. Reduction of isoprostanes and regression of advanced atherosclerosis by apolipoprotein E. J Biol Chem 2001;276:261–6.

71. Pratico D, Tangirala RK, Horkko S, et al. Circulating autoantibodies to oxidized cardiolipin correlate with isoprostane F(2alpha)-VI levels and the extent of atherosclerosis in ApoE-deficient mice: modulation by vitamin E. Blood 2001;97:459–64.

72. Davi G, Alessandrini P, Mezzetti A, et al. In vivo formation of 8-Epi-prostaglandin F2 alpha is increased in hypercholesterolemia. Arterioscler Thromb Vasc Biol 1997;17:3230–5.

73. Reilly MP, Praticó D, Delanty N, et al. Increased formation of distinct F2 isoprostanes in hypercholesterolemia. Circulation 1998;98:2822–8.

74. Davi G, Ciabattoni G, Consoli A, et al. In vivo formation of 8-iso-prostaglandin f2alpha and platelet activation in diabetes mellitus: effects of improved metabolic control and vitamin E supplementation. Circulation 1999;99:224–9.

75. Gopaul NK, Anggard EE, Mallet AI, et al. Plasma 8-epi-PGF2 alpha levels are elevated in individuals with non-insulin dependent diabetes mellitus. FEBS Lett 1995;368:225–9.

76. Morrow JD, Frei B, Longmire AW, et al. Increase in circulating products of lipid peroxidation (F2-isoprostanes) in smokers. Smoking as a cause of oxidative damage. N Engl J Med 1995;332:1198–203.

77. Reilly M, Delanty N, Lawson JA, et al. Modulation of oxidant stress in vivo in chronic cigarette smokers. Circulation 1996;94:19–25.

78. Minuz P, Patrignani P, Gaino S, et al. Increased oxidative stress and platelet activation in patients with hypertension and renovascular disease. Circulation 2002;106:2800–5.

79. Davi G, Di Minno G, Coppola A, et al. Oxidative stress and platelet activation in homozygous homocystinuria. Circulation 2001;104:1124–8.

80. Voutilainen S, Morrow JD, Roberts LJ, et al. Enhanced in vivo lipid peroxidation at elevated plasma total homocysteine levels. Arterioscler Thromb Vasc Biol 1999;19:1263–6.

81. Pratico D, Iuliano L, Mauriello A, et al. Localization of distinct F2-isoprostanes in human atherosclerotic lesions. J Clin Invest 1997;100:2028–34.

82. Gniwotta C, Morrow JD, Roberts LJ, et al. Prostaglandin F2-like compounds, F2-isoprostanes, are present in increased amounts in human atherosclerotic lesions. Arterioscler Thromb Vasc Biol 1997;17:3236–41.

83. Mallat Z, Nakamura T, Ohan J, et al. The relationship of hydroxyeicosatetraenoic acids and F2-isoprostanes to plaque instability in human carotid atherosclerosis. J Clin Invest 1999;103:421–7.

84. Cipollone F, Ciabattoni G, Patrignani P, et al. Oxidant stress and aspirin-insensitive thromboxane biosynthesis in severe unstable angina. Circulation 2000;102:1007–13.

85. Iuliano L, Pratico D, Greco C, et al. Angioplasty increases coronary sinus F2-isoprostane formation: evidence for in vivo oxidative stress during PTCA. J Am Coll Cardiol 2001;37:76–80.

86. Reilly MP, Delanty N, Roy L, et al. Increased formation of the isoprostanes IPF2α-I and 8-epi-prostaglandin F2α in acute coronary angioplasty: evidence for oxidant stress during coronary reperfusion in humans. Circulation 1997;96:3314–20.

87. Delanty N, Reilly MP, Praticó D, et al. 8-Epi PGF2α generation during coronary reperfusion: a potential quantitative marker of oxidant stress in vivo. Circulation 1997;95:2492–9.

88. Witztum JL. To E or not to E – how do we tell? Circulation 1998;98:2785–7.

89. Roberts LJ, Morrow JD. Measurement of F2-isoprostanes as an index of oxidative stress in vivo. Free Rad Biol Med 2000;28:505–13.

90. Aikawa M, Libby P. The vulnerable atherosclerotic plaque: pathogenesis and therapeutic approach. Cardiovasc Pathol 2004;13:125–38.

91. Naruko T, Ueda M, Haze K, et al. Neutrophil infiltration of culprit lesions in acute coronary syndromes. Circulation 2002;106:2894–900.

92. Falk E, Shah PK, Fuster V. Coronary plaque disruption. Circulation 1995;92:657–71.

93. Podrez EA, Poliakov E, Shen Z, et al. A novel family of atherogenic oxidized phospholipids promotes macrophage foam cell formation via the scavenger receptor CD36 and is enriched in atherosclerotic lesions. J Biol Chem 2002;277:38517–23.

94. Podrez EA, Abu-Soud HM, Hazen SL. Myeloperoxidase-generated oxidants and atherosclerosis. Free Rad Biol Med 2000;28:1717–25.

95. Hazell LJ, Stocker R. α-Tocopherol does not inhibit hypochlorite-induced oxidation of apolipoprotein B-100 of low-density lipoprotein. FEBS Lett 1997;414:541–4.

96. Hazen SL. Myeloperoxidase and plaque vulnerability. Arterioscler Thromb Vasc Biol 2004;24:1143–6.

97. Daugherty A, Dunn JL, Rateri DL, et al. Myeloperoxidase, a catalyst for lipoprotein oxidation, is expressed in human atherosclerotic lesions. J Clin Invest 1994;94:437–44.

98. Leeuwenburgh C, Hardy MM, Hazen SL, et al. Reactive nitrogen intermediates promote low density lipoprotein oxidation in human atherosclerotic intima. J Biol Chem 1997;272:1433–6.

99. Hazen SL, Heinecke JW. 3-Chlorotyrosine, a specific marker of myeloperoxidase-catalyzed oxidation, is markedly elevated in low density lipoprotein isolated from human atherosclerotic intima. J Clin Invest 1997;99:2075–81.

100. Abu-Soud HM, Hazen SL. Nitric oxide is a physiological substrate for mammalian peroxidases. J Biol Chem 2000;275:37524–32.

101. Gaut JP, Byun J, Tran HD, et al. Myeloperoxidase produces nitrating oxidants in vivo. J Clin Invest 2002;109:1311–19.

102. Schmitt D, Shen Z, Zhang R, et al. Leukocytes utilize myeloperoxidase-generated nitrating intermediates as physiological catalysts for the generation of biologically active oxidized lipids and sterols in serum. Biochemistry 1999;38:16904–15.

103. Eiserich JP, Baldus S, Brennan ML, et al. Myeloperoxidase, a leukocyte-derived vascular NO oxidase. Science. 2002;296:2391–4.

104. Kutter D, Devaquet P, Vanderstocken G, et al. Consequences of total and subtotal myeloperoxidase

deficiency: risk or benefit? Acta Haematol 2000;104:10–15.

105. Nikpoor B, Turecki G, Fournier C, et al. A functional myeloperoxidase polymorphic variant is associated with coronary artery disease in French-Canadians. Am Heart J 2001;142:336–9.

106. Pecoits-Filho R, Stenvinkel P, Marchlewska A, et al. A functional variant of the myeloperoxidase gene is associated with cardiovascular disease in end-stage renal disease patients. Kidney Int Suppl 2003;S172–6.

107. Asselbergs FW, Tervaert JW, Tio RA. Prognostic value of myeloperoxidase in patients with chest pain. N Engl J Med 2004;350:516–18.

108. Brennan ML, Anderson MM, Shih DM, et al. Increased atherosclerosis in myeloperoxidase-deficient mice. J Clin Invest 2001;107:419–30.

109. Sugiyama S, Okada Y, Sukhova GK, et al. Macrophage myeloperoxidase regulation by granulocyte macrophage colony-stimulating factor in human atherosclerosis and implications in acute coronary syndromes. Am J Pathol 2001;158:879–91.

110. Sugiyama S, Kugiyama K, Aikawa M, et al. Hypochlorous acid, a macrophage product, induces endothelial apoptosis and tissue factor expression: involvement of myeloperoxidase-mediated oxidant in plaque erosion and thrombogenesis. Arterioscler Thromb Vasc Biol 2004;24:1309–14.

111. Vita JA, Brennan ML, Gokce N, et al. Serum myeloperoxidase levels independently predict endothelial dysfunction in humans. Circulation 2004;110:1134–9.

112. Zhang R, Brennan ML, Fu X, et al. Association between myeloperoxidase levels and risk of coronary artery disease. JAMA 2001;286:2136–42.

113. Brennan ML, Penn MS, Van Lente F, et al. Prognostic value of myeloperoxidase in patients with chest pain. N Engl J Med 2003;349:1595–604.

114. Baldus S, Heeschen C, Meinertz T, et al. Myeloperoxidase serum levels predict risk in patients with acute coronary syndromes. Circulation 2003;108:1440–5.

115. Shishehbor MH, Brennan ML, Aviles RJ, et al. Statins promote potent systemic antioxidant effects through specific inflammatory pathways. Circulation 2003;108:426–31.

116. Fukai T, Folz RJ, Landmesser U, et al. Extracellular superoxide dismutase and cardiovascular disease. Cardiovasc Res 2002;55:239–49.

117. Sies H. Glutathione and its role in cellular functions. Free Radic Biol Med 1999;27:916–21.

118. Forgione MA, Cap A, Liao R, et al. Heterozygous cellular glutathione peroxidase deficiency in the mouse: abnormalities in vascular and cardiac function and structure. Circulation 2002;106:1154–8.

119. Forgione MA, Weiss N, Heydrick S, et al. Cellular glutathione peroxidase deficiency and endothelial dysfunction. Am J Physiol Heart Circ Physiol. 2002;282:H1255–61.

120. Blankenberg S, Rupprecht HJ, Bickel C, et al. Glutathione peroxidase 1 activity and cardiovascular events in patients with coronary artery disease. N Engl J Med 2003;349:1605–13.

121. Utermann G. The mysteries of lipoprotein(a). Science. 1989;246:904–10.

122. Scanu AM, Nakajima K, Edelstein C. Apolipoprotein(a): structure and biology. Front Biosci 2001;6:D546–54.

123. Hobbs HH, White AL. Lipoprotein(a): intrigues and insights. Curr Opin Lipidol 1999;10:225–36.

124. Kostner KM, Kostner GM. Lipoprotein(a): still an enigma? Curr Opin Lipidol 2002;13:391–6.

125. Dangas G, Mehran R, Harpel PC, et al. Lipoprotein(a) and inflammation in human coronary atheroma: association with the severity of clinical presentation. J Am Coll Cardiol 1998;32:2035–42.

126. Jürgens G, Chen Q, Esterbauer H, et al. Immunostaining of human autopsy aortas with antibodies to modified apolipoprotein B and apoprotein(a). Arterioscler Thromb 1993;13:1689–99.

127. Cushing GL, Gaubatz JW, Nava ML, et al. Quantitation and localization of apolipoproteins [a] and B in coronary artery bypass vein grafts resected at re-operation. Arteriosclerosis 1989;9:593–603.

128. Utermann G. Genetic architecture and evolution of the lipoprotein(a) trait. Curr Opin Lipidol 1999;10:133–41.

129. Armstrong VW, Cremer P, Eberle E, et al. The association between serum Lp(a) concentrations and angiographically assessed coronary atherosclerosis. Dependence on serum LDL levels. Atherosclerosis 1986;62:249–57.

130. Danesh J, Collins R, Peto R. Lipoprotein(a) and coronary artery disease. Metanalysis of prospective studies. Circulation 2000;102:1082–5.

131. Maher VM, Brown BG, Marcovina SM, et al. Effects of lowering elevated LDL cholesterol on the cardiovascular risk of lipoprotein(a). JAMA 1995;274:1771–4.

132. Schaefer EJ, Lamon-Fava S, Jenner JL, et al. Lipoprotein(a) levels and risk of coronary heart disease in men. The Lipid Research Clinics Coronary Primary Prevention Trial. JAMA 1994;271:999–1003.

133. Ridker PM, Hennekens CH, Stampfer MJ. A prospective study of lipoprotein(a) and the risk of myocardial infarction. JAMA 1993;270:2195–9.

134. Foody JM, Milberg JA, Robinson K, et al. Homocysteine and lipoprotein(a) interact to increase CAD risk in young men and women. Arterioscler Thromb Vasc Biol 2000;20:493–9.

135. Sandkamp M, Funke H, Schulte H, et al. Lipoprotein(a) is an independent risk factor for myocardial infarction at a young age. Clin Chem 1990;36:20–3.

136. Schwartz GG, Olsson AG, Ezekowitz MD, et al. Effects of atorvastatin on early recurrent ischemic events in acute coronary syndromes: the MIRACL study: a randomized controlled trial. JAMA 2001;285:1711–18.

137. McKenney JM, McCormick LS, Weiss S, et al. A randomized trial of the effects of atorvastatin and niacin in patients with combined hyperlipidemia or isolated hypertriglyceridemia. Am J Med 1998;104:137–43.

138. Schaefer EJ, McNamara JR, Tayler T, et al. Effects of atorvastatin on fasting and postprandial lipoprotein subclasses in coronary heart disease patients versus control subjects. Am J Cardiol 2002;90:689–96.

139. Dart A, Jerums G, Nicholson G, et al. A multicenter, double-blind, one-year study comparing safety and efficacy of atorvastatin versus simvastatin in patients with hypercholesterolemia. Am J Cardiol 1997;80:39–44.

140. Bredie SJ, Westerveld HT, Knipscheer HC, et al. Effects of gemfibrozil or simvastatin on apolipoprotein-B-containing lipoproteins, apolipoprotein-CIII and lipoprotein(a) in familial combined hyperlipidaemia. Neth J Med 1996;49:59–67.

141. Slunga L, Johnson O, Dahlen GH. Changes in Lp(a) lipoprotein levels during the treatment of hypercholesterolaemia with simvastatin. Eur J Clin Pharmacol 1992;43:369–73.

142. Klezovitch O, Edelstein C, Scanu AM. Stimulation of interleukin-8 production in human THP-1 macrophages by apolipoprotein(a). Evidence for a critical involvement of elements in its C-terminal domain. J Biol Chem 2001;276:46864–9.

143. Yano Y, Shimokawa K, Okada Y, et al. Immunolocalization of lipoprotein(a) in wounded tissues. J Histochem Cytochem 1997;45:559.

144. Trieu VN, Uckun FM. Apolipoprotein(a), a link between atherosclerosis and tumor angiogenesis. Biochem Biophys Res Commun 1999;257:714–18.

145. Maeda S, Abe A, Seishima M, et al. Transient changes of serum lipoprotein(a) as an acute phase protein. Atherosclerosis 1989;78:145–50.

146. Blencowe C, Hermetter A, Kostner GM, et al. Enhanced association of platelet-activating factor acetylhydrolase with lipoprotein (a) in comparison with low density lipoprotein. J Biol Chem 1995;270:31151–7.

147. Berneis KK, Krauss RM. Metabolic origins and clinical significance of LDL heterogeneity. J Lipid Res 2002;43: 1363–79.

148. Krauss RM, Burke DJ. Identification of multiple subclasses of plasma low density lipoproteins in normal humans. J Lipid Res 1982;23:97–104.

149. Swinkels DW, Hak-Lemmers HL, Demacker PN. Single spin density gradient ultracentrifugation method for the detection and isolation of light and heavy low density lipoprotein subfractions. J Lipid Res 1987;28: 1233–9.

150. Segrest JP, Jones MK, De Loof H, et al. Structure of apolipoprotein B-100 in low density lipoproteins. J Lipid Res 2001;42:1346–67.

151. Otvos JD, Jeyarajah EJ, Bennett DW, et al. Development of a proton nuclear magnetic resonance spectroscopic method for determining plasma lipoprotein concentrations and subspecies distributions from a single, rapid measurement. Clin Chem 1992;38:1632–8.

152. Austin MA, Jarvik GP, Hokanson JE, et al. Complex segregation analysis of LDL peak particle diameter. Genet Epidemiol 1993;10:599–604.

153. Krauss RM, Dreon DM. Low-density-lipoprotein subclasses and response to a low-fat diet in healthy men. Am J Clin Nutr 1995;62:478S–87S.

154. Campos H, Willett WC, Peterson RM, et al. Nutrient intake comparisons between Framingham and rural and Urban Puriscal, Costa Rica. Associations with lipoproteins, apolipoproteins, and low density lipoprotein particle size. Arterioscler Thromb 1991;11:1089–99.

155. Tribble DL, Rizzo M, Chait A, et al. Enhanced oxidative susceptibility and reduced antioxidant content of metabolic precursors of small, dense low-density lipoproteins. Am J Med. 2001;110:103–10.

156. Bjornheden T, Babyi A, Bondjers G, et al. Accumulation of lipoprotein fractions and subfractions in the arterial wall, determined in an in vitro perfusion system. Atherosclerosis 1996;123:43–56.

157. Chait A, Brazg RL, Tribble DL, et al. Susceptibility of small, dense, low-density lipoproteins to oxidative modification in subjects with the atherogenic lipoprotein phenotype, pattern B. Am J Med. 1993;94:350–6.

158. Dejager S, Bruckert E, Chapman MJ. Dense low density lipoprotein subspecies with diminished oxidative resistance predominate in combined hyperlipidemia. J Lipid Res 1993;34:295–308.

159. Tribble DL, Rizzo M, Chait A, et al. Enhanced oxidative susceptibility and reduced antioxidant content of metabolic precursors of small, dense low-density lipoproteins. Am J Med. 2001;110:103–10.

160. Kwiterovich PO. The metabolic pathways of high-density lipoprotein, low-density lipoprotein, and triglycerides: a current review. Am J Cardiol 2000;86:5–10.

161. Campos H, Genest JJ, Jr, Blijlevens E, et al. Low density lipoprotein particle size and coronary artery disease. Arterioscler Thromb 1992;12:187–95.

162. Austin MA, Breslow JL, Hennekens CH, et al. Low-density lipoprotein subclass patterns and risk of myocardial infarction. JAMA 1988;260:1917–21.

163. Griffin BA, Freeman DJ, Tait GW, et al. Role of plasma triglyceride in the regulation of plasma low density lipoprotein (LDL) subfractions: relative contribution of small, dense LDL to coronary heart disease risk. Atherosclerosis 1994;106:241–53.

164. Coresh J, Kwiterovich PO, Jr., Smith HH, et al. Association of plasma triglyceride concentration and LDL particle diameter, density, and chemical composition with premature coronary artery disease in men and women. J Lipid Res 1993;34:1687–97.

165. Gardner CD, Fortmann SP, Krauss RM. Association of small low-density lipoprotein particles with the incidence of coronary artery disease in men and women. JAMA 1996;276:875–81.

166. Lamarche B, St Pierre AC, Ruel IL, et al. A prospective, population-based study of low density lipoprotein particle size as a risk factor for ischemic heart disease in men. Can J Cardiol 2001;17:859–65.

167. St Pierre AC, Ruel IL, Cantin B, et al. Comparison of various electrophoretic characteristics of LDL particles and their relationship to the risk of ischemic heart disease. Circulation 2001;104:2295–9.

168. Campos H, Moye LA, Glasser SP, et al. Low-density lipoprotein size, pravastatin treatment, and coronary events. JAMA 2001;286:1468–74.

169. Krauss RM, Lindgren FT, Williams PT, et al. Intermediate-density lipoproteins and progression of coronary artery disease in hypercholesterolaemic men. Lancet 1987;2:62–6.

170. Krauss RM. Relationship of intermediate and low-density lipoprotein subspecies to risk of coronary artery disease. Am Heart J. 1987;113:578–82.

171. Watts GF, Mandalia S, Brunt JN, et al. Independent associations between plasma lipoprotein subfraction levels and the course of coronary artery disease in the St Thomas' Atherosclerosis Regression Study (STARS). Metabolism 1993;42:1461–7.

172. Phillips NR, Waters D, Havel RJ. Plasma lipoproteins and progression of coronary artery disease evaluated by angiography and clinical events. Circulation 1993;88:2762–70.

173. Mack WJ, Krauss RM, Hodis HN. Lipoprotein subclasses in the Monitored Atherosclerosis Regression Study (MARS). Treatment effects and relation to coronary angiographic progression. Arterioscler Thromb Vasc Biol 1996;16:697–704.

174. Hodis HN, Mack WJ, Dunn M, et al. Intermediate-density lipoproteins and progression of carotid arterial wall intima-media thickness. Circulation 1997;95:2022–6.

175. Miller BD, Alderman EL, Haskell WL, et al. Predominance of dense low-density lipoprotein particles predicts angiographic benefit of therapy in the Stanford Coronary Risk Intervention Project. Circulation 1996;94:2146–53.

176. Manninen V, Tenkanen L, Koskinen P, et al. Joint effects of serum triglyceride and LDL cholesterol and HDL cholesterol concentrations on coronary heart disease risk in the Helsinki Heart Study. Implications for treatment. Circulation 1992;85:37–45.

177. Zambon A, Hokanson JE, Brown BG, et al. Evidence for a new pathophysiological mechanism for coronary artery disease regression: hepatic lipase-mediated changes in LDL density. Circulation 1999;99:1959–64.

178. Caslake MJ, Packard CJ. Lipoprotein-associated phospholipase A2 (platelet-activating factor acetylhydrolase) and cardiovascular disease. Curr Opin Lipidol 2003;14:347–52.

179. Macphee CH. Lipoprotein-associated phospholipase A2: a potential new risk factor for coronary artery disease and a therapeutic target. Curr Opin Pharmacol 2001;1:121–5.

180. Asano K, Okamoto S, Fukunaga K, et al. Cellular source(s) of platelet-activating-factor acetylhydrolase activity in plasma. Biochem Biophys Res Commun 1999;261:511–14.

181. Benitez S, Sanchez-Quesada JL, Ribas V, et al. Platelet-activating factor acetylhydrolase is mainly associated with electronegative low-density lipoprotein subfraction. Circulation 2003;108:92.

182. MacPhee CH, Moores KE, Boyd HF, et al. Lipoprotein-associated phospholipase A2, platelet-activating factor acetylhydrolase, generates two bioactive products during the oxidation of low-density lipoprotein: use of a novel inhibitor. Biochem J 1999;338(Pt 2):479–87.

183. Marathe GK, Zimmerman GA, McIntyre TM. Platelet-activating factor acetylhydrolase, and not paraoxonase-1, is the oxidized phospholipid hydrolase of high density lipoprotein particles. J Biol Chem 2003;278:3937–47.

184. Tjoelker LW, Wilder C, Eberhardt C, et al. Anti-inflammatory properties of a platelet-activating factor acetylhydrolase. Nature 1995;374:549–53.

185. Noto H, Hara M, Karasawa K, et al. Human plasma platelet-activating factor acetylhydrolase binds to all the murine lipoproteins, conferring protection against oxidative stress. Arterioscler Thromb Vasc Biol 2003;23:829–35.

186. Hase M, Tanaka M, Yokota M, et al. Reduction in the extent of atherosclerosis in apolipoprotein E-deficient mice induced by electroporation-mediated transfer of the human plasma platelet-activating factor acetylhydrolase gene into skeletal muscle. Prostaglandins Other Lipid Mediat. 2002;70:107–18.

187. Quarck R, De Geest B, Stengel D, et al. Adenovirus-mediated gene transfer of human platelet-activating

factor-acetylhydrolase prevents injury-induced neointima formation and reduces spontaneous atherosclerosis in apolipoprotein E-deficient mice. Circulation 2001;103:2495–500.

188. Hakkinen T, Luoma JS, Hiltunen MO, et al. Lipoprotein-associated phospholipase A(2), platelet-activating factor acetylhydrolase, is expressed by macrophages in human and rabbit atherosclerotic lesions. Arterioscler Thromb Vasc Biol 1999;19:2909–17.

189. Hiramoto M, Yoshida H, Imaizumi T, et al. A mutation in plasma platelet-activating factor acetylhydrolase (Val279→Phe) is a genetic risk factor for stroke. Stroke 1997;28:2417–20.

190. Yamada Y, Ichihara S, Fujimura T, et al. Identification of the G994→T missense in exon 9 of the plasma platelet-activating factor acetylhydrolase gene as an independent risk factor for coronary artery disease in Japanese men. Metabolism. 1998;47:177–81.

191. Yamada Y, Yoshida H, Ichihara S, et al. Correlations between plasma platelet-activating factor acetylhydrolase (PAF-AH) activity and PAF-AH genotype, age, and atherosclerosis in a Japanese population. Atherosclerosis 2000;150:209–16.

192. Unno N, Nakamura T, Kaneko H, et al. Plasma platelet-activating factor acetylhydrolase deficiency is associated with atherosclerotic occlusive disease in Japan. J Vasc Surg 2000;32:263–7.

193. Caslake MJ, Packard CJ, Suckling KE, et al. Lipoprotein-associated phospholipase A2, platelet-activating factor acetylhydrolase: a potential new risk factor for coronary artery disease. Atherosclerosis 2000;150:413–19.

194. Packard CJ, O'Reilly DSJ, Caslake MJ, et al. Lipoprotein-associated phospholipase A2 as an independent predictor of coronary heart disease. N Engl J Med 2000;343:1148–55.

195. Koenig W, Khuseyinova N, Lowel H, et al. Lipoprotein-associated phospholipase A2 adds to risk prediction of incident coronary events by C-reactive protein in apparently healthy middle-aged men from the general population. Results from the 14-year follow-up of a large cohort from southern Germany. Circulation 2004;01.

196. Blake GJ, Dada N, Fox JC, et al. A prospective evaluation of lipoprotein-associated phospholipase A2 levels and the risk of future cardiovascular events in women. J Am Coll Cardiol 2001;38:1302–6.

197. Ballantyne CM, Hoogeveen RC, Bang H, et al. Lipoprotein-associated phospholipase A2, high-sensitivity C-reactive protein, and risk for incident coronary heart disease in middle-aged men and women in the atherosclerosis risk in communities (ARIC) study. Circulation 2004;109:837–42.

198. Tsimihodimos V, Karabina SA, Tambaki A, et al. Effect of atorvastatin on the concentration, relative distribution, and chemical composition of lipoprotein subfractions in patients with dyslipidemias of type IIA and IIB. J Cardiovasc Pharmacol 2003;42:304–10.

199. Tsimihodimos V, Kakafika A, Tambaki AP, et al. Fenofibrate induces HDL-associated PAF-AH but attenuates enzyme activity associated with apoB-containing lipoproteins. J Lipid Res 2003;44:927–34.

200. Blankenberg S, Stengel D, Rupprecht HJ, et al. Plasma PAF-acetylhydrolase in patients with coronary artery disease: results of a cross-sectional analysis. J Lipid Res 2003;44:1381–6.

201. Winkler K, Abletshauser C, Friedrich I, et al. Fluvastatin slow-release lowers platelet-activating factor acetyl hydrolase activity: a placebo-controlled trial in patients with type 2 diabetes. J Clin Endocrinol Metab 2004;89:1153–9.

202. Kudolo GB, Bressler P, DeFronzo RA. Plasma PAF acetylhydrolase in non-insulin dependent diabetes mellitus and obesity: effect of hyperinsulinemia and lovastatin treatment. J Lipid Mediat Cell Signal 1997;17:97–113.

203. Pratico D, Lawson JA, Rokach J, et al. The isoprostanes in biology and medicine. Trends Endocrinol Metab 2001;12:243–7.

CHAPTER 12

Ultrasonic detection of coronary disease

Mani A Vannan, Chowdhury Ahsan, Johan Verjans, Artiom Petrov & Jagat Narula

Clinical ultrasound imaging approaches of coronary plaques at the present time is limited to catheter-based ultrasound systems, namely intravascular ultrasound (IVUS). The advantages of IVUS are that it is real time and yields information on both plaque and vessel morphology. Another ultrasound approach is to delineate the cellular or molecular markers of plaque instability. This latter approach is experimental at the present time but offers a potential to enhance the role of ultrasound imaging of unstable plaques.

Plaque morphology by intravascular ultrasound

Current IVUS systems are either mechanical or phased array transducer systems which can image at a frequency of 20–50 MHz depending of the depth of the image. The axial resolution of the IVUS is ~150 μm at best and typically about ~200 μm. The lateral resolution is varied and is ~250 μm. During the last 10 years plus of IVUS experience in coronary artery disease, its strengths and weakness have been well established. This experience can be best summarized as, in its ability to identify vulnerable plaques, IVUS is useful but not conclusive or comprehensive. This has partly to do with technical factors and partly to do with the fact that ultrasound per se does not have the capability to image cellular or molecular components of a plaque. IVUS imaging shows three kinds of plaques (Figure 12.1): (i) echolucent; (ii) echobright and echolucent; and (iii) echobright.[1] Plaques which are echolucent are the so-called soft plaques with a large lipid core. However, echolucency can also be due to thrombus and/or necrosis. IVUS is very

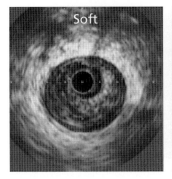 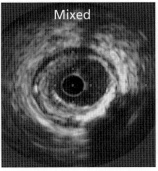 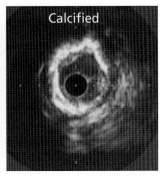

Figure 12.1 Atheroma morphology by IVUS. Soft (left), mixed fibrous and calcified (middle), and heavily calcified (right) atheromas are illustrated. (Reproduced with permission from: Nissen and Yock. Intravascular ultrasound. Novel pathophysiological insights and current clinical applications. Circulation 2001;103: page 606 of 604–616.[1])

Table 12.1 Morphologic markers of vulnerable plaque.

Eccentric and long lesions
Prominent echolucent core
Positive remodeling of the vessel wall
Presence of ulceration and/or thrombus
Presence of calcification
Thin fibrous cap
Presence of inflammation (macrophage accumulation)

limited in its ability to image acute thrombus and the differentiation between necrosis and thrombus is largely subjective. Notwithstanding these limitations, an echolucent plaque is considered to be a vulnerable plaque. The second pattern of IVUS appearance is due to a combination of lipid and fibrous tissue. These plaques are relatively more stable. Echobright plaques contain calcium and often there is acoustic shadowing beyond the plaque which obscures visualization of the vessel wall.

The morphologic hallmarks of unstable plaques are listed in Table 12.1. IVUS is best in imaging the echolucency and calcification. Echolucent plaques are imaged with relative ease, although luceny may be due to necrosis, thrombus, or lipid core (Figure 12.2). From a practical standpoint this differentiation may not be important because all three features reflect plaque instability. IVUS is particularly sensitive to imaging calcium and is in fact superior to angiography in this respect.[2] Remodeling of the vessel is another aspect where IVUS is very useful and unique in its ability (Figure 12.3). Positive or outward remodeling is typical of early atheroma where there is an attempt to preserve vessel lumen size.[3–6] IVUS provides clear images of the intima, media, and external elastic membrane (EEM). The area between the intima and EEM at the lesion is compared to a reference segment either distal or proximal to the lesion. This area has been variously called "plaque area" or "plaque burden." It is a practical index derived from the fact that the leading edge of the intima and the EEM are the two most consistently seen boundaries on IVUS images.[7] Ideally the outer boundary should include the adventitia, but the latter is often not clearly demarcated on ultrasound images. Likewise the inner boundary should be the trailing edge of the intima, but this is also seen distinctly in a significant number of IVUS images. Another shortcoming of this index is that it assumed that the reference segment is normal and the EEM area in this segment is the original size of the vessel. This is not always the case. Despite these limitations, the presence of positive remodeling has been associated with plaque instability[8] (Figure 12.4). On the other hand, negative remodeling occurs relatively late in the atheromatous process and is characterized by luminal narrowing. Negative remodeling is associated with stable coronary syndromes. Plaque

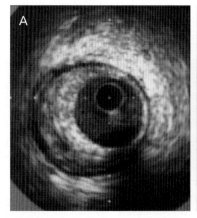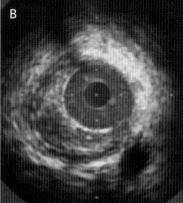

Figure 12.2 Stable and vulnerable plaques. A, Lesion with a thick fibrous cap and small lipid core (stable plaque). B, Lesion with a thin fibrous cap and large lipid core (vulnerable plaque). (Reproduced with permission from Nissen and Yock. Intravascular ultrasound. Novel pathophysiological insights and current clinical applications. Circulation 2001;103: page 610 of 604–616.[1])

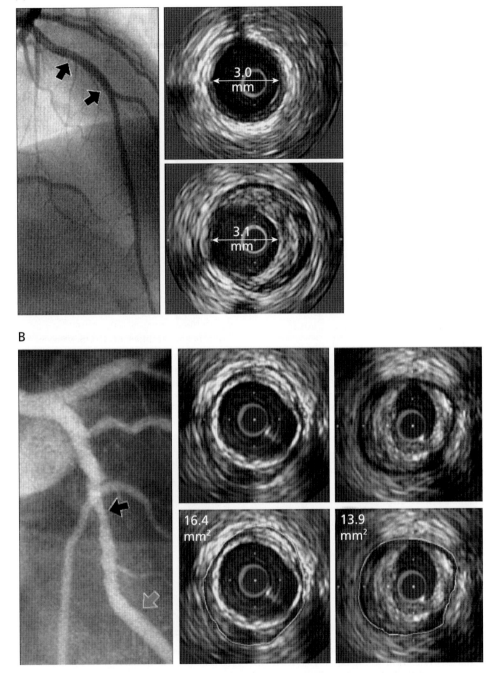

Figure 12.3 A, Example of coronary remodelling. Left: Angiogram is completely normal. However, two sites in left anterior artery (arrows) show a varying extent of atherosclerosis by IVUS. More distal site (top right) has little disease, but more proximal site (bottom right) has a large crescentic atheroma. The lumen size at both sites is similar because of remodeling, resulting in a false-negative angiogram. B, Example of stenosis with negative remodeling. A distal reference segment (gray arrow on right) has EEM area of 16.4 mm² (middle panels). Stenosis (black arrow on left; right panels) has EEM area of 13.9 mm², demonstrating that it is partly due to negative remodeling. (Reproduced with permission from Nissen and Yock. Intravascular ultrasound. Novel pathophysiological insights and current clinical applications. Circulation 2001;103: page 610 of 604–616.[1])

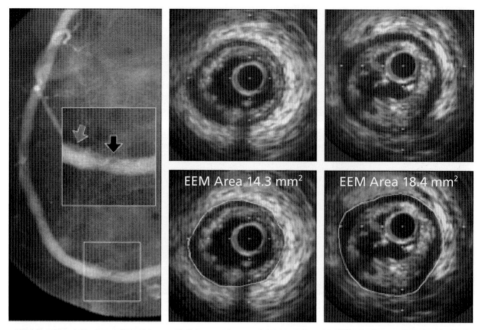

Figure 12.4 Ruptured plaque with positive remodeling. Angiogram (left) was obtained after thrombolysis for acute myocardial infarction. Black arrow indicates occlusion site and gray arrow shows a proximal reference site. At reference site, EEM area is smaller (14.3 mm^2) than area at rupture site (18.4 mm^2), indicating presence of positive remodeling. (Reproduced with permission from Nissen and Yock. Intravascular ultrasound. Novel pathophysiological insights and current clinical applications. Circulation 2001;103: page 610 of 604–616.[1])

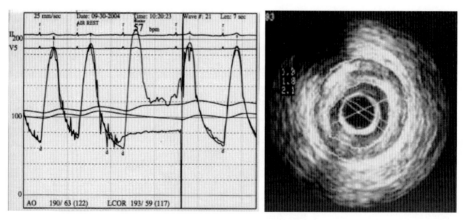

Figure 12.5 IVUS of the LAD from a 76-year-old lady with decreased exertional capacity. Adenosine sestamibi imaging showed equivocal ischemia in the LAD territory. Coronary arteriography showed 60% luminal stenosis. Fractional flow reserve (FFR) was 0.75 (borderline). IVUS images show a significant plaque thickness, positive remodeling, and an eccentric lesion.

eccentricity is another marker of vulnerability (Figure 12.5). The ratio of the longest and shortest distance between the leading edge of the intima and the EEM (plaque thickness) provides an index of eccentricity. IVUS is particularly useful for this purpose. Other IVUS measurements such as circumferential extent of intimal thickening or lesion length are also sometimes reported, but these are not reliable predictors of vulnerability. Plaque fissuring is usually associated with clinically manifest acute coronary syndromes and as such does not strictly fall into the category of vulnerable plaques.

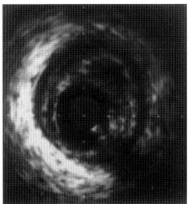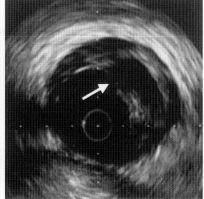

Figure 12.6 IVUS images of a type IV/V lesion (left) and a type VIa lesion (right). Arrow indicates plaque ulceration. (Reproduced with permission from Schmermund A, Erbel R. Unstable coronary plaque and its relation to coronary calcium. Circulation. 2001;104:1682.[14])

However, fissuring and rupture may be accompanied by nonocclusive thrombus and hence may represent unstable lesions. IVUS can image rupture[8,9] and occasionally acute thrombus (Figures 12.6, 12.7), but it is not reliable for visualizing fissures. A number of image processing approaches have been described to improve on the objectivity, reproducibility, and accuracy of the morphological information obtained during IVUS imaging. These are described in detail elsewhere, but all of these remain investigational and are hampered by off-line and often time-consuming algorithms. Nevertheless, some combination of such image analysis is going to be necessary for IVUS to be a serious contender as an imaging modality to delineate plaque vulnerability.

There are two other aspects of unstable plaques where IVUS has either very limited or no role at the present time. The thickness of the fibrous cap is an important predictor of unstable plaque. Thin fibrous cap (~65–150 μm) is a predictor of vulnerability. With its current resolution limits of about ~150 μm at best, IVUS is not useful for this purpose. Imaging modalities will have to have resolution in the order of 10 μm or less to image the fibrous cap reliably, such as optical coherence tomography. The other aspect where IVUS suffers a disadvantage is that it cannot depict the microarchitecture of the plaque. Vulnerable plaques exhibit significant inflammation and macrophage activity beneath the fibrous cap. Imaging these elements would further enhance the accuracy of any imaging modality. IVUS at the present time cannot do this.

Targeted imaging using ultrasound contrast agents

Recent developments in microbubble technology have made them stable for imaging the arterial circulation after intravenous injection. Generally, these microbubbles consist of an inner core of gas surrounded by a shell and sized to pass through capillaries. They behave similar to specular reflectors, and hence can be imaged by ultrasound. Furthermore, because the shells carry an electric charge it is feasible to attach ligands, antibodies, or other molecules aimed specifically image at a phenomenon such as inflammation (Figure 12.8). These targeted microbubbles offer a newer approach to imaging a vulnerable plaque.[10,11] Inflammation affords the most obvious target, since initial work to image activated white blood cells (WBCs) has been encouraging in both cardiac and extracardiac tissue (Figures 12.9, 12.10).

Another method for imaging inflammation is to target the endothelial cell adhesion molecules (ECAMs). Here again the preliminary results are promising.

Despite these encouraging results, imaging inflammation in vulnerable plaque with targeted microbubbles is fraught with significant challenges, some of which are listed in Table 12.2. There are other unresolved issues even if molecular imaging was possible by contrast-enhanced ultrasound. Imaging noninvasively would be best if possible at all. The transducer frequency would be optimal

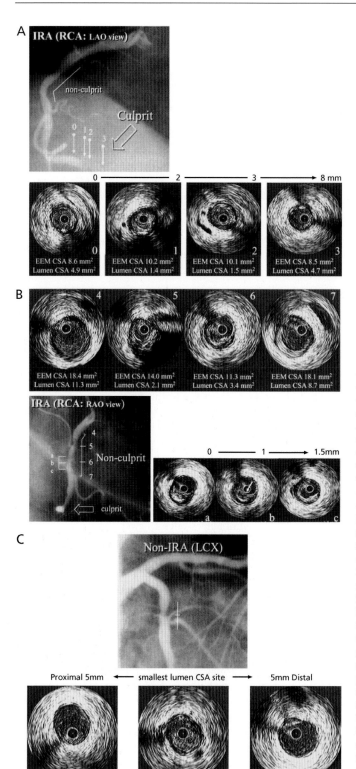

Figure 12.7 This patient presented with acute inferior infarction. Right coronary artery (RCA) is shown in A (left anterior oblique (LAO) projection) and B (right anterior oblique (RAO) projection). Angiography showed total occlusion (open arrow), which presumably was culprit lesion within distal RCA. There was a secondary nonculprit lesion within proximal RCA. Serial IVUS images in A represent culprit lesion. IVUS catheter is surrounded by layered, brightly speckled material (especially seen in IVUS image 1). Although not seen angiographically, lumen beyond occlusion is not obstructed (IVUS image 3). Serial IVUS images in B (4–7) represent proximal nonculprit plaque in IRA. There is plaque rupture (IVUS images a–c, in which arrow indicates ruptured site). Left coronary artery (non-IRA) is shown in C. There is negative remodeling. LCX = left circumflex. (Reproduced with permission from Kotani J, Mintz GS, Castagna MT, Pinnow E, Berzingi CO, Bui AB, Pichard AO, Satler LF, Suddath WO, Waksman R, Laird JR, Jr, Kent KM, Weissman NJ. Intravascular ultrasound analysis of infarct-related and non-infarct-related arteries in patients who presented with an acute myocardial infarction. Circulation 2003:107: 2889–93.[9])

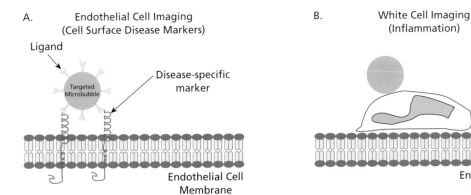

A. Endothelial Cell Imaging
(Cell Surface Disease Markers)

Ligand

Disease-specific
marker

Endothelial Cell
Membrane

B. White Cell Imaging
(Inflammation)

Endothelial Cell
Membrane

Figure 12.8 Mechanisms of microbubble adhesion to endothelium. A, Bubbles bearing a ligand on the shell, such as an antibody, may adhere specifically to a disease-specific epitope on the endothelial cell surface. B, Bubbles not bearing a specific ligand on the surface may adhere to activated leukocytes. Not drawn to scale. (Reproduced with permission from Villanueva FS, Wagner WR, Vannan MA, Narula J. Targeted ultrasound imaging using microbubbles. Cardiol Clin 2004;22: page 285 of 283–298.[15])

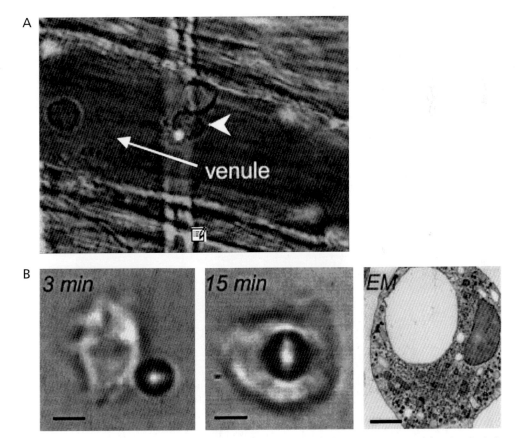

Figure 12.9 Interactions between microbubbles and activated leukocytes. A, Intravital microscopy of the microcirculation of the mouse cremaster muscle treated with tumor necrosis factor – demonstrating attachment of a fluorescently labeled albumin microbubble to an activated leukocyte adherent to the venular surface (arrowhead). The direction of flow is indicated by the arrow. B, Light microscopy demonstrating attachment of a lipid microbubble to the surface of a leukocyte early (3 minutes) after their combination in an in vitro system, followed by phagocytosis at 15 minutes. Electron microscopy (EM) confirmed the intracellular location of the microbubbles. (Reproduced with permission from Lindner JR, Song J, Christiansen J, Klibanov AL, Xu F. Ultrasound assessment of injury and inflammation using microbubbles targeted to P-selectin. Circulation 2001;104:2107–12.[16])

Table 12.2 Challenges in contrast-enhanced imaging of unstable plaques.

Differentiation of microbubbles from other specular reflectors

Overcome aggregation of smaller or submicron bubbles

Imaging smaller or submicron bubbles

Predictable intravascular distribution of microbubbles

Reliability of endovascular binding of targeted microbubbles

Reproducible sonoporation to effect extravascular passage

Imaging intracellular or extravascular microbubbles

for microbubble imaging (lower frequencies), as opposed to invasive intravascular imaging where higher imaging frequency is necessary for visualization of the vessel wall, but these high frequencies may cause excessive microbubble destruction. An alternative may be the use of targeted echo-reflective liposomes[12] which may be imaged at those high frequencies without undue destruction. Preliminary work in imaging atheroma constituents using this approach has shown promising results (Figures 12.11, 12.12). Then there is the question of how to incorporate any imaging modality as a clinical tool.

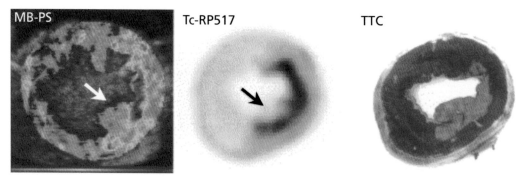

Figure 12.10 Myocardial short-axis images obtained in vivo with CEU and leukocyte-targeted microbubbles (MB-PS) and ex vivo by use of radionuclide imaging with a technetium-labeled neutrophil-avid tracer (Tc-RP517) after ischemia-reperfusion injury of the left circumflex artery territory. The location of inflammation is similar by the two techniques and extends outside of the triphenyltetrazoliumchloride (TTC)-defined infarct region into the noninfarcted risk area. Arrows denote a region of early microvascular no-reflow. (Reproduced with permission from Christiansen JP, Leong-Poi H, Xu F, et al. Noninvasive imaging of myocardial reperfusion injury using leukocyte-targeted contrast echocardiography. Circulation 2002;105:1764–7.[17])

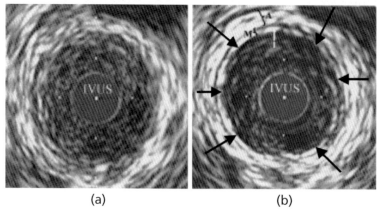

(a)   (b)

Figure 12.11 The intravascular ultrasound (IVUS) images of a right femoral artery showing enhancement of injured endothelium by anti-fibrinogen conjugated echogenic immunoliposome (ELIP). (a) After saline injection and (b) 5 minutes after 8 mg anti-fibrinogen conjugated ELIP. Because of blooming of the endothelium from ELIP enhancement, the media is the black rim and some of the white rim from the intima. Arrows indicate enhanced endothelium. A = dense adventitia; I = intima; M = media. (Reproduced with permission from Hamilton AJ, Huang SL, Warnick D, Rabbat M, Kane B, Nagaraj A, Klegerman M, McPherson DD. J Am Coll Cardiol 2004;43: page 456 of 453–60.[12])

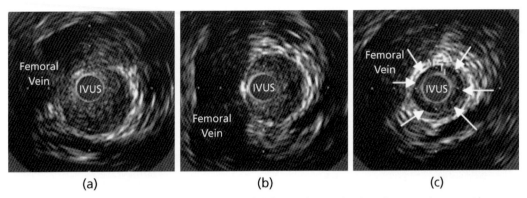

(a) (b) (c)

Figure 12.12 The intravascular ultrasound (IVUS) images of a left carotid artery showing atheroma enhancement by anti-intercellular adhesion molecule (ICAM) conjugated echogenic immunoliposome (ELIP). (a) After saline injection, (b) 5 minutes after 5 mg unconjugated ELIP, and (c) 5 minutes after 5 mg ICAM-conjugated ELIP. Notice the additional enhancement of the adventitia outside the area highlighted by the arrows, indicating adventitial enhancement by ELIP, as confirmed by immunohistochemistry. Arrows indicate enhanced intima/atheroma. (Reproduced with permission from Hamilton AJ, Huang SL, Warnick D, Rabbat M, Kane B, Nagaraj A, Klegerman M, McPherson DD. J Am Coll Cardiol 2004;43: page 457 of 453–60.[12])

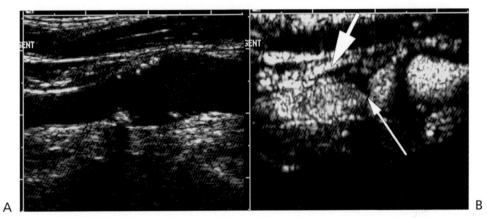

A   B

Figure 12.13 Contrast-enhanced Duplex images of a longitudinal scan of the carotid artery. A, Non-contrast-enhanced view, which shows a suggestion of minimal plaque. B, Contrast was used (this was non-harmonics imaging), which shows large areas of plaque (small, white arrow) that was not visualized on non-contrast imaging. The white arrow on B notes a vessel near the adventitial wall of the carotid (vasa vasorum). (Reproduced with permission from Martin RP, Lerakis S. Contrast for vascular imaging. Cardiol Clin 2004;22: page 316 of 313–20.[18])

This would require a noninvasive approach which means a surrogate site other than the coronary tree may have to be imaged. Here, also, contrast-enhanced ultrasound shows promise in revealing adventitial neovessels in the carotids (Figure 12.13), which are markers of plaque instability. Alternatively, aortic plaques may be imaged noninvasively with targeted microbubbles (Figure 12.14). There is work to be done in this area, but contrast-enhanced ultrasound may enhance the future role of ultrasound imaging of vulnerable plaques.

Conclusion

IVUS is valuable in delineating plaque morphology and identifying some key indicators of instability. It is also the most widely available ultrasound tool although not used extensively. This is both to do with economic issues and also the recognition of the fact that to identify vulnerable plaques, it is invasive and has significant limitations. Advances in targeted ultrasound imaging using microbubbles or echo-reflective liposomes may bridge some of

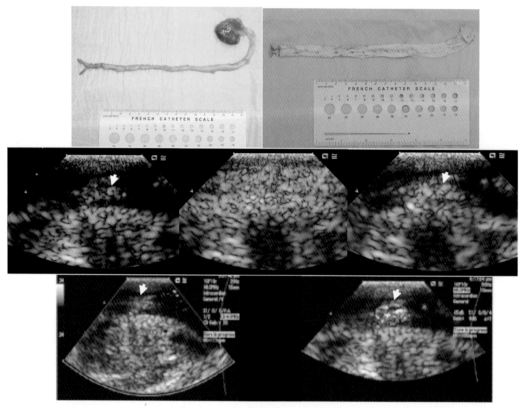

Figure 12.14 Thin fibrous caps and their infiltration by macrophages are obligatory components of atherosclerotic plaques that are vulnerable to rupture.[13] Whereas the plaque thickness can be roughly estimated by intravascular ultrasound, presence of inflammation requires targeted imaging. For this purpose, radiolabeled ligands specifically directed at the receptors for chemoattractant peptides and adhesion molecules have been used by nuclear imaging strategies. We developed a novel ultrasonic method for contrast imaging of these lesions. Since phosphatidylserine (PS) receptors are ubiquitously expressed by macrophages, we developed echogenic liposomes with PS phospholipids excess. The imaging was performed with the premise that these bubbles will be preferentially attracted by the lesions which harbor abundant macrophages (or vulnerable plaque). With this hypothesis, experimental atherosclerotic lesions were developed in rabbits by balloon de-endothelialization of the infradiaphragmatic aorta followed by a 1% cholesterol, 6% peanut oil diet for 4 months. Such animals develop AHA type II (20%), III (30%), and IV (50%) lesions. Intravenous administration of PS-rich microbubbles filled with perfluorocarbon (PFC) was injected intravenously. In the figure the top panel shows the dissected intact aorta (left) and the opened aorta (right) showing yellow plaques. In the middle panel, A shows baseline ultrasound image of the aortic plaque (arrow), B shows microbubbles in the aortic lumen soon after intravenous injection, and C shows microbubble enhancement of the aortic plaque about 25 min after injection. The lumen is free of circulating microbubbles and high mechanical index ultrasound imaging was done after 25 minutes. Note the brighter appearance of the plaque. The lower panel shows another example in which the figure on the left is the baseline image of a plaque and the figure on the right is a color-coded baseline-subtracted videointensity image of the microbubble-enhanced atheroma.

these shortcomings. However, there is still a long way to go before these newer approaches can be clinically used.

References

1. Nissen SE, Yock P. Intravascular ultrasound. Novel pathophysiological insights and current clinical applications. Circulation 2001;103:604–16.

2. Tuzcu EM, Berkalp B, De Franco AC, et al. The dilemma of diagnosing coronary calcification: angiography versus intravascular ultrasound. J Am Coll Cardiol 1996;27: 832–838.

3. Glagov S, Weisenberg E, Zarins C, et al. Compensatory enlargement of human atherosclerotic coronary arteries. N Engl J Med 1987;316:1371–5.

4. Pasterkamp G, Wensing PJ, Post MJ, et al. Paradoxical arterial wall shrinkage may contribute to luminal

narrowing of human atherosclerotic femoral arteries. Circulation 1995;91:1444–9.

5. Mintz GS, Kent KM, Pichard AD, et al. Contribution of inadequate arterial remodeling to the development of focal coronary artery stenoses: an intravascular ultrasound study. Circulation 1997;95:1791–8.

6. Shoenhagen P, Ziada K, Kapadia SR, et al. Extent and direction of arterial remodeling in stable versus unstable coronary syndromes: an intravascular ultrasound study. Circulation 2000;101:598–603.

7. Gussenhoven EJ, Essed CE, Lancee CT, et al. Arterial wall characteristics determined by intravascular ultrasound imaging: an in vitro study. J Am Coll Cardiol. 1989;14: 947–52.

8. Kearney P, Erbel R, Rupprecht HJ, et al. Differences in the morphology of unstable and stable coronary lesions and their impact on the mechanisms of angioplasty: an in vivo study with intravascular ultrasound. Eur Heart J 1996; 17:(5)721–730.

9. Kotani J, Mintz GS, Castagna MT, et al. Intravascular ultrasound analysis of infarct-related and non-infarct-related arteries in patients who presented with an acute myocardial infarction. Circulation 2003:107: 2889–93.

10. Lindner JR. Detection of inflamed plaques with contrast ultrasound. Am J Cardiol 2002;90:32L–35L.

11. Lindner JR. Microbubbles in medical imaging: current applications and future directions. Nature Rev Drug Discov 2004;3 :527–33.

12. Hamilton AJ, Huang SL, Warnick D, et al. Intravascular ultrasound molecular imaging of atheroma components in vivo. J Am Coll Cardiol 2004;43:453–60.

13. Kolodgie FD, Petrov A, Virmani R, et al. Targeting of apoptotic macrophages and experimental atheroma with radiolabeled annexin V: a technique with potential for noninvasive imaging of vulnerable plaque. Circulation 2003;108:3134–9.

14. Schmermund A, Erbel R. Unstable coronary plaque and its relation to coronary calcium. Circulation 2001;104:1682.

15. Villanueva FS, Wagner WR, Vannan MA, Narula J. Targeted ultrasound imaging using microbubbles. Cardiol Clin 2004;22:283–98.

16. Lindner JR, Song J, Christiansen J, Klibanov AL, Xu F. Ultrasound assessment of injury and inflammation using microbubbles targeted to P-selectin. Circulation 2001;104:2107–12.

17. Christiansen JP, Leong-Poi H, Xu F, et al. Noninvasive imaging of myocardial reperfusion injury using leukocyte-targeted contrast echocardiography. Circulation 2002;105:1764–7.

18. Martin RP, Lerakis S. Contrast for vascular imaging. Cardiol Clin 2004;22:313–20.

CHAPTER 13

Intravascular ultrasound for plaque characterization

D Geoffrey Vince & Anuja Nair

Intravascular ultrasound (IVUS) gives accurate information on vessel morphology in the form of a two-dimensional cross-sectional view of the artery (Figure 13.1) and allows real-time assessment of atherosclerotic plaque. In standard IVUS imaging, regions of high reflectance (e.g. calcified areas) appear bright, whereas lipidic areas with low reflectivity are thought to appear dark.[3] However, use of such visual interpretation of IVUS images as the sole diagnostic tool is limited.[4] Previous studies have successfully reported computer-based determination of plaque composition by IVUS image analysis.[5,6] However, these image-based texture analysis methods do not have potential for real-time implementation, as they are expensive in terms of computational time.

More recent studies have demonstrated the capacity of spectral analysis of ultrasound back-scattered radiofrequency (RF) data for differentiating between vessel layers and tissue types.[7,8] Such spectral analysis methods have gained importance, because they are fast and can be employed for real-time applications. In addition, a spectral analysis approach enables a more detailed analysis of tissue composition as compared to image analysis methods. Nair et al. reported that spectra derived from the back-scattered ultrasound pulses show correspondence to the underlying tissue.[9] Factors affecting the nature of backscatter spectra include density, size and shape of scatterers, their spatial orientation and deterministic or random nature of spatial distribution.

Clinical application of IVUS backscatter

Spectral analysis is only commercially available to date on intravascular ultrasound machines produced by volcano therapeutics that utilize a phased-array transducer. These systems have RF spectral analysis built in to the console and require only an additional external ECG input so that data can be collected at the same phase of the cardiac cycle.

Acquisition of RF data

The phased array catheter comprises a static array of transducers positioned circumferentially around a catheter body. The scanner comprises an array of 64 individual transducers contained within a flexible circuit. To maintain an acceptable catheter crossing-profile the individual transducer elements are significantly smaller than the transducers utilized in the rotational devices. These elements are

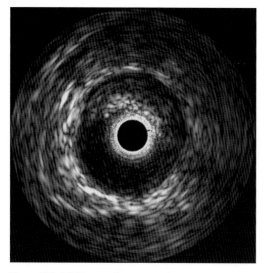

Figure 13.1 IVUS image of coronary artery.

controlled by five multiplexing integrated circuits that are also bonded to the flexible substrate circuit. The transducer array is constructed in such a way that its central portion is hollow, this allows the device to ride over a guide wire rather than adjacent to it as with rotational devices. Unlike the rotating transducer, synthetic aperture transducers have no moving parts and there is therefore less variability in the signal.

The RF signal generated by each of the transducer elements is combined in a process known as synthetic aperture focusing to produce the image. The summed RF signals from each focal position are combined to form a single focused scanline. Each IVUS image comprises 512 scanlines (Figure 13.2). By analyzing the frequencies and amplitudes of the scanline it is possible to determine the plaque composition. This method is known as spectral analysis. During the pullback, the transducers are continuously firing while the catheter is being slowly withdrawn at a constant rate, typically 0.5 mm/s. Thirty images are created per second. An ECG-gating card housed within the console monitors the ECG signal to determine appropriate data acquisition times during the pullback. Upon detection of the peak R-wave, the ECG-gating card instructs the console to save one frame of RF data. The gating card also records the time each frame of data was captured to ensure accurate placement of images when 3D reconstruction is performed. This process is repeated throughout the pullback procedure.

Determining plaque composition

Once the specific areas of plaque have been identified, spectral analysis of the RF signals backscattered from the plaque provides more detailed analysis of the plaque composition. In previous work by our group, a technique for classification of coronary plaque into one of four categories was developed.[10] Mathematical models were used to calculate corresponding spectra from RF signals from within the plaque. These spectra were normalized to remove the catheter/console system response and then several parameters describing the spectra are calculated. These parameters were fed into a statistical classification tree, which is built using a large database of spectral parameters and their corresponding histologic gold-standard. Predictive tissue maps are created using this technique.[9] Figure 13.3 shows an IVUS image and corresponding tissue map where dark green is fibrous tissue, light green is fibro-fatty, red is necrotic core, and white is dense calcium.

Correlation of tissue maps with histology

Previous studies by our group have shown accuracies of 80–93% when the tissue maps are compared to Movat-stained histology sections.[9] Figure 13.4A demonstrates the grayscale IVUS, Movat-stained histology section, and the tissue map of a human plaque. A bright echo with shadow behind can be

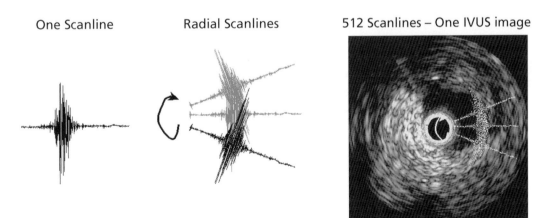

One Scanline   Radial Scanlines   512 Scanlines – One IVUS image

Figure 13.2 Single scan line (left); multiple scan lines (middle); and diagram of how scanlines are arranged to create an IVUS image (right).

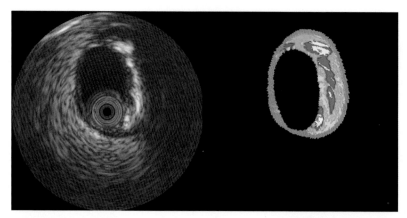

Figure 13.3 IVUS image (left) and corresponding tissue map (right).

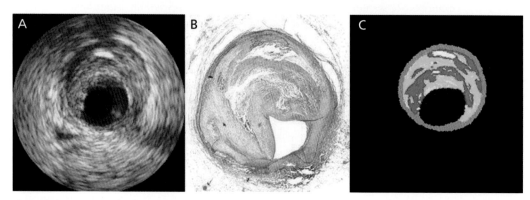

Figure 13.4 IVUS image (A); Movat stained histology section (B); and tissue map (C).

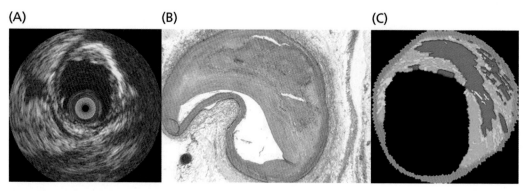

Figure 13.5 IVUS image (A); Movat stained histology section (B); and tissue map (C)

seen in the IVUS image. This feature is typically thought to demonstrate the presence of calcium in the plaque. The remainder of the image is "speckled" and "bright" and would commonly be interpreted as a stable or hard plaque. The corresponding histology image (Figure 13.4B) shows the presence of a dense calcium and a necrotic core deep in the plaque from 11 o'clock to 2 o'clock and a crescent of necrotic core from 7 o'clock to 3 o'clock. Micro-calcifications and pieces of dense calcium can be seen in the necrotic tissue. The tissue map correctly identified the calcific and necrotic regions, both deep in the tissue and circumferentially in the mid region of the lesion (Figure 13.4C). This type of lesion would be classified as fibroatheroma.

Figure 13.5 shows a grayscale IVUS image of an

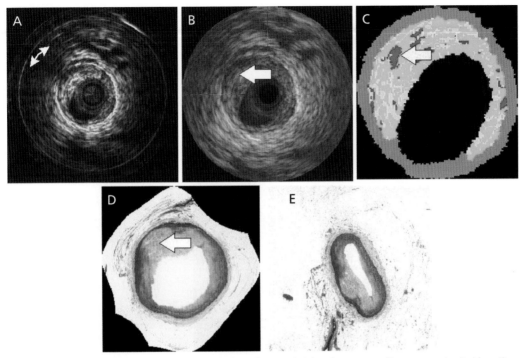

Figure 13.6 Contrast enhanced IVUS image captured from the console (A) and unprocessed image reconstructed from the raw RF data (B). Tissue map (C) and histology (D & E) are also shown.

arc of calcium from 1 o'clock to 3 o'clock. The corresponding histology image demonstrates that this structure is in fact part of a large necrotic core with extensive microcalcification. It can be assumed that the bright echo on the grayscale IVUS was caused by multiple reflections of the ultrasound beam of the signal scattering from the microcalcification. The propagating ultrasound wave would be attenuated by this scattering, but enough signal remained deep in the tissue to extract the frequency information and correctly classify the tissue behind the necrotic core.

Further examples are shown in Figures 13.6 and 13.7. Figure 13.6 shows how the brightness and shadow (marked with an arrow) of an IVUS image is critically dependent on the postprocessing steps used to create the image. Figure 13.6A shows a grayscale IVUS image before image postprocessing. The postprocessing version is shown in Figure 13.6B. Note the change in intensity of the calcific region marked with an arrow. The tissue map presented in Figure 13.6C shows that this region is in fact a necrotic core (with microcalcification) and is validated with reference to the histology image

shown in Figure 13.6D. Figure 13.6E shows the original histology image before "warping" to match the IVUS geometry. Figure 13.7A and B show further examples of correct tissue classification behind calcified regions.

Implications for identification of vulnerable plaques and beyond

Recent publications have documented that vulnerable plaques tend to have a fibrous cap that is 65 to 150 μm thick that covers a large necrotic core. According to the criteria of the American Heart Association Committee on Vascular Lesions, lesion types depend in part on the phase of plaque progression. AHA type II lesion is termed "intimal xanthomas" or "fatty streaks" and corresponds to a lesion with fat-laden macrophages (Figure 13.8). Type III plaques, often termed "pathological intimal thickening," are lesions that comprise mainly fibrous and fibro-fatty tissue, with necrotic core accounting for 0% to less than 3% of the total components. Although these categories of lesions are

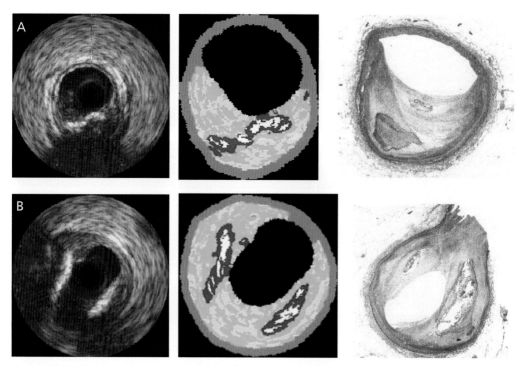

Figure 13.7A and B Demonstrates correct tissue classification behind calcified regions.

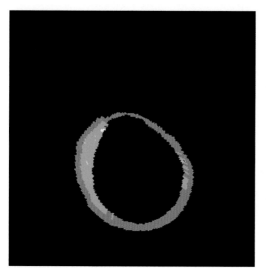

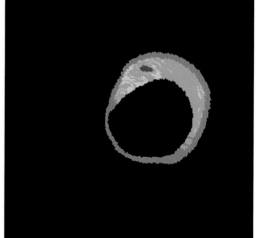

Figure 13.8 Fibrous plaque with focal areas of lipid accumulation.

Figure 13.9 Tissue map demonstrating "Pathological Intimal Thickening".

indicative of disease and possible future progression to risky atheroma, they are not viewed to be acutely dangerous (Figure 13.9).

Coronary "vulnerable" type IV and type Va lesions and the "complicated" type VI lesions are the most relevant to ACS. Type IV and Va lesions, although not necessarily stenotic at angiography, are prone to disruption. Fibroatheroma has a distinct layer of superficial fibrous tissue confining an area of necrosis. The fibrous cap thickness

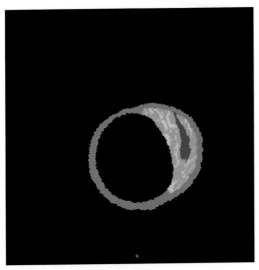

Figure 13.10 Tissue map demonstrating "Fibroatheroma".

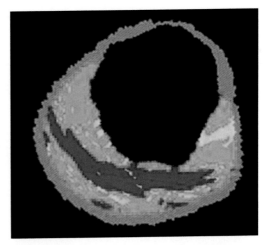

Figure 13.12 Fibroatheroma without presence of dense calcium.

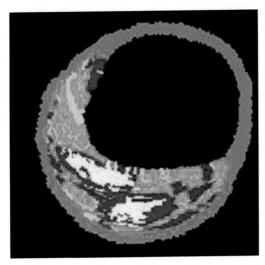

Figure 13.11 Fibroatheroma with dense calcium present in plaque.

primarily distinguishes the fibroatheroma from the classic vulnerable plaque which is called a thin-cap fibroatheroma. With IVUS-based tissue characterization, fibroatheromatous plaque will appear as fibrous/fibro-fatty regions with necrotic cores comprising more than 10% of the lesion area. (Figure 13.10) Fibroatheroma can be further differentiated into three subgroups:

1 Fibroatheroma with dense calcium present in plaque is generally viewed as being more dangerous

than fibroatheroma without dense calcium. Note that here the necrotic core is not displayed as "on" or near the lumen on tissue map. (Figure 13.11).

2 Fibroatheroma without presence of dense calcium. Note that here necrotic core is also not displayed as "on" or near the lumen on tissue map. (Figure 13.12).

3 Thin cap fibroatheroma (TICFA) or vulnerable plaque. Necrotic core is significant (>10% of total plaque volume) and located on or near the lumen at tissue map. Note that tissue map is limited by the inherent resolution of IVUS, which is approximately 100 μm. Therefore, the fibrous cap, which is most certainly present, covers the atheroma, is not visualized by IVUS or the tissue map. (Figure 13.13).

(a) TICFA with narrowing where narrowing is defined as greater than 50% reduction in cross-sectional area on IVUS, or stenosis of 25% or greater on angiogram. Data from Virmani et al. (see Chapter 1) suggests that TICFA with significant narrowing represents the highest risk of all plaques (Figure 13.14).

(b) TICFA without significant narrowing is defined as a cross-sectional area reduction of less than 50% on IVUS or less than 25% narrowing on angiogram. These plaques are considered to have a lower probability of rupture. (Figure 13.15). Due to the inability of IVUS to display plaques other than as grayscale renderings, interventional cardiologists have not been able to draw

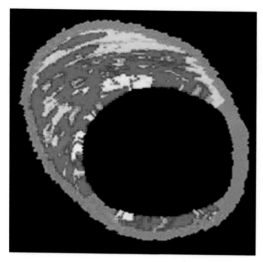

Figure 13.13 Thin cap fibroatheroma (TCFA) or vulnerable plaque.

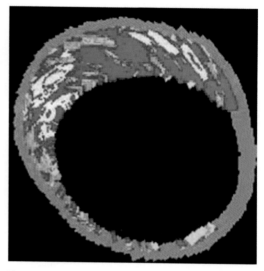

Figure 13.15 TCFA with less than 50% narrowing. These plaques are considered to have a lower probability of rupture.

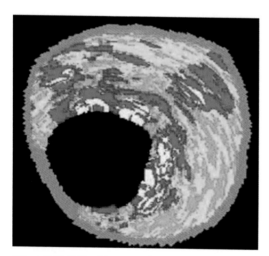

Figure 13.14 TCFA with greater than 50% narrowing. These plaques represent the highest risk of all plaques.

conclusions about the plaque type or disease type seen in individual lesions or patients. IVUS provides little information as to the composition of lesions and is unable to assess their potential vulnerability on a consistent basis.

IVUS-based tissue characterization may eventually (with supporting clinical outcomes data) be able to provide plaque composition in real time in the catheterization laboratory in such a way that interventional cardiologists can easily and quickly gain

important new information about each patient. Specifically, it is envisaged that it will provide information on intermediate or ambiguous lesions that will assist the physician in making his or her treatment decision. For example, if VH can provide plaque type information on 40–60% lesions, the knowledge of whether a plaque comprises purely fibrous/fibro-fatty tissue (typifying pathological intimal thickening) versus a significant necrotic core may add to the diagnostic/therapeutic guidance value of IVUS.

References

1. American Heart Association. Statistical Fact Book, 2004.
2. Virmani R, Kolodgie FD, Burke AP, Farb A, Schwartz SM. Lessons from sudden coronary death: a comprehensive morphological classification scheme for atherosclerotic lesions. Arterioscler Thromb Vasc Biol 2000;20:1262–75.
3. Nissen SE, Yock P. Intravascular ultrasound: novel pathophysiological insights and current clinical applications. Circulation 2001;103:604–16.
4. Palmer ND, Northridge D, Lessells A. In vitro analysis of coronary atheromatous lesions by intravascular ultrasound; reproducibility and histological correlation of lesion morphology. Eur Heart J 1999;20:1701–6.
5. Dixon KJ, Vince DG, Cothren RM, Cornhill JF. Characterization of coronary plaque in intravascular

ultrasound using histological correlation. Annu Int Conf IEEE Eng Med Biol Proc 1997;2:530–3.

6. Vince DG, Dixon KJ, Cothren RM. Comparison of texture analysis methods for the characterization of coronary plaques in intravascular ultrasound images. Comput Med Imag Graphics 2000;24:221–9.

7. Bridal S, Fornes P, Brunevar P, Berger G. Parametric (integrated backscatter and attenuation) images constructed using backscattered radio frequency signals (25–56 MHz) from human aortae in-vitro. Ultrasound Med Biol 1997;23:215–29.

8. Lizzi FL, Ostromogilsky M, Feleppa EJ, Rorke MC, Yaremko MM. Relationship of ultrasonic spectral parameters to features of tissue microstructure. IEEE Trans Ultrason Ferroelec Freq Control 1987;33:319–28.

9. Nair A, Kuban BD, Tuzcu EM, Schoenhagen P, Nissan SE, Vince DG. Coronary plaque classification using intravascular ultrasound radiofrequency data analysis. Circulation 2002;106:2200–6.

10. Nair A, Kuban BD, Obuchowski N, Vince DG. Assessing spectral algorithms to predict atherosclerotic plaque composition with normalized and raw intravascular ultrasound data. Ultrasound Med Biol 2001;27:(10):1319–31.

CHAPTER 14

Magnetic resonance imaging and intravascular magnetic resonance imaging

Hee Kwon Song, Ronald L Wolf, Jacob Schneiderman & Robert L Wilensky

Magnetic resonance imaging (MRI) is ideally suited for the assessment of vascular plaque burden and lesion composition for several reasons.[1] First, it is a noninvasive technique. Second, MRI is able to visualize and characterize the composition of the atherosclerotic wall. Angiography effectively measures the degree of vessel stenosis only when luminal narrowing has occurred. Angiography cannot detect lesions at the early stages when the luminal area is left relatively unaffected due to positive vascular remodeling and compensatory dilatation.[2] Although a high-degree stenosis is more likely to produce symptoms of stable predictable ischemia, often lesser stenoses are more vulnerable and cause unstable disease, such as myocardial infarction or death when present in the coronary vasculature.[3,4] The lack of sufficient agreement between angiography and clinical progression of coronary artery disease has been demonstrated[5–7]. The lack of agreement between angiography and surgical findings was demonstrated by Streifler et al.,[8] who showed in a report on 500 patients included in the North American Symptomatic Carotid Endar-terectomy study that the diagnostic accuracy of carotid angiography for detecting plaque ulceration was only 61%. Finally, MRI is the only technique currently available that can determine the various components of atherothrombotic plaque including lipid, fibrous tissue, calcium, and thrombus formation.[9]

The use of MR to evaluate the composition of the underlying atherosclerotic plaque takes advantage of several biophysical and biochemical properties of the lesion that result in differential responses to the application of an electromagnetic radiofrequency (RF) pulse in a strong static magnetic field. A high external magnetic field causes a net alignment of the proton spins within the body along the direction of the field. A short RF pulse is then applied, causing absorption of energy and nutation of the spins onto the transverse plane. The absorbed RF energy is subsequently released as the excited protons return to their original equilibrium state at a rate determined by the spin-lattice relaxation time (called T_1). In addition, the spins dephase with a specific relaxation time determined by the spin-spin relaxation time (called T_2). Both T_1 and T_2 relaxation times are dependent on tissue composition and the local spin environment. The signal produced by the relaxing spins are detected with RF receiver coils, and the level of T_1 and T_2 contrasts in the reconstructed image can be controlled with imaging parameters such as the sequence repetition time TR or the echo time TE. Finally, a proton-density weighted image can also be obtained by reducing the contribution from T_1 and T_2, and leaving only the differences in water or lipid proton densities for image contrast. These three different imaging contrasts, along with a time-of-flight (TOF) scan, can be exploited to determine plaque composition (see below).

Technical advances in high-resolution carotid plaque magnetic resonance imaging

One of the challenges in high-resolution *in-vivo* imaging is the achievable signal-to-noise ratio (SNR). Recent advances in both hardware and imaging techniques for plaque imaging have improved the image SNR, allowing the assessment of the morphology of plaque development, as well as its composition. In addition, new techniques have been developed to improve the lumen-wall contrast critical for lesion delineation and to increase the overall scanning efficiency. The following summarizes some of the recent advances.

Black-blood pulse sequences

An important requirement for visualization of atheromatous lesions is a pulse sequence that provides high contrast between the lumen and the vessel wall. Previously, the most common methods involved the use of spatial presaturation pulses[10] along with multi-line data acquisition such as the fast spin-echo sequence (FSE, RARE). Adequate suppression of the blood signal requires sufficiently fast flow and replacement of the blood in the imaging slice by the presaturated blood. This condition is not always satisfied, particularly in the region of the carotid bulb where recirculation can lead to residual signal that could mimic plaque.[11]

An alternative technique that is more robust to slow or recirculating blood flow is the double inversion black-blood technique.[12] It is essentially an inversion recovery sequence, in which a non-selective inversion pulse is applied, followed by a delay time TI (inversion time) and data acquisition. The period TI is optimally chosen such that the blood signal is nulled when the data collection begins. A second, slice-selective inversion pulse is applied immediately after the first to preserve the tissue signal in the imaging slice (thus the term "double inversion"), while any blood in that slice would flow out during TI. The double-inversion technique has been shown to perform better for blood signal nulling than spatial presaturation.[13] The improved nulling is in part due to the longer period between inversion and acquisition, allowing more time for the nulled blood to replace the unaffected blood in the imaging region. This additional time is particularly important in the presence of slow-flowing or recirculating blood, as in regions of turbulence or disturbed flow like the carotid bulb. Figure 14.1 shows a comparison of the performance of the spatial presaturation and double inversion sequences, demonstrating the superiority of the latter technique.

Although highly effective for black-blood imaging, one of the drawbacks of the original double inversion technique is its inefficiency since the method is inherently a single-slice technique. Study protocols that include multiple scans with different contrast weightings (proton density, T_1- or T_2-weighted, with or without fat saturation) can therefore become prohibitively long. Several different multiple-slice double inversion pulse sequences have been recently developed to improve scanning

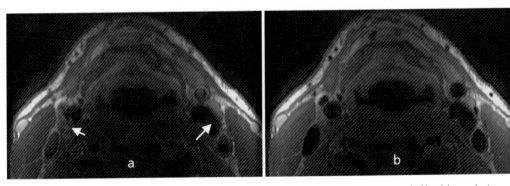

Figure 14.1 *In-vivo* carotid vessel wall imaging near the bulb region using an FSE sequence preceded by: (a) superior/inferior spatial presaturation pulses; (b) double inversion preparation. In a, flow-related artifacts are visible both within and outside the lumen (arrows).

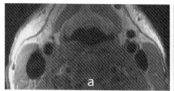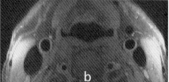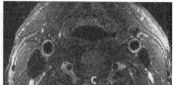

Figure 14.2 Carotid vessel images acquired with the double-inversion sequence and phased array receiver coils (one pair for each side of the neck): (a) proton-density weighted image; (b) proton-density weighted image with fat saturation; (c) T_2-weighted image with fat saturation. The vessel walls are clearly delineated, particularly with fat suppression.

efficiency.[14–16] Efficiency factors of two or greater can be achieved with these techniques depending on the exact imaging parameters.

Phased array receiver coils

For a reliable analysis of the various components of an atherosclerotic lesion in the carotid arteries, the image resolution should be sufficiently high, ideally less than 400–500 μm in plane and 2–3 mm slice thickness. At these dimensions, the standard head and neck coils cannot provide adequate SNR in a reasonable amount of time.

Near the bifurcation the carotid artery is located at a depth of approximately 30–50 mm from the surface of the neck. Hence, a surface coil reception results in higher SNR than imaging with a head or neck coil. The approximate cylindrical geometry of the neck further allows multiple receiver coils to be circumferentially aligned in close proximity to the artery, increasing the overall detection sensitivity and ultimately image SNR. Several studies of vessel wall imaging using receive – only phased arrays, including the optimization of coil size and geometry, have been reported in the literature.[17–19] Compared to conventional 3-inch single surface coils, gains of 37%[17] and 100%[18] have been achieved with various size two-coil arrays. With

such coil arrays, high-resolution images of the carotid arteries are now routinely obtained, and multiple scans with different contrast weightings can be achieved with sufficient image quality (Figure 14.2).

Multiple contrast magnetic resonance imaging for plaque characterization

The possible role of MRI for noninvasive assessment of plaque morphology and content has been addressed in several investigations.[20–26] Martin et al.[21] showed that the transverse relaxation time T_2 can be used to discriminate between medial and adventitial layers of the arterial wall, as well as to detect intimal thickening at early stages of the atherosclerotic process. Toussaint et al.[23] found T_2 to discriminate between the collagenous cap and lipid core of atherosclerotic lesions. Further they found that the T_2 values measured *in-vivo* correlate well with *in-vitro* T_2 measurements. For plaque tissue characterization, a combination of TOF, and proton-density, T_2-, and T_1-weighted scans, can help determine the lesion make up, including calcifications, necrotic cores, and recent hemorrhage[25] (Table 14.1).

Table 14.1 Plaque characterization based on multiple contrast weightings. Intensities are relative to that of the sternocleidomastoid muscle. (Modified from Yuan et al. Radiology 2001;221:285–99.[25])

Component	TOF	T_1-weighted	PD/intermediate-weighted	T_2-weighted
Hemorrhage (recent)	High	High-moderate	Variable	Variable
Lipid-rich necrotic core	Moderate	High	High	Variable
Calcification	Low	Low	Low	Low
Fibrous tissue	Moderate-low	Moderate	High	Variable

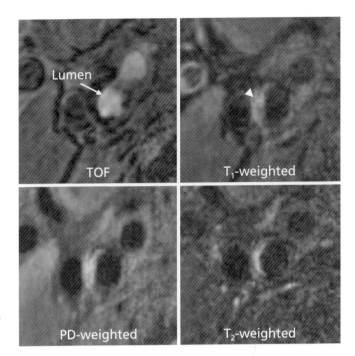

Figure 14.3 Small eccentric plaque (arrowhead) without calcification (dark on TOF, moderate increased intensity on black-blood images), most consistent with Type III plaque.

Figures 14.3–14.6 show *in-vivo* images of the carotid arteries with different contrast weightings, including TOF and T_1-, T_2-, and PD-weighted black-blood images of several different plaque types. Different components of the plaque at various stages of lesion development can be detected, demonstrating the potential for MR imaging for *in-vivo* carotid plaque characterization.

Detection of coronary lesions

Double inversion black-blood techniques have also been used for imaging the coronary arteries. Coronary wall MRI is considerably more difficult than imaging the carotids for various reasons, including the need to employ both respiratory and cardiac gating to prevent motion artifacts. Although images can be acquired during one or more breath-holds (Figure 14.7), prospective navigator gating for coronary imaging has recently been shown to be effective, allowing data acquisition during free-breathing.[27,28] Spiral acquisition schemes, which are more robust to motion and have shorter data acquisition windows, have also been implemented for improved image quality[28] and for efficient multi-slice acquisitions.[29] With dedicated phased array cardiac receiver coils and further optimization of black-blood pulse sequences, high resolution imaging of coronary lesions has been shown to be possible (Figure 14.8).[30]

In spite of the recent progress, because of the deeper location of the coronary arteries from the surface of the chest (4–10 cm), and the difficulty of close receiver coil placement, attaining sufficient SNR remains a major challenge for coronary MRI. The smaller dimensions of the arterial wall (on the order of 1 mm thick) further exacerbates the problem, since higher spatial resolution is required for accurate plaque volume quantification and classification. Partial volume effects from relatively thick slices or large in-plane pixel widths can cause an overestimation of the wall thickness and lesion size. Thus, current techniques are limited primarily to the major coronary arteries, and additional studies are needed to validate the accuracy and repeatability of the current strategies. However, with the increasing availability of high field scanners and improved coil design, including the possibility of intravascular coils,[31] *in-vivo* coronary MRI may soon be a viable option for plaque characterization.

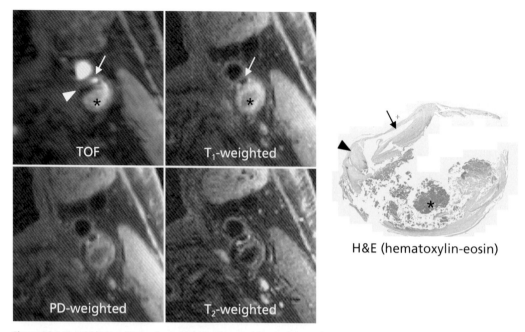

Figure 14.4 Type VI lesion. Hemorrhage (denoted by asterisk) was detected with MRI (bright relative to muscle on T$_1$-weighted and TOF, decreased intensity on PD-weighted and especially T$_2$-weighted images) and confirmed by histology. Arrow indicates the internal carotid artery lumen and arrowhead indicates mineral.

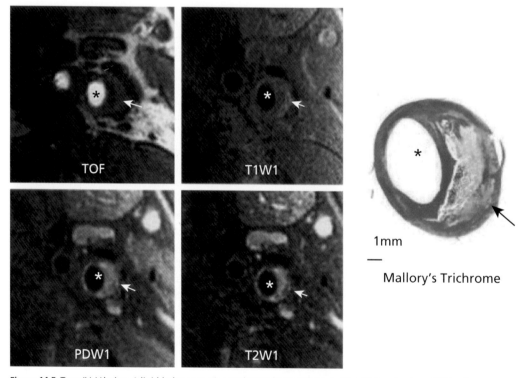

Figure 14.5 Type IV–V lesion. A lipid-laden necrotic core (arrows) was detected with MRI (moderate on TOF and T$_1$-weighted, PD and T$_2$-weighted) and confirmed by histology. Asterisk (*) indicates lumen. (From Cai et al. Circulation 2002;106:1368–73, with permission.[26])

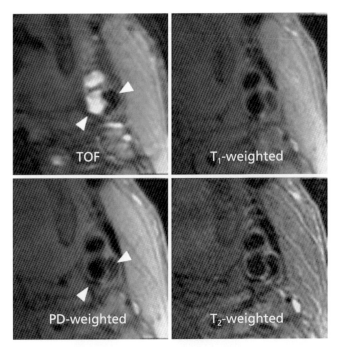

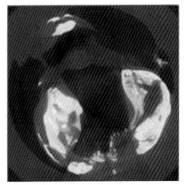

Specimen Micro-CT

Figure 14.6 Type VII lesion with heavy calcification (arrowheads) detected by MRI (decreased intensity on all sequences). The presence of calcification was confirmed by micro-CT of the specimen.

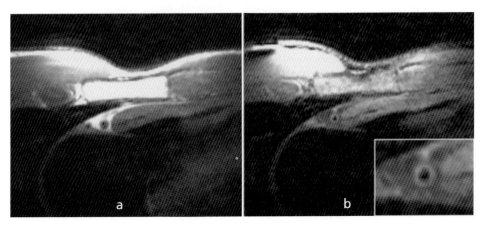

Figure 14.7 Double-inversion FSE black-blood images of the RCA: (a) without fat suppression; (b) with fat saturation applied (inset: magnified). The RCA wall is more clearly visible in the fat-saturated images. Each image was acquired from a 36-year-old healthy volunteer during a single 20-second breath-held scan using a single 3-inch surface receiver coil. Imaging parameters: TR = 1 × RR; slice thickness = 5 mm; 18 × 18 cm² FOV; 256 × 256 matrix size; receiver bandwidth = 128 kHz; echo spacing = 6.5 ms; echo train length = 16.

Use of intravascular coils

As distance between the MRI coil and the interrogated structure increases, the SNR decreases, necessitating the reduction in the image resolution. One approach used to interrogate deeper lying arteries, such as coronary arteries, is the placement of an intravascular coil. Early studies with such coils have shown improved resolution. Correia et al.[32] evaluated isolated human thoracic segments and showed an 80% agreement between histology and MRI with an excellent correlation between MRI and luminal area. Fibrous cap recognition was observed in 20/24 plaques and a necrotic core in 23/24.

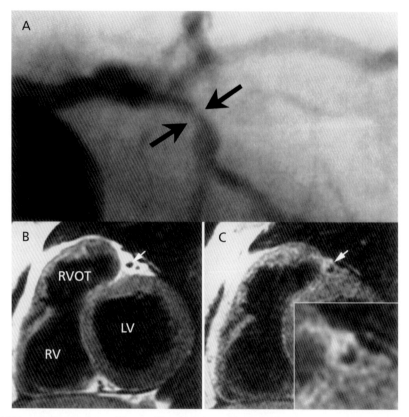

Figure 14.8 (A) X-ray angiogram from a 76-year-old male patient with stenosis in the proximal LAD (arrows). A partially obstructed lumen could be seen in the black-blood FSE images acquired without (B) and with (C) fat saturation (arrows). A four-element (two anterior, two posterior) phased array coil was used for signal reception. Imaging parameters: TR = 2 × RR; TE = 40 ms; 4 mm slice thickness; 29 × 21.75 cm^2 FOV; 384 × 256 matrix size; echo train length = 32; 125 kHz receiver bandwidth. RVOT = right ventricular outflow tract; RV = right ventricle; LV = left ventricle. (From Fayad et al. Circulation 2000;102:506–10, with permission.[30])

Others have shown in examination of human carotid plaques that signal property differences between fibrous cap, lipid, and calcium can be detected with an intravascular coil.[33] At the current time, however, the use of intravascular coils is limited by the invasive nature of the diagnostic approach, size of the catheter, and the time-consuming imaging protocols. Nonetheless, this is an area of active investigation.

Use of magnetic resonance imaging to evaluate changes in plaque composition and size

Several studies in animals and humans have demonstrated that MRI can be utilized to diagnose and follow *in-vivo* atherosclerotic lesions. In diet-induced atherosclerosis in rabbits T_2-weighted MR images were used to document regression in aortic atherosclerosis following withdrawal of the atherosclerotic diet.[34] Changes in wall thickness and percent stenosis were observed. A decrease in the lipid components of the atherosclerotic plaque has also been shown with MRI. In animals continued on a high-cholesterol diet, progression of disease and increased lipid deposition was shown.[35] Botnar et al.[36] offered evidence that molecular imaging using a fibrin-specific binding contrast agent detected acute and subacute thrombi in a rabbit atherosclerotic model.

In humans Corti et al.[37] demonstrated a decrease in cross-sectional arterial wall area in atherosclerotic segments of the aorta and carotid artery following treatment with a statin. Of interest was that there was no change in the luminal area in the setting of a decrease in plaque size and negative remodeling resulting from the reduction in plaque dimensions. Finally, Zhao and colleagues[38] used MRI to demonstrate that patients treated with intensive lipid-lowering therapy had less lipid within the carotid arteries compared to patients without such treatment over a 10-year follow-up period. The results showed that patients treated with intensive lipid-lowering therapy had a smaller lipid core area and decreased lipid composition of the carotid plaque. Decreased lipid plaque content has been associated with more stable atherosclerotic lesions. The sum of these studies would indicate that MRI is a very acceptable noninvasive approach to evaluating plaque size and composition in reaction to treatment strategies.

Intravascular magnetic resonance imaging

As discussed above, magnetic resonance imaging is a potential approach to determine plaque composition in human coronary arteries. MRI can be used to determine the presence of lipid within the arterial wall or, in combination with local delivery of contrast agents, MRI can determine the presence of specific cell types associated with plaque instability or thrombus. Previous studies using external magnet MRI in patients with carotid artery disease have shown that high resolution multi-contrast MRI is capable of assessing atherosclerotic lesions based on lesion composition[39] and has been shown clinically to identify the presence of ruptured fibrous caps that are associated with transient ischemic attacks or stroke.[40] However, cardiac and respiratory motion inhibits adequate data acquisition thereby limiting the application to the coronary vasculature. The intravascular MRI catheter (Topspin Medical, Lod, Israel) was designed for intravascular interrogation of the arterial wall and is unencumbered by cardiac motion. As such this technology holds promise in the *in-vivo* evaluation of lipid-rich unstable coronary artery lesions.

Technical properties of the intravascular MRI catheter

The MRI system consists of a self-contained intravascular MRI probe integrated at the tip of a vascular catheter, and a portable control unit. The MR probe contains the components necessary for MR analysis, including the magnets, radiofrequency (RF) coil, and electronics that allow transmission of echo train, and reception of signals. It is independent of external magnets and coils; hence the system can be used within the cardiac catheterization laboratory. The probe creates a sector-shaped sensitive region with radial evaluation of the vessel wall. Strong static magnetic field gradients are locally generated at the site of measurement, and are highly responsive to the diffusion properties of the analyzed tissue (Figure 14.9). Lipid-rich tissue, abundant within the necrotic core of thin-cap fibroatheromas, can be readily detected by diffusion coefficient measurements.[41] Preliminary experiments evaluating human carotid endarterectomy plaques with MR microscopy demonstrated the effectiveness of diffusion coefficient parameter in diagnosing lipid-rich tissue (Figure 14.10). In addition, multi-contrast MRI such as T1, T2, and proton density are readily obtained with this catheter.

The MRI probe assesses a 2 mm tissue slice, providing a lateral view of 60°, and radial resolution of 250 μ field of view (FOV). Within each FOV two bands are defined simultaneously: a shallow luminal band (0–100 μ in depth) and a deeper band, 100–250 μ in depth. In order to interrogate the circumference of the arterial wall, MRI measurements are performed in 3 or 4 quadrants of 60° each and the data is integrated to produce a color-coded display. The resulting image, therefore, represents the sum of 2 superficial and deep FOV bands in each of the 4 quadrants. To achieve high resolution MRI the catheter is stabilized against the arterial wall by a low-pressure side balloon (Figure 14.11). Each subsequent MRI measurement yields a time constant that relates specifically to the diffusion coefficient of the tissue and is the basis for determination of the lipid fraction (LF). The LF represents the percentage of lipid within the

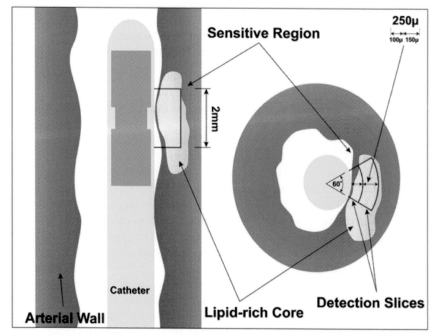

Figure 14.9 The self-contained MRI catheter is shown placed inside an artery with a 2 mm window in close proximity to the arterial wall containing a lipid-rich core. On the right panel a cross-section of the artery is seen showing the resulting MRI image in the two detection slices.

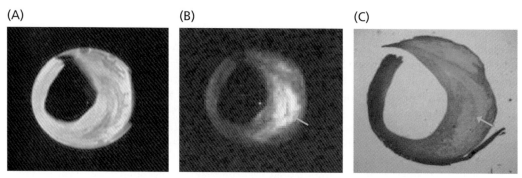

Figure 14.10 MR microscopy used for the analysis of sliced carotid plaque. Proton density (A) as well as diffusion coefficient contrast (B) are demonstrated next to photomicroscopy (Hematoxylin & eosin staining) of the tissue. Note the correlation between diffusion coefficient and histopathology (C) in regard to lipid-rich tissue diagnosis (arrows).

evaluated tissue volume. An increased LF is yellow in the MRI display while a decreased LF is displayed in blue.

Previous histologic studies have shown that "vulnerable plaques" deemed thin-cap fibroatheromas have a fibrous cap thickness of less than 75 µ. Hence, the MRI determinates of a thin-cap fibroatheroma were defined as the presence of an increased LF in the shallow luminal band of the FOV. An increased LF in turn indicates the *absence* of fibrous tissue; hence, a thin-cap fibroatheroma presumed to be an unstable lesion. Conversely, the absence of lipid within the superficial FOV denotes a fibrous cap >100 µ deemed to be a thick fibrous cap atheromas, generally observed in more stable lesions. Increased lipid in the deep FOV in turn indicates the presence of a necrotic core or increased foam cells.

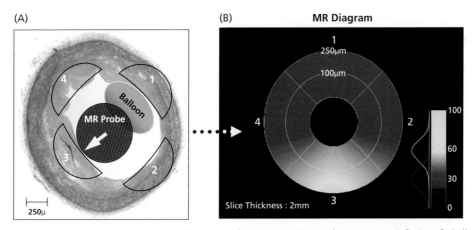

Figure 14.11 (A) Coronary artery cross-section with MRI sampling sites superimposed. Low pressure inflation of a balloon fixes the MRI probe to the arterial wall allowing for adequate sampling. (B) Resulting MRI image with one sector lipid rich (yellow) and the other sectors fibrous rich (blue).

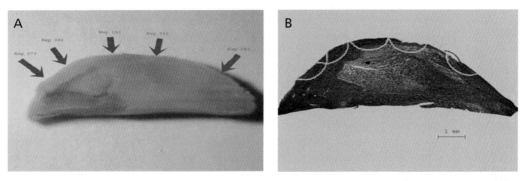

Figure 14.12 Sliced carotid endarterectomy plaques that were analyzed by the MR probe. The plaque is shown in A, while in B the pathologist's delineation of the lipid-rich areas are shown. Also highlighted in blue are the sectors undergoing MR analysis.

Preliminary experiments with the MRI probe

The diagnostic capabilities of the MR probe were initially tested on formalin fixed carotid endarterectomy plaques obtained from symptomatic and asymptomatic patients. To account for tissue fixation, parallel experiments were performed on unfixed samples. Although formalin fixation lowers the tissue's MR signal by 30–50% in comparison to fresh unfixed tissue, the detectable tissue property was not abolished. The tissues were dissected according to the plaque's morphology, to allow direct application of the probe to the tissue surface. Both lipid-rich, as well as fibrous tissue

were analyzed at multiple loci with precise registration of the interrogated sites (Figure 14.12). A pathologist unaware of the MR results reviewed the histologic slides and delineated areas containing high lipid, low lipid, and no lipid tissue, prior to superposition of the map of analyzed loci. The correlation of MR results vs histological diagnosis yielded a sensitivity of 90% (Figure 14.13). The results showed that the MR probe was capable of differentiating lipid from fibrous tissue.

In-vivo preclinical studies

In order to assess the MRI functional capacity of the IVMRI catheter an *in-vivo* porcine femoral

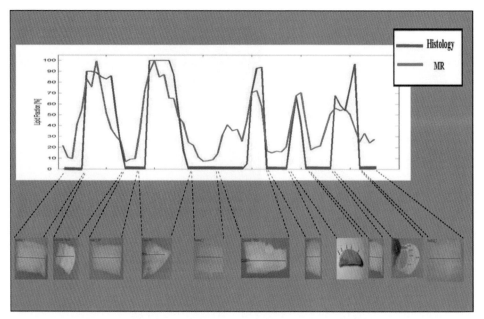

Figure 14.13 Plot comparing the MR diagnoses of increased lipid fraction against the histopathologic diagnosis. Each tissue slice was interrogated at multiple sites along a registered line.

artery model was designed which mimics lipid-rich atherosclerotic lesions. The superficial femoral artery was dissected in the thigh. The vessel, approximately 4 mm in diameter, was wrapped intermittently with 1 cm rings of subcutaneous fat, involving either the entire circumference or 180° of the circumference (Figure 14.14). The IVMRI catheter was inserted into the vessel and positioned alternatively within bare or fat-wrapped arterial segments. Precise positioning of the probe was accomplished by direct visualization through the thin-walled vessel as well as by external electrical stimulation which identified the probe's coil. The MRI results demonstrated an excellent correlation with an "all blue" display for bare-segment bands or a superficial blue and deep sector yellow display in the fat-wrapped segments.

Subsequent studies were performed in 14 non-atherosclerotic domestic swine to assess the maneuverability and safety of the IVMRI catheter in coronary vessel wall investigation. In each pig one coronary artery underwent interrogation in two locations within the proximal 6 cm of the vessel. The full circumferential assessment of the vessel

wall was achieved by performing measurements at 4 quadrants (90° apart). The pigs were randomized to euthanasia at 24 hours after interrogation (acute group, n = 7) and after 30 days in the chronic group (n = 7). Two additional pigs were utilized to compare the histologic effects of the IVMRI catheter placement compared to an intravascular ultrasound (IVUS) catheter. Angiography at the end of the procedure and at the completion of the study (24 hours or 30 days) revealed no vascular damage. Histopathology of the vessels demonstrated minimal scattered endothelial denudation, comparable to the effect of placement of the IVUS catheter. These experiments demonstrated the *in-vivo* safety of the IVMRI catheter.

Intravascular MRI studies in human postmortem vascular tissues

To assess the functional capacity of the IVMRI catheter in human vascular tissues, the device was used to analyze fresh postmortem human aortas and coronary arteries. Sixteen segments of proximal

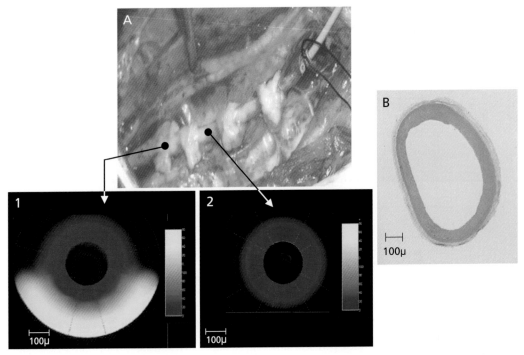

Figure 14.14 The *in-vivo* porcine femoral artery model designed to mimics deep lipid-rich atherosclerotic lesions (A): 1) MRI image of an area of 180° fat wrapping around the femoral artery while 2) shows an area without fat wrapping. Yellow indicates the presence of an increased lipid fraction, in this case >100 μ from the arterial surface while areas of a low lipid fraction are noted in blue. A cross-section of the non-atherosclerotic femoral artery is shown (B).

aorta, exhibiting a variety of atherosclerotic lesions (by morphology), were selected for analysis and placed in a saline bath at 37°C. The MR probe was applied to the tissue at the site of interest and MR measurements were obtained (Figure 14.15). An experienced cardiovascular pathologist blinded to the MRI results then evaluated the samples. The aortic specimens were diagnosed by histology as follows: Ulcerated plaques (absence of fibrous cap, n = 4), thin cap fibroatheromas (n = 2), thick fibrous cap atheromas (n = 2), intimal xanthomas (n = 2), and adaptive intimal thickening (n = 6). There was a strong correlation of the MRI data with histological diagnosis at each site of measurement demonstrated with MRI correctly predicting the histologic results in 15 of 16 cases (95% sensitivity, 100% specificity).[41] In one case MRI incorrectly diagnosed a single thick fibrous cap atheroma as a vulnerable lesion.

Further studies were performed in *ex-vivo*, in-situ coronary arteries. Fourteen hearts underwent post-mortem selective coronary arteriography to confirm the presence of atherosclerotic disease. Eighteen moderately stenotic proximal and mid lesions (30–60% in diameter reduction) were selected. MR analysis using the IVMRI catheter were performed within the whole heart whilst immersed in saline solution at 37°C and undergoing coronary perfusion with saline. Prior to MR analysis the location of the intermediate coronary lesion determined by angiography was marked on the epicardial surface, and the position of the MR probe was validated electronically. MR acquisition was performed at 4 quadrants per location. Immediately following MRI evaluation the examined arteries were dissected and 5 mm segments containing the lesions were processed for histological evaluation. The tissues were serially sectioned through the area of interest at 6 μ intervals and sections every 100 μ were stained with

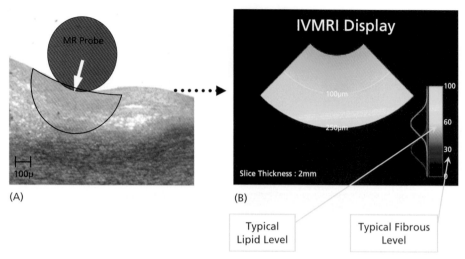

Figure 14.15 (A) Human *ex-vivo* aortic segment with cartoon depiction of the MRI catheter on the surface. (B) Corresponding MRI image showing the presence of both superficial and deep lipids.

hematoxylin & eosin and Movat's pentachrome stains. The presence of macrophages was determined by immunohistochemistry. A trained cardiovascular pathologist, blinded to the MR data, evaluated the tissue slides and lesions were classified according to the recently published classification.[43] Thin cap fibroatheroma (vulnerable plaques) were defined by histology as lesions containing necrotic cores and thin (<75 μ) fibrous caps. Lesions abundant with foam cells containing lipid-laden macrophages, regardless of the thickness of the fibrous cap. Fibrous lesions contained few foam cells and no necrotic cores. Histology results were then compared to results obtained with the MRI catheter.

Coronary artery lesions were classified as: adaptive intimal thickening, n = 1; fatty streak (intimal xanthoma), n = 2; thick fibrous cap atheroma, n = 4; thin cap fibroatheroma (vulnerable plaque), n = 3; ruptured plaque with intra-plaque hemorrhage, n = 1; plaque hemorrhage, n = 1; healed plaque rupture, n = 1; and fibrocalcific plaque, n = 5. MRI diagnosis for every specimen was obtained by integrating lipid fraction data, which was assessed within both bands simultaneously, within each quadrant. MRI diagnosis of lesion characteristics correlated with histologic diagnosis

in 16 out of 18 lesions (89%) including the diagnosis of 3 thin cap fibroatheromas.[42]

In vivo human study with the IVMRI

Clinical studies with the IVMRI catheter have been initiated and are continuing. Both peripheral, as well as coronary arteries have been analyzed, primarily to establish safety of the device. Moderately stenotic lesions (30–60% luminal narrowing) in the superficial femoral artery or lesions within the proximal segment (5–6 cm) of the coronary arteries were identified by angiography (Figure 14.16). There were no procedure-related complications noted.[44]

Future directions

With the increasing availability of high field whole-body scanners (3T or greater), investigators have only recently began to study the potential for SNR gains for carotid vessel wall imaging.[38–40] Higher field strength increases the achievable SNR (approximately linearly), and this gain can be utilized to achieve higher spatial resolution for improved measurement accuracy or detection sensitivity. Alternatively, the SNR gain can be used to

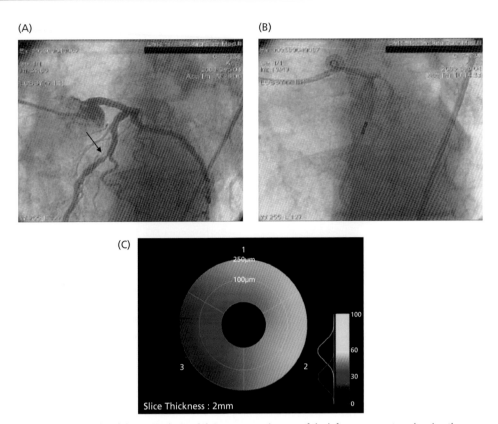

Figure 14.16 *In-vivo* results of the IVMRI device. (A) Coronary angiogram of the left coronary artery showing the presence of an intermediate lesion in the mid left anterior descending artery (arrow). (B) Placement of the IVMRI catheter into the lesion. (C) The corresponding MRI display at the bottom indicating an increased lipid fraction, both superficial and deep in 3 of 4 sectors.

reduce the scan time. An SNR improvement of 2, for example, could potentially be used to lower the scan time by a factor of 4 or, alternatively, increase the in-plane resolution by a factor of √2. Any expected gains, however, will be affected by the lengthening of T_1 and the reduction of T_2 at higher fields, factors which will tend to reduce the SNR gain. Recent comparisons between 1.5 and 3T systems have shown improvements on the order of 1.5–2 in the carotid vessel wall at the higher field.[45–47]

Advances in MR scanner hardware have also led to the consideration of alternative imaging strategies. Ultra-fast imaging strategies such as steady-state free precession techniques have recently been proposed for lumen and vessel wall imaging.[48,49] The performance of this method, which is sensitive to off-resonance effects from magnetic field inhomogeneity, has improved as a result of faster and higher gradient amplitudes allowing for ultra-short TR. This approach had been shown recently to provide images with high lumen/plaque contrast in the aorta.[42] Additional studies are necessary, however, to determine the utility of these techniques for high resolution *in-vivo* plaque characterization.

A self-contained MRI probe will allow detection of thin fibrous cap atheromas that are postulated to be the major cause of unstable angina, myocardial infarction or ischemic sudden death. Future developments may result in the ability to target through MRI contrast solutions the presence of macrophages and/or thrombus formation allowing for more directed diagnosis of coronary lesions with the increased propensity to become unstable and lead to clinical symptoms. Hence, targeted evaluation of patients with increased risk of myocardial infarction may be possible leading to focal prophylactic treatment of such lesions. Whether intravascular MRI will be used alone or in conjunction with other intravascular technologies remains to be examined. In addition, outcomes studies evaluating all technologies with regard to predicting clinical course of such possible "vulnerable lesions" is also necessary.

References

1. Yuan C, Lin E, Millard J, Hwang JN. Closed contour edge detection of blood vessel lumen and outer wall boundaries in black-blood MR images. Magn Reson Imaging 1999;17:257–66.

2. Glagov S, Weisenberg E, Zarins CK, Stankunavicius R, Kolettis GJ. Compensatory enlargement of human atherosclerotic coronary arteries. N Engl J Med 1987;316:1371–5.

3. Schaar JA, Muller JE, Falk E, et al. Terminology for high-risk and vulnerable coronary artery plaques. Report of a meeting on the vulnerable plaque, June 17 and 18, 2003, Santorini, Greece. Eur Heart J 2004;25(12): 1077–82.

4. Varnava AM, Mills PG, Davies MJ. Relationship between coronary artery remodeling and plaque vulnerability. Circulation 2002;105:939–43.

5. Ambrose JA, Tannenbaum MA, Alexopoulos D, et al. Angiographic progression of coronary artery disease and the development of myocardial infarction. J Am Coll Cardiol 1988;12:56–62.

6. Little WC, Constantinescu M, Applegate RJ, et al. Can coronary angiography predict the site of a subsequent myocardial infarction in patients with mild-to-moderate coronary artery disease? Circulation 1988;78:1157–1166.

7. Giroud D, Li JM, Urban P, et al. Relation of the site of acute myocardial infarction to the most severe coronary arterial stenosis at prior angiography. Am J Cardiol 1992;69:729–732.

8. Streifler JY, Eliasziw M, Fox AJ, Benavente OR, Hachinski VC, Ferguson GG, Barnett HJ. Angiographic detection of carotid plaque ulceration. Comparison with surgical observations in a multicenter study. North American Symptomatic Carotid Endarterectomy Trial. Stroke 1994;25:1130–2.

9. Fuster V, Corti R, Fayad ZA, Schwitter J, Badimon JJ. Integration of vascular biology and magnetic resonance imaging in the understanding of atherothrombosis and acute coronary syndromes. J Thromb Haemost 2003;1:1410–21.

10. Felmlee JP, Ehman RL. Spatial presaturation: a method for suppressing flow artifacts and improving depiction of vascular anatomy in MR imaging. Radiology 1987;164: 559–64.

11. Steinman DA, Rutt BK. On the nature and reduction of plaque-mimicking flow artifacts in black blood MRI of the carotid bifurcation. Magn Reson Med 1998;39: 635–41.

12. Edelman RR, Chien D, Kim D. Fast selective black blood MR imaging. Radiology 1991;181:655–60.

13. Nayak KS, Rivas PA, Pauly JM, Scott GC, Kerr AB, Hu BS, Nishimura DG. Real-time black-blood MRI using spatial presaturation. J Magn Reson Imaging 2001;13: 807–12.

14. Song HK, Wright AC, Wolf RL, Wehrli FW. Multislice double inversion pulse sequence for efficient black-blood MRI. Magn Reson Med 2002;47:616–20.

15. Parker DL, Goodrich KC, Masiker M, Tsuruda JS, Katzman GL. Improved efficiency in double-inversion fast spin-echo imaging. Magn Reson Med 2002;47: 1017–21.

16. Itskovich VV, Mani V, Mizsei G, et al. Parallel and non-parallel simultaneous multislice black-blood double inversion recovery techniques for vessel wall imaging. J Magn Reson Imaging 2004;19:459–67.

17. Hayes CE, Mathis CM, Yuan C. Surface coil phased arrays for high-resolution imaging of the carotid arteries. J Magn Reson Imaging 1996;6:109–12.

18. Ouhlous M, Lethimonnier F, Dippel DW, van Sambeek MR, van Heerebeek LC, Pattynama PM, van Der Lugt A. Evaluation of a dedicated dual phased-array surface coil using a black-blood FSE sequence for high resolution MRI of the carotid vessel wall. J Magn Reson Imaging 2002;15:344–51.

19. Liffers A, Quick HH, Herborn CU, Ermert H, Ladd ME. Geometrical optimization of a phased array coil for high-resolution MR imaging of the carotid arteries. Magn Reson Med 2003;50:439–43.

20. Yuan C, Tsuruda JS, Beach KN, et al. Techniques for high-resolution MR imaging of atherosclerotic plaque. J Magn Reson Imaging 1994;4:43–9.

21. Martin AJ, Gotlieb AI, Henkelman RM. High-resolution MR imaging of human arteries. J Magn Reson Imaging 1995;5:93–100.

22. Toussaint JF, Southern JF, Fuster V, Kantor HL. T_2-weighted contrast for NMR characterization of human atherosclerosis. Arterioscler Thromb Vasc Biol 1995;15:1533–42.

23. Toussaint JF, LaMuraglia GM, Southern JF, Fuster V, Kantor HL. Magnetic resonance images lipid, fibrous,

calcified, hemorrhagic, and thrombotic components of human atherosclerosis in vivo. Circulation 1996;94: 932–8.

24. Yuan C, Mitsumori LM, Ferguson MS, et al. In vivo accuracy of multispectral magnetic resonance imaging for identifying lipid-rich necrotic cores and intraplaque hemorrhage in advanced human carotid plaques. Circulation 2001;104:2051–6.

25. Yuan C, Mitsumori LM, Beach KW, Maravilla KR. Carotid atherosclerotic plaque: noninvasive MR characterization and identification of vulnerable lesions. Radiology 2001;221:285–99.

26. Cai JM, Hatsukami TS, Ferguson MS, Small R, Polissar NL, Yuan C. Classification of human carotid atherosclerotic lesions with in vivo multicontrast magnetic resonance imaging. Circulation 2002;106:1368–73.

27. Botnar RM, Stuber M, Kissinger KV, Kim WY, Spuentrup E, Manning WJ. Noninvasive coronary vessel wall and plaque imaging with magnetic resonance imaging. Circulation 2000;102:2582–7.

28. Botnar RM, Kim WY, Börnert P, Stuber M, Spuentrup E, Manning WJ. 3D coronary vessel wall imaging utilizing a local inversion technique with spiral image acquisition. Magn Reson Med 2001;46:848–54.

29. Song HK. Highly efficient double-inversion spiral technique for coronary vessel wall imaging [Abstract]. In: Proceedings of the 12th Annual Meeting of ISMR Honolulu. 2002, p. 1566.

30. Fayad ZA, Fuster V, Fallon JT, et al. Noninvasive in vivo human coronary artery lumen and wall imaging using black-blood magnetic resonance imaging. Circulation 2000;102:506–10.

31. Botnar RM, Bucker A, Kim WY, Viohl I, Gunther RW, Spuentrup E. Initial experiences with in vivo intravascular coronary vessel wall imaging. J Magn Reson Imaging 2003;17:615–19.

32. Correia LC, Atalar E, Kelemen MD, et al. Intravascular magnetic resonance imaging of aortic atherosclerotic plaque composition. Arterioscler Thromb Vasc Biol 1997;17:3626–32.

33. Rogers WJ, Prichard JW, Hu YL, et al. Characterization of signal properties in atherosclerotic plaque components by intravascular MRI. Arterioscler Thromb Vasc Biol 2000;20:1824–30.

34. McConnell MV, Aikawa M, Maier SE, Ganz P, Libby P, Lee RT. MRI of rabbit atherosclerosis in response to dietary cholesterol lowering. Arterioscler Thromb Vasc Biol 1999;19:1956–9.

35. Helft G, Worthley SG, Fuster V, et al. Progression and regression of atherosclerotic lesions: monitoring with serial noninvasive magnetic resonance imaging. Circulation 2002;105:993–8.

36. Botnar RM, Perez AS, Witte S, et al. In vivo molecular imaging of acute and subacute thrombosis using a fibrin-binding magnetic resonance imaging contrast agent. Circulation 2004;109:2023–9.

37. Corti R, Fayad ZA, Fuster V, et al. Effects of lipid-lowering by simvastatin on human atherosclerotic lesions: a longitudinal study by high-resolution, non-invasive magnetic resonance imaging. Circulation 2001; 104:249–52.

38. Zhao XQ, Yuan C, Hatsukami TS, Frechette EH, Kang XJ, Maravilla KR, Brown BG. Effects of prolonged intensive lipid-lowering therapy on the characteristics of carotid atherosclerotic plaques in vivo by MRI: a case-control study. Arterioscler Thromb Vasc Biol 2001;21: 1623–9.

39. Cai JM, Hatsukami TS, Ferguson MS, et al. Classification of human carotid atherosclerotic lesions with in vivo multicontrast magnetic resonance imaging. Circulation 2002;106:1368–73.

40. Yuan C, Zhang SX, Polissar NL, et al. Identification of fibrous cap rupture with magnetic resonance imaging is highly associated with recent transient ischemic attack or stroke. Circulation 2002;105:181–5.

41. Toussaint JF, Southern JF, Fuster V, et al. Water diffusion properties of human atherosclerosis and thrombosis measured by pulse field gradient nuclear magnetic resonance. Arterioscler Thromb Vasc Biol 1997;17: 542–6.

42. Schneiderman J, Wilensky RL, Weiss A, et al. Diagnosis of thin-cap fibroatheromas by a self-contained intravascular magnetic resonance imaging probe in ex-vivo human aorta and in-situ coronary arteries. J Am Coll Cardiol 2005;45:1961–9.

43. Virmani R, Kolodgie FD, Burke AP, et al. Lessons from sudden coronary death: a comprehensive morphological classification scheme for atherosclerotic lesions. Arterioscler Thromb Vasc Biol 2000;20:1262–75.

44. Regar E, Hennen B, Grube E, et al. First in man application of a minature self-contained intracoronary magnetic resonance imaging probe. A multi-center safety and feasibility trial. Euro Intervent 2006;2:77–83.

45. Terashima M, Nguyen PKP, Yarnykh VL, et al. Carotid plaque imaging at 1.5T and 3T: Systematic SNR comparison [Abstract]. In: Proceedings of the 12th Annual Meeting of ISMRM, Kyoto. 2004, 1910.

46. Anumula S, Song HK, Wright AC, Wehrli FW. Carotid vessel wall imaging: a comparison between 1.5T and 3T [Abstract]. In: Proceedings of the 12th Annual Meeting of ISMRM, Kyoto. 2004, p. 911.

47. Yarnykh VL, Hayes CE, Shimakawa A, et al. High-resolution black-blood MRI of carotid atherosclerotic

plaque at 3T: optimization of clinical protocol [Abstract]. In: Proceedings of the 12th Annual Meeting of ISMRM Kyoto, 2004, p. 1912.

48. Washington E, Simonetti O, Chiou A, Finn JP. A novel true FISP technique for visualizing vascular plaque.

Denver [Abstract]. In: Proceedings of the 8th Annual Meeting of ISMRM, 2000, p. 1666.

49. Spuentrup E, Katoh M, Stuber M, Botnar R, Schaeffter T, Buecker A, Gunther RW. Coronary MR imaging using free-breathing 3D steady-state free precession with radial k-space sampling. Rofo 2003;175:1330–4.

CHAPTER 15

Radionuclide imaging

Johan Verjans & Jagat Narula

As discussed in the earlier chapters, the likelihood of development of acute coronary syndromes including sudden cardiac death is determined by the histomorphologic substrate of the atherosclerotic plaques. Therefore, various imaging techniques have attempted to characterize fibrous cap thickness, necrotic cores, and the severity of the inflammatory component in the lesions. Limited success has been achieved by the use of angioscopy[1] and intravascular ultrasonography,[2,3] or more recently with optical coherence tomography,[4,5] thermography,[6,7] elastography,[8,9] and magnetic resonance imaging.[10] Since plaques that are vulnerable to rupture or erosion have a distinct molecular morphology, appropriate targeting of the predominant cellular population and biochemistry of the atherosclerotic plaque may help predict the likelihood of clinical events with radionuclide imaging techniques.[11]

Plaques that are vulnerable to rupture harbor intense macrophage infiltration.[12,13] Macrophages at the site of rupture are often apoptotic and are associated with matrix metalloproteinases upregulation and activation within the neointima;[14] inflammation may also contribute to the release of prothrombotic substances such as tissue factor.[15] The presence of inflammation has been indirectly supported by the increase in serum levels of C-reactive protein levels and myeloperoxidase and glutathione-1 peroxidase enzymes in acute coronary syndromes.[16–20] On the other hand, inflammation within the plaque has been localized with the help of temperature probes and the demonstration of paramagnetic iron particle deposition in macrophage population by magnetic resonance.[21] Since the monocyte-macrophage cells that transgress to the neointima develop a wide range of adhesion molecules and receptors, ligands to these neoexpressions have also been successfully used for developing radionuclide imaging techniques.[22]

Plaques vulnerable to erosions, in contrast to those prone to rupture, demonstrate significant alterations in the proportional distribution of neointimal ground substance; there is relatively higher expression of proteoglycans, such as hyaluranon. This hyaluranon-rich neointima has thrombogenic properties which are further amplified by its inability to stabilize the covering endothelial cells. Sloughing of the endothelial cells exposes hyaluranon, to which platelets harbor distinct receptors. Targeting of interstitial alterations may therefore offer an opportunity to target lesions vulnerable to erosion.[23]

Targeting atherosclerotic lesions vulnerable to rupture

Since inflammation is the most important feature of plaque vulnerability, and is often associated with programmed cell death and abundance of various metalloproteinases at the site of rupture, novel characteristics of noncirculating resident macrophages, the process of apoptosis, and expression of metalloproteinases have been proposed as potential targets for noninvasive radionuclide detection of vulnerable plaques.

Potential molecular targets of infiltrating macrophages

Macrophage infiltration in the vessel wall follows a systematic process that includes phases such

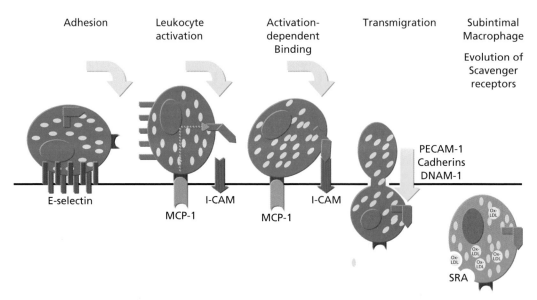

Figure 15.1 Representation of leukocyte infiltrating the vessel wall. The initial phase of leukocyte infiltration consists of reversible binding of selectin molecules expressed as a result of endothelial activation. With subsequent expression of chemotactic peptides such as MCP-1, the leukocyte adheres firmly to the vessel wall. Ultimate expression of integrins is followed by transmigration. Intimal leukocytes express scavenger receptors, enabling them to take up modified LDL.

as leukocyte rolling, leukocyte-adhesion, and leukocyte-transmigration (Figure 15.1).[24,25] The initial endothelial cell injury results in expression of selectin molecules, such as E- or P-selectin, corresponding to monocyte selectins such as L-selectin. The resulting monocyte–endothelial interaction induces a potentially reversible monocyte "rolling" on the endothelial cell surface and slows the otherwise rapidly moving circulating monocytes providing a greater opportunity for subsequent monocyte arrest. Monocytes adhere firmly to the endothelium if chemotactic peptides such as monocyte chemoattractant protein-1 (MCP-1) are expressed on the endothelial surface. If the chemoattractants have not been expressed the monocytes roll back to the blood stream as the selectins get shed. The chemoattractant-based interaction leads to activation of G protein-coupled receptors of β_1- or β_2-integrins (such as VLA-4, LFA-1, or Mac-1).[26] The integrins lock in with endothelial adhesion molecules of the immunoglobulin gene superfamily such as vascular cell adhesion molecule 1 (VCAM-1) and intercellular adhesion molecule (ICAM) 1 2, as the monocytes probe the interen-

dothelial cell junctions. The migration of monocytes is a dynamic process which is mediated partly by endothelial cell junctional molecules including platelet–endothelial cell adhesion molecule 1 (PECAM-1), cadherins, and the newly described β_2 integrin ligand DNAM-1.[27,28]

Radionuclide imaging of inflammation

As a first proof of principle for imaging of inflammatory component of atherosclerotic plaques, indium-111 oxine-labeled autologous monocytes were used in patients with angiographic evidence of peripheral vascular disease. After transition through the lungs during dynamic acquisition, radiolabeled monocytes predominantly accumulated in the spleen. Focal sites of uptake were visible over the carotid or femoral arteries only in 40% of patients with proven atherosclerotic disease.[29]

Since the receptors for chemoattractants or adhesion molecules are only expressed by infiltrating monocytes, radiolabeled MCP-1 and VCAM have been used for the noninvasive detection of atherosclerotic lesions. Iodine-131 or [99mTc]-labeled MCP-1 has been shown to selectively accumulate in

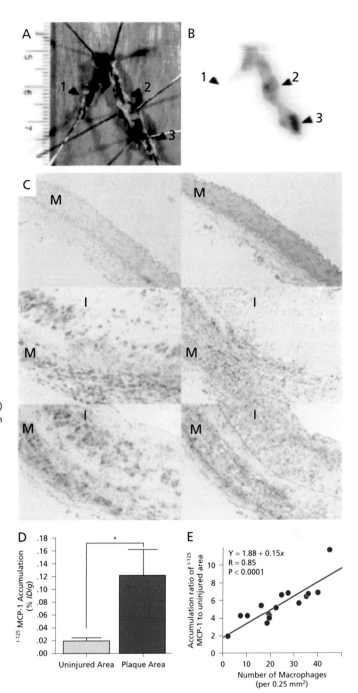

Figure 15.2 Detection of monocyte chemoattractant protein-1 receptor expression in experimental atherosclerotic lesions. Pictures represent iliac arteries stained with Evans blue dye (A) with the corresponding autoradiograph (B) and immune-stained sections (C, left column) and H&E sections (C, right column) taken from a control area (1), denuded area (2), and plaque area (3). I = Intima; M = media. Most pronounced areas of radioactivity correspond to plaque area (3), which had highest concentration of RAM-11-stained cells. Medium pronounced areas correspond to the de-endothelialized area (2). The areas of lowest activity corresponded to noninjured areas (1). D, Activity per gram in uninjured and plaque region of artery. Accumulation of ^{125}I-MC-1 in re-endothelialized areas was greater than that in de-endothelialized area (6.55 ± 2.26 vs 4.34 ± 1.43 counts/pixel, $P < 0.05$). E, Relationship of ^{125}I-MC-1 lesion/normal accumulation ratio to number of macrophages per unit area ($r = 0.85$, $P < 0.0001$). (From Ohtsuki K et al. Circulation 2001;104:203–8.[30])

lipid-rich, macrophage-rich regions of experimental atherosclerosis model in rabbits by macroautoradiography (Figure 15.2).[30] The macroautoradiographic results closely correlated with the severity of lesions, with no uptake in the uninjured part of aorta, moderate uptake in the atherosclerotic lesions, and maximum uptake in the area with significant lesions. The histopathologic and immunohistochemical characterization of the aortic specimens demonstrated increasing prevalence of macrophages in proportion to the increasing radiotracer uptake. The percent injected dose per gram uptake of the radiolabeled MCP-1 was significantly higher in the diseased aorta as compared to the nonatherosclerotic regions.[31] Further, quantitative estimates of the number of macrophages per unit area correlated with percent injected dose per gram accumulation of ^{125}I-MCP-1 in the atherosclerotic lesions ($r = 0.85$, $P < 0.0001$). Similar to role of chemoattractants, antibodies to adhesion molecules have been used for noninvasive detection of vascular imaging in skin transplantation.[32] The uptake offers a proof of concept and can be extrapolated for applicability in atherosclerotic imaging.

After subendothelial migration, monocytes develop scavenger receptors that allow ingestion of oxidized LDL more avidly (than native LDL), and are not downregulated with an increase in the cholesterol content of the cell.[33] The scavenger receptors for oxidized LDL uptake in subintimal macrophages include SRA I or II, CD36, CD68, and FcγRII. Since these receptors are not borne by circulating monocytes, the radiolabeled ligands for these receptors may constitute attractive ligands for noninvasive imaging. The scavenger receptors have been targeted with radiolabeled LDL[34] and nonspecific immunoglobulin G (IgG)[35] in multiple clinical trials. The potential of these radiolabeled agents has not been fully investigated. It is relatively simple to use radiolabeled IgG, which is currently available for clinical use for noninvasive detection of occult inflammatory foci.

Association of macrophages with plaque vulnerability

Although the inflammatory component of the atherosclerotic plaque renders the lesion susceptible to rupture, the putative mechanisms that link inflammation to plaque rupture are not well understood. Recent literature supports that cell death in the neointima may contribute to actual plaque rupture. In a study in the hearts of victims of sudden death secondary to plaque rupture,[36] there was a strikingly high prevalence of apoptotic nuclei at the rupture sites by in situ end-labeling. Further characterization demonstrated that the apoptotic cells in the culprit lesions suggested exclusive apoptosis of macrophages, these macrophages expressed

caspase-1 or ICE. Immunoblot studies of the plaques demonstrated cleaved active band of ICE in the ruptured plaques; whereas only unprocessed ICE was present in stable plaques, both processed and unprocessed ICE bands were not seen in normal vessel wall. On quantitative analysis of the prevalence of cells and incidence of apoptosis in various cell types, apoptotic cells were predominantly observed at the rupture site and only occasionally encountered in the regions of the same plaque remote from the site of rupture; apoptosis was most prevalent in macrophages. Stable plaques demonstrated minimal evidence of apoptotic cells, which was predominantly confined to smooth muscle cells (SMC).

In addition to actual association with an acute event, slow process of cell death of macrophages and smooth muscle cells contributes to gradual evolution of an unstable plaque.[13] In a study of nonulcerated atheromatous plaques,[37] a high incidence of apoptosis was observed in inflammatory cells predominantly in macrophages surrounding the lipid core, a finding that has been corroborated by numerous other studies of human plaques.[36,38,39] These studies have suggested that macrophage cell death is perhaps responsible for core formation and expansion. Other studies have proposed that the chronic loss of SMC in atherosclerotic plaques in human aorta may lead to fibrous cap attenuation and vulnerability.[40] In addition to direct cap thinning, SMC apoptosis may also contribute to plaque vulnerability by recruitment of inflammation in the fibrous cap, by induction of expression of MCP-1 and IL-8.[41]

Noninvasive detection of apoptosis of macrophages in atherosclerotic plaques

Since Annexin-V can identify the cell membrane alterations associated with apoptosis and the process of apoptosis may contribute to plaque vulnerability and rupture, radiolabeled Annexin-V has been employed for the detection of atherosclerotic lesions, both in experimental and clinical settings.[11,42] Radiolabeled Annexin-V has a high affinity for the aberrantly expressed phosphatidyl serine on the apoptotic cells, and the proof of concept of its use in the detection of apoptotic macrophages was demonstrated in apo E$^{-/-}$ mice with simultaneous administration of fluorescent

Figure 15.3 Feasibility of noninvasive imaging of apoptosis by radiolabeled annexin-V. Left lateral oblique gamma images of an experimental atherosclerotic (A–C) and control (D–F) rabbit injected with ^{99m}Tc-annexin-V; L and K mark liver and kidney activities, respectively. Images at the time of injection (A, D) and at 2 hours after injection (B, E) are shown. While blood pooling is seen at the time of injection, tracer uptake is clearly visible in the abdominal aorta at 2 hours (B). C, Ex vivo image of B shows intense ^{99m}Tc-annexin-V uptake in the arch and abdominal region. The annexin-positive areas were confirmed to contain atherosclerotic plaque by histology. D–F, Demonstration of corresponding images in the control animals. Note the aorta is indistinguishable from background at 2 hours after injection. F, Ex vivo aortic image of E demonstrates the absence of ^{99m}Tc-annexin-V uptake. G, Box plot representing a quantitative analysis of ^{99m}Tc-annexin-V uptake in the various lesion types. The uptake or radiolabel was significantly higher in AHA type IV lesions; no differences were noted between type II and III lesions. H, Simple regression analyses of SMC- (white) and macrophage-burden (black) with ^{99m}Tc-annexin-V uptake, demonstrated no significant relationship between SMC (E, $r = 0.08$, $P = 0.73$), but directly proportional relationship to macrophage burden (F, $r = 0.47$, $P = 0.04$). %ID/g = percent injected per gram wet weight of tissue. (From Kolodgie et al. Circulation 2003;108:3134–9.[11])

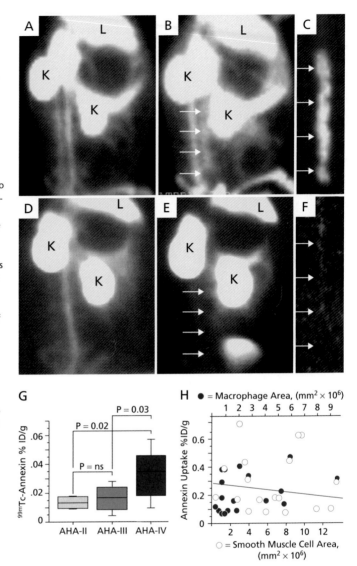

Annexin-V. The green Annexin-V localized clearly in the arterial lesions with abundant macrophages lesions.[43] Annexin-V, both radiolabeled and fluorescein-labeled, were injected in 50-week-old ApoE-deficient mice. Autoradiographically identified regions of ^{99m}Tc-Annexin-V uptake in ascending aorta and carotid arteries demonstrated localization of fluorescent tracer in macrophage-rich regions of AHA type IV lesions, which were subsequently determined to harbor apoptotic cells.

To investigate the feasibility of noninvasive detection, atherosclerotic lesions were induced in NZW rabbits by de-endothelialization of the infradiaphragmatic aorta followed by 12 weeks of a high fat, high cholesterol diet (Figures 15.3, 15.4).[11] All animals received 0.5–1 mg of Annexin-V labeled with 7–10 mCi of technetium-99 m intravenously for in vivo imaging studies. The left lateral decubitus gamma images showed clear delineation of radiolabel within the abdominal aorta 2 hours after Annexin administration. Ex vivo images showed a robust uptake of radiotracer in the infradiaphragmatic aorta within the lesion distribution corresponding to the in vivo images. By contrast, the uptake of radiolabel was absent in areas without grossly visible atherosclerotic lesions; these areas

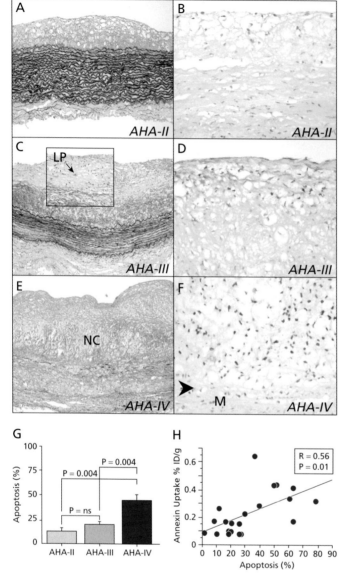

Figure 15.4 Pathologic characterization of annexin-V uptake and DNA fragmentation in experimental atherosclerotic lesions, and the relationship of the prevalence of apoptosis with ^{99m}Tc-annexin-V uptake. Lesion type was assigned using an American Heart Association classification scheme: A and B, AHA type II lesion. C and D, AHA type III lesion (inset in B shows lipid pools, LP). E and F, AHA type IV lesion. The black nuclei in B, D, and F represent positive DNA fragment staining while methyl green is the counterstain (bluish-green nuclei). G, Bar graph showing apoptotic index relative to lesion type; there was a significant increase in the prevalence of apoptosis in AHA type IV lesions. H, Simple regression analysis of ^{99m}Tc-annexin-V uptake with apoptotic index; the prevalence of apoptosis was related to annexin-V uptake; $r = 0.56$, $P = 0.01$. NC = necrotic core; M = media; arrowhead in F = internal elastic lamina. (From Kolodgie et al. Circulation 2003;108:3134–9.[11])

were predominantly localized to the nondenuded descending thoracic aorta. In contrast to vessels with plaques, there was no localization of radiotracer within the presumably normal vessel wall; ex vivo imaging confirmed the lack of radiotracer uptake. The accumulation of ^{99m}Tc-Annexin-V in atherosclerotic lesions in the balloon-denuded region of the aorta was approximately 9.3-fold greater than in the corresponding control abdominal aortic region. The mean ± SEM percent-injected dose per gram uptake in the specimens with lesions

$(0.054 ± 0.0095\%)$ was significantly higher than the background activity in the normal specimens $(0.0058 ± 0.001, P < 0.000)$. Histopathologic correlation of the severity of atherosclerotic lesions and the radiotracer uptake demonstrated that Annexin accumulation predominantly occurred in AHA type IV lesions with only minimal uptake in type II and III lesions. A large proportion of the cells stained positively for the presence of apoptosis in type IV lesions, which had shown the maximal radiotracer uptake. Further, there was a modest direct relationship of Annexin-V uptake with total macrophage burden ($r = 0.47$, $P = 0.04$); no association was observed between SMC burden and radiotracer uptake ($r = 0.08$, $P = 0.73$).

We have recently used Annexin-V for the detection of vulnerable atherosclerotic lesions in patients with carotid vascular disease.[42] Of the four patients, two had recent transient ischemic episodes and the remaining two patients had remote episodes. All of them underwent carotid endarterectomy after imaging. The positive uptake correlated with macrophage apoptosis in the neointima which represented vulnerability of the plaque. One of the two patients with a recent transient ischemic attacks (TIA) had a severe lesion on the contraleteral carotid, but without an Annexin uptake. The two patients with remote TIA and statin therapy had negative scans and endarterectomy specimens demonstrated quiet, SMC-rich atherosclerotic lesions.

Fluorine-18-labeled FDG (Figure 15.5) and Indium-III-labeled immunoglobulin have been used for non-specific but effective targeting of plaque inflammation.

Radionuclide detection of matrix metalloproteinase upregulation in atherosclerotic lesions

Inflammation within the atherosclerotic plaque may further perpetuate plaque instability by production of matrix metalloproteinase (MMP) (Figure 15.5). When activated by cytokines (TNF-γ, IL-1), macrophages secrete inactive MMP, including interstitial collagenases (MMP-1), gelatinase B (MMP-9), stromolysins 1–3 (MMP-3, -10, -11), and a membrane type. When activated by plasmin or by inactivation of intrinsic inhibitors in tissue, MMP can degrade the connective tissue matrix.[44] Mechanical testing in vitro of cap tissue shows that an increase in the number of macrophages and a reduction in collagen and glycosaminoglycans content reduce the amount of stress needed to fracture the tissue.[45] Sections of plaques laid on a gelatin substrate in vitro show active degeneration of collagen in lipid-rich plaques.[46] Plaque cap rupture can therefore be seen resulting from a destructive process initiated by macrophages that gains ascendancy over the repair process of collagen deposition by SMC.

The MMP production is predominantly seen in the vicinity of macrophage predominance in human coronary atherosclerotic lesions. Since active digestion of fibrous cap by MMP upregulation and activation may be an important event in plaque instability, noninvasive detection of MMP should allow better prediction of clinical outcomes in CAD patients. To prove the principle, a broad-spectrum MMP inhibitor (specificity for MMPs 1–3, 7–9, and 13, Ki 1–15 nM (Bristol-Myers Squibb, North Billerica, MA)) radiolabeled with indium-111 was used for imaging experimental

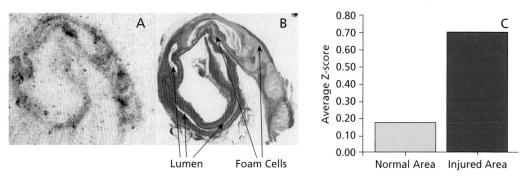

Figure 15.5 Detection of atherosclerosis using a novel positron-sensitive probe and 18-fluorodeoxyglucose (FDG). Microautoradiography (A) of ^{3}H-glucose uptake and corresponding photomicrograph (B). This injured artery was coiled longitudinally and underwent autoradiography before H&E staining. The lumen falls in and out of plane on this two-dimensional section. Accumulations of foam cells appear as uniform light pink areas between the intima and the darker staining fibrous tissue lining the lumen. Highest uptake is demonstrated in this subintimal tissue. C, Positron-sensitive probe counts of normal and injured artery segments. A total of 93 arterial segments were probed in nine animals at a detector LLD = 0.5. Mean probe Z-scores were 4.8-fold higher over injury atherosclerosis compared with uninjured normal iliac artery segments ($P < 0.001$). (From: Lederman RJ, et al. Nucl Med Commun 2001;22(7):747–53.[51])

atherosclerotic lesions in NZW rabbits.[47] Lesions were induced by balloon de-endothelialization of the infradiaphragmatic aorta and diets were manipulated by feeding 0.5% high cholesterol either continuously or interrupted with normal chow. Animals were randomized as follows: group I (control group) animals were unmanipulated rabbits and received normal chow for 4 months; group IV animals received continuous high cholesterol diet for 4 months (test group); group III (diet-interrupted group) received high cholesterol diet for 2 months/normal chow for 1 month/ high cholesterol diet again for 1 month; group II (diet withdrawal group) received high cholesterol diet for 2 months/normal chow for 2 months. By noninvasive gamma imaging, the abdominal atherosclerotic lesions were visualized best at 3 hours in group IV. The percent injected dose per gram uptake of radiolabeled MMP inhibitor was maximum in group IV lesions (0.033 ± 0.019; lesion-to-nonlesion ratio 11 : 1), and significantly higher than the interrupted diet group III (0.015 ± 0.005, $P = 0.01$). Uptake in group I control animals (0.003 ± 0.001) was minimum and similar to the diet withdrawal group II (0.01 ± 0.003, $P =$ ns). Threshold analysis of histologic sections after immunostaining showed a significant increase of MMP in plaque segments demonstrating a high radiolabeled MMP inhibitor uptake (MMP-1 = 12.5 ± 2.1, MMP-3 = 14.3 ± 1.8, MMP-9 = 1.3 ± 0.5 mm^2) relative to those with low uptake (MMP-1 = 7.7 ± 0.2, MMP-3 = 9.1 ± 1.5, MMP-9 = 0.2 ± 0.05 mm^2; $P < 0.03$). These preliminary observations suggest that in vivo quantitation of MMP in atherosclerotic plaques is feasible, and correlates with their pathologic distribution in the plaque. The observations have also confirmed the previous belief[48–50] that withdrawal of the hyperlipidemic diet (and use of statins) abrogates MMP upregulation in the plaque.[47]

Targeting atherosclerotic lesions vulnerable to erosion

Unlike rupture of the atherosclerotic plaques, the culprit lesions in smokers demonstrate a relatively stable atherosclerotic base. Men and women, even premenopausal, are equally affected and may not necessarily demonstrate the abundance of common coronary risk factors. Such lesions demonstrate significant alteration in the plaque ground substance which is not able to firmly retain the endothelial cells, and contributes to neointimal SMC migration, and thrombogenecity if denuded. The study of accumulation and distribution of specific proteoglycans, hyaluronan and cell surface receptor for hyaluronan (CD44) was recently undertaken. Proteoglycans and hyaluronan accumulated in distinct patterns depending on plaque type. The fibrous cap of stable lesions was enriched in versican and biglycan, with considerably less staining for decorin and hyaluronan, whereas picrosirius red revealed a heavy accumulation of collagen type I. By contrast, intense staining for hyaluronan and versican was found in erosions at the plaque/thrombus interface, with weak staining for biglycan and decorin; collagen content was predominantly type III. Rupture sites showed little immunoreactivity for proteoglycans or hyaluronan. CD44 was localized along the plaque/thrombus interface in erosions, whereas in ruptures and stable plaques, it was mostly confined to inflammatory cells. Positive immunostaining for immature SM cells (SM myosin heavy chain SM1 and SMemb) was present in stable and eroded plaques, whereas the presence of SM2 and smoothelin was weak or nonexistent. Although no imaging attempt has been made for the detection of erosive atherosclerotic lesions, the upregulation of hyaluronon theoretically allows the possibility of development of imaging strategy.

Future directions

The future of vascular imaging by radionuclide means is dependent upon the development of new radioligands with the capability to target distinct histopathologic characteristics in the atherosclerotic lesions, and the development of new technology for the intravascular detection of atherosclerotic lesions. Although appropriate targeting agents have been well identified, detection of radioligand uptake in small vascular lesions is a significant undertaking technologically. It is likely that such a challenge will be best met by higher resolution imaging cameras or by intravascular radiation detectors comparable to intravascular ultrasound.

References

1. Mizuno K, Satomura K, Miyamoto A, et al. Angioscopic evaluation of coronary-artery thrombi in acute coronary syndromes. N Engl J Med 1992;326:287–91.

2. Waller BF, Pinkerton CA, Slack JD. Intravascular ultrasound: a histological study of vessels during life. The new "gold standard" for vascular imaging. Circulation 1992;85:2305–10.

3. Hodgson JM, Reddy KG, Suneja R, Nair RN, Lesnefsky EJ, Sheehan HM. Intracoronary ultrasound imaging: correlation of plaque morphology with angiography, clinical syndrome and procedural results in patients undergoing coronary angioplasty. J Am Coll Cardiol 1993;21:35–44.

4. Yabushita H, Bouma BE, Houser SL, et al. Characterization of human atherosclerosis by optical coherence tomography. Circulation 2002;106:1640–5.

5. Brezinski ME, Tearney GJ, Weissman NJ, et al. Assessing atherosclerotic plaque morphology: comparison of optical coherence tomography and high frequency intravascular ultrasound. Heart 1997;77:397–403.

6. Stefanadis C, Diamantopoulos L, Vlachopoulos C, et al. Thermal heterogeneity within human atherosclerotic coronary arteries detected in vivo: a new method of detection by application of a special thermography catheter. Circulation 1999;99:1965–71.

7. Casscells W, Hathorn B, David M, et al. Thermal detection of cellular infiltrates in living atherosclerotic plaques: possible implications for plaque rupture and thrombosis. Lancet 1996;347:1447–51.

8. de Korte CL, Pasterkamp G, van der Steen AF, Woutman HA, Bom N. Characterization of plaque components with intravascular ultrasound elastography in human femoral and coronary arteries in vitro. Circulation 2000;102:617–23.

9. de Korte CL, Carlier SG, Mastik F, Doyley MM, van der Steen AF, Serruys PW, Bom N. Morphological and mechanical information of coronary arteries obtained with intravascular elastography; feasibility study in vivo. Eur Heart J 2002;23:405–13.

10. Skinner MP, Yuan C, Mitsumori L, Hayes CE, Raines EW, Nelson JA, Ross R. Serial magnetic resonance imaging of experimental atherosclerosis detects lesion fine structure, progression and complications in vivo. Nat Med 1995;1:69–73.

11. Kolodgie FD, Petrov A, Virmani R, et al. Targeting of apoptotic macrophages and experimental atheroma with radiolabeled annexin V: a technique with potential for noninvasive imaging of vulnerable plaque. Circulation 2003;108:3134–9.

12. Burke AP, Farb A, Malcom GT, Liang YH, Smialek J, Virmani R. Coronary risk factors and plaque morphology in men with coronary disease who died suddenly. N Engl J Med 1997;336:1276–82.

13. Kolodgie FD, Burke AP, Farb A, et al. The thin-cap fibroatheroma: a type of vulnerable plaque: the major precursor lesion to acute coronary syndromes. Curr Opin Cardiol 2001;16:285–92.

14. Lee RT, Libby P. The unstable atheroma. Arterioscler Thromb Vasc Biol. 1997;17:1859–67.

15. Jander S, Sitzer M, Wendt A, et al. Expression of tissue factor in high-grade carotid artery stenosis: association with plaque destabilization. Stroke 2001;32:850–4.

16. Liuzzo G, Biasucci LM, Gallimore JR, Grillo RL, Rebuzzi AG, Pepys MB, Maseri A. The prognostic value of C-reactive protein and serum amyloid a protein in severe unstable angina. N Engl J Med 1994;331:417–24.

17. Berk BC, Weintraub WS, Alexander RW. Elevation of C-reactive protein in "active" coronary artery disease. Am J Cardiol 1990;65:168–72.

18. de Beer FC, Hind CR, Fox KM, Allan RM, Maseri A, Pepys MB. Measurement of serum C-reactive protein concentration in myocardial ischaemia and infarction. Br Heart J 1982;47:239–43.

19. Blankenberg S, Rupprecht HJ, Bickel C, et al. Glutathione peroxidase 1 activity and cardiovascular events in patients with coronary artery disease. N Engl J Med 2003;349:1605–13.

20. Brennan ML, Penn MS, Van Lente F, et al. Prognostic value of myeloperoxidase in patients with chest pain. N Engl J Med 2003;349:1595–604.

21. Ruehm SG, Corot C, Vogt P, Kolb S, Debatin JF. Magnetic resonance imaging of atherosclerotic plaque with ultrasmall superparamagnetic particles of iron oxide in hyperlipidemic rabbits. Circulation 2001;103:415–22.

22. Narula J, Virmani R, Iskandrian AE. Strategic targeting of atherosclerotic lesions. J Nucl Cardiol 1999;6:81–90.

23. Kolodgie FD, Burke AP, Farb A, Weber DK, Kutys R, Wight TN, Virmani R. Differential accumulation of proteoglycans and hyaluronan in culprit lesions: insights into plaque erosion. Arterioscler Thromb Vasc Biol 2002;22:1642–8.

24. Butcher EC. Leukocyte-endothelial cell recognition: three (or more) steps to specificity and diversity. Cell 1991;67:1033–6.

25. Osterud B, Bjorklid E. Role of monocytes in atherogenesis. Physiol Rev 2003;83:1069–112.

26. Springer TA. Traffic signals for lymphocyte recirculation and leukocyte emigration: the multistep paradigm. Cell 1994;76:301–14.

27. Shibuya A, Campbell D, Hannum C, et al. DNAM-1, a novel adhesion molecule involved in the cytolytic function of T lymphocytes. Immunity 1996;4:573–81.

28. Bogen S, Pak J, Garifallou M, Deng X, Muller WA. Monoclonal antibody to murine PECAM-1 (CD31)

blocks acute inflammation in vivo. J Exp Med 1994;179:1059–64.

29. Virgolini I, Muller C, Fitscha P, Chiba P, Sinzinger H. Radiolabelling autologous monocytes with 111-indium-oxine for reinjection in patients with atherosclerosis. Prog Clin Biol Res 1990;355:271–80.

30. Ohtsuki K, Hayase M, Akashi K, Kopiwoda S, Strauss HW. Detection of monocyte chemoattractant protein-1 receptor expression in experimental atherosclerotic lesions: an autoradiographic study. Circulation 2001; 104:203–8.

31. Petrov A, Hartung D, Kolodgie F, et al. Imaging inflammation in atherosclerotic lesions by radiolabeled chemotactic peptide: would identification of vulnerable plaques become feasible? J Am Coll Cardiol 2003; 41(suppl):II-445.

32. Sadeghi M, Schechner J, Sinusas A, Narula J, Zaret B, Bender J. Noninvasive detection of endothelial activation. Orlando: 50th American College of Cardiology, 2001;37:424A.

33. Steinberg D, Witzum JL. Lipoproteins, lipoprotein oxidation, and atherogenesis. In: Cheien KR, ed. Molecular basis of cardiovascular disease. Philadelphia: WB Saunders, 1998:458–76.

34. Lees AM, Lees RS, Schoen FJ, Isaacsohn JL, Fischman AJ, McKusick KA, Strauss HW. Imaging human atherosclerosis with ^{99m}Tc-labeled low density lipoproteins. Arteriosclerosis 1988;8:461–70.

35. Fischman AJ, Rubin RH, Khaw BA, et al. Radionuclide imaging of experimental atherosclerosis with non-specific polyclonal immunoglobulin G. J Nucl Med 1989;30:1095–100.

36. Geng YJ, Henderson LE, Levesque EB, Muszynski M, Libby P. Fas is expressed in human atherosclerotic intima and promotes apoptosis of cytokine-primed human vascular smooth muscle cells. Arterioscler Thromb Vasc Biol 1997;17:2200–8.

37. Bjorkerud S, Bjorkerud B. Apoptosis is abundant in human atherosclerotic lesions, especially in inflammatory cells (macrophages and T cells), and may contribute to the accumulation of gruel and plaque instability. Am J Pathol 1996;149:367–80.

38. Cai W, Devaux B, Schaper W, Schaper J. The role of Fas/APO 1 and apoptosis in the development of human atherosclerotic lesions. Atherosclerosis 1997;131: 177–86.

39. Crisby M, Kallin B, Thyberg J, Zhivotovsky B, Orrenius S, Kostulas V, Nilsson J. Cell death in human atherosclerotic plaques involves both oncosis and apoptosis. Atherosclerosis 1997;130:17–27.

40. Geng YJ, Libby P. Evidence for apoptosis in advanced human atheroma. Colocalization with interleukin-1 beta-converting enzyme. Am J Pathol 1995;147:251–66.

41. Schaub FJ, Han DK, Liles WC, et al. Fas/FADD-mediated activation of a specific program of inflammatory gene expression in vascular smooth muscle cells. Nat Med 2000;6:790–6.

42. Kietselaer B, Reutelingsperger C, Heidendal G, Daemen M, Mess W, Hofstra L, Narula J. Non-invasive detection of plaque instability using radiolabeled Annexin-V in patients with atherosclerotic carotid artery disease. N Eng J Med 2004;**350**:1472–3.

43. Mari C, Blankenberg F, Narula N, Narula J, Ghazarossian V, Tait J, Strauss H. Atherosclerotic plaque identification in ApoE$^{-/-}$ mice: radiolabeled MCP-1 vs. annexin-V. Presented at the Annual Scientific Sessions of the Society of Nuclear Medicine, Los Angeles, CA, June 2002.

44. Galis ZS, Sukhova GK, Lark MW, Libby P. Increased expression of matrix metalloproteinases and matrix degrading activity in vulnerable regions of human atherosclerotic plaques. J Clin Invest 1994;94:2493–503.

45. Lendon CL, Davies MJ, Born GV, Richardson PD. Atherosclerotic plaque caps are locally weakened when macrophages density is increased. Atherosclerosis 1991; 87:87–90.

46. Sukhova GK, Schonbeck U, Rabkin E, Schoen FJ, Poole AR, Billinghurst RC, Libby P. Evidence for increased collagenolysis by interstitial collagenases-1 and -3 in vulnerable human atheromatous plaques. Circulation 1999;99:2503–9.

47. Kolodgie FD, Edwards S, Petrov A, et al. Noninvasive detection of matrix metalloproteinase upregulation in experimental atherosclerotic lesions and its abrogation by dietary modification. Circulation 2001;104:II-694.

48. Fukumoto Y, Libby P, Rabkin E, et al. Statins alter smooth muscle cell accumulation and collagen content in established atheroma of watanabe heritable hyperlipidemic rabbits. Circulation 2001;103:993–9.

49. Aikawa M, Rabkin E, Sugiyama S, et al. An HMG-CoA reductase inhibitor, cerivastatin, suppresses growth of macrophages expressing matrix metalloproteinases and tissue factor in vivo and in vitro. Circulation 2001;103:276–83.

50. Aikawa M, Rabkin E, Okada Y, et al. Lipid lowering by diet reduces matrix metalloproteinase activity and increases collagen content of rabbit atheroma: a potential mechanism of lesion stabilization. Circulation 1998;97:2433–44.

51. Lederman RJ, Raylman RR, Fischer SJ, et al. Detection of atherosclerosis using a positron-sensitive probe and 18-fluorodeoxyglucose (FDG). Nucl Med Commun 2001;22:747–53.

CHAPTER 16

Near-infrared spectroscopy

Pedro R Moreno, Barbara Marshik & James E Muller

Light travels fast at 186 000 miles per second and always in straight direction. As an example, the daily light we get every sunrise travels 9 million miles to reach the earth in only 8 minutes. In addition, light travels in waves composed by photons, the energy unit of light. Scientists do not yet fully understand the true nature of light, but its behavior and properties have been extensively studied. A clear working idea of these "wave motions" can be visualized similar to the undulations seen on the surface of water after a stone is dropped. Maxwell (1855) first pointed out that light can be classified according to its wavelength. The shorter the wavelength, the greater the energy of individual photons. The electromagnetic spectrum classifies light according to its wavelength including γ-rays,

X-rays, ultraviolet light, near, mid and thermal infrared light, microwave, and TV/radio light (Figure 16.1). Infrared light lies between visible (color) and radar rays.

Spectroscopy is defined as the analysis of emission, absorption, or scattering of electromagnetic radiation or light from matter to provide quantitative or qualitative information about the atoms or molecules contained in the substance. Light interacts with matter at different intensities and wavelengths, which are specific to the material properties, creating what is known as "spectra," forming the basis for spectroscopy. For example, echocardiography deals with ultrasound, which is spectroscopy performed in the audio region of the electromagnetic chart (Figure 16.1) that uses the reflection of sound

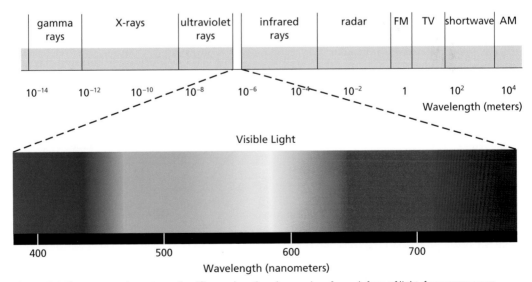

Figure 16.1 Electromagnetic spectrum. Specific wavelength scales are given for each form of light, from gamma rays to TV/radio light (see text for details). (Reproduced with permission from Kaiser PK. The joy of visual perception. Web book. www.yorku.ca/eye/how-to.htm.)

waves to create visual images of body organs. Using spectroscopy to study advanced atherosclerotic lesions in the near infrared (NIR) wavelength region, spectra from diseased vessels can be analyzed using diffuse reflectance NIR spectroscopy.

Light can be manipulated in a variety of ways. When totally blocked, light can be reflected back and produces a shadow. Light can also be deviated, changing its pathway on a symmetric angle. This is called reflection as shown in Figure 16.2. Mirrors have the ability to do this and therefore are frequently used in spectroscopy. Passing light through a media with different density, like from water to air, will deviate the light photons from their original pathway and produce a different image regarding the location of the object. This is called refraction. For instance, a flat surface will produce symmetric reflections (Figure 16.3A), however, irregular surfaces, like skins or diseased vessels will produce diffuse reflections (Figure 16.3B).

When photons strike a tissue, molecules become excited and begin to vibrate. Light can be emitted, absorbed, and/or reflected by tissue. Combinations of carbon–hydrogen, nitrogen–hydrogen, oxygen–hydrogen, and other bonds in tissue result in characteristic absorbance at specific wavelengths that can be used for sample identification and tissue characterization. The distribution of light within tissue is determined by the intrinsic properties of the tissue being illuminated. If photons are absorbed,

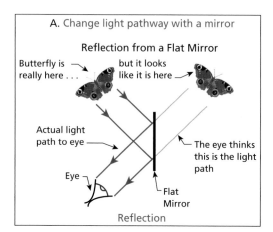
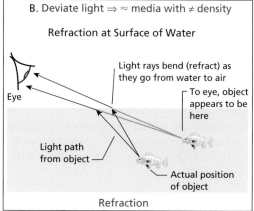

Figure 16.2 The light pathway can be changed. If a mirror is used, light can be directed in specific angulation. This is called reflection. (Adapted with permission from http://www.opticalres.com/kidoptx_f.html.)

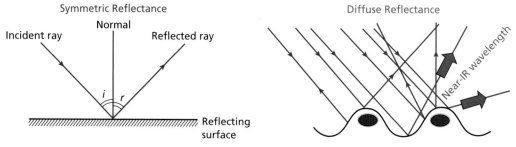

Figure 16.3 Two different forms of reflection are illustrated in this figure. A, Symmetric reflection is produced when a mirror is used on a flat surface. Reflected photons will exit at the same angle as the incident photons. B, Diffuse reflection is produced when irregular surfaces are encountered. Reflected photons will exit in different angles as the incident photons. When studying advanced atherosclerotic lesions in the near infrared wavelength region, light spectra can be analyzed using diffuse reflectance near-infrared spectroscopy. (Adapted with permission from Kaiser PK. The joy of visual perception. Web book. www.yorku.ca/eye/how-to.htm.)

the energy will cause the molecules to vibrate if the energy was in the infrared region. If the excitation energy is great enough the atom or molecule is excited to a higher energy level and will decay back to the steady-state energy level by emitting light. Depending upon the excitation source, the process will result in emission or fluorescence energy.[1]

While a portion of the light may be absorbed by the tissue, most of the light passes through the tissue with a small fraction of light being scattered. This scattering may produce reflectance of photons at the same or slightly different energy of the incident photons. Light that is scattered right back at the same wavelength is known as elastic collision or scattering and the reflected photons are classified as Raleigh scattering. If the scattering is inelastic and is due to the vibrations of the molecules, the reflected photons will have either higher or lower energy than the incident photons and are classified as Raman scattering.[1] Far more photons undergo Raleigh than Raman scattering.

Several forms of spectroscopy have been adapted for atherosclerosis research.[2] This review will focus on diffuse reflectance NIR spectroscopy for detection of vulnerable atherosclerotic plaques.

Diffuse reflectance near-infrared spectroscopy

Diffuse reflectance NIR spectroscopy is based on analysis of light at different wavelengths in the NIR region from 750 to 2500 nm. In this wavelength region, hemoglobin – the main chromophore in the visible range – has relatively low absorbance, making NIR an attractive technique for evaluation of plaque composition through blood. Every organic compound has a measurable spectrum that can be identified in the NIR window. Photons can penetrate into tissues relatively well providing simultaneous, multicomponent, nondestructive chemical analysis of biological tissue with acquisition times of less than 1 second.[3] No sample preparation is required, and physical and biological properties as well as molecular information can be derived from spectra. As a result, diffuse reflectance NIR spectroscopy has been successfully used to quantify systemic and cerebral oxygenation, and to identify multiple plasma constituents including glucose, total protein, triglycerides, cholesterol, urea, creatinine, uric acid, and human metalloproteins.[4–8]

Atherosclerotic plaque characterization using diffuse reflectance NIR spectroscopy was performed by Cassis and Lodder using a novel NIR fiber-optic probe in the hypercholesterolemic rabbit more than a decade ago. A vectorized 3-D cellular automaton-based algorithm using quantile bootstrap error-adjusted single-sample theory (BEST) technique was used to analyze the spectra in hyperspace.[9] A few years later, Dr. Dempsey successfully performed diffuse reflectance NIR spectroscopy in human carotid plaque plaques at the time of surgery prior to endarterectomy. After surgery, the excised plaque was examined by a pathologist and frozen in liquid nitrogen for *in vitro* NIR scanning followed by validation of lipoprotein composition by ultracentrifugation and gel electrophoresis.[10]

Near-infrared spectra of vulnerable atherosclerotic plaques

Following histological criteria for vulnerable atherosclerotic plaques, spectra from 199 human aortic samples were obtained using an InfraAlyzer 500 spectrophotometer.[11] An algorithm, constructed with 50% of the samples (reference set) predicted high-risk features as determined by histology. Absorbance values were obtained as log $(1/R)$ data from 1100 to 2200 nm at 10-nm intervals as shown in Figure 16.4. Principal component regression analysis was used for prediction. Sensitivity and specificity of NIR were 90% and 93% for lipid pool, 77% and 93% for thin cap, and 84% and 91% for inflammatory cells, respectively.[11] These findings were consistent with data obtained by Jarros et al. in human aortic plaques with high correlation coefficient between cholesterol contents determined by NIR spectroscopy and by reversed-phase, high-pressure liquid chromatography was 0.96.[12] In addition, Wang et al. also found high correlation of ex-vivo lipid/protein ratios in human carotid plaques using an NIR spectrometry fitted with a fiber-optic probe.[13] The same promising results were also obtained in human coronary autopsy specimens *in-vitro*.[14]

All these experiments using human tissue were performed without blood, and in some cases the

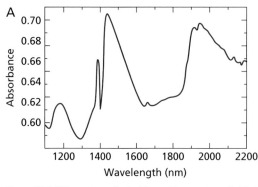
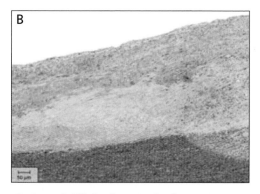

Figure 16.4 NIR spectra collected from atheromatous, lipid-rich aortic plaque. A, NIR absorbance tracing from spectra collected with an InfraAlyzer 500 spectrophotometer. Absorbance values were collected from a 1100- to 2200-nm wavelength window at 10-nm intervals (see text for details). B, Lipid-rich aortic plaque (elastic trichrome staining). (Adapted with permission from Moreno PR, et al., Circulation 2002;105:923–7.[11])

tissue was formalin-fixed or paraffin-embedded. Despite of the low absorbance of hemoglobin in the NIR wavelength, proper identification of human atherosclerotic plaques needed to be tested in fresh tissue, through blood. Marshik et al. acquired NIR spectra from 751 fresh human aortic specimens using the a Foss 6500 NIRSystem spectrometer with a fiber optic probe (SmartProbe™) classified by histology into lipid-rich, fibrotic, calcific, and normal tissue as shown in Figure 16.5. Specimens were pinned to a 5 × 5 × 0.5 cm black rubber sheet and immersed in bovine blood pre-warmed to 37 ± 1 degree centigrade. NIR spectra were subsequently acquired at various probe-to-tissue separations of 0.0, 0.25, 0.5, 1.0, 1.5, 2.0, 2.5 and 3.0 mm with blood intervening. Prediction algorithms were constructed as previously reported[15] using partial least squares discrimination analysis with bootstrapping which was then used for blind identification of tissue composition as shown in Figure 16.6. The results indicated that NIR spectroscopy was able to distinguish a lipid filled lesion 3.0 mm from the tissue sample through blood.

A system was then developed for the measurement of intracoronary NIR spectra in living patients. The first generation catheter a 3.2 French monorail system developed by MedVenture Technologies, Louisville, KY was successfully tested for safety in swine coronaries and patients scheduled for percutaneous coronary intervention for stable angina pectoris. Substantial motion artifact was observed, which guided the development of a second-generation all-optical system for testing in 2004. Such a system is likely to be capable of identifying the chemical composition of coronary plaques in patients already undergoing catheterization for the treatment of stenosis.

Perspectives

Multiple technological advances will provide information about plaque composition and vulnerability. Nevertheless, the clinical significance need to be tested in clinical trials. Such trials will determine if it is possible to identify a "vulnerable or high-risk plaque" matched with a "vulnerable or high-risk patient" – a combination that will risk-stratify thrombosis and acute coronary events. The trials will determine a "vulnerability index" composed by both plaque composition and clinical markers. If high-risk areas of an artery can be detected, both systemic and local therapy should be evaluated. Local therapy with coronary stents is an attractive option, though it may not be sufficient considering the multi-focal nature of the disease. Stenting is associated with significant reductions in total plaque and lipid core areas, increased collagen III and most importantly, with a dramatic increase in fibrous cap thickness.[16] While drug-eluting stents offer promise for the treatment of non-stenotic, high-risk plaques, such therapy should not be adopted until proven to be safe and effective in a randomized clinical trial.

Normal 　　　　　　　1 mm 　　　Fibrotic

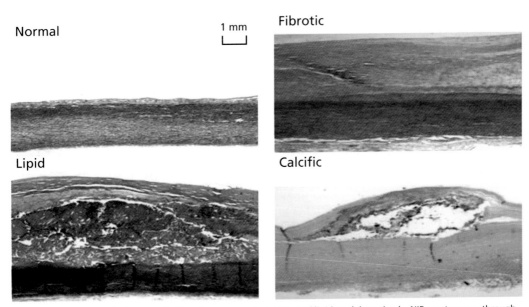

Lipid 　　　　　　　　　　　　Calcific

Figure 16.5 Human aortic tissue studied for plaque characterization and lipid pool detection by NIR spectroscopy through blood using elastic trichrome staining for the normal, fibrotic, and lipid pool tissue, and hemotaxylin and eosin staining for the calcific sample. (Adapted with permission from Marshik B, et al., from Am J Cardiol 2002;90:129H.[15])

Figure 16.6 Diffuse reflectance NIR spectroscopy of fresh human atherosclerotic plaques through blood. The left hand panel illustrates the set-up of the experiments. The NIR probe and tissue were placed within a darkened chassis to minimize the effect of stray light and spectra obtained through bovine blood held at 37°C. The NIR probe was lowered to the surface of the tissue until touched using a z-stage positioner. NIR spectra were subsequently acquired at various probe-to-tissue separations of 0.0, 0.25, 0.5, 1.0, 2.0, 2.5, and 3.0 mm through blood. The right hand panel displays sensitivity and specificity for lipid pool detection at various probe to tissue separation distances, from 0 to 3.0 mm. (Adapted with permission from Marshik B, et al., from Am J Cardiol 2002;90:129H.[15])

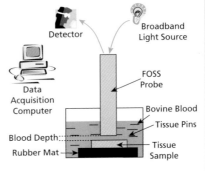

	Sensitivity	Specificity
0 mm	86%	88%
0.5 mm	92%	87%
1.0 mm	94%	90%
1.5 mm	92%	87%
2.0 mm	83%	85%
2.5 mm	81%	77%
3.0 mm	86%	72%

References

1. Chang R. Basic Principles of Spectroscopy. New York (NY): McGraw-Hill, Inc; 1971.
2. Moreno PR, Muller JE. Identification of high-risk atherosclerotic plaques: a survey of spectroscopic methods. Curr Opin Cardiol. 2002;(6):638–47.
3. Dempsey RJ, Cassis LA, Davis DG, Lodder RA. Near-infrared imaging and spectroscopy in stroke research: lipoprotein distribution and disease. Ann N Y Acad Sci. 1997;820:149–69.

4. McKinley BA, Marvin RG, Cocanour CS, et al. Tissue hemoglobin O_2 saturation during resuscitation of traumatic shock monitored using near infrared spectrometry. J Trauma. 2000;48:637–42.

5. Spielman AJ, Zhang G, Yang C, et al. Intracerebral hemodynamics probed by near infrared spectroscopy in the transition between wakefulness and sleep. Brain Res. 2000;866:313–325.

6. Gabriely I, Wozniak R, Mevorach M, et al. Transcutaneous glucose measurement using near-infrared spectroscopy during hypoglycemia. Diabetes Care. 1999;12:2026–32.

7. Shaw RA, Kotowich S, Leroux M, et al. Multianalyte serum analysis using mid-infrared spectroscopy. Ann Clin Biochem. 1998;35:624–32.

8. Shaw RA, Mansfield JR, Kupriyanov VV, et al. In vivo optical/near-infrared spectroscopy and imaging of metalloproteins. J Inorg Biochem. 2000;79:285–93.

9. Cassis LA, Lodder RA. Near-IR imaging of atheromas in living arterial tissue. Anal Chem. 1993;65:1247–56.

10. Dempsey RJ, Davis DG, Buice RG, Lodder RA. Biological and medical applications of near-infrared spectroscopy. Applied Spectroscopy. 1996;50:18A–34A.

11. Moreno PR, Lodder RA, Purushothaman KR, Charash WE, O'Connor WN, Muller JE. Detection of lipid pool, thin fibrous cap, and inflammatory cells in human aortic atherosclerotic plaques by near-infrared spectroscopy. Circulation. 2002;105:923–7.

12. Jarros W, Neumeister V, Lattke P, et al. Determination of cholesterol in atherosclerotic plaques using near infrared diffuse reflection spectroscopy. Atherosclerosis. 1999; 147:327–337.

13. Wang J, Geng YJ, Guo B, et al. Near-infrared spectroscopic characterization of human advanced atherosclerotic plaques. J Am Coll Cardiol. 2002;39:1305–1313.

14. Moreno PR, S. Eric Ryan, David Hopkins, K-Raman Purushothaman, William E. Charash, William O'Connor, James E. Muller. Identification of Lipid-Rich Plaques in Human Coronary Artery Autopsy Specimens by Near-Infrared Spectroscopy. J. Am Coll Cardiol. 2001; 37:356A:1219–90.

15. Marshik D, Tan H, Tang J, Zuluaga A, Moreno PR, Purushothaman KR, O'Connor W, Tearney G. Discrimination of lipid-rich plaques in human aorta specimens with NIR spectroscopy through blood. Am J Cardiol 2002;90:129H.

16. Moreno PR, Kilpatrick D, Purushothaman KR, Coleman L, O'Connor WN. Stenting vulnerable plaque improves fibrous cap thickness and reduces lipid content: Understanding alternatives for plaque stabilization. Am J Cardiol 2002;90:50H.

CHAPTER 17

Intravascular thermography

Mohammad Madjid, Morteza Naghavi, Silvio Litovsky,
Samuel Ward Casscells, & James T Willerson

Atherosclerosis is a disease of antiquity. It was discovered in Egyptian mummies dating back as far as 1580 BC.[1] Despite its clinical manifestations later in life, pathological studies have shown that atherosclerotic changes can be observed early in life. Osler described slight foci of vascular fatty degeneration in children and stated that it is "exceptional to find no patches of arterial degeneration in any arteries at body post mortem examination".[2] Atherosclerosis begins during the very early years of life. Oxidation of LDL cholesterol and formation of fatty streaks have even been reported at the fetal stage.[3]

In their landmark study, Enos et al.[4] showed the presence of coronary artery disease in young US soldiers killed during the Korean War. Findings were confirmed during autopsies of young soldiers killed in Vietnam[5] and later in the Pathobiological Determinants of Atherosclerosis in Youth (PDAY) and the Bogalusa studies, which showed that atherosclerosis originates in childhood and is related to the presence of risk factors.[6,7] This pattern has been observed in other countries as well.[8] In addition to postmortem studies, intravascular ultrasonography (IVUS) has shown a high prevalence of atherosclerotic disease in coronary arteries of asymptomatic young transplant donors.[9] Tuzcu et al. found coronary atheromas in 17% of donors younger than 20 years, 37% of those aged 20–29 years, and 60% of those aged 30–39 years, while angiographic results failed to find lesions in 97% of these individuals.

Thermography as a method for detection of vulnerable plaques

Given the central role of inflammation in the pathogenesis of acute coronary syndromes, our group (SWC and JTW) began to explore the utility of heat detection to find inflamed loci in the arterial wall, thus locating vulnerable plaques.

In the period 1993–1996, Casscells, Willerson, and coworkers[10] investigated the possibility of measuring heat (a sign of inflammation) to predict presence of inflammation in the arterial wall. Casscells and Willerson[10] postulated that inflamed plaques may release more heat due to the metabolic activity of the activated macrophages and T-cells and an increase in angiogenesis.

Macrophages are metabolically active cells and consume increased amounts of energy.[11] Their high metabolic rate leads to increased heat production in areas of macrophage accumulation. This effect may be aggravated by the fact that many portions of plaques may be ischemic. Lack of oxygen may lead to ineffective metabolism of nutrients and greater loss of energy in the form of heat. Kockx et al.[12] have shown increased expression of mitochondrial uncoupling proteins (UCP) 2 and 3 in macrophages obtained from atherosclerotic plaques. UCPs are homologs of thermogenin (UCP-1, responsible for thermogenesis in brown fat tissue) and may contribute to heat production in plaques.

In addition, vulnerable plaques demonstrate increased neoangiogenesis.[13] Neovessel formation increases blood flow inside plaques with resulting higher temperature (Table 17.1).

Thermal heterogeneity of atherosclerotic plaques

In the period 1993–1996, Casscells and coworkers[10] measured the intimal surface temperatures of carotid

Table 17.1 Hypothetical mechanisms of heat production in plaque.

Inflammation
Activated macrophages, T-cells
Infections
Increased neovessel formation
Ineffective energy metabolism
Thermogenesis (UCPs)

artery plaques obtained after their removal with endarterectomy in patients (Figure 17.1). They used a needle thermistor to measure the surface temperature of multiple sites on each plaque and found significant temperature variations of 0.2–2.2°C. Temperature heterogeneity may also be observed with infrared cameras. The measured temperature showed direct correlation with cell density ($r = 0.68$; $P = 0.0001$) and an inverse correlation with the depth of the cell clusters ($r = -0.38$; $P = 0.0006$) (Figure 17.2). Although the temperature correlated with the density of macrophages/monocytes and activated T-cells (which have a high metabolic rate), it did not correlate with the density of smooth muscle cells, which have a lower metabolic rate.

In separate studies, we observed positive correlation of temperature with the macrophages density ($r = 0.66$; $P = 0.0001$) (Figure 17.3A), and an inverse correlation with the smooth muscle cell density ($r = -0.41$; $P = 0.0001$) (Figure 17.3B).[14] Temperature heterogeneity did not correlate with the presence of *Chlamydia pneumoniae* nor with the gross color of the luminal surface of human atherosclerotic carotid plaques.[14]

Foci of inflammation in the body are characterized by an increased temperature and a relatively low pH. pH and temperature heterogeneity result from inflammation at foci of macrophage and activated T-cell accumulation. Thickness of plaque and the resultant low oxygen diffusion rate contribute to anaerobic metabolism.[11,15]

We have also found a lower pH in vulnerable plaques in human carotid endarterectomy specimens, atherosclerotic rabbit aortas, and ApoE-deficient mice aortas. In these studies, we noted a lower pH was associated with a higher temperature ($r = 0.7$; $P < 0.0001$), lipid-rich areas had lower pHs and higher temperatures, whereas calcified areas had higher pHs and lower temperatures (Figure 17.4).[16] Temperature and pH were markedly and inversely correlated ($r = 0.94$; $P < 0.001$) (Figure 17.5). Fluorescent microscopic imaging confirmed pH heterogeneity in both human and rabbit plaques, but was not found in human umbilical artery samples that served as control.[16]

The above proof-of-concept studies demonstrate the presence of thermal and pH heterogeneity in vulnerable atherosclerotic plaques, and pave the way to investigate the utility of thermography in identifying inflamed vulnerable plaques in humans.

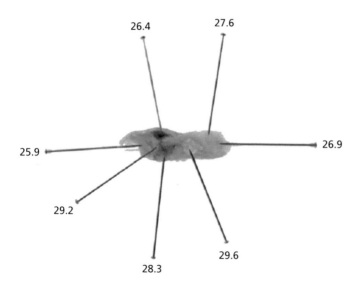

Figure 17.1 Endarterectomized carotid plaques showing temperature heterogeneity. (Reprinted with permission from Madjid et al. In Fuster V, ed. Assessing and modifying the vulnerable atherosclerotic plaque. Armonk, NY: Futura Publishing Company, 2002.[17])

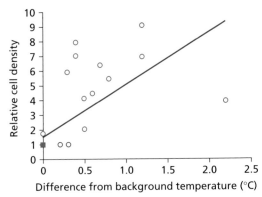

Figure 17.2 Surface temperature in relation to cell density. (Reproduced with permission from Casscells W, et al. Lancet 1996;347:1447–51.[10])

In vivo thermography

Infrared camera for detection of thermal heterogeneity

Infrared photography can be used to detect thermal heterogeneity in vivo and ex vivo. Casscells et al. used an infrared camera to detect temperature differences over endarterectomized carotid atherosclerotic plaques.[10] The same group used this method for detection of a heterogeneous pattern of heat emission over the atherosclerotic coronary arteries of dogs while undergoing open heart surgery, and over the arteriovenous grafts of hemodialysis patients, where the thermal heterogeneity was correlated with graft blood flow (QB_{max}) and venous

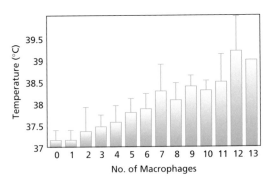
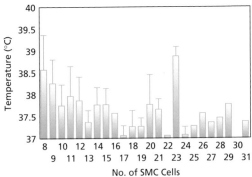

Figure 17.3 A, Close correlation between surface temperature (intimal surface temperatures of carotid artery plaques taken at endarterectomy) and the density of monocyte-macrophages. B, Inverse relation between temperature and the density of the smooth muscle cells. (Reprinted with permission from Madjid et al. Am J Cardiol 2002;90(10C):36L–9L.[14])

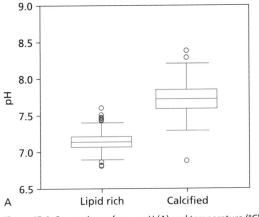
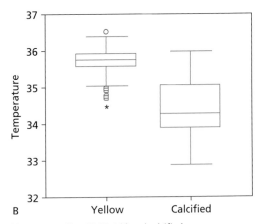

Figure 17.4 Comparison of mean pH (A) and temperature (°C), (B) between yellow (lipid-rich) and calcified areas. (Reprinted with permission from Madjid et al. In Fuster V, ed. Assessing and modifying the vulnerable atherosclerotic plaque. Armonk, NY: Futura Publishing Company, 2002.[17])

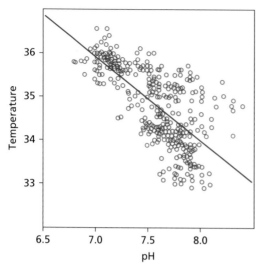

Figure 17.5 Inverse correlation of pH and temperature (°C) in human carotid artery plaques. (Reprinted with permission from Madjid et al. In Fuster V, ed. Assessing and modifying the vulnerable atherosclerotic plaque. Armonk, NY: Futura Publishing Company, 2002.[17])

resistance at QB_{250} (VR_{250}).[17] However, it should be noted that the patterns observed by the infrared camera images over intact arteries may be influenced by the circulatory flow rather than inflammation in the arterial wall.

Photonic-based catheters for detection of thermal heterogeneity – ex vivo studies

An infrared angiothermography catheter has been developed for the coronary system.[18] This 4F side-viewing fiberoptic catheter can measure vascular wall temperature in a 180 degree scope. This catheter has 19 chalcogenide fibers (each 100 μm in diameter) and a 1-mm-wide, wedge-shaped mirror at its tip, which is transparent to infrared radiation and reflects heat from the side of the catheter. The catheter is connected to a focal plane array cooled infrared camera. It has a thermal resolution of 0.01°C and a spatial resolution of 100 μm. The catheter has been tested ex vivo in a phantom model using a continuous flow of normal saline in a silicon tube system which simulates blood vessels and "hot" plaques. The catheter was able to detect temperature heterogeneity accurately along the lumen of the tube, with heated spots simulating "hot" plaques.[18]

Contact-based catheters for detection of thermal heterogeneity – animal studies

Naghavi et al.[19] have developed a "thermo-basket" catheter for measuring the in vivo temperature over the arterial wall. This is a thermocouple-based catheter with nitinol small, flexible thermocouples. The 3F catheter has an expandable, externally controllable basket and four highly flexible wires with built-in thermocouples. A personal computer with a special computer board and customized software allow real-time high-speed data acquisition, tracking, and thermographic imaging. The basket catheter has a thermal sensor in its central wire, allowing simultaneous monitoring of the blood temperature. The dive has a thermal resolution of 0.02°C and has a sampling rate of 20 temperature readings per second. It detected temperature heterogeneity over the atherosclerotic plaques in the femoral arteries of inbred atherosclerotic dogs (Figure 17.6) and the aortas of Watanabe rabbits.[17,19]

Verheye et al.[20] devised an over-the-wire thermography catheter with four thermistors and a retractable covering sheath. They used their catheter in 20 New Zealand rabbits randomized to receive either a normal diet ($n = 10$) or a cholesterol-rich (0.3%) diet ($n = 10$) for 6 months. They euthanized the control rabbits and half of the hypercholesterolemic rabbits at 6 months, and placed the five remaining hypercholesterolemic rabbits on a normal diet for 3 months. They studied the aortas with

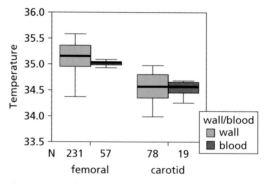

Figure 17.6 Studies with thermobasket catheter showing higher absolute temperature as well as temperature heterogeneity in femoral arteries of atherosclerotic dogs compared to their carotid arteries which are free of disease.

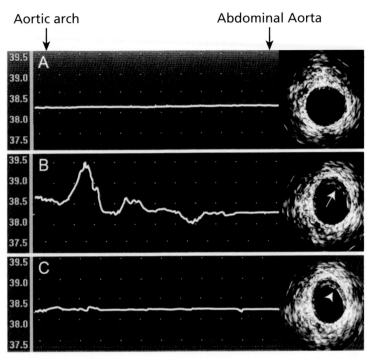

Aortic arch   Abdominal Aorta

Figure 17.7 In vivo temperature measurements of the endoaortic surface in rabbits. A, In control rabbits at 6 months, temperature differences are absent along the aortic wall. IVUS image illustrates the absence of plaque formation. B, In atherosclerotic rabbits at 6 months, marked temperature variations up to > 1°C are apparent along the endoluminal surface of the aortic wall. IVUS demonstrates plaque formation at the level of the proximal descending aorta just distal from the arch (arrow). C, In atherosclerotic rabbits after 3 months of dietary cholesterol lowering, temperature heterogeneity is absent, although IVUS (taken at the same level as in B) demonstrates the presence of a similar plaque (arrowhead). (Reprinted with permission from Verheye S, et al. Circulation 2002;105:1596.[20])

IVUS and thermography catheter (Figure 17.7) and found marked temperature heterogeneity (up to 1°C) in the hypercholesterolemic rabbits at sites of thick plaques with a high macrophage density. They did not see temperature heterogeneity in plaques with a low macrophage density. In rabbits receiving 3 months of a low-cholesterol diet after the high-cholesterol diet period, plaque thickness remained unchanged, whereas the macrophage content decreased significantly. In ex vivo studies, these same researchers showed a relationship between the local temperature and local total macrophage mass.

Intravascular thermal detection – human studies

Stefanadis and colleagues[21] were the first to perform human thermographic studies in 1999. By using a single-channel, thermistor-based catheter, they found that temperature differences (ΔT)

between atherosclerotic plaque and healthy vascular wall was lowest in patients with stable angina (ΔT: 0.106 ± 0.110°C) and highest in those with unstable angina (ΔT: 0.683 ± 0.347°C) and acute myocardial infarction (ΔT: 1.472 ± 0.691°C) (Figure 17.8). They found plaque temperature heterogeneity in 20%, 40%, and 67% of the patients with stable angina, unstable angina, and acute myocardial infarction, respectively. They did not observe temperature heterogeneity in control subjects. In their studies, thermal heterogeneity was not correlated with the degree of stenosis.

In humans, lesser degrees of temperature heterogeneity have been reported by Webster,[22] Verheye,[23] and Erbel (R Erbel, 2003, personal correspondence) and their colleagues. Differences in these observations may be explained in part by the discrepancies in use of medications, such as aspirin and/or statins, as well as different effects

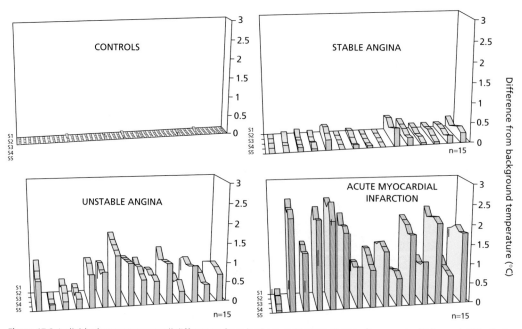

Figure 17.8 Individual temperature wall differences from background temperature in four groups. S1 through S5 indicate sites of measurement from proximal (S1) to distal (S5) parts of regions of interest. (Reproduced from Stefanadis C, et al. Circulation 1999;99:1965–71.[21])

of thermography catheters on blood flow. For example, in contrast to the devices used by the latter investigators that did not obstruct flow, the larger thermistor used by Stefanadis et al. often "wedged" the lesion and obstructed blood flow. It is well known that blood flow can affect the measured temperature heterogeneity over the atherosclerotic plaque.[24]

In recent studies, Webster,[22] Erbel and coworkers from New Zealand and Europe have studies six-patients with unstable angina and 14 patients with stable angina. A cutoff temperature of ≥ 0.1°C yielded 10 patients with no temperature hetero-geneity, 4 patients with a single hot spot, three patients with two hot spots, and three patients with three hot spots. An alternative cutoff temperature of ≥ 0.2°C resulted in only two of 17 patients with a hot spot, and one patient with two such lesions.

A thermography catheter (ThermoCoil Guidewire, Imetrx, CA) has been recently used in human subjects.[25] This guidewire consists of a 0.014-inch wire with an angled tip rotating at 0.5 Hz at a pullback scanning rate of 0.5 mm/s, inscribing a helix on the lumen. The wire has a temperature sensor in the distal tip with sensitivity of 0.03°C. Of the 13

patients in this study, two had unstable angina, one had non-ST elevation MI, one had ST elevation MI, and nine had stable angina. Fifteen lesions were evaluated and no device-related adverse effects or system failures were reported. Investigators could detect intraarterial temperature rises (0.1–0.3°C) in four subjects. Mean CRP level in patients with temperature elevation was higher than in patients without elevated temperature (14.0 mg/L vs. 6.2 mg/L, P = not reported).[25]

Schmermund have used a thermography catheter (Volcano Therapeutics, Orange County, California) in 10 patients. They used a 3.3F catheter equipped with a self-expanding basket with five arms and a thermocouple on each arm, as well as a central thermocouple with a sensitivity of 0.05°C. Patients were 60 ± 11 years old (11 men, eight women) and needed coronary intervention. Eleven patients had stable angina, and eight had unstable angina. Intracoronary thermography was per-formed before intervention in the vessel with the culprit lesion (diameter stenosis, 55–90%). Focal increases (0.14° to 0.36°C) in arterial wall temper-ature were observed in seven patients at the site of the culprit lesion. The authors reported presence of "hot plaques" in four patients (50%) with unstable angina and three patients (27%) with stable angina.[26]

Temperature heterogeneity and systemic inflammation

Stefanadis and colleagues[27] studied 60 patients with coronary artery disease, including patients with stable angina, unstable angina, and acute myocardial infarction, as well as 20 sex- and age-matched control subjects without coronary artery disease. They found a strong correlation between C-reactive protein (CRP) and serum amyloid A levels with ΔTs values ($r = 0.796$, $P = 0.01$ and $r = 0.848$, $P = 0.01$, respectively).

By contrast, in the studies by Webster,[22] Erbel and colleagues most patients had normal serum CRP levels, and the number of "hot" spots did not correlate with the percentage of luminal stenosis or the CRP level. The difference in results may be due to a higher use of statins and anti-inflammatory medications in the studies by Weber and Erbel.

Temperature heterogeneity and arterial remodeling

Toutouzas and coauthors[28] investigated a relationship between temperature heterogeneity and vascular remodeling (a marker of plaque vulnerability associated with local inflammation in plaque[29]). They observed a strong and positive correlation between the coronary remodeling index (defined as the ratio of the external elastic membrane area at the lesion, to that at the proximal site, as determined by IVUS) and the ΔT between the atherosclerotic plaque and healthy vascular wall in patients with acute coronary syndromes. In addition, they found a correlation between the serum matrix metalloproteinase-9 concentration and ΔT values.[30] Matrix metalloproteinases (MMPs) play important roles in vascular remodeling[31]; however, the strength of the relationship between serum levels of MMPs and focal activity of such enzymes at the plaque level has not been determined.

Recently, Toutouzas et al. used direct coronary atherectomy to obtain samples from coronary lesions after performing intravascular thermography in eight patients. They found a significant increase in presence of matrix metalloproteinases 1, 3, and 9 (on immunohistochemistry studies) in samples which showed high temperature differences.[32]

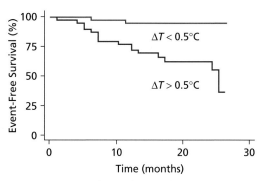

Figure 17.9 Estimated survival among the study group according to temperature difference (ΔT). The risk of an adverse cardiac event in patients with $\Delta T > 0.5°C$ is significantly increased, as compared with that in patients with $\Delta T < 0.5°C$. (Reprinted from Stefaniadis et al. J Am Coll Cardiol 2001;37:1277–83, with permission from the American College of Cardiology.[33])

Temperature heterogeneity and clinical prognosis

Stefanadis et al.[33] studied 86 patients undergoing successful percutaneous intervention and followed them up for 17 ± 7 months. They found that ΔT strongly predicts adverse cardiac events on follow-up. The cut off point for the risk of an adverse cardiac event was $> 0.5°C \Delta T$. The risk of adverse cardiac events was 41% in patients with a ΔT of $\geq 0.5°C$, compared with 7% in those with a ΔT of $< 0.5°C$ (Figure 17.9).

Temperature heterogeneity and use of statins

Animal studies have shown that statins reduce the number of inflammatory cells and increase the collagen content in atherosclerotic plaques, leading to a more "stabilized" plaque.[34] Stefanadis et al. randomized 72 patients to a statin or placebo[35] and found that statins significantly decreased the ΔT in patients stable angina, unstable angina, and acute myocardial infarction (ΔT: 0.29 ± 0.33 vs. $0.56 \pm 0.41°C$). This change in ΔT was independent of the serum cholesterol level at hospital admission.

Coronary sinus thermography

A thermography catheter has been deployed in the coronary sinus to measure blood temperature.[36] In 60 patients, the ΔT between the coronary sinus and the right atrium was increased in patients with significant left anterior descending coronary artery atherosclerotic lesions, but not in subjects who lacked lesions. The researchers concluded that coronary sinus thermography may be used to detect inflamed atherosclerotic plaques in the left anterior descending artery.[36] Further trials are needed to confirm the reproducibility of these findings and their possible clinical utility.

Future research

Several basic and technical issues need to be resolved before extensive use of this method can be recommended. The measured surface temperature will be related to the number of macrophages at the proximity of the plaque cap; however, the correlation with macrophages deep inside the plaque may not be as strong. In addition, temporal changes in temperature in plaques and the prospective intraplaque reproducibility of heat measurements need to be determined.

Coronary temperature readings are influenced by coronary flow (which has a "cooling effect" on measured temperature). It has been shown that complete obstruction of blood flow may increase the degree of detected temperature heterogeneity (up to 60–76%).[24] Therefore, proximal occlusion of the artery by use of a balloon may be utilized to avoid this "cooling effect." However, this method has the obvious shortcoming of obstructing the flow for a short time.

Vulnerable plaques are determined by a combination of several histopathological and functional characteristics. Combining anatomic imaging methods (e.g. IVUS, elastography, optical coherence tomography) with functional imaging methods, such as thermography, should provide comprehensive insight into the structure and activity of plaques.[37]

Conclusions

In an accompanying editorial of the 1996 report by Casscells, Willerson, and their colleagues in the *Lancet*, the late Michael J Davies predicted that thermal detection systems are likely be developed within a short time and may find clinical value for detection of "hot" plaques in clinical settings.[38] This method, since its conception in 1996 in ex vivo studies, has followed a rather fast track. It is currently being investigated in human clinical trials in New Zealand, Europe, and the USA (after receiving FDA approval for being tested in human subjects). Human clinical trials need to determine if this method is safe, reproducible, and beneficial. Once approved, it may be used to detect vulnerable plaques and to predict the risk of vulnerable lesions and vulnerable patients.

Acknowledgment

Supported in part by DOD Grant #DAMD 17–01–2–0047.

References

1. Ruffer M. On arterial lesions found in Egyptian mummies. J Path Bact 1911;15:453–65.
2. Arteriosclerosis. Br Med J 1909:1800.
3. Napoli C, D'Armiento FP, Mancini FP, et al. Fatty streak formation occurs in human fetal aortas and is greatly enhanced by maternal hypercholesterolemia. Intimal accumulation of low density lipoprotein and its oxidation precede monocyte recruitment into early atherosclerotic lesions. J Clin Invest 1997;100:2680–90.
4. Enos WF, Holmes RH, Beyer J. Landmark article, July 18, 1953: Coronary disease among United States soldiers killed in action in Korea. Preliminary report. By William F. Enos, Robert H. Holmes and James Beyer. JAMA 1986;256:2859–62.
5. McNamara JJ, Molot MA, Stremple JF, Cutting RT. Coronary artery disease in combat casualties in Vietnam. JAMA 1971;216:1185–7.
6. Natural history of aortic and coronary atherosclerotic lesions in youth. Findings from the PDAY Study. Pathobiological Determinants of Atherosclerosis in Youth (PDAY) Research Group. Arterioscler Thromb 1993;13:1291–8.
7. Berenson GS, Srinivasan SR, Bao W, Newman WP, 3rd, Tracy RE, Wattigney WA. Association between multiple cardiovascular risk factors and atherosclerosis in children and young adults. The Bogalusa Heart Study. N Engl J Med 1998;338:1650–6.
8. Imakita M, Yutani C, Strong JP, et al. Second nationwide study of atherosclerosis in infants, children and young adults in Japan. Atherosclerosis 2001;155:487–97.
9. Tuzcu EM, Kapadia SR, Tutar E, et al. High prevalence of coronary atherosclerosis in asymptomatic teenagers and

young adults: evidence from intravascular ultrasound. Circulation 2001;103:2705–10.

10. Casscells W, Hathorn B, David M, et al. Thermal detection of cellular infiltrates in living atherosclerotic plaques: possible implications for plaque rupture and thrombosis. Lancet 1996;347:1447–51.

11. Newsholme P, Newsholme EA. Rates of utilization of glucose, glutamine and oleate and formation of end-products by mouse peritoneal macrophages in culture. Biochem J 1989;261:211–18.

12. Kockx MK, Knaapen MWM, Martinet W, De Meyer GRY, Verheye S, Herman AG. Expression of the uncoupling protein UCP-2 in macrophages of unstable human atherosclerotic plaques. Circulation 2000;102:II-12.

13. Tenaglia AN, Peters KG, Sketch MH, Jr, Annex BH. Neovascularization in atherectomy specimens from patients with unstable angina: implications for pathogenesis of unstable angina. Am Heart J 1998;135:10–14.

14. Madjid M, Naghavi M, Malik BA, Litovsky S, Willerson JT, Casscells W. Thermal detection of vulnerable plaque. Am J Cardiol 2002;90:36L–9L.

15. Bjornheden T, Bondjers G. Oxygen consumption in aortic tissue from rabbits with diet-induced atherosclerosis. Arteriosclerosis 1987;7:238–47.

16. Naghavi M, John R, Naguib S, et al. pH heterogeneity of human and rabbit atherosclerotic plaques; a new insight into detection of vulnerable plaque. Atherosclerosis 2002;164:27–35.

17. Madjid M, Naghavi N, Willerson JT, Casscells W. Thermography: a novel approach for identification of plaques at risk of rupture and/or thrombosis. In: Fuster V, ed. Assessing and modifying the vulnerable atherosclerotic plaque. Armonk, NY: Futura Publishing Company, 2002:107–27.

18. Naghavi M, Melling M, Gul K, et al. First prototype of a 4 French 180 degree side-viewing infrared fiber optic catheter for thermal imaging of atherosclerotic plaque. J Am Coll Cardiol 2001;37:3A.

19. Naghavi M, Madjid M, Gul K, et al. Thermography basket catheter: In vivo measurement of the temperature of atherosclerotic plaques for detection of vulnerable plaques. Catheter Cardiovasc Interv 2003;59:52–9.

20. Verheye S, De Meyer GRY, Van Langenhove G, Knaapen MWM, Kockx MM. In vivo temperature heterogeneity of atherosclerotic plaques is determined by plaque composition. Circulation 2002;105:1596–601.

21. Stefanadis C, Diamantopoulos L, Vlachopoulos C, et al. Thermal heterogeneity within human atherosclerotic coronary arteries detected in vivo: a new method of detection by application of a special thermography catheter. Circulation 1999;99:1965–71.

22. Webster M, Stewart J, Ruygrok P, et al. Intracoronary thermography with a multiple thermocouple catheter: initial human experience (abstract). Am J Cardiol 2002;90:24H.

23. Verheye S, Van Langenhove G, Diamantopoulos L, Serruys PW, Vermeersch P. Temperature heterogeneity is nearly absent in angiographically normal or mild atherosclerotic coronary segments: interim results from a safety study (abstract). Am J Cardiol 2002;90:24H.

24. Stefanadis C, Toutouzas K, Tsiamis E, et al. Thermal heterogeneity in stable human coronary atherosclerotic plaques is underestimated in vivo: the "cooling effect" of blood flow. J Am Coll Cardiol 2003;41:403–8.

25. Wainstein MV, Ribierro JP, Zago AJ, et al. Coronary plaque theromography: heterogeneity detected by Imetrx thermocoil guidewire. Am J Cardiol 2003;92:5L.

26. Schmermund A, Rodermann J, Boese D, et al. Heterogenous coronary arterial wall temperature and hot spots detected by novel thermography system with self-expanding basket. Am J Cardiol 2003;92:6L.

27. Stefanadis C, Diamantopoulos L, Dernellis J, et al. Heat production of atherosclerotic plaques and inflammation assessed by the acute phase proteins in acute coronary syndromes. J Mol Cell Cardiol 2000;32:43–52.

28. Toutouzas MK, Stefanadis CM, Vavuranakis MM, et al. Arterial remodeling in acute coronary syndromes: correlation of IVUS characteristics with temperature of the culprit lesion. Circulation 2000;102:II-707.

29. Varnava AM, Mills PG, Davies MJ. Relationship between coronary artery remodeling and plaque vulnerability. Circulation 2002;105:939–43.

30. Toutouzas K, Stefanadis C, Tsiamis E, et al. The temperature of atherosclerotic plaques is correlated with matrix metalloproteinases concentration in patients with acute coronary syndromes. J Am Coll Cardiol 2001;37:356A.

31. Shah PK. Mechanisms of plaque vulnerability and rupture. J Am Coll Cardiol 2003;41:15S–22S.

32. Toutouzas K, Spanos V, Ribichini F, et al. Correlation of coronary plaque temperature with inflammatory markers obtained from atherectomy specimens in human. Am J Cardiol 2003;92:198L.

33. Stefanadis C, Toutouzas K, Tsiamis E, et al. Increased local temperature in human coronary atherosclerotic plaques: an independent predictor of clinical outcome in patients undergoing a percutaneous coronary intervention. J Am Coll Cardiol 2001;37:1277–83.

34. Sukhova GK, Williams JK, Libby P. Statins reduce inflammation in atheroma of nonhuman primates independent of effects on serum cholesterol. Arterioscler Thromb Vasc Biol 2002;22:1452–8.

35. Stefanadis C, Toutouzas K, Vavuranakis M, et al. Statin treatment is associated with reduced thermal hetero-

geneity in human atherosclerotic plaques. Eur Heart J 2002;23:1664–9.

36. Stefanadis C, Toutouzas K, Vaina S, Vavuranakis M, Toutouzas P. Thermography of the cardiovascular system. J Interv Cardiol 2002;15:461–6.

37. Naghavi M, Madjid M, Khan MR, Mohammadi RM, Willerson JT, Casscells SW. New developments in the detection of vulnerable plaque. Curr Atheroscler Rep 2001;3:125–35.

38. Davies MJ. Detecting vulnerable coronary plaques. Lancet 1996;347:1422–3.

CHAPTER 18

Optical coherence tomography

Paul Magnin & Evelyn Regar

In 1990, David Huang was in his fourth year of an MD–PhD program at Massachusetts Institute of Technology (MIT). He had been studying optical coherence domain reflectometry (OCDR) to perform ranging measurements in the eye. The OCDR project was an offshoot of femtosecond ranging projects that had been ongoing in Professor James Fujimoto's laboratory. The retinal OCDR scans, however, were very hard to interpret. The thought occurred to Dr Huang that by adding transverse scanning to OCDR graphs one would create an image that would be much easier for a human to interpret than a set of OCDR waveforms. What was required was to add a translation stage and a software package to convert a data matrix into an image. "The first time we got an OCT image was during a late night session where we scanned the retina of a cadaver eye for many hours. But the late night work was well worth the excitement of seeing a new type of imaging demonstrated for the first time," according to Huang, "I got very excited about the potential for imaging in all parts of the body and the next morning visited several clinicians in the Harvard/MIT system to get various tissue samples to scan."

The concept of using an interferometer to overcome measurement difficulties caused by the incredibly fast speed of light actually first arose over 100 years earlier. It was an interferometer that was used to make the first accurate measurements of the speed of light by the American Physicist, Albert Michelson in 1881. This was eventually used to verify a central conclusion of Einstein's theory of relativity; that the speed of light is a constant in all reference frames. An interferometer operates by comparing two light beams with each other. This can be done most simply by combining light beams that impinge on different faces of a half-silvered mirror.

The central problem in making tomographic images using light was to develop a technique that would permit reflections from various depths to be measured and recorded in a fashion analogous to ultrasonic imaging. In the case of sound, electronic circuits are fast enough to separate the echoes from structures that are within the resolution cell of the ultrasonic transducer. By using an interferometer, for the first time it was possible to record light reflections from various depths in a biological tissue also.

Since 1990, OCT technology has generated over 570 articles in academic journals. The first paper from MIT, published in *Science* in November of 1991,[1] describes the basic concept of an OCT imaging system and discusses its possible applications in both retinal and arterial imaging. It became clear early on that OCT could contribute to the diagnosis of ocular diseases. It was believed that the new technology had the potential to serve as an in vivo microscope that could obtain non-excisional biopsy information from locations at which a conventional biopsy was either impossible or impractical to perform. A second research thrust from the MIT group was to push the resolution of the technology to increasingly higher levels using wider bandwidth optical sources. With sufficiently wide bandwidth sources, one may be able to resolve subcellular structures and measure the ratio of the nuclear volume to the total cell volume in a manner similar to what a pathologist does when diagnosing cancer.

In the days since the initial discussion in Professor Fujimoto's office, several members of the MIT OCT team have gone on to start academic OCT research programs throughout the USA. Joseph Izatt, a former postdoctoral researcher in

Dr Fujimoto's lab, left MIT to start the Case Western OCT program and later started a second program at Duke University. Brett Bouma and Gary Tearney left MIT to start the OCT research effort at Massachusetts General Hospital (MGH), where they have been doing ground-breaking work in coronary imaging, among other applications. David Huang went on to do research in OCT and ophthalmology at the Cleveland Clinic, Mark Brezinski does research at Brigham and Women's hospital, and Steven Boppart left to do OCT research at the University of Illinois.

Physics and technology

Principle

An OCT system for intravascular imaging is analogous to a mechanically scanned IVUS imaging system. The fundamental difference is that the OCT system employs infrared light, while the IVUS system employs ultrasonic waves in the 20–40 MHz range. Simple electronic time-gating techniques, that are capable of identifying ultrasonic echoes from different depths, are far too slow to gate reflections that return at the speed of light. In OCT imaging, time gating is accomplished using a special form of interferometry called low coherence or white-light interferometry.

In an OCT simple system (Figure 18.1), a light beam that reflects from a tissue in the sample arm of an interferometer mixes with a second light beam that reflects from a reference mirror located inside the imaging system. The light from the source enters a beam splitter that consists of a half silvered mirror or a fiberoptic coupler. One output of the beam splitter travels through an optical fiber in the imaging catheter. At the distal end of the catheter, the beam enters a tiny microscope, the first stage of which diverges the light from the core of the optical fiber to expand the imaging system aperture. It then passes through an objective lens to focus the light at the desired point in the tissue and finally passes through a prism that steers the beam 90 degrees to the axis of the catheter and sends the light through the sheath of the catheter onto the wall of the artery.

The reference beam travels in an optical fiber with a length approximately equal to that of the optical fiber in the sample arm. According to the principles of low-coherence interferometry, interference occurs only when the distances the light travels in the sample and reference arms match to within a coherence length of the light source. The position of the mirror in the reference arm determines the position of the range gate in the tissue. When the light reflected from the tissue and the light reflected from the moving mirror return to detector, only the sample arm reflections that come from a tissue depth that is identical to the length of the reference arm can interfere coherently. Reflections from all other depths do not interfere and wash out incoherently. A number of

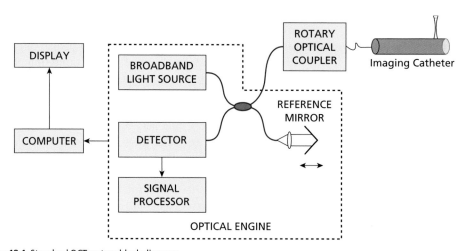

Figure 18.1 Standard OCT system block diagram.

means have been employed to vary the length of the reference path. The simplest is a moving mirror at the distal end of the reference arm, as shown in Figure 18.1. If one wished to scan in depth over a 4-mm range, for example, the reference mirror would need to vibrate over a distance of 4 mm. In fact, the relationship between the moving mirror travel in the reference arm and the range gate travel in the sample arm and tissue is scaled by the ratio of the speed of light in the air to the speed of light in the tissue, which is typically 1.35–1.4 times slower.

If the moving mirror travels over its 4-mm range in a millisecond, all of the range information from a single image line can be collected in that time. By rotating the optical fiber and the tiny microscope inside the catheter, adjacent lines are recorded to form a circular image. Typically the reference arm is varied over a 4-mm range at a rate of about 1–10 kHz. The inertia of the reference arm mirror itself becomes a significant limitation at those rates and consequently more efficient methods for varying the length of the reference arm have been devised. In Figure 18.2, the simple moving mirror has been replaced by a rotating series of cam-shaped (retro-reflecting) mirrored surfaces. The rotating cam approach has the advantage that it requires no change in momentum and therefore can produce higher image line rates. All of the lines that are collected during a complete rotation of the optical fiber and microscope are stored and converted into an image in real time. To accommodate the rotation of the optical fiber in the catheter, a rotary

optical coupler is connected on the proximal end of the catheter. The system shown in Figure 18.2 also incorporates dual detectors for recording signals from two overlapping beams at the output of the interferometer. These two detectors can be preceded by filters that pass specific wavelengths or specific polarizations. One may wish to create images at two specific areas in the optical frequency spectrum, if the absorption or scattering properties of the light in these parts of the spectrum help to characterize different tissue types. One might wish to precede the two detectors with orthogonal polarization filters and then display the sum of the square of the detector outputs in order to remove polarization artifacts that can arise from stresses in the optical fibers or to measure the birefringence of the tissue.

It is important to note that the light source is not a laser but rather a low-coherence light source. Although the source can be a pulsed laser, for cost reasons, a superluminescent diode is typically used. In either case, the source must have must have a broad spectral bandwidth to enable high-resolution range gating.

The absorption curves for protein, lipid, water and hemoglobin are shown in Figure 18.3. From these graphs, one can see that an absorption window exists around 1300 nm where all the four absorption coefficients are all low. One can also see a second available window between 1600 nm and 1800 nm at which imaging can take place. Beyond 1800 nm the absorption caused by water becomes

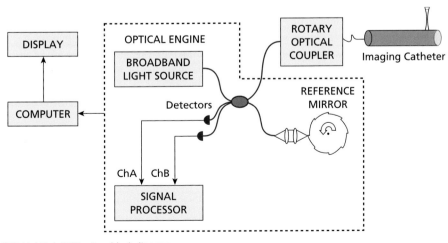

Figure 18.2 LightLab OCT system block diagram.

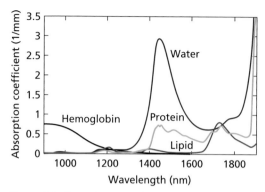

Figure 18.3 Absorption curves for biological tissues in the infrared region.

very high. This graph however does not show the attenuative effect of multiple scattering, which in most cases is more significant that the losses due to absorption. Multiple scattering losses tend to decrease as the wavelength increases.

Technology tradeoffs

As with all imaging technologies, tradeoffs must be made in the design of the imaging system. Primary amongst these is the interrelationship between the line rate and the signal-to-noise ratio. The fidelity of the OCT signal at any point in the image is proportional to the number of photons that are collected from that point. To increase the number of photons collected, one can increase the power of the source to only a limited degree. When the power gets too high, the heating produced by the light will cause damage to the tissue. Another way to increase the number of photons collected at a point is to spend more time interrogating the point. If the system dwells twice as long on each point in the line, the signal-to-noise ratio doubles, but the line acquisition rate halves. The dwell time is primarily determined by the speed at which the moving mirror in Figure 18.1 sweeps through the range of desired depths.

At a fixed line rate, the frame rate and line density vary in inverse proportion. For example, if the system collects 4000 image lines each second, and uses 256 lines to display one complete revolution of the catheter, a frame rate of 15.6 Hz will result. A line rate this high is typically adequate for coronary artery imaging; however, to display the maximum possible lateral resolution in large arteries, more

lines may be necessary in each frame. The lateral resolution at the focal point of a typical OCT imaging catheter used in the coronaries is about 25 μm. In a 3-mm artery, for example, the focal point would typically be 1.5 mm beyond the catheter wall which is approximately 2.0 mm from the center of the image. To display the maximum resolution in the lateral dimension, the system must generate about 1000 lines in a single frame. At a line rate of 4000 lines per second, this results in a frame rate of 4 frames per second. Given typical coronary artery motion, such a low frame rate would cause severe motion artifacts and geometrical distortions. The compromise usually made for coronary imaging is to undersample the image (spatially) in exchange for higher frame rates.

Limitations for coronary artery imaging

The major difficulty of OCT for coronary applications is the need to remove the red blood cells from the field of view. This is because red blood cells are very strong scattering sites and the coherence of the light is rapidly reduced by multiple scattering in the blood. Unlike IVUS, the dominant mode of attenuation for OCT imaging in the 1300-nm wavelength range is scattering. For IVUS the attenuation is mostly caused by absorption. One can get a sense of this by trying to shine a flashlight through the palm of a hand. Indeed, the light (at least, in the red portion of the spectrum) will pass completely through the hand. There will not, however, be any observable shadowing behind the bones in the hand. This is because the light is not traveling in straight lines but rather it is being scattered from one scattering site to another along a serpentine path.

If the blood remains in the path of the infrared light, after about 0.25–0.5 mm the light has been scattered from so many red blood cells that the signal that is returned to the catheter is completely incoherent with respect to the signal from the same distance in the reference arm. When the two signals are combined at the half silvered mirror, they cannot add constructively and instead get washed out.

There are many approaches to removing the red blood cells from the path to the vessel wall. The simplest is to inject saline, Ringer's solution, or an X-ray contrast agent through the guide catheter. In proximal, slow flow situations a 10-ml saline injection can provide a clear image for a few seconds. If the point at which the image is to be made is more distal or if there are significant bifurcations between the distal end of the guide catheter and the image point, the 10-ml injection will usually not clear the blood field sufficiently to make an image.

A second approach is to use an angiography catheter to deliver a flush more distally, which effectively eliminates the fluid loss to intervening bifurcations. Flush through a 4.2F angiography catheter is adequate for a 1F OCT imaging device. Commercially available delivery or transit catheters are also suitable for this approach. The advantage is that, for a given flush volume, a longer imaging time will result. The disadvantage is that if therapy is contemplated, it will be necessary to use the diagnostic/delivery catheter in conjunction with a standard guide catheter, adding extra time and cost to the procedure. If still longer image times are desired, one can image distal to an occlusion balloon. In this situation the imaging catheter is passed through the guidewire lumen of the balloon. The balloon is inflated with low pressure so as not to damage the artery wall and a small amount of flush is injected into the distal artery through the guidewire lumen. This is particularly useful for situations that require long image times to acquire three-dimensional data by pulling back the imaging catheter or the imaging fiber within the imaging catheter. A fourth approach is to image through the balloon itself. For example, the guidewire in an over-the-wire balloon can be exchanged for an OCT imaging catheter but, rather than exiting the balloon distally as in the previous example, the imaging catheter can remain inside the balloon. The moment the balloon touches the artery wall, a clear image will result. This can be particularly useful if one wishes to monitor the deployment of a stent in real-time.

The flush can also be incorporated into an imaging catheter. In such a device, the imaging catheter has one lumen for the optical fiber and a second lumen for the flush. This incorporates into a single catheter both the flush delivery and the image catheter. One does not need to be concerned with the optimal placement of the flush delivery catheter with respect to the imaging catheter since the two are integrated into a single unit. Furthermore, this integrated catheter is amenable to monorail

delivery on a guidewire, whereas delivery devices based on balloons require guidewire exchanges.

Another limitation of the technology is the depth of penetration. Assuming that most of the blood has been removed by one of the above techniques, OCT images can be acquired from depths up to about 1.5 mm into the artery wall from the surface. This limits the utility of OCT in research applications that measure the total plaque burden, volume, or mass. It is likely that IVUS will remain the technology of choice for such applications. Interestingly, there is one exception to the penetration limitation. Calcium nodules are relatively transparent to infrared light whereas they cast large shadows in IVUS images. The difference can cause some confusion because operators familiar with IVUS, at first, have difficulty identifying calcium in OCT images.

Resolution

Assuming the power spectrum of the light source is Gaussian in shape, the resolution of an OCT system in the range (radial) direction is inversely proportional to the bandwidth of the light source according to the equation:

$$\text{Axial res.} = 0.44 * \lambda^2 / \Delta\lambda \qquad \text{(eqn 18.1)}$$

where λ is the center wavelength and $\Delta\lambda$ (or bandwidth) is the full width at half maximum of the optical spectrum of the light source.

From this relationship we see that the resolution in the range dimension is proportional to the square of the wavelength and inversely proportional to the bandwidth of the light source. To increase the resolution, it is necessary to employ a wider bandwidth light source. To date, state of the art OCT images have been obtained with resolutions near the 0.75 µm level.[2] At such dimensions, subcellular structures can be resolved. The technology for these wider bandwidth sources will be driven by the telecommunications industry in which bandwidth is critical for permitting transmission of more information in a given amount of time. Significant effort is being aimed at producing such sources at reasonable costs and much progress is being made. This challenge at these resolutions is to match the lateral resolution to the increased axial resolution.

The lateral resolution is determined by the diffraction pattern in the same way that the lateral resolution of a camera or an ultrasonic imaging system is determined:

Lateral res. = $1.27^*\lambda(f/a)$ (eqn 18.2)

where *a* is the aperture diameter and *f* is the focal distance.

As with camera optics, the square of the lateral resolution and the depth of focus are also inversely related.

Depth of field = $2.54^*\lambda^*(f/a)^2$ (eqn 18.3)

This results in the tradeoff between a tight focus at a particular point near the catheter or a wider focus over longer depth further from the catheter.

Device description

The imaging system that produced the images that follow was developed by LightLab Imaging, Inc. The system is a portable tool for use in the cardiac catheterization laboratory (Figure 18.4). It is composed of four major components: the OCT imaging engine, the computer, the probe interface unit, and the imaging catheters. It is capable of imaging in real-time using video scanning rates up to 30 frames per second. The range resolution is 15–20 μm and the lateral and out of plane resolution are 25 μm at the focus.

The OCT imaging engine

The imaging engine is responsible for emitting and receiving the infrared signals. The broadband light source is housed in the engine, along with the interferometer, the reference arm, and the detection circuitry. The optical engine contains the fiberoptic interferometer coupled to the near-IR (1300 nm), broad-bandwidth light source and the reference arm. The optical interference signals with orthogonal polarizations are detected by a pair of photodiodes and digitized. They are then digitally filtered and sent to the computer for processing into an image.

The computer

The computer consists of a computer processor running an embedded operating system. The computer processes the OCT information and converts it to a displayable format. The computer also controls the optical engine and the patient interface

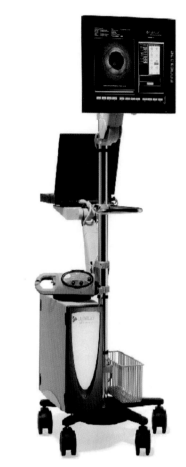

Figure 18.4 The LightLab OCT system for use in the cardiac catheterization laboratory.

unit and serves as the image storage device for both still-frame images and video images.

The patient interface unit

The probe interface unit (Figure 18.5) serves as the human interface for the interventional cardiologist and the location where the imaging catheter plugs into the system. It starts and stops the imaging, and selects whether the catheter is to be automatically pulled back inside the catheter sheath or moved manually by the operator. The probe interface unit provides the motor drive that spins the imaging core to create the circular image and performs the automated pullback to collect the third dimension of image information if that mode is selected by the operator. Inside of the probe interface unit is a rotary coupler that connects the stationary optical

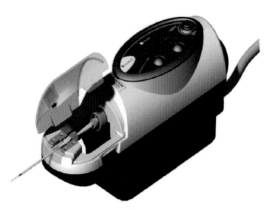

Figure 18.5 The probe interface unit.

fiber to the rotating catheter imaging core. There is also a foot switch that mirrors the two buttons on the probe interface unit to make operation more convenient for the operator in the sterile field.

The catheter system

The LightLab Imaging catheter or ImageWire is a single lumen catheter (Figure 18.6). The small lumen holds the imaging fiber that consists of the optical fiber, the lenses, and the prism. The imaging core is made of glass with a polymer coating on the outside to strengthen it both in torsion and in flexion. The diameter of the imaging core is 140 μm. At the proximal end of the catheter is a tapered section of tubing that captures the imaging core and allows it to move along the catheter axis to perform an "automated pullback" while spinning.

The outside of the imaging catheter is stationary with respect to the vessel wall. The imaging core is rotated and translated inside of the external catheter sheath. The distal end of the ImageWire has an atraumatic spring tip to prevent vessel injury when it exits the delivery catheter. The proximal end of the catheter is designed to allow for both rotational and translational movement of the probe tip.

In the distal tip of the catheter, the light passes through a tiny microscope consisting of three optical components, as shown in Figure 18.7. The first is a diverging lens which expands the light from the optical core where it travels for most of the length of the catheter. This lens effectively increases the aperture of the imaging system from the 9 μm optical fiber core where the light is carried to the entire width of the fiber, to the outer dimension of the glass part of the fiber itself which is 125 μm. The second lens is the focusing or objective lens that creates the focus in the tissue, and the third is a prism that steers the light at an angle 90 degrees to the axis of the catheter. After the light passes through the microscope it passes through the catheter sheath and into the tissue. In the body, the light is reflected from the microstructures in the tissue and returns through the microscope into the optical fiber core, through the rotary coupler, and back into the interferometer. The optical core, inside the catheter, is rotated through 360 degrees to provide the second dimension in the 2D image, in a manner identical to mechanically scanned IVUS

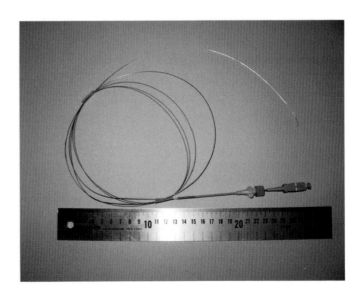

Figure 18.6 The OCT imaging catheter (ImageWire).

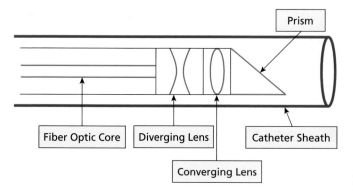

Figure 18.7 Catheter tip microscope.

systems. The information from each line is then combined into a 2D representation of the tissue and displayed on the imaging system monitor.

The ImageWire is delivered to the imaging site through the lumen of the delivery catheter. The delivery catheter can be either a balloon or just a simple single lumen catheter that delivers a modest amount of contrast or lactated Ringer's solution to the imaging location while the image is being collected. The purpose of the flush is to clear the red blood cells from the ImageWire's field of view. In the current design, the guidewire is exchanged for the ImageWire when the delivery catheter is in a location proximal to the imaging site. If an occlusion balloon is to be employed to increase the imaging time, the inflation pressure in the balloon can be kept low to minimize stretching of the artery wall or it can be undersized to avoid stretching the artery at all.

Potential applications in interventional cardiology

Detailed analysis of the coronary artery structure was up to now restricted to histology, and thus, postmortem analysis. Intravascular optical coherence tomography offers the unique possibility to study the coronary artery micro-structure in vivo. Potential clinical applications include the assessment of angiographic ambiguous lesions, and the selection and guidance of a therapeutic approach. These applications are the current domains of intravascular ultrasound imaging; however, intravascular optical coherence tomography might be an alternative approach that offers specific advantages in the clinical scenario.

Assessment of angiographic ambiguous lesions

Coronary angiography represents the standard modality for visualization of coronary arteries.[3] It provides a unique overview of the coronary tree, anatomy, and topography. However, angiography has limitations. Angiographic "ambiguous" lesions are a result of methodological limitations in the detection of coronary artery disease or in the assessment of lesion severity.

Angiography is restricted to visualize blood pool in the lumen and not the vessel wall itself. As a consequence, atherosclerotic lesions can only be detected if they cause lumen obstructions or expansions. This yields to a systematic and significant underestimation of plaque burden.[4,5] Comparison to postmortem histology revealed only moderate sensitivity for atherosclerotic lesions in the range of 60%.[6–8] Similarly, angiography shows a relatively low sensitivity (24–28%) and specificity (49–100%) in detecting atherosclerotic lesions as compared to IVUS,[9] which is to date considered the gold-standard for the in vivo detection of atherosclerotic lesions.

Another limitation of angiography affects the judgement of lesion severity. It consists in the fact that projection of the coronary lumen is dependent on anatomical and technical issues. Correct lesion projection can be hampered by lesion eccentricity,[10] side branch overlap, geometric distortion, and foreshortening.[11] Thus, the error in diameter measurements in two orthogonal views is dependent on lesion geometry up to 25%.[12,13] Intravascular optical coherence tomography offers in principal the same advantage of direct visualization of the vessel wall as IVUS.

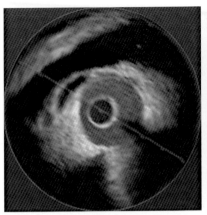

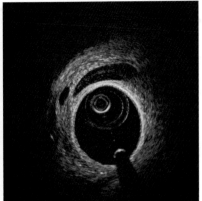

IVUS Image 40 MHz Center
Frequency IVUS

OCT Image 1300 nm
Wavelength

Figure 18.8 Comparison of IVUS and OCT in vivo images of porcine coronary.

Lumen dimension and lesion severity as well as vessel wall architecture and extent of atherosclerotic disease can be directly assessed. The considerably higher image resolution of OCT allows for detection of much smaller structural changes (Figure 18.8).

Early descriptive in vitro studies of sections of the human abdominal aorta ($n = 5$ patients)[14] and coronary arteries[15] suggested superior detail resolution of plaque structures that were close to the luminal surface with OCT as compared with a 30-MHz IVUS system. In vivo animal studies confirmed that OCT can detect both normal and pathologic artery structures and that OCT is superior in visualizing intimal tears and fissures[16,17] (Figure 18.9).

Such type of very detailed information allows overcoming classical limitations of angiography and will improve our understanding of coronary artery pathophysiology. These findings are of particular interest in patients presenting with chest pain that is typical for angina pectoris, but who do not show significant coronary artery disease by angiography.

Selection and guidance of therapeutic approach

Similar to IVUS, optical coherence tomography can provide qualitative and quantitative information that might be helpful for clinical decision making and the selection and guidance of a thera-

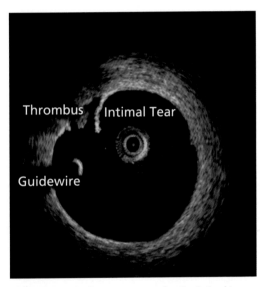

Figure 18.9 In vivo human coronary showing intimal tear and micro-thrombus. (Courtesy of LightLab.)

peutic approach. It seems likely that the choice of not treating certain plaques may also be facilitated by OCT, as suggested by Figure 18.10 where two plaques that might appear indistinguishable in an angiogram in fact appear very different in the OCT image. The plaque on the left appears to be a very fibrous and presumably stable plaque whereas the plaque on the right is a thin-capped fibroatheroma with a mixture of lipid, necrotic cells and calcium in the plaque. Since the blood pools are approximately

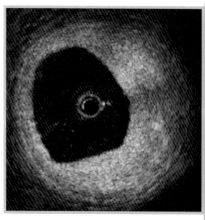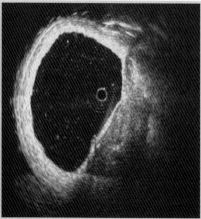

Figure 18.10 Comparison of two OCT images demonstrating the ability to differentiate plaque types. Left: a fibrous and presumed stable plaque; right: a thin-capped fibroatheroma.

the same in size and shape these lesions would appear identical in the angiogram. It is at least possible that the treatment for these two lesions should be quite different and it seems likely that the plaque on the left is relatively benign.

Plaque characterization

The capability of OCT for plaque characterization has been analyzed in an in vitro study of more than 300 human atherosclerotic artery segments (aorta, carotid and coronary arteries). Plaque types were defined by OCT as follows: fibrous plaques were characterized by homogeneous, signal-rich regions; fibrocalcific plaques by well-delineated, signal-poor regions with sharp borders; and lipid-rich plaques by signal-poor regions with diffuse borders. Independent validation of these criteria by two OCT readers demonstrated high sensitivity and specificity with high interobserver and intra-observer reliabilities of OCT assessment (κ values of 0.88 and 0.91, respectively).[18]

In vitro data suggest further that OCT is able to overcome two classical shortcomings of IVUS imaging: detection of lipid-rich lesions and assessment of calcified lesions. While IVUS can classify fibrotic plaques with high sensitivity (89%) and specificity (97%),[19] the detection of lipid-rich lesions is more difficult with a reported sensitivity as low as 50%.[20] Recent data on OCT suggest a considerably higher sensitivity (90–94%) and specificity (90–92%) for the detection of lipid-rich lesions.[18]

OCT can penetrate calcified plaques; it is not hampered by shadowing and allows for tissue analysis behind the calcification. Furthermore, analysis of structures in front of calcium is not impeded by reverberations[16,17] (Figure 18.11).

Guidance of tissue ablative therapies

The small size of the optical imaging fibers makes OCT attractive for application in combined devices. This would allow morphologic assessment during therapeutic intervention without the somewhat cumbersome need to exchange catheters during the procedure. Such an approach might be particularly interesting for guided atherectomy or for newer therapies such as cryoablation. In the latter case, OCT is not only able to document the therapeutic tissue defect but also the freeze penetration depth, and thus might allow for titration of the applied cryoenergy.

Assessment of stent deployment

OCT might be applied for stent assessment at baseline and during long-term follow-up. OCT allows the assessment of stent expansion, visualization of periprocedural thrombus formation (Figure 18.12), and the delicate interaction between stent struts and vessel wall (Figure 18.13).[21]

Long-term follow-up of drug-eluting stents have shown to significantly limit neointimal growth to such an extent that the neointima tissue might consist of only a few cell layers that can not be

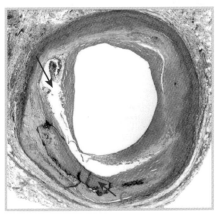

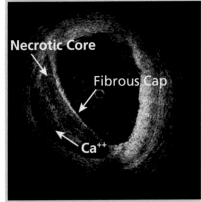

Figure 18.11 Postmortem analysis of human coronary artery. Calcified plaque – left: histology, Movat's pentachrome staining; right: corresponding OCT image. (Courtesy of LightLab.)

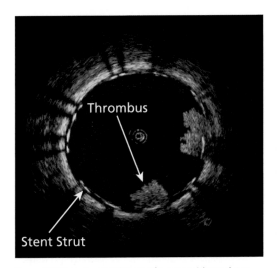

Figure 18.12 In vivo OCT image of a stent with two large thrombi.

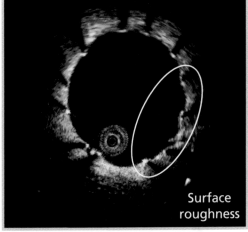

Figure 18.13 Rough intimal surface after stent deployment.

accurately visualized with IVUS. The high image resolution capability of OCT offers the possibility to assess late stent expansion and neointima growth patterns (Figure 18.14).[22]

Diagnosis of vulnerable plaque

For more than 40 years, coronary angiography has represented the universal, standard modality for visualization of the coronary arteries.[7] The prognostic relevance for subsequent cardiac events, however, is limited. The percentage diameter stenosis of a lesion does not provide reliable

information concerning the risk for myocardial infarction and death.[23–27]

These observations triggered the hypothesis that the identification of unstable or "vulnerable" plaques that are at high risk for rupture might allow risk stratification for subsequent life-threatening adverse cardiac events.

Vulnerable coronary plaques have been analyzed in autopsy series. Classical pathognomonic features include the presence of a thin fibrous cap that covers a necrotic lipid core,[28,29] local inflammation, macrophage accumulation,[30] and increased activity.[31] Disruption of the thin fibrous cap with

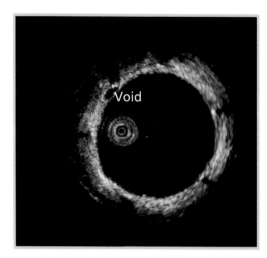

Figure 18.14 Slight neointimal growth after stent implantation and tissue void.

consecutive intraluminal thrombosis causes acute lumen obstruction. In addition, two other pathophysiologic mechanisms have been suggested: First, local plaque neovascularization[32] that causes intraplaque hemorrhage with consecutive plaque disruption and coronary thrombosis,[33] and second erosion of plaques with calcified nodules that causes thrombosis.[34]

Requirements for a technology to diagnose vulnerable plaque

Up to now, there is no validated method for the in vivo detection of vulnerable plaque available. The ideal tool should allow the detection of the described morphologic characteristics with high sensitivity and specificity. It should allow one to assess the mechanical properties of the fibrous cap and vasa vasorum, and it should also allow for physiologic assessment, e.g. macrophage and thrombocyte activation, inflammation. Furthermore, it should be accurate, easy to apply, repeatable, noninvasive, and inexpensive.

Potential of OCT for the detection of vulnerable plaque

In theory, the morphologic features of vulnerable plaque that have been described in autopsy series are accessible to OCT. For the following features the concept is underlined by a body of technical and experimental evidence.

Thin fibrous cap

The in vivo visualization of a thin fibrous cap is missed by angiography and angioscopy because it is limited to the visualization of the lumen and it is missed by intravascular ultrasound by its limited image resolution (axial resolution 150–200 mm, lateral resolution 200–400 mm). OCT produces, in a manner similar to IVUS, real-time imaging of the arterial wall but offers ten times higher resolution and thus the possibility of detecting thin fibrous caps (Figure 18.15). In vitro quantitative analysis of fibrous cap thickness in atherosclerotic specimen suggests high agreement ($r = 0.91$, $P = 0.0001$) compared to histomorphometry.[35]

Necrotic/lipid core

OCT offers a much higher sensitivity in the detection necrotic/lipid cores within coronary atheromas than IVUS. OCT can detect lipid-rich lesions with a sensitivity of 90–94% and a specificity of 90–92%,[18] whereas the sensitivity of IVUS has been reported considerably lower (50–83%).[20] In theory, sophisticated signal processing or combination with other techniques such as spectroscopy might allow even more detailed plaque characterization.

Macrophage accumulation

Recently, in vitro data propose the possibility to detect macrophage accumulation within atherosclerotic plaques by OCT.[36] Detection of macrophage accumulation with OCT is based on the hypothesis that plaques containing macrophages have a high heterogeneity of optical refraction indices that exhibit strong optical scattering. Optical scattering results in a relatively high variance of the OCT signal intensity that can be expressed as normalized standard deviation (NSD) of the OCT signal.

Tearney and coworkers compared, in vitro, the correlation between NSD of the OCT signal and immunohistochemical detection of macrophages in 26 human atherosclerotic aortic and carotid arteries. OCT was performed using an OCT microscope in a pre-set region of interest within the plaque. NSD of both, the conventional, compressed (base 10 logarithm) OCT images and of the uncompressed raw OCT data images was calculated. The NSD of OCT raw data showed a high degree of positive correlation between OCT and fibrous

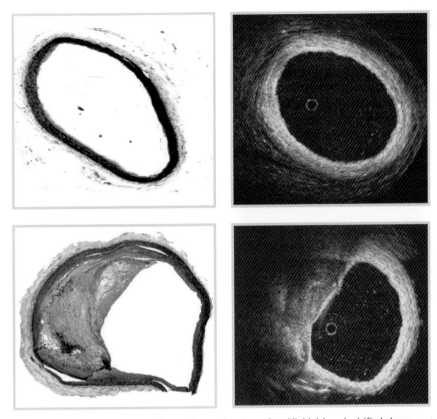

Figure 18.15 Histology and OCT comparison of normal artery (top image) and lipid rich and calcified plaque areas (bottom image). (Movat's pentachrome stain.) (Courtesy of LightLab.)

cap macrophage density ($r = 0.84$, $P < 0.0001$). Additionally, a negative correlation between OCT and histological measurements of smooth muscle actin density ($r = -0.56$, $P < 0.005$) was found.

Clinical experience

Clinical studies

To date, there is only limited experience with intravascular OCT in the clinical setting. Two different systems for intravascular optical coherence tomography are currently used clinically; the MHG researchers in Boston use a modified IVUS catheter,[18] the LightLab system is described above.

A first clinical study proofed the concept of in vivo intravascular OCT using a modified 3.2F IVUS catheter. In 10 patients scheduled for coronary stent implantation, mild to moderate coronary lesions that were remote from the target stenosis were investigated. Most coronary structures that were detected by IVUS could also been visualized with OCT. All fibrous plaques, macrocalcifications, and echolucent regions identified by IVUS were visualized in corresponding OCT images. Intimal hyperplasia and echolucent regions, which may correspond to lipid pools, were identified more frequently by OCT than by IVUS.[37]

We performed a pilot study using dedicated OCT imaging wires and OCT imaging catheters.[38] Patients scheduled for percutaneous coronary intervention in a native coronary artery underwent pre-interventional OCT imaging. OCT with motorized catheter pullback was successfully performed in all vessels and well tolerated in all patients.

OCT analysis of coronary artery wall was possible in all patients and the entire vessel circumference was visualized. OCT allowed for differentiation of the normal artery wall and a wide spectrum of different plaque morphologies. Normal arteries show a clear demarcation between tunica intima

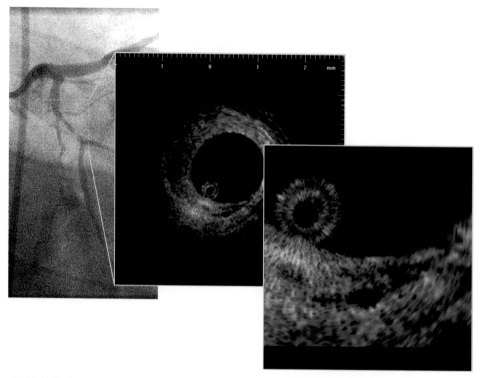

Figure 18.16 In vivo human coronary artery image showing a thin-cap fibroatheroma and lipid accumulation.

(high reflective), tunica media (low reflective), and tunica adventitia (high reflective). Lipid-rich, necrotic plaques are visualized as low reflective structures within the artery wall, predominantly fibrous plaque shows a highly reflective, uniform pattern, calcified lesions appear as low reflective structures with relatively sharp boundaries.

OCT is able to clearly identify thin fibrous cap atheromas in vivo. Thin-cap fibroatheromas consisted of inhomogeneous, low reflecting necrotic cores, covered by highly reflecting fibrous caps with a thickness in the range of 50 μm (Figure 18.16).

This pilot study demonstrates the clinical feasibility of intracoronary OCT. Thin-cap fibroatheroma can be visualized in vivo. The very promising data justify further clinical investigation. Future trials will have to address the incidence of thin-cap fibroatheromas, their "natural course," and their prognostic relevance.

Safety

The applied energies in intravascular OCT are relatively low (output power in the range of 5.0–8.0 mW)

and are not considered to cause functional or structural damage to the tissue.

Safety issues, thus, seem mainly dependent on the OCT catheter mechanical design and the extent of ischemia caused by flow obstruction from the catheter itself and the displacement of blood. Representative safety data for intravascular OCT are not yet available, as there is only preliminary clinical experience in a small number of patients. These data are difficult to interpret as all patients underwent angioplasty before or after the OCT imaging procedure.

In our series, the most frequent complications were transient ECG changes indicative for ischemia (58%) and chest pain (38%). These data match well with large IVUS registries that reported transient coronary ischemia, caused by the imaging catheter in 67% and angina in 22% of patients.[39,40]

Future directions

At present, intracoronary OCT has proven its potential to visualize coronary artery structures that are associated with plaque vulnerability and has proven clinical feasibility in relatively small patient cohorts. Future developments will aim at extending the information that can be gained by near infrared light in order to improve tissue characterization, e.g. birefringence and spectroscopy.

The degree of birefringence in a tissue may be helpful in determining its structure, since highly oriented tissue fibers are birefringent, while randomly oriented fibers or amorphous constituents of tissue are not. Technically, this can be realized as infrared light is a transverse wave that can be polarized and the polarization axis can be determined from two transversely polarized receiving channels.

Spectroscopy analysis would allow insight into the size, orientation, and even chemical content of the arterial structures. A change in the signal processing could be introduced into the OCT system that would extract spectral parameters that are indicative of particular chemical bonds or microanatomic structures. The spectroscopic image could then be color coded and presented simultaneous with the reflection image.

Another future application would be Doppler flow assessment. It is possible to introduce into the signal processing channel a Doppler shift detector. This would allow the creation of a Doppler image simultaneous with the reflection (or anatomic) image. This would permit color flow mapping in real time, in a manner analogous to Doppler flow mapping in echocardiology systems.

Conclusions

Optical coherence tomography shows promise for use in the coronary arteries. It has the potential to provide a new level of anatomic detail and a new dimension of chemical and structural information for the diagnosis of coronary artery disease and specifically for the diagnosis of vulnerable plaques.

References

1. Huang D, Swanson EA, Lin CP, et al. Optical coherence tomography. Science 1991;254:1178–81.
2. Drexler W, Morgner U, Kärtner FX, et al. In vivo ultra-high resolution optical coherence tomography. Optics Lett 1999;24:1221–3.
3. Sones F, Shirey E, Proufit W, Westcott R. Cine-coronary angiography. Circulation 1959;20:773.
4. Arnett EN, Isner JM, Redwood DR, et al. Coronary artery narrowing in coronary heart disease: comparison of cineangiographic and necropsy findings. Ann Intern Med 1979;91:350–6.
5. Goldberg RK, Kleiman NS, Minor ST, Abukhalil J, Raizner AE. Comparison of quantitative coronary angiography to visual estimates of lesion severity pre and post PTCA. Am Heart J 1990;119:178–84.
6. Vlodaver Z, Frech R, Van Tassel RA, Edwards JE. Correlation of the antemortem coronary arteriogram and the postmortem specimen. Circulation 1973;47:162–9.
7. Grondin CM, Dyrda I, Pasternac A, Campeau L, Bourassa MG, Lesperance J. Discrepancies between cineangiographic and postmortem findings in patients with coronary artery disease and recent myocardial revascularization. Circulation 1974;49:703–8.
8. Murphy ML, Galbraith JE, de Soyza N. The reliability of coronary angiogram interpretation: an angiographic–pathologic correlation with a comparison of radiographic views. Am Heart J 1979;97:578–84.
9. Mintz GS, Painter JA, Pichard AD, et al. Atherosclerosis in angiographically "normal" coronary artery reference segments: an intravascular ultrasound study with clinical correlations. J Am Coll Cardiol 1995;25:1479–85.
10. Saner HE, Gobel FL, Salomonowitz E, Erlien DA, Edwards JE. The disease-free wall in coronary atherosclerosis: its relation to degree of obstruction. J Am Coll Cardiol 1985;6:1096–9.
11. Topol EJ, Nissen SE. Our preoccupation with coronary luminology. The dissociation between clinical and angiographic findings in ischemic heart disease [see comments]. Circulation 1995;92:2333–42.
12. Spears JR, Sandor T, Baim DS, Paulin S. The minimum error in estimating coronary luminal cross-sectional area from cineangiographic diameter measurements. Cathet Cardiovasc Diagn 1983;9:119–28.
13. Serruys PW, Reiber JH, Wijns W, et al. Assessment of percutaneous transluminal coronary angioplasty by quantitative coronary angiography: diameter versus densitometric area measurements. Am J Cardiol 1984;54:482–8.
14. Brezinski ME, Tearney GJ, Weissman NJ, et al. Assessing atherosclerotic plaque morphology: comparison of optical coherence tomography and high frequency intravascular ultrasound. Heart 1997;77:397–403.
15. Patwari P, Weissman NJ, Boppart SA, et al. Assessment of coronary plaque with optical coherence tomography and high-frequency ultrasound. Am J Cardiol 2000;85:641–4.

16. Fujimoto JG, Boppart SA, Tearney GJ, Bouma BE, Pitris C, Brezinski ME. High resolution in vivo intra-arterial imaging with optical coherence tomography. Heart 1999;82:128–33.

17. Tearney GJ, Jang IK, Kang DH, et al. Porcine coronary imaging in vivo by optical coherence tomography. Acta Cardiol 2000;55:233–7.

18. Yabushita H, Bouma BE, Houser SL, et al. Characterization of human atherosclerosis by optical coherence tomography. Circulation 2002;106:1640–5.

19. Kostamaa H, Donovan J, Kasaoka S, Tobis J, Fitzpatrick L. Calcified plaque cross-sectional area in human arteries: correlation between intravascular ultrasound and undecalcified histology. Am Heart J 1999;137:482–8.

20. Hiro T, Leung CY, Russo RJ, Karimi H, Farvid AR, Tobis JM. Variability of a three-layered appearance in intravascular ultrasound coronary images: a comparison of morphometric measurements with four intravascular ultrasound systems. Am J Card Imaging 1996;10:219–27.

21. Jang IK, Tearney G, Bouma B. Visualization of tissue prolapse between coronary stent struts by optical coherence tomography: comparison with intravascular ultrasound. Circulation 2001;104:2754.

22. Grube E, Gerckens U, Buellesfeld L, Fitzgerald PJ. Images in cardiovascular medicine. Intracoronary imaging with optical coherence tomography: a new high-resolution technology providing striking visualization in the coronary artery. Circulation 2002;106:2409–10.

23. Holmes DR, Jr, Davis K, Gersh BJ, Mock MB, Pettinger MB. Risk factor profiles of patients with sudden cardiac death and death from other cardiac causes: a report from the Coronary Artery Surgery Study (CASS). J Am Coll Cardiol 1989;13:524–30.

24. Ambrose JA, Tannenbaum MA, Alexopoulos D, et al. Angiographic progression of coronary artery disease and the development of myocardial infarction. J Am Coll Cardiol 1988;12:56–62.

25. Little WC, Constantinescu M, Applegate RJ, et al. Can coronary angiography predict the site of a subsequent myocardial infarction in patients with mild-to-moderate coronary artery disease? Circulation 1988;78:1157–66.

26. Brensike JF, Levy RI, Kelsey SF, et al. Effects of therapy with cholestyramine on progression of coronary arteriosclerosis: results of the NHLBI Type II Coronary Intervention Study. Circulation 1984;69:313–24.

27. Brown WV. Review of clinical trials: proving the lipid hypothesis. Eur Heart J 1990;11(Suppl H):15–20.

28. Falk E. Plaque rupture with severe pre-existing stenosis precipitating coronary thrombosis. Characteristics of coronary atherosclerotic plaques underlying fatal occlusive thrombi. Br Heart J 1983;50:127–34.

29. Burke AP, Farb A, Malcom GT, Liang YH, Smialek J, Virmani R. Coronary risk factors and plaque morphology in men with coronary disease who died suddenly. N Engl J Med 1997;336:1276–82.

30. Kolodgie FD, Narula J, Burke AP, et al. Localization of apoptotic macrophages at the site of plaque rupture in sudden coronary death. Am J Pathol 2000;157:1259–68.

31. Lendon CL, Davies MJ, Born GV, Richardson PD. Atherosclerotic plaque caps are locally weakened when macrophages density is increased. Atherosclerosis 1991;87:87–90.

32. Barger AC, Beeuwkes R 3rd, Lainey LL. Hypothesis: vasa vasorum and neovascularization of human coronary arteries. A possible role in the pathophysiology of atherosclerosis. N Engl J Med 1984;310:175–7.

33. Jeziorska M, Woolley D. Neovascularization in early atherosclerotic lesions of human carotid arteries: its potential contribution to plaque development. Hum Pathol 1999;30:919–25.

34. Virmani R, Burke A, Kolodgie F, Farb A. Vulnerable plaque: the pathology of unstable coronary lesions. J Interv Cardiol. 2002;15:439–46.

35. Jang IK. Cardiovascular optical coherence tomography. Ex-vivo results, The 4th Vulnerable Plaque Satellite Sympsium at TCT 2002, Chicago, 2002. Association for the Eradication of Heart Attack.

36. Tearney GJ, Yabushita H, Houser SL, et al. Quantification of macrophage content in atherosclerotic plaques by optical coherence tomography. Circulation 2003;107:113–19.

37. Jang IK, Bouma BE, Kang DH, et al. Visualization of coronary atherosclerotic plaques in patients using optical coherence tomography: comparison with intravascular ultrasound. J Am Coll Cardiol 2002;39:604–9.

38. Regar E, Schaar J, van der Giessen W, van der Steen A. Real-time, in vivo optical coherence tomography of human coronary arteries using a dedicated imaging wire. Am J Cardiol 2002;90(suppl 6A):129H.

39. Hausmann D, Erbel R, Alibelli-Chemarin MJ, et al. The safety of intracoronary ultrasound. A multicenter survey of 2207 examinations. Circulation 1995;91:623.

40. Batkoff BW, Linker DT. Safety of intracoronary ultrasound: data from a Multicenter European Registry. Cathet Cardiovasc Diagn 1996;38:238–41.

CHAPTER 19

Intravascular palpography

Johannes A Schaar, Chris L de Korte, Frits Mastik,
Pim de Feyter, Cornelis J Slager, Anton FW van der Steen
& Patrick W Serruys

Although a vast number of techniques are under development for the detection of vulnerable plaque,[1–3] no clinically available technique is able to identify these plaques. All techniques focus on detection of one of the pathological aspects of these plaques. Using thermography, the heat production of the macrophages may be measured. Optical coherence tomography has a very high resolution and is capable of measuring the thickness of the fibrous cap. Additionally, fibrous and fatty tissue can be discriminated. Near infrared spectroscopy has a high sensitivity and specificity to identify lipid pools and a moderate sensitivity and high specificity to detect thin caps and inflammation. With Raman spectroscopy calcium salts and cholesterol can be detected.

The question that remains is "Why does the vulnerable plaque rupture?" Therefore, it is not only important to identify the composition and geometry of the plaques but also the response of the tissue on the pulsating force applied by the blood pressure. The plaque is supposed to be rupture prone if the cap is unable to withstand the stress applied on it. All the stress that is applied on the plaque by the blood pressure is concentrated in the cap, since the lipid pool is unable to withstand forces on it.[4,5] As a result, the stress in a thin cap will be higher than the stress in a thicker cap. Furthermore, the strength of the cap is affected by inflammation: fibrous caps with inflammation by macrophages were locally weakened.[6] Therefore, the strength of a cap seems to be a more important parameter than the thickness of the cap.

Intravascular palpography is a technique based on intravascular ultrasound (IVUS). IVUS is currently the only commercially available clinical technique providing real-time cross-sectional images of the coronary artery.[7] Using IVUS, the morphology of the coronary wall and plaque are obtained. Furthermore, calcified and noncalcified plaque components can be identified. However, the sensitivity to identify fatty plaque components remains low.[8,9] Recent radiofrequency-based tissue identification strategies appear to have a better performance.[9,10] With palpography, the local strain of the tissue is obtained. This strain is directly related to the mechanical properties. It is known that the mechanical properties of fibrous and fatty plaque components are different,[11–13] and therefore palpography has the potential to differentiate between different plaque components. An even more promising feature of palpography is the detection of high stress regions. Using computer simulations, concentrations of circumferential tensile stress were more frequently found in unstable plaque than in stable plaques.[5,14] A local increase in circumferential stress in tissue is directly related to an increase of radial strain.

Intravascular palpography

Ophir and colleagues[15,16] have developed an imaging technique called elastography, which is based on deformation of tissue. The rate of deformation (strain) of the tissue is directly related to the mechanical properties. The tissue under inspection is deformed and the strain between pairs of ultrasound signals with and without deformation is determined.[17] For intravascular purposes, the compression can be obtained from the systemic

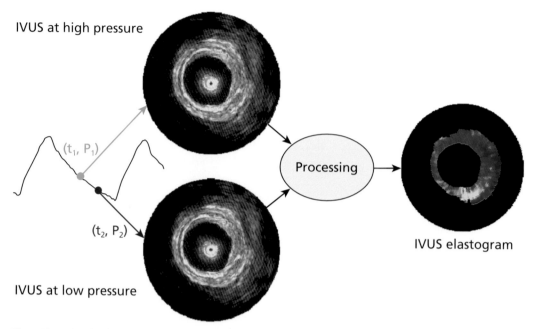

IVUS at high pressure

(t_1, P_1)

Processing

IVUS elastogram

(t_2, P_2)

IVUS at low pressure

Figure 19.1 Principle of intravascular elastography measurement procedure. An IVUS echogram is acquired with a low and a high intraluminal pressure. Using cross-correlation analysis on the high frequency radiofrequency data, the radial strain in the tissue is determined. This information is plotted as an additional image to the IVUS echogram. In this example an eccentric soft lesion is visible between 6 and 12 o'clock in the elastogram where this lesion cannot be identified from the IVUS echogram.

pressure difference. Additionally, well-controlled deformation is possible by using a compliant intravascular balloon.[18]

The principle of intravascular elastography is illustrated in Figure 19.1. An ultrasound image of a human coronary artery is acquired at a high intracoronary pressure. After a short time interval, a second acquisition at a slightly lower pressure (approx. 5 mmHg) is performed. The strain is determined by correlating the signals of the two IVUS echograms. For a detailed description of different methods see de Korte et al.[19] The elastogram (image of the radial strain) is plotted as a complimentary image to the IVUS echogram. The elastogram reveals the presence of an eccentric region with increased strain values at the shoulders of the eccentric plaque.

Plaque characterization

Elastographic experiments were performed in excised human coronary ($n = 4$) and femoral ($n = 9$) arteries. Data were acquired at room temperature

at intraluminal pressures of 80 and 100 mmHg. Coronary arteries were measured using a solid state 20-MHz array catheter (EndoSonics, Rancho Cordova, CA, USA). Femoral arteries were investigated using a single element 30-MHz catheter (DuMed/ EndoSonics, Rijswijk, The Netherlands). The radiofrequency data was stored and processed off-line. The visualized segments were stained for the presence of collagen, smooth muscle cells, and macrophages. Matching of elastographic data and histology was performed using the IVUS echogram. The cross-sections were segmented in regions ($n = 125$) based on the strain value on the elastogram. The dominant plaque types in these regions (fibrous, fibro-fatty, or fatty) were obtained from histology and correlated with the average strain and echo-intensity.

Mean strain values of 0.27%, 0.45%, and 0.60% were found for fibrous, fibro-fatty, and fatty plaque components. The strain for the three plaque types as determined by histology differed significantly ($P = 0.0002$). This difference was independent of the type of artery (coronary or femoral) and was mainly evident between fibrous and fatty tissue ($P = 0.0004$). The plaque types did not reveal echo-intensity differences in the IVUS echogram ($P = 0.992$). Conversion of the strain into Young's modulus values resulted in 493 kPa, 296 kPa, and 222 kPa for fibrous, fibro-fatty, and fatty plaques. Although these values are higher than values measured by Lee et al.,[13] the ratio between fibrous and fatty material is similar. Since fibrous and fatty tissue demonstrated a different strain value and high strain values were often colocalized with increased concentrations of macrophages, these results reveal the potential of identification of the vulnerable plaque features.

Vulnerable plaque detection

Although plaque vulnerability is associated with the plaque composition, detection of a lipid or fibrous composition does not directly warrant identification of the vulnerable plaque. Therefore, a study to evaluate the predictive power of elastography to identify the vulnerable plaque was performed.

Diseased coronary arteries ($n = 24$) were measured in vitro. Elastographic data was acquired at intracoronary pressures of 80 and 100 mmHg using a standard IVUS catheter (JOMED). After the ultrasound experiments, the cross-sections were stained for collagen and fat, smooth muscle cells (SMC), and macrophages. In histology, a vulnerable plaque was defined as a lesion with a large atheroma (>40%), and a thin fibrous cap with moderate to heavy infiltration of macrophages. A plaque was considered vulnerable in elastography when a high strain region was present at the lumen–plaque boundary that was surrounded by low strain values. Using this definition, the instability of the region is assessed.

Figure 19.2 shows a typical example of a vulnerable elastogram. High strain regions are present at 6 and 12 o'clock and these regions are surrounded by low strain values. These regions correspond to the shoulders of this eccentric plaque. The histology reveals a large lipid pool (absence of collagen and SMC) that is covered by a thin fibrous cap. The cap

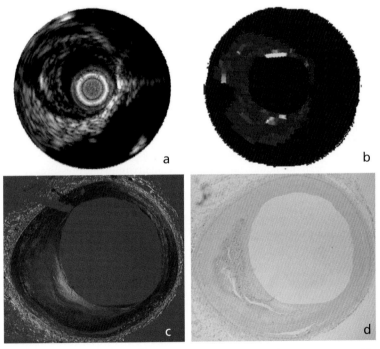

Figure 19.2 IVUS echogram (a) and elastogram (b) with corresponding histology of a coronary artery with a vulnerable plaque. The echogram reveals an eccentric plaque between 6 and 12 o'clock. The elastogram shows high strain regions (yellow) at the shoulders of the plaque surrounded by low strain values (blue). The histology reveals a plaque with a typical vulnerable appearance: a thin cap with a lack of collagen (c) at the shoulders, a large atheroma, and heavy infiltration of macrophages (d).

lacks collagen at the shoulder regions. Inflammation by macrophages is found in the lipid pool and in the cap.

Vulnerable plaques ($n = 23$) were correctly identified by elastography in 20 cases. Nonvulnerable plaques ($n = 31$) were detected 27 times but diagnosed as false positives vulnerable in four cases. This corresponds to a sensitivity and a specificity that are both 87%, and an 83% positive predictive value and a 90% negative predictive value.[20]

In vivo validation

IVUS elastography was validated in vivo using an atherosclerotic Yucatan minipig.[21,22] External iliac and femoral arteries were made atherosclerotic by endothelial Fogarty denudation and subsequent atherosclerotic diet for 7 months. Balloon dilatation was performed in the femoral arteries and the diet was discontinued. Before termination, 6 weeks after balloon dilatation and discontinuation of the diet, data were acquired in the external iliac and femoral artery in six Yucatan pigs. In total, 20 cross-sections were investigated with a 20 MHz Visions catheter (Jomed, Rancho Cordova, CA, USA). The tissue was strained by the pulsatile blood pressure. Two frames acquired at end diastole with a pressure differential of approx. 4 mmHg were taken to determine the elastograms.

After the ultrasound experiments and before dissection, X-ray was used to identify the arterial segments that had been investigated by ultrasound. The specimens were frozen in liquid nitrogen. The cross-sections (7 μm) were stained for collagen (picro Sirius red and polarized light) and macrophages (alcalic phosphatase). Plaques were classified as absent, as early fibrous lesion, as early fatty lesion, or as advanced fibrous plaque. The mean strain in these plaques and normal cross-sections was determined to assess the tissue characterization properties of the technique. Furthermore, the instability of the elastogram was correlated with the presence of fat and macrophages. The instability was characterized by the presence of a high strain region (strain is higher than 1%) at the lumen vessel–wall boundary.

Strains were similar in the plaque free arterial wall and the early and advanced fibrous plaques.

Univariate analysis of variance revealed significantly higher strain values in cross-sections with early fatty lesions than in fibrous plaques ($P = 0.02$) independently of the presence of macrophages. Although a higher strain value was found in plaques with macrophages than in plaques without macrophages, this difference was not significant after correction for fatty components. However, the presence of a high strain region had a high sensitivity (92%) and specificity (92%) to identify the presence of macrophages. Therefore, it was concluded that the mean strain value is dominated by the tissue type. Localized high strain values are related to local phenomena like inflammation.

Patient studies

Preliminary acquisitions were performed in patients during percutaneous transluminal coronary angioplasty (PTCA) procedures.[23,24] Data were acquired in patients ($n = 12$) with an EndoSonics InVision echoapparatus equipped with a radiofrequency output. For obtaining the radiofrequency data, the machine was working in ChromaFlo mode resulting in images of 64 angles with unfocussed ultrasound data. The systemic pressure was used to strain the tissue. This strain was determined using cross-correlation analysis of sequential frames. A likelihood function was determined to obtain the frames with minimal motion of the catheter in the lumen, since motion of the catheter prevents reliable strain estimation. Minimal motion was observed near end-diastole. Reproducible strain estimates were obtained within one pressure cycle and over several pressure cycles. Validation of the results was limited to the information provided by the echogram. Strain in calcified material (0.20%) was lower ($P < 0.001$) than in noncalcified tissue (0.51%).

High-resolution elastograms were acquired using an EndoSonics InVision echoapparatus.[25] The beam-formed image mode (512 angles) ultrasound data ($f_c = 20$ MHz) was acquired with a PC-based acquisition system. Frames acquired at end-diastole with a pressure difference of approx. 5 mmHg were taken to determine the elastograms.

The elastogram of a patient with unstable angina pectoris reveals high strain values in the plaque with very high strain values (up to 2%) at the shoulders of this plaque (Figure 19.3). This

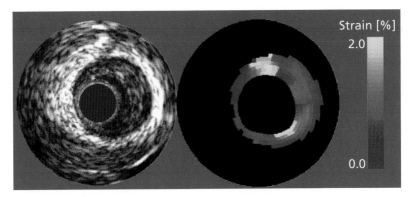

Figure 19.3 In vivo intravascular echogram and elastogram of a human coronary artery. The elastogram reveals that the plaque has soft edges with adjacent hard tissue.

geometry and strain distribution was also found in the vitro studies. The corresponding histology revealed in that study a plaque with a large lipid core covered from the blood by a thin cap. This cap had a lack of collagen at the shoulders and increased inflammation by macrophages. Calcified material, as identified from the echogram, shows strain values of $0-0.2\%$.

Three-dimensional palpography

In the previous studies, elastograms revealed information of one cross-section. However, the distribution of the strain in the 3D geometry of an artery is an important tool to identify the presence of high strain spots, the amount, and the distribution. Especially, since the correlation between plaque vulnerability and parameters provided by the echogram is low,[8,9] selection of cross-sections based on the IVUS echogram introduces selection bias and increases the chance to miss the vulnerable spot. Additionally, during longitudinal monitoring of patients it is extremely difficult to find back the same spot after some months. Therefore, it would be a big step forward to have strain information of the full 3D coronary artery. Since the rupture of a plaque happens in the superficial area of the plaque the elastic information of the surface is displayed as a palpogram.

In palpography, out-of-plane motion is considered as one of the main sources for decorrelation of the signals and thus decreasing the quality of the strain estimate.[26,27] Therefore, for palpographic acquisitions, the position of the transducer is kept

as stable as possible and only motion in the direction of the beam is allowed.[16,28] As a consequence, it is unlikely that valid intravascular strain palpograms can be obtained while performing a continuous pullback of the catheter. However, if the pullback speed is only 1 mm/s and the strain is determined using two subsequent frames, the motion introduced by the pullback is minimal. Furthermore, it is known that due to the contraction of the heart, in diastole the catheter will move distally in the coronary if the catheter is kept at a steady position. Therefore, performing a pullback will decrease out of plane in this phase of the heart cycle. Since elastography uses data acquired in the diastolic phase, performing a pullback and thus obtaining 3D data seems feasible.

Preliminary experiments in rabbit aortas reveal that 3D palpography is feasible in vivo. Despite the introduction of out-of-plane motion by the continuous pullback of the catheter, the similarity between successive frames acquired in the diastolic phase is high enough to calculate several palpograms per heart cycle. By combining these palpograms, one compound palpogram per heart cycle is determined.[29] Strain measurements give an indication of the mechanical properties of the plaque, without taking the shear forces into account, which may be responsible for activation of biological processes, which induce instabilities. Assessment of shear stress is feasible by obtaining high-resolution reconstruction of 3D coronary lumen and wall morphology using the combination of angiography and IVUS.[30] Briefly, a biplane angiogram of a sheath-based IVUS catheter taken at end-diastole allows reconstruction of the 3D pullback trajectory of the catheter. Combining this path with lumen and wall information derived from IVUS images that are successively acquired during catheter pullback at end-diastole gives accurate 3D lumen and wall reconstruction with resolution determined by IVUS. Filling the 3D lumen space with a high-resolution 3D mesh allows calculation of the detailed blood velocity profile in the lumen.[31] For this purpose absolute flow and blood viscosity need to be provided as boundary conditions. From the blood velocity profile local wall shear stress on the endothelium can be accurately derived. Wall shear stress is the frictional force, normalized to surface area that is induced by the blood passing the wall. Although from a mechanical point of view shear stress is of a very small magnitude compared to blood pressure-induced tensile stress, it has a profound influence on vascular biology[32] and explains the localization of atherosclerotic plaque in the presence of systemic risk factors.[33] Many of these biological processes also influence the stability of the vulnerable plaque including inflammation, thrombogenicity, vessel remodeling, intimal thickening or regression, and smooth muscle cell proliferation. Therefore, the assessment of shear stress in combination with strain measurements is of utmost importance.

Clinical application of palpography

Identification of plaque components and the proneness of a lesion to rupture is a major issue in interventional cardiology. Intravascular ultrasound echography is a real-time, clinically available technique capable of providing cross-sectional images and identifying calcified plaque components. Since palpography only requires ultrasound data sets that are acquired at different levels of intraluminal pressure, it can be realized using conventional catheters. It has been shown that palpograms can be produced in vitro and in vivo.

The question still not answered is the relevance of the information given by the palpogram. A palpogram is an image of the strain and is therefore a representation of the Young's modulus. This artifactual presentation can be observed in Figure 19.3. Although the plaque contains a large lipid core, the elastogram does not reveal high strain values in the core of the plaque. This is caused by the geometry of this plaque. The fibrous cap is protecting the lipid pool for large deformation. However at the shoulder regions a larger strain than expected is observed. This example indicates that the strain cannot always be directly translated into a Young's modulus. Nevertheless, using finite element analysis, an image of the Young's modulus can be reconstructed using the strain and/or displacement information (also known as solving the inverse problem).[34,35] Analysis of these complex geometries has to be performed to identify the differences between and the similarities of strain and modulus images. Currently, the inverse problem is being solved for strain images acquired from human artery specimens in vitro. The resulting Young's modulus images and the strain images will be related to the histology.

Identification of vulnerable plaques is of paramount importance in investigating the underlying principle of plaque rupture, the effectiveness of pharmaceutical treatments, and in the long-term prevention of sudden cardiac deaths. For detecting these vulnerable plaques, a Young's modulus image seems not necessary. The presence of a high strain spot that is surrounded by low strain has a high predictive power to identify the rupture-prone plaque in vitro with high sensitivity and specificity. Since there is currently no clinically available technique capable of identifying the rupture-prone plaque, IVUS palpography may be one of the first techniques that can be applied in patients to assess the vulnerability of plaques. With the development of 3D palpography, identification of weak spots over the full length of a coronary artery becomes available. A prospective study in patients that correlates clinical events with the distribution of these weak spots is currently being performed and will reveal the power of elastography as a clinical tool.

Conclusions

Intravascular palpography is a technique that assesses the local strain of the vessel wall and plaque. Both in vitro and in vivo studies revealed that the strain is higher in fatty than in fibrous plaques. Additionally, the presence of a high strain region has a high sensitivity and specificity to detect the vulnerable plaque. With the introduction of

3D palpography a technique becomes available that may develop into a clinically available tool to identify the rupture-prone plaque.

Acknowledgments

Supported by the Dutch Technology Foundation (STW) and the Netherlands Organization for Scientific Research (NWO), the Dutch Heart Foundation (NHS), and the German Heart Foundation (DHS).

References

1. Falk E, Shah P, Fuster V. Coronary plaque disruption. Circulation 1995;92:657–71.
2. Fuster V, Stein B, Ambrose J, et al. Atherosclerotic plaque rupture and thrombosis. Evolving concepts. Circulation 1990;82:II.47–59.
3. Moreno PR, Falk E, Palacios IF, et al. Macrophage infiltration in acute coronary syndromes: implcations for plaque rupture. Circulation 1994;90:775–8.
4. Loree HM, Kamm RD, Stringfellow RG, et al. Effects of fibrous cap thickness on peak circumferential stress in model atherosclerotic vessels. Circ Res 1992;71:850–8.
5. Richardson PD, Davies MJ, Born GVR. Influence of plaque configuration and stress distribution on fissuring of coronary atherosclerotic plaques. Lancet 1989;21: 941–4.
6. Lendon CL, Davies MJ, Born GVR, et al. Atherosclerotic plaque caps are locally weakened when macrophage density is increased. Atherosclerosis 1991;87:87–90.
7. Mintz GS, Nissen SE, Anderson WD, et al. ACC Clinical Expert Consensus Document on Standards for Acquisition, Measurement and Reporting of Intravascular Ultrasound Studies (IVUS). A report of the American College of Cardiology Task Force on Clinical Expert Consensus Documents. J Am Coll Cardiol 2001;37: 1478–92.
8. Prati F, Arbustini E, Labellarte A, et al. Correlation between high frequency intravascular ultrasound and histomorphology in human coronary arteries. Heart 2001;85:567–70.
9. Komiyama N, Berry G, Kolz M, et al. Tissue characterization of atherosclerotic plaques by intravascular ultrasound radiofrequency signal analysis: an in vitro study of human coronary arteries. Am Heart J 2000; 140:565–74.
10. Hiro T, Fujii T, Yasumoto K, et al. Detection of fibrous cap in atherosclerotic plaque by intravascular ultrasound by use of color mapping of angle-dependent echo-intensity variation. Circulation 2001;103:1206–11.
11. Loree HM, Tobias BJ, Gibson LJ, et al. Mechanical properties of model atherosclerotic lesion lipid pools. Arteriscler Thromb 1994;14:230–4.
12. Loree HM, Grodzinsky AJ, Park SY, et al. Static circumferential tangential modulus of human atherosclerotic tissue. J Biomech 1994;27:195–204.
13. Lee RT, Richardson G, Loree HM, et al. Prediction of mechanical properties of human atherosclerotic tissue by high-frequency intravascular ultrasound imaging. Arteriscler Thromb 1992;12:1–5.
14. Cheng GC, Loree HM, Kamm RD, et al. Distribution of circumferential stress in ruptured and stable atherosclerotic lesions. A structural analysis with histopathological correlation. Circulation 1993;87:1179–87.
15. Céspedes EI, Ophir J, Ponnekanti H, et al. Elastography: elasticity imaging using ultrasound with application to muscle and breast in vivo. Ultras Imag 1993;17:73–88.
16. Ophir J, Céspedes EI, Ponnekanti H, et al. Elastography: a method for imaging the elasticity in biological tissues. Ultras Imag 1991;13:111–34.
17. Céspedes EI, Huang Y, Ophir J, et al. Methods for estimation of subsample time delays of digitized echo signals. Ultras Imag 1995;17:142–71.
18. Sarvazyan AP, Emelianov SY, Skovorada AR. Intracavity device for elasticity imaging. US patent; 1993.
19. de Korte CL, van der Steen AFW. Intravascular ultrasound elastography: an overview. 2002;40:859–65.
20. Schaar J, de Korte CL, Mastik F, et al. Vulnerable plaque detection with intravascular elastography: a sensitivity and specificity study. Circulation 2001;104:II-459.
21. de Korte CL, Sierevogel M, Mastik F, et al. Intravascular elastography in Yucatan pigs: validation in vivo. Eur Heart J 2001;22:251.
22. de Korte CL, Sierevogel M, Mastik F, et al. Identification of atherosclerotic plaque components with intravascular ultrasound elastography in vivo: a Yucatan pig study. Circulation 2002;105:1627–30.
23. de Korte CL, Carlier SG, Mastik F, et al. Intracoronary elastography in the catheterisation laboratory: preliminary patient results. In: IEEE Ultrasonics Symposium. Lake Tahoe, CA, USA; 1999:1649–52.
24. de Korte CL, Carlier SG, Mastik F, et al. Morphological and mechanical information of coronary arteries obtained with intravascular elastography: a feasibility study in vivo. Eur Heart J 2001;23:349–51.
25. de Korte CL, Doyley MM, Carlier SG, et al. High resolution IVUS elastography in patients. In: IEEE Ultrasonics Symposium. Puerto Rico, USA; 2000:1767–1770.
26. Konofagou E, Ophir J. A new elastographic method for estimation and imaging of lateral displacements, lateral strains, corrected axial strains and Poissons ratios in tissues. 1998;24:1183–99.

27. Kallel F, Ophir J. Three dimensional tissue motion and its effect on image noise in elastography. IEEE Trans UFFC 1997;44:1286–96.
28. Ophir J, Yazdi Y. Method and apparatus for measurement and imaging of tissue compressibility or compliance. In; 1992.
29. Doyley M, Mastik F, de Korte CL, et al. Advancing intravascular ultrasonic palpation towards clinical applications. Ultras Med Biol. 2001;27:1471–80.
30. Slager, CJ, Wentzel JJ, Schuurbiers JCH, et al. True 3-dimensional reconstruction of coronary arteries in patients by fusion of angiography and IVUS (ANGUS) and its quantitative validation. Circulation 2000;102: 511–16.
31. Thury A, Wentzel JJ, Schuurbiers JC, et al. Prominent role of tensile stress in propagation of a dissection after coronary stenting: computational fluid dynamic analysis on true 3D-reconstructed segment. Circulation 2001; 104:E53–4.
32. Malek AM, Alper SL, Izumo S. Hemodynamic shear stress and its role in atherosclerosis. JAMA 1999;282:2035–42.
33. Asakura, T. and T. Karino, Flow patterns and spatial distribution of atherosclerotic lesions in human coronary arteries. Circ Res, 1990;66:1045–66.
34. de Korte CL, Céspedes EI, van der Steen AFW, et al. Image artifacts in intravascular elastography. In: IEEE EMBS. Amsterdam, The Netherlands, 1996:paper no. 685.
35. Soualmi L, Bertrand M, Mongrain R, et al. Forward and inverse problems in endovascular elastography. In: Lees S, Ferrari LA, eds. Acoustical imaging. New York: Plenum, 1997:203–9.

CHAPTER 20

Coronary computed tomography for the detection of atherosclerotic plaque burden

Allen J Taylor & Irwin M Feuerstein

Coronary computed tomography (CT) comprises one of several different methodologies, most commonly electron beam computed tomography (EBCT) or multidetector computed tomography (MDCT) for the detection of coronary artery calcium (CAC). This review will discuss the prognostic and diagnostic implication of CAC (Figure 20.1).

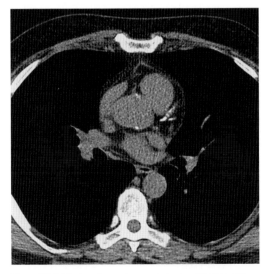

Figure 20.1 Electron beam tomography in a 59-year-old man with extensive multivessel calcifications. Total calcium score was 1101, exceeding the 90th percentile for age and gender. Calcification is shown in the mid-portion of the left anterior descending coronary artery (arrowhead) and ostium of the right coronary artery (arrow).

Coronary plaque burden

Pathology studies have demonstrated a modest direct relationship between the presence and quantity of CAC and atheromatous plaque.[1-3] The strategy of coronary CT lies within the radiographic detection of CAC which indicates the presence of atherosclerosis.[4] Thus the noninvasive detection of coronary calcium with radiological techniques is a potentially useful means of detecting the presence and quantification of both early and advanced coronary atherosclerosis.[5-7]

Technical aspects of coronary computed tomography for coronary artery calcium detection

Although the manner of image production is different for EBCT and MDCT, each form of technology is used to generate a sequence of "slices" through the heart, of variable thickness. Scanner technology continues to improve, with the latest generation of 64-slice MDCT and 50-millisecond EBCT scanners leading to improved image quality and fewer technical constraints (e.g. heart rate). Thus, the studies detect both the presence of coronary calcium as well as the location, extent, and density of calcific deposits. Based on the detection of discrete coronary calcium in specific epicardial coronary vessels, a "calcium score" is measured from the product of the area of calcification (in mm^2) and the density score (each segment of detected calcium is rated on a scale from 1 to 4 based on the maximal CT density in Hounsfield units). Typically, coronary CT results are reported as a composite calcium score for the entire epicardial coronary system (range 0 to >1000). Any score above zero indicates the presence of coronary calcification. Coronary calcification is always associated with atheromatous plaque. The prevalence of coronary calcification increases with age.[8] Calcium score results obtained with EBCT and MDCT in general show good intermethod agreement, with some divergence at the lower range of calcium score severity.[9,10] An alternative reporting system evaluates the volume of CAC. The scan takes approximately 10 minutes (actual scanning requires 20–40 seconds), requires minimal patient cooperation, and there is no need for intravenous contrast medium. Radiation exposure does occur, and is several-fold greater for MDCT than EBCT. For EBCT, the exposure integrated over the thorax is approximately 82 milliRem (mR) for men and 150 mR for women (compared to 10 milliRem for PA and lateral chest film, and 35 mR for screening two-view mammogram). It is comparable to about one-half the radiation exposure to the average person living the USA in 1 year and is an order of magnitude less than coronary arteriography.[11]

Relationship of coronary artery calcium to obstructive coronary lesions

The promise of coronary CT as a diagnostic and prognostic test lies within the current paradigm of acute ischemic coronary syndromes whereby these events arise most commonly as a result of plaque rupture or erosion of mild, nonobstructive arterial stenoses. Assuming that calcification is a sensitive marker for all atheromatous disease, regardless of degree of obstruction, these tests offers a noninvasive way of detecting subclinical disease earlier, and intervening accordingly, in order to prevent acute coronary events.

Diagnosis of coronary artery disease by coronary CT

Janowitz et al.[12] used EBCT to scan the hearts of 1396 men and 502 women (14–88 years of age) to determine the prevalence of coronary calcifications. In this study, there was a good correlation with autopsy studies of coronary calcium prevalence in accidental deaths. Two large studies, including one from Chicago in predominantly Caucasian Americans[13] and another from the Military Health Care System,[14] provide estimates on the relationships between gender, age, and calcium score.

Clinical utility of coronary computed tomography

Asymptomatic populations

Current evidence suggests that coronary CT may be a useful aid to predicting which asymptomatic patients are at risk for cardiovascular events.[15–17] Whether coronary calcium is a superior marker of cardiovascular risk than traditional risk factors has been controversial,[16,18] although the most recent data appears to support an incremental prognostic value over standard risk factor measurements. Furthermore, because silent myocardial ischemia is an important predictor of prognosis, patients with a calcium score of 400 should be referred for stress imaging procedures.[19] Almost half of such patients will have abnormalities on myocardial perfusion studies, indicating the presence of myocardial ischemia. In most cases, these patients would be appropriate for consideration of ischemia suppression, for example with beta blockers, to improve prognosis. Finally, a negative or lower risk coronary CT does not confer the complete absence of risk for cardiovascular events, and proper consideration must be given to standard cardiovascular risk factors and their treatment.

Symptomatic patients

The presence and extent of coronary calcification is related to the severity of angiographic coronary artery disease[6,20–25] (Figure 20.2) and has been related to coronary prognosis in a fashion similar to that observed in asymptomatic patients.[26] Coronary CT has a sensitivity of 81–94% and a specificity of 72–86% for the diagnosis of any angiographic coronary artery disease.[24,25] For obstructive coronary artery disease (>50% stenosis of any epicardial vessel) the sensitivity and specificity are approximately 95% and 50% respectively.[23,24,27] Thus,

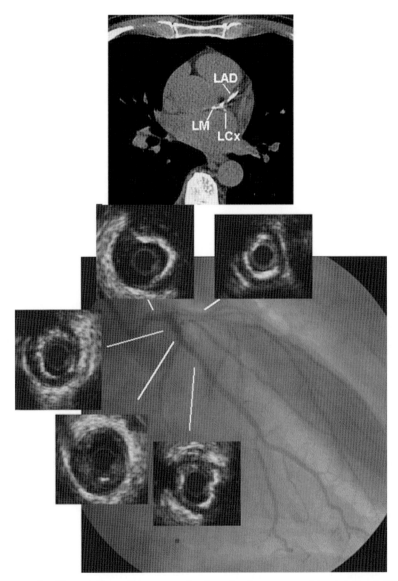

Figure 20.2 EBCT scan in a 61-year-old marathon runner, showing extensive coronary calcium in left main (LM), proximal anterior descending (LAD), and left circumflex (LCx) coronary artery (top panel). CT image at the base of the heart. The total Agatston coronary calcium score was 1105, which was more than in 94% of men of the same age (94th percentile). Because ECG and laboratory analyses showed silent acute myocardial infarction, the patient underwent coronary angiography, revealing severe coronary three-vessel disease. The lower panel shows the left coronary angiogram, demonstrating high-grade left main and proximal left anterior descending coronary artery stenoses. In addition, ICUS (inserts) showed massive calcified and – in one section in the left circumflex artery – noncalcified plaque formation. (Reproduced from Schmermund et al. Cardiol Clin 2003;21:521–34, with permission Elsevier Inc.[34])

coronary CT may be used to "rule out" obstructive coronary artery disease in patients with atypical symptoms and a low-intermediate pretest probability. A value of 123 for the coronary calcium score has been proposed as a "cutoff" at which the sensit-

ivity and specificity for detection of a 70% stenosis is 82%.[28] False negative studies may be more common in young patients due to the presence of early, noncalcified atherosclerosis. The higher the calcium score, the greater the likelihood of obstructive

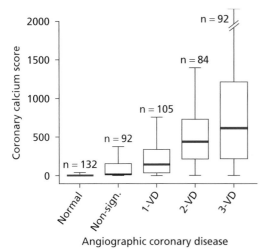

Figure 20.3 Coronary calcium score (Agatston method) as a function of angiographic disease in 505 patients. The median calcium scores in the five categories of angiographic coronary disease (normal, non-sign: 1-VD, 2-VD, 3-VD) were 1.3, 21.1, 146.7, 439.5, and 611.4 ($P < 0.0001$, Kruskal–Wallis test) with addition of 182 more recently examined patients. 1-VD = one-vessel disease; 2-VD = two-vessel disease; 3-VD = three-vessel disease; non-sign = wall irregularities; normal = smooth vessel contours. (Data from Schmermund et al. Cardiol Clin 2003;21:521–34, with permission Elsevier Inc.[34])

coronary artery disease (Figure 20.3). The accuracy of exercise testing, myocardial perfusion imaging, and coronary CT for the identification of patients with obstructive coronary artery disease are comparable.[29] But, because the intertest agreement of these tests is limited, these methods are best considered as complementary.

Although generally used as a method of finding calcified plaque, an emerging application of coronary CT is the detection of soft plaque. This achieves importance as several studies have suggested that the presence of calcified plaques on EBCT is more predictive of soft events, such as coronary revascularization procedures, than hard events, such as cardiac death and myocardial infarction.[15,30] For example, Secci et al. found that EBCT is only a weak predictor of coronary death and infarction, but predicts revascularization well among high risk, older patients.[31] Advanced plaques containing fibrocalcific elements are most likely to be detected with coronary CT and are also more resistant to rupture than soft, lipid-rich plaques. Consistent with these data, Schmermund

et al. found CAC in only one of eight patients who had either mildly stenotic plaques at a single site or nonatherosclerotic causes of an unstable coronary syndrome.[32] These patients were significantly younger than other patients in the same study with acute coronary events and CAC. Using contrast-enhanced coronary CT, MDCT in particular is now being investigated as a means to differentiate calcified and noncalcified plaque in the arterial wall (Figure 20.4). Arterial wall plaques outside of the contrast-opacified lumen are discriminated on the basis of radiographic density. A recent study by Achenbach and colleagues[33] showed a moderate correlation between MDCT-defined plaque volume using intravascular ultrasound as a gold standard, however there was limited sensitivity (53%) for the detection of noncalcified plaque. Future improvements in scanner spatial and temporal resolution should lead to increased accuracy of this application, which then will require prospective study to determine the prognostic implications of the data.

References

1. Rumberger JA, Simons DB, Fitzpatrick LA, et al. Coronary artery calcium area by electron-beam computed tomography and coronary atherosclerotic plaque area. A histopathologic correlative study [see comments]. Circulation 1995;92:2157–62.
2. Sangiorgi G, Rumberger JA, Severson A, et al. Arterial calcification and not lumen stenosis is highly correlated with atherosclerotic plaque burden in humans: a histologic study of 723 coronary artery segments using nondecalcifying methodology. J Am Coll Cardiol 1998;31: 126–33.
3. Eggen DA, Strong JP, McGill HCJ. Coronary calcification. Relationship to clinically significant coronary lesions and race, sex, and topographic distribution. Circulation 1965;32:948–55.
4. Mautner GC, Mautner SL, Froehlich J, et al. Coronary artery calcification: assessment with electron beam CT and histomorphometric correlation. Radiology 1994;192:619–23.
5. Kaufmann RB, Peyser PA, Sheedy PF, et al. Quantification of coronary artery calcium by electron beam computed tomography for determination of severity of angiographic coronary artery disease in younger patients. J Am Coll Cardiol 1995;25:626–32.
6. Fallavollita JA, Brody AS, Bunnell IL, et al. Fast computed tomography detection of coronary calcification in

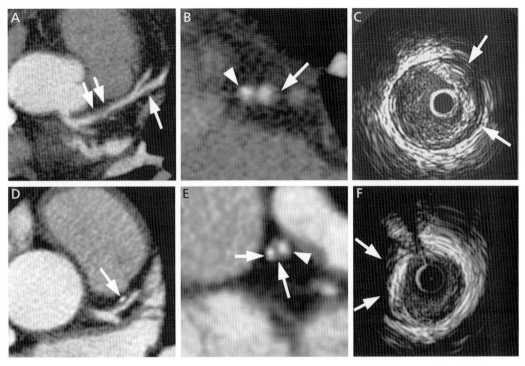

Figure 20.4 A–C, Patient with noncalcified plaque in segments 6 and 7 of left anterior descending coronary artery (LAD). A, Axial MDCT image showing noncalcified plaque in segments 6 (proximal LAD; small arrows) and 7 (LAD distal to diagonal branch; large arrow). B, Multiplanar reconstructed MDCT image showing cross-section of LAD segment 7 with plaque (arrow). Arrowhead indicates diagonal branch. C, IVUS image showing noncalcified plaque in segment 7 (arrows). D–F, Patient with calcified and noncalcified plaque components in proximal LAD (segment 6). D, Axial MDCT image showing partly calcified plaque in proximal LAD (arrow). E, Multiplanar reconstructed MDCT image showing cross section of proximal LAD with plaque (large arrow), including calcification (small arrow). Arrowhead indicates contrast-enhanced lumen. F, IVUS image showing partly calcified plaque in proximal LAD (arrows). (Reproduced from Achenbach et al. *Circulation* 2004;109:14–17, with permission (American Heart Association).[33])

the diagnosis of coronary artery disease. Comparison with angiography in patients <50 years old. Circulation 1994;89:285–90.

7. Guerci AD, Spadaro LA, Popma JJ, et al. Relation of coronary calcium score by electron beam computed tomography to arteriographic findings in asymptomatic and symptomatic adults. Am J Cardiol 1997;79:128–33.

8. Hoff JA, Daviglus ML, Chomka EV, et al. Conventional coronary artery disease risk factors and coronary artery calcium detected by electron beam tomography in 30 908 healthy individuals. Ann Epidemiol 2003;13:163–9.

9. Horiguchi J, Nakanishi T, Ito K. Quantification of coronary artery calcium using multidetector CT and a retrospective ECG-gating reconstruction algorithm. AJR Am J Roentgenol 2001;177:1429–35.

10. Becker CR, Jakobs TF, Aydemir S, et al. Helical and single-slice conventional CT versus electron beam CT

for the quantification of coronary artery calcification. AJR Am J Roentgenol 2000;174:543–7.

11. Rumberger JA, Sheedy PF, Breen JF, et al. Electron beam computed tomography and coronary artery disease: scanning for coronary artery calcification. Mayo Clin Proc 1996;71:369–77.

12. Janowitz WR, Agatston AS, Kaplan G, et al. Differences in prevalence and extent of coronary artery calcium detected by ultrafast computed tomography in asymptomatic men and women. Am J Cardiol 1993;72:247–54.

13. Hoff JA, Chomka EV, Krainik AJ, et al. Age and gender distributions of coronary artery calcium detected by electron beam tomography in 35 246 adults. Am J Cardiol 2001;87:1335–9.

14. Feuerstein IM, Brazaitis MP, Zoltick JM, et al. Electron beam computed tomography screening of the coronary arteries: experience with 3263 patients at Walter Reed Army Medical Center. Mil Med 2001;166:432–42.

15. O'Malley PG, Taylor AJ, Jackson JL, et al. Prognostic value of coronary electron-beam computed tomography for coronary heart disease events in asymptomatic populations. Am J Cardiol 2000;85:945–8.

16. Shaw LJ, Raggi P, Schisterman E, et al. Prognostic value of cardiac risk factors and coronary artery calcium screening for all-cause mortality. Radiology 2003;228:826–33.

17. Grover SA, Coupal L, Hu XP. Identifying adults at increased risk of coronary disease. How well do the current cholesterol guidelines work? JAMA 1995;274:801–6.

18. Greenland P, LaBree L, Azen SP, et al. Coronary artery calcium score combined with Framingham score for risk prediction in asymptomatic individuals. JAMA 2004;291:210–15.

19. Yao Z, Liu XJ, Shi R, et al. A comparison of ^{99m}Tc-MIBI myocardial SPET with electron beam computed tomography in the assessment of coronary artery disease. Eur J Nucl Med 1997;24:1115–20.

20. Mautner SL, Mautner GC, Froehlich J, et al. Coronary artery disease: prediction with in vitro electron beam CT [see comments]. Radiology 1994;192:625–30.

21. Bielak LF, Kaufmann RB, Moll PP, et al. Small lesions in the heart identified at electron beam CT: calcification or noise? [see comments]. Radiology 1994;192:631–6.

22. Devries S, Wolfkiel C, Fusman B, et al. Influence of age and gender on the presence of coronary calcium detected by ultrafast computed tomography. J Am Coll Cardiol 1995;25:76–82.

23. Rumberger JA, Sheedy PF, Breen JF, et al. Coronary calcium, as determined by electron beam computed tomography, and coronary disease on arteriogram. Effect of patient's sex on diagnosis [see comments]. Circulation 1995;91:1363–7.

24. Budoff MJ, Georgiou D, Brody A, et al. Ultrafast computed tomography as a diagnostic modality in the detection of coronary artery disease: a multicenter study. Circulation 1996;93:898–904.

25. Kaufmann RB, Sheedy PF, Maher JE, et al. Quantity of coronary artery calcium detected by electron beam computed tomography in asymptomatic subjects and angiographically studied patients. Mayo Clin Proc 1995;70:223–32.

26. Mohlenkamp S, Lehmann N, Schmermund A, et al. Prognostic value of extensive coronary calcium quantities in symptomatic males – a 5-year follow-up study. Eur Heart J 2003;24:845–54.

27. Mautner GC, Mautner SL, Froehlich J, et al. Coronary artery calcification: assessment with electron beam CT and histomorphometric correlation [see comments]. Radiology 1994;192:619–23.

28. Rumberger JA, Sheedy PF, Breen JF, et al. Electron beam computed tomographic coronary calcium score cutpoints and severity of associated angiographic lumen stenosis. J Am Coll Cardiol 1997;29:1542–8.

29. Kajinami K, Seki H, Takekoshi N, et al. Noninvasive prediction of coronary atherosclerosis by quantification of coronary artery calcification using electron beam computed tomography: comparison with electrocardiographic and thallium exercise stress test results. J Am Coll Cardiol 1995;26:1209–21.

30. Arad Y, Spadaro LA, Goodman K, et al. Predictive value of electron beam computed tomography of the coronary arteries. 19-month follow-up of 1173 asymptomatic subjects [see comments]. Circulation 1996;93: 1951–3.

31. Secci A, Wong N, Tang W, et al. Electron beam computed tomographic coronary calcium as a predictor of coronary events: comparison of two protocols. Circulation 1997;96:1122–9.

32. Schmermund A, Baumgart D, Gorge G, et al. Coronary artery calcium in acute coronary syndromes: a comparative study of electron-beam computed tomography, coronary angiography, and intracoronary ultrasound in survivors of acute myocardial infarction and unstable angina. Circulation 1997;96:1461–9.

33. Achenbach S, Moselewski F, Ropers D, et al. Detection of calcified and noncalcified coronary atherosclerotic plaque by contrast-enhanced, submillimeter multidetector spiral computed tomography: a segment-based comparison with intravascular ultrasound. Circulation 2004;109:14–17.

34. Schmermund A, Mohlenkamp S, Erbel R. Coronary artery calcium and its relationship to coronary artery disease. Cardiol Clin 2003;21:521–34.

5 PART 5
Management

CHAPTER 21

New developments in treatment of vulnerable plaques

Mohammad Madjid, Silvio Litovsky, James T Willerson,
& Samuel Ward Casscells

Although the pathogenesis of plaque development, progression, and complication are not identical, the risk factors for myocardial infarction, stable angina pectoris, and sudden cardiac death are similar. Therefore, the need for an individualized treatment for vulnerable plaques does not seem to be pressing. There are new data that suggest some interventions may selectively or preponderantly affect the vulnerable plaque, i.e. the plaque(s) most likely to rupture or fissure leading to a luminal thrombus. For example, the need for focal (vs. systemic) treatment becomes more urgent in acute situations, such as with the development of unstable angina or after an acute myocardial infarction when the patient is at the highest risk for another event(s) in the short term. In this situation, there is often "a cluster of vulnerable plaques," which also may undergo destabilization, leading to rupture and the risk of thrombosis and inflammation. While aspirin acts within a few hours to reduce mortality, statins do not begin to effect mortality for weeks to months, thus immediate focal therapies may be needed to stabilize the patient and "bridge" him/her until systemic therapies exert their full potential.

In this paper, we suggest that a practical approach to treatment of vulnerable plaques consists of risk factor(s) modification to prevent the formation of unstable plaques (or even regress inflammation), systemic therapeutic measures aimed at decreasing the overall burden of disease, and a change to a more benign phenotype and focal therapies in high-risk patients.

Control of risk factors

The first approach to plaque stabilization – control of classic risk factors – leads to a decrease in the toll of cardiovascular disease – albeit modestly – in most primary and secondary prevention studies by acting on hypertension,[5–7] hypercholesterolemia,[5,8–11] cigarette smoking,[12] and the use of aspirin.[13] Some of the benefit is believed to be due to a slowing of atherogenesis and some to a stabilization of vulnerable plaques.

Some patients continue to experience coronary thrombosis despite adequate control of risk factors, underscoring the need for additional therapeutic approaches. However, the fact that so many patients have yet to reach a desirable level of blood pressure, cholesterol, blood sugar, and body weight makes the traditional risk factors a good place to begin discussing the treatment of vulnerable plaques. Indeed, once vulnerable plaques can be identified, it will be important to test the hypothesis that vulnerable patients benefit from more aggressive treatment of risk factors.

Lifestyle modification

Diet and dietary supplements

Diet is an effective approach to control several risk factors both as a primary approach for control and as adjunct to drug treatments. Multiple controlled studies have shown benefits from dietary restriction of salt for control of hypertension. Dietary control is not only used as a first line therapy, but also increases the efficacy of antihypertensive therapies.[14,15] The same holds true for lipid-lowering diets for control of hyperlipidemia.[16]

Consumption of fish lowers the risk of sudden cardiac death independent of any effect on cholesterol.[17] Reducing trans fatty acids may also reduce the risk of sudden cardiac death.[18,19]

Moderate (not heavy) consumption of alcohol, especially red wine, reduces the risk of cardiovascular death.[20–22] Vitamin B supplements (i.e. folic acid, B_6 and B_{12}) can lower serum homocysteine levels, improve endothelial function, and may reduce the risk of subsequent coronary events.[23,24] Supplements of antioxidants, such as vitamin E and beta carotene, have been tried in multiple trials. However, despite a strong theoretical basis, they do not efficiently protect against infarction or sudden cardiac death, and the benefits of alpha tocopherol remains to be proved.[25–28] It is not known whether consumption of antioxidants actually leads to a reduction in the oxidative burden in atherosclerotic plaques.

The Mediterranean diet (or Indo-Mediterranean diet) has been tried in multiple clinical trails with significant success in reduction of cardiovascular mortality.[29–32] This diet, rich in olive and canola oil, wholegrain cereals, fish, and vegetables, reduces the risk of myocardial infarction (MI) and cardiac death by approximately 50%, without a major change in LDL and HDL cholesterol levels or body weight.

Smoking cessation

Smoking is one of the most important coronary artery disease (CAD) risk factors for both genders.[12] Smoking increases the risk of MI both in men and women, probably even more notably in the latter.[33] In the Nurses' Health Study, the risk of an initial MI in women who smoke increased by threefold.[34] The risk of MI decreases rapidly after smoking cessation and by 1 or 2 years, the risk of MI in ex-smokers is lowered to that of those that have never smoked.[35] This suggests that effects on coagulation factors and platelet aggregation are the main mechanisms responsible for the risk associated with smoking.

Pharmacologic therapies

Although no clear standard is yet available for diagnosing vulnerable plaques and evaluating the effect of therapies on them in vivo, potential therapies have been proposed. These therapies consist of systemic and focal approaches. For investigators who champion the idea of multiple vulnerable plaques, the most logical approach to the problem is systemic treatment aimed at plaque stabilization. However, as discussed before, in acute conditions, focal therapies may be needed to achieve more rapid stabilization of plaques.

Several pharmacologic therapies have been shown to reduce risks in randomized clinical trials.

Lipid-lowering medications

HMG CoA reductase inhibitors (statins)

The relationship between CAD and LDL cholesterol has been well documented.[36,37] The risk of coronary events increases 1% with each 2–3% increase in total serum cholesterol level.[38] Clinical trials of statins have shown that coronary mortality and morbidity are decreased with a reduction in LDL cholesterol level in both primary and secondary randomized, controlled studies (Figure 21.1).[9,39,10,40,41] Statin therapy is one of the most effective methods of plaque stabilization.[8–10,42] Statins lower the level of LDL cholesterol and increase HDL cholesterol levels. However, the non-lipid-lowering effects of statins are also an important focus of cardiovascular medicine. Numerous studies have suggested that statins affect systemic markers of immune activation and reduce plaque inflammation independent of LDL level.[43,44] These pleiotropic (non-lipid-related) effects of statins potentially broaden the original indications for these drugs.[44,45] Potential mechanisms include lipid-lowering inhibition of: (i) inflammation; (ii) smooth muscle cell activation, proliferation, and migration; and (iii) decreased collagenolytic and thrombotic activity. Emerging data suggest that effects on small G proteins may be a significant factor in the anti-inflammatory and antithrombotic actions of statins.[42,46] It is of interest that C-reactive protein (CRP), an inflammation marker that has emerged as a powerful predictor of coronary heart disease (CHD), is reduced by statins. This risk reduction parallels the decrease in CRP independent of lipid levels.[47–51] Even the rebound in adverse clinical events after statins are discontinued is independent of cholesterol levels.[52] A point often

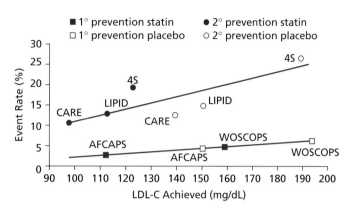

Figure 21.1 Reduction in clinical events in primary- and secondary-prevention statin trials. 4S = Scandinavian Simvastatin Survival Study; AFCAPS = Air Force/Texas Coronary Atherosclerosis Prevention Study; CARE = Cholesterol and Recurrent Events trial; LIPID = Long-term Intervention with Pravastatin in Ischaemic Disease study; WOSCOPS = West of Scotland Coronary Prevention Study. (Reprinted with permission from Ballantyne CM. Am J Cardiol 1998;82:3Q–12Q.[187])

overlooked is that reductions in mortality do not even begin until 6–12 months after statin treatment has begun. Combinations with niacin may work faster than statins alone.[53]

Other lipid-lowering medications

Before statins became widely available, small randomized trials of niacin and of fibrates each reported modest reductions in mortality.[54–56] Drugs that block intestinal fat absorption by inhibiting the cholesterol transport system located within intestinal cell walls (e.g. ezetimibe) have become available recently.[57] Ezetimibe 10 mg/day has been shown to reduce cholesterol absorption by >50%, reduce low-density lipoprotein cholesterol (LDL-C) by approximately 18%, enhance the LDL-C-lowering effect of statin medications by an additional 15–20%, and decrease CRP level.[58] Ezetimibe may be used concurrently with statins to allow for a lower statin dosage, thus avoiding statin-related complications, or used as monotherapy when statin use is poorly tolerated.[57,59]

Statins only modestly raise levels of HDL. The recent success of an HDL mimetic drug (apo A-I Milano) has increased interest in therapies for raising HDL.[60] Candidates include inhibitors of cholesteryl ester transfer protein (CETP) and nuclear orphan receptor agonists that mediate the expression of ATP-binding cassette transporter 1 (ABC1).[61] Several combination therapies have been suggested.[58,62,63]

Finally, fibrates reduce cardiovascular events more than would be predicted by their elevation of HDL and reduction of triglycerides,[64] suggesting that some of the benefit is attributable to fibrates' stimulation of PPAR alpha which not only induces

apo AI and apo AII, but also represses nuclear factor kappa B (NFκB) and thus interleukins (IL) 1 and 6, and CRP.[65]

Anti-inflammatory agents

The inflammatory nature of atherosclerosis and plaque vulnerability provides a strong basis for use of anti-inflammatory drugs in these conditions. The aspirin-related reduction in the risk of a first myocardial infarction appears to be directly related to the level of serum CRP (and its antithrombotic properties), supporting the hypothesis that anti-inflammatory agents may have clinical benefits in preventing cardiovascular disease.[66] Inflammation promotes coagulation and vice versa; therefore, an anti-inflammatory agent may have indirect antithrombotic effects and vice versa.[67] In LDL-receptor-deficient mice, aspirin reduces plaques macrophage infiltration.[68]

In the Clopidogrel in Unstable angina trial to prevent Recurrent Events (CURE), clopidogrel benefit (when added to aspirin) was greatest in those with elevated serum CRP levels and may have reflected recently described anti-inflammatory actions of clopidogrel.[69,70] Likewise, abciximab, the monoclonal anti-glycoprotein IIb IIIa, also has anti-inflammatory properties in addition to inhibiting platelet aggregation.[71] And its benefit is greatest in patients with elevated levels of the inflammatory marker CD40L.[72]

In another recent trial, in patients with an elevated CRP after stenting, prednisone improved event-free survival.[73] Also worth noting are the anti-inflammatory effect of NO[74] and the fact that low molecular weight heparin-enaxoparin inhibits neutrophil and complement activation.[75]

Given the key role of inflammation in atherosclerosis, it is no surprise that more effective and specific anti-inflammatory agents are being sought. The complex control of inflammatory processes opens numerous possibilities. Potential candidates include blockers of monocyte chemoattractant peptide 1 (MCP-1), CD 40 and its ligand, intercellular adhesion molecule 1 (ICAM-1), vascular cell adhesion molecule 1 (VCAM-1), IL-1, IL-6, multiple matrix metalloproteinase (MMP), CRP, and, in particular, NFκB, whose activation is one of the most important molecular controls of the inflammatory process.[76] Inhibitors of tumor necrosis factor alpha (TNF-α) have been used in patients with heart failure, but they produced a nonsignificant, but unexpected, increase in cardiovascular mortality.[77] It should be remembered, however, that heart failure has different mechanisms and follows a different course than that of atherosclerosis. A pilot clinical trial of an inhibitor of TNF-α in unstable angina is currently under way.

Angiotensin-converting enzyme (ACE) inhibitors

Numerous studies have suggested pleiotropic roles, including anti-oxidation, for ACE inhibitors in both cardiac and vascular systems.[74,78] ACE is expressed in culprit atherosclerotic human coronary plaques.[79,80] A strong co-localization of IL-6 and angiotensin II (ANGII) has been found at the shoulder region of plaques.[81] Moreover, there are several reports of inflammatory actions of ANGII, and of anti-inflammatory effects of ACE inhibitors and ANGII receptor antagonists.[82,83]

Large scale clinical trials reported that administration of ACE inhibitors after MI, or in patients with documented coronary artery disease (CAD), reduced not only the cumulative incidence of heart failure, but also the incidence of cardiovascular events, such as stroke, unstable angina, and MIs. Moreover, the HOPE study revealed that the ACE inhibitor ramipril reduces the rates of death, MI, and stroke in high-risk patients without low ejection fraction, hypertension, or heart failure.[28] Recent findings of the EUROPA study demonstrate a significantly improved outcome in patients with stable coronary heart disease, without apparent heart failure, who use perindopril.[84] The ACE genotype DD, which is associated with high circulating levels of ACE, was more frequent in patients with a prior history of MI than in control subjects.[85] Potential mechanisms for the effect of ACE inhibitors on plaque stabilization include a reduction in arterial wall stress caused by lower blood pressure, anti-inflammatory, anti-oxidant and growth-inhibiting effects, and reduced levels of neurohumoral activation.[86,87]

Beta-adrenergic blockers

These drugs were shown several decades ago to reduce mortality after MI. Some of this effect may be due to treatment of coexisting hypertension, heart failure, or arrhythmia.[88] Beta-adrenergic blockade reduces blood pressure, cardiac contractility, vulnerability to arrhythmias of ischemic origin, and increases diastolic filling time. It also reduces the risks of reinfarction and mortality in congestive heart failure. The mechanism by which beta blockers reduce the risk of infarction is not clear, but may in part relate to the reduced number of heartbeats and the reduced rate of pressure rise in the coronary arteries.[89]

Control of hyperglycemia

Diabetes is a major risk factor for acute coronary syndromes. Diabetic patients have a two- to sixfold increased risk of CAD.[90,91] The exact mechanism by which diabetes exerts its deleterious effect is not completely understood. Glycosylation of multiple proteins may be partially responsible for the risk. A deficiency in body insulin increases blood glucose levels and risk of CAD, and a high insulin level is associated with increased risk of CAD as well.[92–94] There is a suggested U-shaped risk relation between insulin level and CAD. Diabetes is associated with increased macrophage infiltration, lipid volume, and thrombi in atherosclerotic plaques.[95]

By 2010, the number of people with type 2 diabetes is expected to double (over 1990) and it is estimated that this, in conjunction with the rise in obesity and smoking in young women, may counteract the reduction in CAD achieved by control of other risk factors.[96,97] Despite the fact that the mortality rate of patients from CAD without type 2 diabetes has declined in the past 20 years, the mortality of men with type 2 diabetes has not changed, and in women it appears to have increased.

The Diabetes Control and Complications Trial (DCCT)[98] and the smaller Stockholm Diabetes Intervention Study[99] showed unequivocally that in type 1 diabetes, lowering blood glucose delays the onset and slows the progression of microvascular complications. But better control of glucose did not decrease the risk of fatal CAD in these patients. Many observational studies have shown a correlation between glycemic control and diabetic complications in patients with type 2 diabetes. Three randomized controlled trials have addressed the benefit of lowering blood glucose on the incidence of complications. The small (200 subjects) University Group Diabetes Program (UGDP) showed no benefit of glycemic control in new-onset type 2 diabetic patients. The second small controlled trial in type 2 diabetes was conducted in 110 lean Japanese subjects and showed that multiple insulin injections resulting in better glycemic control significantly reduced the microvascular complications of diabetes.[100] The third trial in type 2 diabetic patients randomized 153 men to intensive or conventional therapy and failed to show a significant difference in cardiovascular events in a 27-month follow-up.[101] The United Kingdom Prospective Diabetes Study (UKPDS) is the largest and longest study on type 2 diabetic patients to date. UKPDS recruited 5102 patients with newly diagnosed type 2 diabetes in 23 centers within the UK between 1977 and 1991 and followed them for an average of 10 years. UKPDS showed that good diabetic control decreases the risk of microvascular complications, but fails to prevent cardiovascular events.[102] However, aggressive control of other risk factors (e.g. hyperlipidemia, hypertension, and prothrombotic state) in these patients reduces their CAD risk, emphasizing the need for focus on preventive measures in these patients.[103,104] Metformin is one drug which has been shown to reduce the risk of MI in diabetic patients.[105]

The metabolic stage between normal glucose levels and diabetes is known as impaired glucose tolerance (IGT) and is defined as a fasting blood glucose level between 110 and 126 mg/dl. There is a continuous association between the risk of cardiovascular complications and glycemia which follows a J curve.[106,107] Recent clinical trials have shown a significant benefit from use of acarbose in patients with impaired glucose tolerance.[106] Acarbose, an alpha-glucosidase inhibitor, which delays postprandial hyperglycemia, reduces the risk of overt clinical MI and silent MI in patients with impaired glucose tolerance.

Peroxisome proliferator-activated receptor (PPAR) agonists

PPARs are nuclear receptors reported to play a role in atherosclerosis and inflammation, including regulation of lipid metabolism, glucose homeostasis, and cellular differentiation.[108–110] PPAR agonists modulate recruitment and adhesion of leukocytes and monocytes to atherosclerotic plaques and display prominent anti-inflammatory effects. Macrophage lipid homeostasis is influenced by the action of PPAR agonists on the scavenger receptor and the reverse cholesterol transport pathway. Genes that control thrombogenicity are also favorably affected by these agents. Their importance to the cardiovascular complications of diabetes is highlighted by the fact that the synthetic antidiabetic thiazolidinediones (TZDs) are ligands for PPAR gamma.[109] Thus, there is considerable interest in PPAR gamma agonists like pioglitazone for CAD patients without frank diabetes, especially those with insulin resistance and/or elevated inflammatory markers.

Emerging pharmacologic therapies

Several classes of experimental drugs have shown great therapeutic potential for treatment of vulnerable plaque.

Reverse cholesterol transport agents

HDL/apolipoprotein A-I Milano

In cholesterol-fed rabbits, administration of homologous HDL very high density lipoprotein (VHDL) fraction dramatically inhibited the extent of aortic fatty streaks and reduced lipid deposition in the arterial wall and liver without modifying plasma lipid levels.[111] HDL plasma fractions also induced the regression of established aortic fatty streaks and lipid deposits.[112]

Apolipoprotein (apo) A-I Milano is a mutant form of human apoA-I, which results from arginine 173 to cysteine substitution. This structural modification is associated with a high affinity of apoA-I Milano for lipids in lipid–protein complexes, and results in their easy removal. Antiplatelet and antioxidant effects have also been suggested.[113,114] Recombinant A-I Milano/phospholipid complex (A-I Milano/PC) prevented the progression of aortic atherosclerosis and reduced the lipid and macrophage content of plaques in the short term.[27,115] A single direct infusion of recombinant apoA-I Milano into localized carotid atheromatous plaques in the rabbit rapidly reduced the plaque area and lipid content.[116–120] Nissen et al. recently reported a significant regression of coronary atherosclerosis – measured by IVUS – following intravenous administration of recombinant apoA-I Milano/phospholipid complex (ETC-216) in 123 patients.[60]

In addition to apolipoproteins, lipids associated with HDL display certain anti-atherogenic properties. For example, lysosphingolipids, such as sphingosine-1-phosphate and sphingosine-phosphorylcholine, were reported to counteract endothelial dysfunction and apoptosis.[121]

Navab and associates have recently developed a stable oral form of apoA-I mimetic peptides (D-4F) which has been shown to decrease the lesions by 79% in LDL receptor-null mice on a Western diet and in apoE-null mice.[122] Transfer of the apolipoprotein A-I gene to induce regression of atherosclerosis is currently under investigation.[118,119,120,123]

Reverse cholesterol transport modulators

The apparent protective effect of HDL with respect to CHD is thought to be a function of its anti-inflammatory effects and its ability to transport cholesterol from peripheral cells to the liver for excretion from the body. The membrane proteins, scavenger receptor class B, type 1 (SR-B1), and the ATP-binding cassette 1 (ABC1), have been strongly implicated in cholesterol efflux. Lecithin cholesterol acyltransferase (LCAT) esterifies the effluxed cholesterol to form cholesteryl esters, which are then transferred to apoB-containing lipoproteins by cholesteryl ester transfer protein (CETP).[124,125] Drugs that affect these components are under investigation with respect to their potential effect on atherosclerosis and plaque stability.[126]

Inhibition of neovascularization

The atherosclerotic plaque and the underlying vessel wall are highly vascularized tissues. It has been proposed that inhibition of neovacularization could contribute to plaque stabilization. Moulton et al.[127] used the recombinant murine angiogenesis inhibitors, endostatin and TNP-470 in apolipoprotein E-deficient (apoE[−/−]) mice and demonstrated a marked decrease in plaque progression despite no changes in serum cholesterol levels.

Antimicrobial therapy

A role for infections in atherosclerosis has been suggested since the early 20th century.[128] In the past two decades, there has been renewed interest in the role of infection in the pathogenesis of atherosclerosis and in the potential role of antibiotics in the prevention and control of the disease. Several agents have been implicated in the disease process, namely, *Chlamydia pneumoniae*, herpes simplex viruses, *Helicobacter pylori*, *Porphyria gingivalis*, and influenza.[129–133] Despite early encouraging results from preliminary small clinical trials, subsequent large-scale, randomized trials of antibiotics for *Chlamydia pneumoniae* have thus far failed to reduce the incidence of MI or cardiac death.[134–137]

Vaccination

Upper respiratory infections may trigger heart attacks and actually precede approximately one-third of acute MIs.[138] Influenza vaccination has been reported to reduce the risk of secondary MI in patients with chronic coronary disease by 66%, while other groups have reported a 50% reduction in the risk of sudden cardiac death, and similar reduction in the risk of stroke.[131,139–141] A small randomized trial has shown significant reduction in cardiovascular death and risk of stroke in acute MI patients and in patients undergoing percutaneous interventions.[142] A recent large, community cohort study showed a 19% decrease in risk of hospitalization for reasons due to cardiovascular disease in elderly subjects (Figure 21.2).[143]

Specific vaccination against atherosclerosis

Several antigens have been suggested to trigger the immune response in atherosclerosis. These include oxidized LDL, heat shock proteins, β_2 glycoprotein, and several microbial agents, including *C. pneumoniae*, CMV, HSV, and *H. pylori*. Oxidized LDL is a prime candidate, in part because it combines the

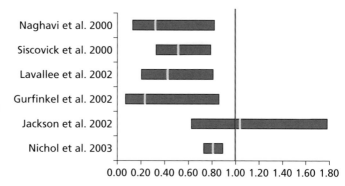

Figure 21.2 Studies of influenza vaccination and cardiovascular outcomes 95% confidence interval of each study's primary cardiovascular outcome. (Madjid M. et al., Texas Heart Inst J 2004;31:4–13. Copyright 2004, Texas Heart Institute.[188])

lipid and inflammatory hypothesis. Evidence for immunogenicity of oxidized LDL is overwhelming and includes high titers of autoantibodies in patients with severe atherosclerosis, activation of T-cells from human atherosclerotic plaques by oxidized LDL, amelioration of disease burden on immunization with oxLDL in the experimental animal.[20–22,144–146] The most likely mechanism for the deleterious effect of oxidized LDL involves the production of reactive aldehydes, which are products of LDL oxidation and form covalent adducts with portions of apoB, becoming targets for the immune system, which can lead to cell damage and inflammation.[147,148]

Several groups have reported that immunizing mice with either homologous or MDA-modified LDL has consistently shown that these compounds reduce atherosclerosis.

Fredrikson et al. (joint effort from UCLA and University of Lund, Drs Shah's and Nilsson's labs, respectively) have devised a strategy of inoculating apoE-deficient mice with peptide sequences (with high degree of homology) with apo B-100, the main protein component of LDL. One of their peptides was able, in spite of even greater hypercholesterolemia, to have a very atheroprotective immune response. This was associated with decrease in plaque burden and inflammation, and an increase in plaque collagen.[149] Other approaches that have been tried include immunization by mucosal administration of heat shock protein-65 in low density lipoprotein receptor-deficient mice.[150]

In summary, although still experimental, there is a significant body of evidence in animal models that the atherosclerotic process could be reduced in terms of total plaque burden and its phenotype rendered less vulnerable by selected immunogens.

Prevention of thrombosis

Antithrombotic therapy has been used for primary prevention most often in patients admitted with acute coronary syndromes. Aspirin is a mainstay in the treatment of coronary artery disease.[13,151] Since aspirin reduces the risk of MI and death by 20–30%, it was proposed to combine aspirin with other antiplatelet agents, such as ticlopidine or clopidogrel. Adding clopidogrel to aspirin reduced the incidence of MI in patients with unstable angina.[152] Clopidogrel also shows greater protective efficacy than aspirin when used alone.[153]

In patients with cardiovascular risk factors without MI or angina, warfarin (alone or combined with aspirin therapy) reduces the event rate compared to aspirin alone.[154,155] Several large trials in patients with acute coronary syndrome have shown an important beneficial effect of coumadin in combination with aspirin.[156,157] It has been proposed to add a third antithrombotic in these conditions because of the low rate of hemorrhagic complications when the INR is kept below 3 (proposed agents are clopidogrel and novel agents, such as thrombin inhibitors, tissue factor inhibitors, and GP1b). Patients at high risk of thrombosis (e.g. high D-dimer, polymorphisms of genes predisposing to thrombosis) could be candidates for this aggressive approach.[158,159] As discussed earlier, aspirin, clopidogrel, and heparins also have a variety of anti-inflammatory effects (beyond that due to preventing thrombosis and thereby preventing infiltration of the thrombus).

Emerging local therapies

Drug-eluting stents

Probably no field has revolutionized the practice

of cardiology as much as coronary stenting. Improvements in polymer science and localized drug delivery have contributed to the development of stents coated with antiproliferative drugs (such as the anti-inflammatory agent sirolimus, and the antimitotic agent paclitaxel), which can potentially abolish in-stent restenosis. The large number of publications and trials, however, have evaluated success as a marked reduction of stenosis and low rate of restenosis. Only lately, have some authors wondered whether it would be advantageous to stent lesions that are not significantly stenotic, but have variables suggestive of vulnerability, such as high temperature, thin fibrous cap on optical coherence tomography (OCT) or ultrasound, large lipid core in a proximal vessel on MRI or ultrasound, remodeling, etc.

Articles involving studies of drug-eluting stents have only dealt with stenotic lesions, as the underlying plaques' composition are largely unknown.

Liistro et al.[160] performed the first clinical study of a paclitaxel-eluting stent (7-hexanoyltaxol (QP2)-eluting polymer stent system (QuaDS)) on 15 patients. Good short-term results were shown, but restenosis in 8 of 13 patients was seen at 12 months.

The TAXUS I trial[161] used the TAXUS NIRx stent compared with bare stents in 61 patients with de novo or restenotic lesions. It showed a marked reduction in major adverse cardiac events (MACE) and restenosis in patients with the drug-eluting stents, compared with the bare stent group. The randomized, controlled, blinded ELUTES trial (European evaluation of PacliTaxel-Eluting Stent) studied 192 patients and showed that the positive results obtained at 6 months were largely maintained by 12 months.[162]

Preliminary results from ASian Paclitaxel-Eluting Stent Clinical Trial (ASPECT) of 177 patients at 6 months showed a significant reduction in MACE and restenosis by intravascular ultrasound.[163] Moreover, the authors also observed a stepwise reduction in intimal hyperplasia with increasing doses.

The TAXUS III trial was designed to study the feasibility and safety of a paclitaxel-eluting stent (TAXUS NIRx) for treatment of in-stent restenosis (a difficult complication to treat). Although one patient in 28 developed late total occlusion, and three showed angiographic restenosis, the authors

believed the results were promising because of the severity of the underlying condition.[164]

RAVEL (Randomized Study with the Sirolimus-Coated Bx Velocity Balloon-Expandable Stent in the Treatment of Patients with De Novo Native Coronary Artery Lesions) showed absence of restenosis at 6 months and of target-lesion revascularization at 1 year after the implantation of sirolimus-eluting stents in a multicenter randomized trial.[165] Of great importance, the efficacy and safety of sirolimus-eluting stents persisted 2 years after implantation in humans with essentially unchanged in-stent luminal dimensions.[166]

Antiproliferating drugs administered orally following stent implantation are a potential therapy for preventing restenosis. Farb et al. used oral everolimus (related to sirolimus) to successfully inhibit in-stent neointimal growth in the iliac arteries of rabbits.[167] Stenting has also been used to deliver controlled gene therapy, such as anti-sense c-Myc oligonucleotides, to prevent restenosis (see below).[168]

Gene therapy

Theoretically, gene therapy could stabilize a vulnerable plaque by reducing its lipid and macrophage content (e.g. ABCA1 gene). Alternatively, by introducing genes that encode for thrombolytic proteins, the physiologic antithrombotic functions of endothelial cells into the plaque, one might be able to inhibit thrombus formation should plaque rupture occur. Alternative approaches may be represented by transfecting the arterial wall with the genes for NO synthase or prostaglandin H (PGH) synthase (to overexpress prostacyclin) or natural inhibitors of tissue factor:factor VIIa complex, such as tissue factor pathway inhibitor (TFPI), which may result in complete inhibition of local thrombosis without incurring potentially harmful systemic effects.[169] Although many technical challenges lie ahead (especially gene delivery and regulation), recent developments indicate that these goals may be reachable in the not too distant future.[170,171] Intrapericardial gene or drug delivery can potentially provide a comprehensive solution for treatment of vulnerable coronary arteries (pan-arterial approach). However, the available techniques for pericardial drug delivery are not suitable to maintain long term effects.[172,173]

Photodynamic therapy

Photodynamic therapy (PDT) is being evaluated for the treatment of atherosclerosis and prevention of restenosis.[174] The ability of PDT to destroy target tissues selectively is especially appealing for treating vulnerable plaques. The agent most commonly used is motexafin lutetium (MLu, Antrin), an expanded porphyrin (texaphyrin) that accumulates in plaques. The combination of the motexafin lutetium and endovascular illumination, or Antrin phototherapy, has been shown to reduce plaque volume in animal models, probably by inducing apoptosis in macrophages and smooth muscle cells.[175] However, chemical destruction of vulnerable plaques with optical firing of photodynamic agents that produce cytotoxic singlet oxygen raises the concerns of future restenosis. Intracoronary stent implantation has been suggested in conjunction with photodynamic therapy.[176]

Thermal stabilization

Gentle local heating of plaques (up to 43°C for 15 minutes) has been shown in ex vivo and animal studies to reduce macrophages density by inducing apoptosis and downregulation of inflammatory genes.[177] Cooling vulnerable plaques has also been suggested as an alternative for plaque stabilization. The value of thermal therapy for vulnerable plaques in coronary arteries remains to be further investigated.

Other new interventions

Patented new therapies include brachytherapy, local chemical treatments (e.g. to dissolve lipids with drugs such as diethylether or dissolve calcium by means of lowering pH), and inhibition of matrix metalloproteinases (MMPs).[175,178,179] A particularly exciting potential treatment is the use of the patient's own bone marrow stem cells – several types of which can give rise to endothelial cells – to restore a healthy anti-thrombotic, anti-inflammatory, vasodilating endothelium.[180–182]

Finally, it can be speculated that future therapies will be guided by the patient's genotype or even by a genomic and proteomic analysis of the atherectomized plaque. In the Framingham Heart Study, individuals with the common *ESR1 c.454−397CC* genotype have a substantial increase in risk of MI.[183]

An example of the potential is seen in a study in which women with the *ER-alpha IVS1−401 C/C* genotype had greater reductions in E-selectin but no further increases in CRP with hormone replacement therapy.[184] Also, in the Estrogen Replacement and Atherosclerosis trial, postmenopausal women with coronary disease who have the *ER-alpha IVS1−401 C/C* genotype, or several other closely related genotypes, showed an augmented response of HDL cholesterol to hormone-replacement therapy.[185,186]

Conclusions

The underlying mechanism of atherosclerosis is under heavy investigation. Better knowledge of the disease can lead to development of more efficient methods to prevent and control it. Given the multifactorial nature of atherosclerotic disease, a comprehensive approach including control of risk factors and specific lipid-lowering, anti-inflammatory, antioxidant, and anti-thrombotic treatments can considerably reduce the risk of fatal and nonfatal outcomes. The development of new imaging techniques will allow locating individual vulnerable plaques, hence enabling physicians to direct local therapy to foci of highest risk. Focal therapy may "buy time" to rapidly reduce the risk of acute coronary syndromes until systemic therapies begin to exert their protective effects.

Acknowledgment

Supported in part by DOD Grant #DAMD 17-01-2-0047.

References

1. American Heart Association. 2002 Heart and Stroke Statistical Update. Dallas, TX: American Heart Association, 2002.
2. Yusuf S, Reddy S, Ounpuu S, Anand S. Global burden of cardiovascular diseases: part I: general considerations, the epidemiologic transition, risk factors, and impact of urbanization. Circulation 2001;104:2746–53.
3. Zipes DP, Wellens HJ. Sudden cardiac death. Circulation 1998;98:2334–51.
4. Ambrose JA, Tannenbaum MA, Alexopoulos D, et al. Angiographic progression of coronary artery disease and the development of myocardial infarction. J Am Coll Cardiol 1988;12:56–62.

5. Major outcomes in moderately hypercholesterolemic, hypertensive patients randomized to pravastatin vs usual care: The Antihypertensive and Lipid-Lowering Treatment to Prevent Heart Attack Trial (ALLHAT-LLT). JAMA 2002;288:2998–3007.

6. Messerli FH, Grossman E. Beta-blockers and diuretics: to use or not to use. Am J Hypertens 1999;12:157S–63S.

7. Chobanian AV, Bakris GL, Black HR, et al. The Seventh Report of the Joint National Committee on Prevention, Detection, Evaluation, and Treatment of High Blood Pressure: the JNC 7 report. JAMA 2003;289:2560–72.

8. Sacks FM, Pfeffer MA, Moye LA, et al. The effect of pravastatin on coronary events after myocardial infarction in patients with average cholesterol levels. Cholesterol and Recurrent Events Trial investigators. N Engl J Med 1996;335:1001–9.

9. Randomised trial of cholesterol lowering in 4444 patients with coronary heart disease: the Scandinavian Simvastatin Survival Study (4S). Lancet 1994;344: 1383–9.

10. Prevention of cardiovascular events and death with pravastatin in patients with coronary heart disease and a broad range of initial cholesterol levels. The Long-Term Intervention with Pravastatin in Ischaemic Disease (LIPID) Study Group. N Engl J Med 1998;339: 1349–57.

11. Downs JR, Clearfield M, Weis S, et al. Primary prevention of acute coronary events with lovastatin in men and women with average cholesterol levels: results of AFCAPS/TexCAPS. Air Force/Texas Coronary Atherosclerosis Prevention Study. JAMA 1998;279:1615–22.

12. Kuller LH, Ockene JK, Meilahn E, Wentworth DN, Svendsen KH, Neaton JD. Cigarette smoking and mortality. MRFIT Research Group. Prev Med 1991;20: 638–54.

13. Moncada S, Palmer RM, Higgs EA. Biosynthesis of nitric oxide from l-arginine. A pathway for the regulation of cell function and communication. Biochem Pharmacol 1989;38:1709–15.

14. Suter PM, Sierro C, Vetter W. Nutritional factors in the control of blood pressure and hypertension. Nutr Clin Care 2002;5:9–19.

15. Appel LJ, Moore TJ, Obarzanek E, et al. A clinical trial of the effects of dietary patterns on blood pressure. DASH Collaborative Research Group. N Engl J Med 1997;336:1117–24.

16. Executive Summary of The Third Report of The National Cholesterol Education Program (NCEP) Expert Panel on Detection, Evaluation, and Treatment of High Blood Cholesterol in Adults (Adult Treatment Panel III). JAMA 2001;285:2486–97.

17. Hu FB, Willett WC. Optimal diets for prevention of coronary heart disease. JAMA 2002;288:2569–78.

18. Siscovick DS, Lemaitre RN, Mozaffarian D. The fish story: a diet-heart hypothesis with clinical implications: n-3 polyunsaturated fatty acids, myocardial vulnerability, and sudden death. Circulation 2003;107:2632–4.

19. Perez-Jimenez F, Lopez-Miranda J, Mata P. Protective effect of dietary monounsaturated fat on arteriosclerosis: beyond cholesterol. Atherosclerosis 2002;163: 385–98.

20. Rimm EB, Giovannucci EL, Willett WC, et al. Prospective study of alcohol consumption and risk of coronary disease in men. Lancet 1991;338:464–8.

21. Rimm EB, Williams P, Fosher K, Criqui M, Stampfer MJ. Moderate alcohol intake and lower risk of coronary heart disease: meta-analysis of effects on lipids and haemostatic factors. BMJ 1999;319:1523–8.

22. Mukamal KJ, Conigrave KM, Mittleman MA, et al. Roles of drinking pattern and type of alcohol consumed in coronary heart disease in men. N Engl J Med 2003;348:109–18.

23. Selhub J, Jacques PF, Bostom AG, et al. Association between plasma homocysteine concentrations and extracranial carotid-artery stenosis. N Engl J Med 1995;332:286–91.

24. Jacques PF, Selhub J, Bostom AG, Wilson PW, Rosenberg IH. The effect of folic acid fortification on plasma folate and total homocysteine concentrations. N Engl J Med 1999;340:1449–54.

25. Moss AJ, Zareba W, Hall WJ, et al. Prophylactic implantation of a defibrillator in patients with myocardial infarction and reduced ejection fraction. N Engl J Med 2002;346:877–83.

26. MRC/BHF Heart Protection Study of antioxidant vitamin supplementation in 20,536 high-risk individuals: a randomised placebo-controlled trial. Lancet 2002;360: 23–33.

27. Shah PK, Yano J, Reyes O, et al. High-dose recombinant apolipoprotein A-I(milano) mobilizes tissue cholesterol and rapidly reduces plaque lipid and macrophage content in apolipoprotein e-deficient mice. Potential implications for acute plaque stabilization. Circulation 2001;103:3047–50.

28. Yusuf S, Sleight P, Pogue J, Bosch J, Davies R, Dagenais G. Effects of an angiotensin-converting-enzyme inhibitor, ramipril, on cardiovascular events in high-risk patients. The Heart Outcomes Prevention Evaluation Study Investigators. N Engl J Med 2000;342:145–53.

29. de Lorgeril M, Renaud S, Mamelle N, et al. Mediterranean alpha-linolenic acid-rich diet in secondary prevention of coronary heart disease. Lancet 1994;343: 1454–9.

30. de Lorgeril M, Salen P, Martin JL, Monjaud I, Delaye J, Mamelle N. Mediterranean diet, traditional risk factors, and the rate of cardiovascular complications after

myocardial infarction: final report of the Lyon Diet Heart Study. Circulation 1999;99:779–85.

31. Singh RB, Rastogi SS, Verma R, et al. Randomised controlled trial of cardioprotective diet in patients with recent acute myocardial infarction: results of one year follow up. Bmj 1992;304:1015–19.

32. Singh RB, Dubnov G, Niaz MA, et al. Effect of an Indo-Mediterranean diet on progression of coronary artery disease in high risk patients (Indo-Mediterranean Diet Heart Study): a randomised single-blind trial. Lancet 2002;360:1455–61.

33. Hansen EF, Andersen LT, Von Eyben FE. Cigarette smoking and age at first acute myocardial infarction, and influence of gender and extent of smoking. Am J Cardiol 1993;71:1439–42.

34. Willett WC, Green A, Stampfer MJ, et al. Relative and absolute excess risks of coronary heart disease among women who smoke cigarettes. N Engl J Med 1987; 317:1303–9.

35. Hermanson B, Omenn GS, Kronmal RA, Gersh BJ. Beneficial six-year outcome of smoking cessation in older men and women with coronary artery disease. Results from the CASS registry. N Engl J Med 1988;319:1365–9.

36. Jacobs D, Blackburn H, Higgins M, et al. Report of the Conference on Low Blood Cholesterol: Mortality Associations. Circulation 1992;86:1046–60.

37. Chen Z, Peto R, Collins R, MacMahon S, Lu J, Li W. Serum cholesterol concentration and coronary heart disease in population with low cholesterol concentrations. Br Med J 1991;303:276–82.

38. Superko HR, Krauss RM. Coronary artery disease regression. Convincing evidence for the benefit of aggressive lipoprotein management. Circulation 1994;90:1056–69.

39. West of Scotland Coronary Prevention Study: identification of high-risk groups and comparison with other cardiovascular intervention trials. Lancet 1996;348: 1339–42.

40. Lewis SJ, Moye LA, Sacks FM, et al. Effect of pravastatin on cardiovascular events in older patients with myocardial infarction and cholesterol levels in the average range. Results of the Cholesterol and Recurrent Events (CARE) trial. Ann Intern Med 1998;129:681–9.

41. Goldberg RB, Mellies MJ, Sacks FM, et al. Cardiovascular events and their reduction with pravastatin in diabetic and glucose-intolerant myocardial infarction survivors with average cholesterol levels: subgroup analyses in the cholesterol and recurrent events (CARE) trial. The Care Investigators. Circulation 1998;98: 2513–19.

42. Libby P, Aikawa M. Mechanisms of plaque stabilization with statins. Am J Cardiol 2003;91:4B–8B.

43. Pitsavos CE, Aggeli KI, Barbetseas JD, et al. Effects of pravastatin on thoracic aortic atherosclerosis in patients with heterozygous familial hypercholesterolemia. Am J Cardiol 1998;82:1484–8.

44. Rosenson RS. Non-lipid-lowering effects of statins on atherosclerosis. Curr Cardiol Rep 1999;1:225–32.

45. Libby P, Ridker PM, Maseri A. Inflammation and atherosclerosis. Circulation 2002;105:1135–43.

46. Veillard NR, Mach F. Statins: the new aspirin? Cell Mol Life Sci 2002;59:1771–86.

47. Albert MA, Danielson E, Rifai N, Ridker PM. Effect of statin therapy on C-reactive protein levels: the pravastatin inflammation/CRP evaluation (PRINCE): a randomized trial and cohort study. JAMA 2001;286: 64–70.

48. Ridker PM, Rifai N, Clearfield M, et al. Measurement of C-reactive protein for the targeting of statin therapy in the primary prevention of acute coronary events. N Engl J Med 2001;344:1959–65.

49. Ridker PM. Should statin therapy be considered for patients with elevated C-reactive protein? The need for a definitive clinical trial. Eur Heart J 2001;22:2135–7.

50. Bermudez EA, Ridker PM. C-reactive protein, statins, and the primary prevention of atherosclerotic cardiovascular disease. Prev Cardiol 2002;5:42–6.

51. Takeda T, Hoshida S, Nishino M, Tanouchi J, Otsu K, Hori M. Relationship between effects of statins, aspirin and angiotensin II modulators on high-sensitive C-reactive protein levels. Atherosclerosis 2003;169:155–8.

52. Heeschen C, Hamm CW, Laufs U, Snapinn S, Bohm M, White HD. Withdrawal of statins increases event rates in patients with acute coronary syndromes. Circulation 2002;105:1446–52.

53. Schwartz GG, Olsson AG, Ezekowitz MD, et al. Effects of atorvastatin on early recurrent ischemic events in acute coronary syndromes: the MIRACL study: a randomized controlled trial. JAMA 2001;285:1711–18.

54. Canner PL, Berge KG, Wenger NK, et al. Fifteen year mortality in Coronary Drug Project patients: long-term benefit with niacin. J Am Coll Cardiol 1986;8:1245–55.

55. McKenney JM, Proctor JD, Harris S, Chinchili VM. A comparison of the efficacy and toxic effects of sustained- vs immediate-release niacin in hypercholesterolemic patients. JAMA 1994;271:672–7.

56. Carlson LA, Rosenhamer G. Reduction of mortality in the Stockholm Ischaemic Heart Disease Secondary Prevention Study by combined treatment with clofibrate and nicotinic acid. Acta Med Scand 1988;223: 405–18.

57. Bruckert E, Giral P, Tellier P. Perspectives in cholesterol-lowering therapy: the role of ezetimibe, a new selective inhibitor of intestinal cholesterol absorption. Circulation 2003;107:3124–8.

58. Ballantyne CM, Houri J, Notarbartolo A, et al. Effect of ezetimibe coadministered with atorvastatin in 628 patients with primary hypercholesterolemia: a prospective, randomized, double-blind trial. Circulation 2003;107:2409–15.

59. Sudhop T, Lutjohann D, Kodal A, et al. Inhibition of intestinal cholesterol absorption by ezetimibe in humans. Circulation 2002;106:1943–8.

60. Nissen SE, Tsunoda T, Tuzcu EM, et al. Effect of recombinant ApoA-I Milano on coronary atherosclerosis in patients with acute coronary syndromes: a randomized controlled trial. JAMA 2003;290:2292–300.

61. Barter PJ, Brewer HB, Jr, Chapman MJ, Hennekens CH, Rader DJ, Tall AR. Cholesteryl ester transfer protein: a novel target for raising HDL and inhibiting atherosclerosis. Arterioscler Thromb Vasc Biol 2003; 23:160–7.

62. Kastelein J. What future for combination therapies? Int J Clin Pract Suppl 2003:45–50.

63. Davidson MH. Niacin: a powerful adjunct to other lipid-lowering drugs in reducing plaque progression and acute coronary events. Curr Atheroscler Rep 2003; 5:418–22.

64. Rubins HB, Robins SJ, Collins D, et al. Gemfibrozil for the secondary prevention of coronary heart disease in men with low levels of high-density lipoprotein cholesterol. Veterans Affairs High-Density Lipoprotein Cholesterol Intervention Trial Study Group. N Engl J Med 1999;341:410–18.

65. Kleemann R, Gervois PP, Verschuren L, Staels B, Princen HM, Kooistra T. Fibrates down-regulate IL-1-stimulated C-reactive protein gene expression in hepatocytes by reducing nuclear p50-NFkappa B-C/EBP-beta complex formation. Blood 2003;101:545–51.

66. Blake GJ, Ridker PM. C-reactive protein and other inflammatory risk markers in acute coronary syndromes. J Am Coll Cardiol 2003;41:37S–42S.

67. Libby P, Simon DI. Inflammation and thrombosis: the clot thickens. Circulation 2001;103:1718–20.

68. Cyrus T, Sung S, Zhao L, Funk CD, Tang S, Pratico D. Effect of low-dose aspirin on vascular inflammation, plaque stability, and atherogenesis in low-density lipoprotein receptor-deficient mice. Circulation 2002; 106:1282–7.

69. Chew DP, Bhatt DL, Robbins MA, et al. Effect of clopidogrel added to aspirin before percutaneous coronary intervention on the risk associated with C-reactive protein. Am J Cardiol 2001;88:672–4.

70. Quinn MJ, Fitzgerald DJ. Ticlopidine and clopidogrel. Circulation 1999;100:1667–72.

71. Lincoff AM, Kereiakes DJ, Mascelli MA, et al. Abciximab suppresses the rise in levels of circulating inflammatory markers after percutaneous coronary revascularization. Circulation 2001;104:163–7.

72. Heeschen C, Dimmeler S, Hamm CW, et al. Soluble CD40 ligand in acute coronary syndromes. N Engl J Med 2003;348:1104–11.

73. Versaci F, Gaspardone A, Tomai F, et al. Immuno-suppressive therapy for the prevention of restenosis after coronary artery stent implantation (IMPRESS Study). J Am Coll Cardiol 2002;40:1935–42.

74. Granger DN, Kubes P. Nitric oxide as antiinflammatory agent. Methods Enzymol 1996;269:434–42.

75. Gikakis N, Khan MM, Hiramatsu Y, et al. Effect of factor Xa inhibitors on thrombin formation and complement and neutrophil activation during in vitro extracorporeal circulation. Circulation 1996;94:II341–6.

76. Valen G, Yan ZQ, Hansson GK. Nuclear factor kappa-B and the heart. J Am Coll Cardiol 2001;38:307–14.

77. Anker SD, Coats AJ. How to RECOVER from RENAIS-SANCE? The significance of the results of RECOVER, RENAISSANCE, RENEWAL and ATTACH. Int J Cardiol 2002;86:123–30.

78. Gibbons GH. Vasculoprotective and cardioprotective mechanisms of angiotensin-converting enzyme inhibition: the homeostatic balance between angiotensin II and nitric oxide. Clin Cardiol 1997;20:II-18–25.

79. Diet F, Pratt R, Berry G, Momose N, Gibbons G, Dzau V. Increased accumulation of tissue ACE in human atherosclerotic coronary artery disease. Circulation 1996;94:2756–67.

80. Hoshida S, Kato J, Nishino M, et al. Increased angiotensin-converting enzyme activity in coronary artery specimens from patients with acute coronary syndrome. Circulation 2001;103:630–3.

81. Schieffer B, Schieffer E, Hilfiker-Kleiner D, et al. Expression of angiotensin II and interleukin 6 in human coronary atherosclerotic plaques: potential implications for inflammation and plaque instability. Circulation 2000;101:1372–8.

82. Soejima H, Ogawa H, Yasue H, et al. Angiotensin-converting enzyme inhibition reduces monocyte chemoattractant protein-1 and tissue factor levels in patients with myocardial infarction. J Am Coll Cardiol 1999;34:983–8.

83. Tummala PE, Chen XL, Sundell CL, et al. Angiotensin II induces vascular cell adhesion molecule-1 expression in rat vasculature: a potential link between the renin-angiotensin system and atherosclerosis. Circulation 1999;100:1223–9.

84. Efficacy of perindopril in reduction of cardiovascular events among patients with stable coronary artery disease: randomised, double-blind, placebo-controlled, multicentre trial (the EUROPA study). Lancet 2003; 362:782–88.

85. Taniguchi I, Yamazaki T, Wagatsuma K, et al. The DD genotype of angiotensin converting enzyme polymorphism is a risk factor for coronary artery disease and

coronary stent restenosis in Japanese patients. Jpn Circ J 2001;65:897–900.

86. Dandona P, Kumar V, Aljada A, et al. Angiotensin II receptor blocker valsartan suppresses reactive oxygen species generation in leukocytes, nuclear factor-kappa B, in mononuclear cells of normal subjects: evidence of an antiinflammatory action. J Clin Endocrinol Metab 2003;88:4496–501.

87. Hernandez-Presa M, Bustos C, Ortego M, et al. Angiotensin-converting enzyme inhibition prevents arterial nuclear factor-kappa B activation, monocyte chemoattractant protein-1 expression, and macrophage infiltration in a rabbit model of early accelerated atherosclerosis. Circulation 1997;95:1532–41.

88. Frishman WH, Lazar EJ. Reduction of mortality, sudden death and nonfatal reinfarction with beta-adrenergic blockers in survivors of acute myocardial infarction: a new hypothesis regarding the cardio-protective action of beta-adrenergic blockade. Am J Cardiol 1990;66:66G–70G.

89. Waeber B, Brunner HR, Burnier M, Cohn JN. Hypertention. In: Cohn JN, ed. Cardiovascular medicine. Edinburgh: Churchill Livingstone, 2000: 1518.

90. Krolewski AS, Kosinski EJ, Warram JH, et al. Magn-itude and determinants of coronary artery disease in juvenile-onset, insulin-dependent diabetes mellitus. Am J Cardiol 1987;59:750–5.

91. Krolewski AS, Warram JH, Valsania P, Martin BC, Laffel LM, Christlieb AR. Evolving natural history of coronary artery disease in diabetes mellitus. Am J Med 1991;90:56S–61S.

92. Jouven X, Charles MA, Desnos M, Ducimetiere P. Circulating nonesterified fatty acid level as a predictive risk factor for sudden death in the population. Cir-culation 2001;104:756–61.

93. Fagot-Campagna A, Balkau B, Simon D, Ducimetiere P, Eschwege E. Is insulin an independent risk factor for hypertension? The Paris Prospective Study. Int J Epidemiol 1997;26:542–50.

94. Charles MA, Fontbonne A, Thibult N, Warnet JM, Rosselin GE, Eschwege E. Risk factors for NIDDM in white population. Paris prospective study. Diabetes 1991;40:796–9.

95. Moreno PR, Murcia AM, Palacios IF, et al. Coronary composition and macrophage infiltration in atherec-tomy specimens from patients with diabetes mellitus. Circulation 2000;102:2180–4.

96. Peter P, Nuttall SL, Kendall MJ. Insulin resistance – the new goal! J Clin Pharm Ther 2003;28:167–74.

97. Fisher M. Diabetes: can we stop the time bomb? Heart 2003;89(suppl 2):ii28–30;discussion ii35–7.

98. The Diabetes Control and Complications Trial Research Group. The effect of intensive treatment of diabetes on the development and progression of long-term complications in insulin-dependent diabetes mellitus. N Engl J Med 1993;329:977–86.

99. Reichard P, Nilsson B-Y, Rosenqvist U. The effect of long-term intensified insulin treatment on the develop-ment of microvascular complications of diabetes melli-tus. N Engl J Med 1993;329:304–9.

100. Ohkubo Y, Kishikawa H, Araki E, et al. Intensive insulin therapy prevents the progression of diabetic microvascular complications in Japanese patients with non-insulin-dependent diabetes mellitus: a random-ized prospective 6-year study. Diabetes Res Clin Pract 1995;28:103–117.

101. Abraira C, Colwell J, Nuttall F, et al. Cardiovascular events and correlates in the Veterans Affairs Diabetes Feasibility Trial. Veterans Affairs Cooperative Study on Glycemic Control and Complications in Type II Diabetes. Arch Intern Med 1997;157:181–8.

102. Prospective Diabetes Study (UKPDS) Group U. Intensive blood-glucose control with sulphonylureas or insulin compared with conventional treatment and risk of complications in patients with type 2 diabetes (UKPDS 33). The Lancet 1998;352:837–53.

103. UK Prospective Diabetes Study Group. Efficacy of atenolol and captopril in reducing risk of macrovascu-lar and microvascular complications in type 2 diabetes: UKPDS 39. Br Med J 1998;317:713–20.

104. UK Prospective Diabetes Study Group. Tight blood pressure control and risk of macrovascular and microvascular complications in type 2 diabetes: UKPDS 38. Br Med J 1998;317:703–13.

105. Prospective Diabetes Study (UKPDS) Group U. Effect of intensive blood-glucose control with metformin on complications in overweight patients with type 2 diabetes (UKPDS 34). Lancet 1998;352:854–65.

106. Chiasson JL, Josse RG, Gomis R, Hanefeld M, Karasik A, Laakso M. Acarbose treatment and the risk of cardio-vascular disease and hypertension in patients with impaired glucose tolerance: the STOP-NIDDM trial. JAMA 2003;290:486–94.

107. Borch-Johnsen K. The new classification of diabetes mellitus and IGT: a critical approach. Exp Clin Endocrinol Diabetes 2001;109(suppl 2):S86–93.

108. Marx N, Kehrle B, Kohlhammer K, et al. PPAR activators as antiinflammatory mediators in human T-lymphocytes: implications for atherosclerosis and transplantation-associated arteriosclerosis. Circ Res 2002;90:703–10.

109. Takano H, Komuro I. Roles of peroxisome proliferator-activated receptor gamma in cardiovascular disease. J Diabetes Complications 2002;16:108–14.

110. Duez H, Fruchart JC, Staels B. PPARS in inflammation, atherosclerosis and thrombosis. J Cardiovasc Risk 2001;8:187–94.

111. Badimon JJ, Badimon L, Galvez A, Dische R, Fuster V. High density lipoprotein plasma fractions inhibit aortic fatty streaks in cholesterol-fed rabbits. Lab Invest 1989;60:455–61.

112. Badimon JJ, Badimon L, Fuster V. Regression of atherosclerotic lesions by high density lipoprotein plasma fraction in the cholesterol-fed rabbit. J Clin Invest 1990;85:1234–41.

113. Li D, Weng S, Yang B, et al. Inhibition of arterial thrombus formation by ApoA1 Milano. Arterioscler Thromb Vasc Biol 1999;19:378–83.

114. Bielicki JK, Oda MN. Apolipoprotein A-I(Milano) and apolipoprotein A-I(Paris) exhibit an antioxidant activity distinct from that of wild-type apolipoprotein A-I. Biochemistry 2002;41:2089–96.

115. Shah PK, Nilsson J, Kaul S, et al. Effects of recombinant apolipoprotein A-I(Milano) on aortic atherosclerosis in apolipoprotein E-deficient mice. Circulation 1998;97:780–5.

116. Chiesa G, Monteggia E, Marchesi M, et al. Recombinant apolipoprotein A-I(Milano) infusion into rabbit carotid artery rapidly removes lipid from fatty streaks. Circ Res 2002;90:974–80.

117. Ameli S, Hultgardh-Nilsson A, Cercek B, et al. Recombinant apolipoprotein A-I Milano reduces intimal thickening after balloon injury in hypercholesterolemic rabbits. Circulation 1994;90:1935–41.

118. Tangirala RK, Tsukamoto K, Chun SH, Usher D, Pure E, Rader DJ. Regression of atherosclerosis induced by liver-directed gene transfer of apolipoprotein A-I in mice. Circulation 1999;100:1816–22.

119. Tsukamoto K, Hiester KG, Smith P, Usher DC, Glick JM, Rader DJ. Comparison of human apoA-I expression in mouse models of atherosclerosis after gene transfer using a second generation adenovirus. J Lipid Res 1997;38:1869–76.

120. Benoit P, Emmanuel F, Caillaud JM, et al. Somatic gene transfer of human ApoA-I inhibits atherosclerosis progression in mouse models. Circulation 1999;99:105–10.

121. Assmann G, Nofer JR. Atheroprotective effects of high-density lipoproteins. Annu Rev Med 2003;54:321–41.

122. Navab M, Anantharamaiah GM, Hama S, et al. Oral administration of an Apo A-I mimetic peptide synthesized from D-amino acids dramatically reduces atherosclerosis in mice independent of plasma cholesterol. Circulation 2002;105:290–2.

123. Rader DJ. Gene therapy for atherosclerosis. Int J Clin Lab Res 1997;27:35–43.

124. Krause BR, Auerbach BJ. Reverse cholesterol transport and future pharmacological approaches to the treatment of atherosclerosis. Curr Opin Invest Drugs 2001;2:375–81.

125. Yamashita S, Sakai N, Hirano K, et al. Roles of plasma lipid transfer proteins in reverse cholesterol transport. Front Biosci 2001;6:D366–87.

126. Kawashiri MA, Maugeais C, Rader DJ. High-density lipoprotein metabolism: molecular targets for new therapies for atherosclerosis. Curr Atheroscler Rep 2000;2:363–72.

127. Moulton KS, Heller E, Konerding MA, Flynn E, Palinski W, Folkman J. Angiogenesis inhibitors endostatin or TNP-470 reduce intimal neovascularization and plaque growth in apolipoprotein E-deficient mice. Circulation 1999;99:1726–32.

128. Nieto FJ. Infections and atherosclerosis: new clues from an old hypothesis? Am J Epidemiol 1998;148:937–48.

129. Higuchi ML, Sambiase N, Palomino S, et al. Detection of *Mycoplasma pneumoniae* and *Chlamydia pneumoniae* in ruptured atherosclerotic plaques. Braz J Med Biol Res 2000;33:1023–6.

130. Haraszthy VI, Zambon JJ, Trevisan M, Zeid M, Genco RJ. Identification of periodontal pathogens in atheromatous plaques. J Periodontol 2000;71:1554–60.

131. Naghavi M, Barlas Z, Siadaty S, Naguib S, Madjid M, Casscells W. Association of influenza vaccination and reduced risk of recurrent myocardial infarction. Circulation 2000;102:3039–45.

132. Chmiela M, Kowalewicz-Kulbat M, Miszczak A, et al. A link between *Helicobacter pylori* and/or *Chlamydia* spp. infections and atherosclerosis. FEMS Immunol Med Microbiol 2003;36:187–92.

133. Ott NT, Tarhan S, McGoon DC. Circulatory effects of vagal inflation reflex in man. Z Kardiol 1975;64:1066–70.

134. Gupta S, Leatham EW, Carrington D, Mendall MA, Kaski JC, Camm AJ. Elevated *Chlamydia pneumoniae* antibodies, cardiovascular events, and azithromycin in male survivors of myocardial infarction. Circulation 1997;96:404–7.

135. Gupta S, Camm AJ. Chronic infection in the etiology of atherosclerosis – the case for *Chlamydia pneumoniae*. Clin Cardiol 1997;20:829–36.

136. Muhlestein JB, Anderson JL, Carlquist JF, et al. Randomized secondary prevention trial of azithromycin in patients with coronary artery disease: primary clinical results of the ACADEMIC Study. Circulation 2000;102:1755–60.

137. Girard SE, Temesgen Z. Emerging concepts in disease management: a role for antimicrobial therapy in coronary artery disease. Expert Opin Pharmacother 2001;2:765–72.

138. Spodick DH, Flessas AP, Johnson MM. Association of acute respiratory symptoms with onset of acute myocardial infarction: prospective investigation of 150 consecutive patients and matched control patients. Am J Cardiol 1984;53:481–2.

139. Madjid M, Naghavi M, Litovsky S, Casscells SW. Influenza and cardiovascular disease: a new opportunity for prevention and the need for further studies. Circulation 2003;108:2730–6.

140. Siscovick DS, Raghunathan TE, Lin D, et al. Influenza vaccination and the risk of primary cardiac arrest. Am J Epidemiol 2000;152:674–7.

141. Lavallee P, Perchaud V, Gautier-Bertrand M, Grabli D, Amarenco P. Association between influenza vaccination and reduced risk of brain infarction. Stroke 2002;33:513–18.

142. Gurfinkel EP, de la Fuente RL, Mendiz O, Mautner B. Influenza vaccine pilot study in acute coronary syndromes and planned percutaneous coronary interventions: the FLU Vaccination Acute Coronary Syndromes (FLUVACS) Study. Circulation 2002;105:2143–7.

143. Nichol KL, Nordin J, Mullooly J, Lask R, Fillbrandt K, Iwane M. Influenza vaccination and reduction in hospitalizations for cardiac disease and stroke among the elderly. N Engl J Med 2003;348:1322–32.

144. Meraviglia MV, Maggi E, Bellomo G, Cursi M, Fanelli G, Minicucci F. Autoantibodies against oxidatively modified lipoproteins and progression of carotid restenosis after carotid endarterectomy. Stroke 2002; 33:1139–41.

145. Palinski W, Miller E, Witztum JL. Immunization of low density lipoprotein (LDL) receptor-deficient rabbits with homologous malondialdehyde-modified LDL reduces atherogenesis. Proc Natl Acad Sci USA 1995;92:821–5.

146. Zhou X, Caligiuri G, Hamsten A, Lefvert AK, Hansson GK. LDL immunization induces T-cell-dependent antibody formation and protection against atherosclerosis. Arterioscler Thromb Vasc Biol 2001;21:108–14.

147. Freigang S, Horkko S, Miller E, Witztum JL, Palinski W. Immunization of LDL receptor-deficient mice with homologous malondialdehyde-modified and native LDL reduces progression of atherosclerosis by mechanisms other than induction of high titers of antibodies to oxidative neoepitopes. Arterioscler Thromb Vasc Biol 1998;18:1972–82.

148. Palinski W, Witztum JL. Immune responses to oxidative neoepitopes on LDL and phospholipids modulate the development of atherosclerosis. J Intern Med 2000; 247:371–80.

149. Fredrikson GN, Soderberg I, Lindholm M, et al. Inhibition of atherosclerosis in ApoE-Null Mice by immunization with ApoB-100 peptide sequences. Arterioscler Thromb Vasc Biol 2003;23:879–84.

150. Maron R, Sukhova G, Faria AM, et al. Mucosal administration of heat shock protein-65 decreases atherosclerosis and inflammation in aortic arch of low-density lipoprotein receptor-deficient mice. Circulation 2002; 106:1708–15.

151. Hennekens CH, Dyken ML, Fuster V. Aspirin as a therapeutic agent in cardiovascular disease: a statement for healthcare professionals from the American Heart Association. Circulation 1997;96:2751–3.

152. Budaj A, Yusuf S, Mehta SR, et al. Benefit of clopidogrel in patients with acute coronary syndromes without ST-segment elevation in various risk groups. Circulation 2002;106:1622–6.

153. A randomised, blinded, trial of clopidogrel versus aspirin in patients at risk of ischaemic events (CAPRIE). CAPRIE Steering Committee. Lancet 1996; 348:1329–39.

154. Thrombosis prevention trial: randomised trial of low-intensity oral anticoagulation with warfarin and low-dose aspirin in the primary prevention of ischaemic heart disease in men at increased risk. The Medical Research Council's General Practice Research Framework. Lancet 1998;351:233–41.

155. Rudnicka AR, Ashby D, Brennan P, Meade T. Thrombosis prevention trial: compliance with warfarin treatment and investigation of a retained effect. Arch Intern Med 2003;163:1454–60.

156. van Es RF, Jonker JJ, Verheugt FW, Deckers JW, Grobbee DE. Aspirin and coumadin after acute coronary syndromes (the ASPECT-2 study): a randomised controlled trial. Lancet 2002;360:109–13.

157. Brouwer MA, van den Bergh PJ, Aengevaeren WR, et al. Aspirin plus coumarin versus aspirin alone in the prevention of reocclusion after fibrinolysis for acute myocardial infarction: results of the Antithrombotics in the Prevention of Reocclusion In Coronary Thrombolysis (APRICOT)-2 Trial. Circulation 2002; 106:659–65.

158. Psaty BM, Smith NL, Lemaitre RN, et al. Hormone replacement therapy, prothrombotic mutations, and the risk of incident nonfatal myocardial infarction in postmenopausal women. JAMA 2001;285:906–13.

159. Yamada Y, Izawa H, Ichihara S, et al. Prediction of the risk of myocardial infarction from polymorphisms in candidate genes. N Engl J Med 2002;347:1916–23.

160. Liistro F, Stankovic G, Di Mario C, et al. First clinical experience with a paclitaxel derivate-eluting polymer stent system implantation for in-stent restenosis: immediate and long-term clinical and angiographic outcome. Circulation 2002;105:1883–6.

161. Grube E, Silber S, Hauptmann KE, et al. TAXUS I: six- and twelve-month results from a randomized, double-blind trial on a slow-release paclitaxel-eluting stent for de novo coronary lesions. Circulation 2003;107:38–42.

162. Gershlik A, De Scheerder I, Chevalier B. Long-term follow-up in the ELUTES clinical study. Am J Cardiol 2002;90:1H.

163. Hong MK, Mintz GS, Lee CW, et al. Paclitaxel coating reduces in-stent intimal hyperplasia in human coronary arteries: a serial volumetric intravascular ultrasound analysis from the Asian Paclitaxel-Eluting Stent Clinical Trial (ASPECT). Circulation 2003;107:517–20.

164. Tanabe K, Serruys PW, Grube E, et al. TAXUS III Trial: in-stent restenosis treated with stent-based delivery of paclitaxel incorporated in a slow-release polymer formulation. Circulation 2003;107:559–64.

165. Morice MC, Serruys PW, Sousa JE, et al. A randomized comparison of a sirolimus-eluting stent with a standard stent for coronary revascularization. N Engl J Med 2002;346:1773–80.

166. Sousa JE, Costa MA, Sousa AG, et al. Two-year angiographic and intravascular ultrasound follow-up after implantation of sirolimus-eluting stents in human coronary arteries. Circulation 2003;107:381–3.

167. Farb A, John M, Acampado E, Kolodgie FD, Prescott MF, Virmani R. Oral everolimus inhibits in-stent neointimal growth. Circulation 2002;106:2379–84.

168. Khurana R, Martin JF, Zachary I. Gene therapy for cardiovascular disease: a case for cautious optimism. Hypertension 2001;38:1210–16.

169. Serruys PW, Degertekin M, Tanabe K, et al. Intravascular ultrasound findings in the multicenter, randomized, double-blind RAVEL (RAndomized study with the sirolimus-eluting VElocity balloon-expandable stent in the treatment of patients with de novo native coronary artery Lesions) trial. Circulation 2002;106:798–803.

170. Feldman LJ, Isner JM. Gene therapy for the vulnerable plaque. J Am Coll Cardiol 1995;26:826–35.

171. Zoldhelyi P, Chen ZQ, Shelat HS, McNatt JM, Willerson JT. Local gene transfer of tissue factor pathway inhibitor regulates intimal hyperplasia in atherosclerotic arteries. Proc Natl Acad Sci USA 2001;98:4078–83.

172. Waxman S, Pulerwitz TC, Rowe KA, Quist WC, Verrier RL. Preclinical safety testing of percutaneous transatrial access to the normal pericardial space for local cardiac drug delivery and diagnostic sampling. Catheter Cardiovasc Interv 2000;49:472–7.

173. Baek SH, Hrabie JA, Keefer LK, et al. Augmentation of intrapericardial nitric oxide level by a prolonged-release nitric oxide donor reduces luminal narrowing after porcine coronary angioplasty. Circulation 2002;105:2779–84.

174. Rockson SG, Lorenz DP, Cheong WF, Woodburn KW. Photoangioplasty: an emerging clinical cardiovascular role for photodynamic therapy. Circulation 2000;102:591–6.

175. Chou TM, Woodburn KW, Cheong WF, et al. Photodynamic therapy: applications in atherosclerotic vascular disease with motexafin lutetium. Catheter Cardiovasc Interv 2002;57:387–94.

176. Rockson SG, Kramer P, Razavi M, et al. Photoangioplasty for human peripheral atherosclerosis: results of a phase I trial of photodynamic therapy with motexafin lutetium (Antrin). Circulation 2000;102:2322–4.

177. Lal BN, Casscells SW, Willerson JT, Geng Y. Short term thermal treatment enhances apoptosis, reduces cytokine expression in atherosclerotic plaques, and inactivates NF-Kappa B in cultured macrophages. Circulation 2001;104:II-294.

178. Williams DO. Intracoronary brachytherapy: past, present, and future. Circulation 2002;105:2699–700.

179. Sangiorgi G, Carbone GL, Oxvig C, et al. Plaque sealing with stenting is associated with marked reduction of biologic markers of vulnerability. Am J Cardiol 2003;92:5L.

180. Yeh ET, Zhang S, Wu HD, Korbling M, Willerson JT, Estrov Z. Transdifferentiation of human peripheral blood CD34+-enriched cell population into cardiomyocytes, endothelial cells, and smooth muscle cells in vivo. Circulation 2003;108:2070–3.

181. Goldschmidt-Clermont PJ. Loss of bone marrow-derived vascular progenitor cells leads to inflammation and atherosclerosis. Am Heart J 2003;146:S5–12.

182. Xu Q, Zhang Z, Davison F, Hu Y. Circulating progenitor cells regenerate endothelium of vein graft atherosclerosis, which is diminished in ApoE-deficient mice. Circ Res 2003;93:e76–86.

183. Shearman AM, Cupples LA, Demissie S, et al. Association between estrogen receptor alpha gene variation and cardiovascular disease. JAMA 2003;290:2263–70.

184. Herrington DM, Howard TD, Brosnihan KB, et al. Common estrogen receptor polymorphism augments effects of hormone replacement therapy on E-selectin but not C-reactive protein. Circulation 2002;105:1879–82.

185. Herrington DM, Howard TD, Hawkins GA, et al. Estrogen-receptor polymorphisms and effects of estrogen replacement on high-density lipoprotein cholesterol in women with coronary disease. N Engl J Med 2002;346:967–74.

186. Braunstein JB, Kershner DW, Bray P, et al. Interaction of hemostatic genetics with hormone therapy: new insights to explain arterial thrombosis in postmenopausal women. Chest 2002;121:906–20.

187. Ballantyne CM. Low-density lipoproteins and risk for coronary artery disease. Am J Cardiol 1998;82:3Q–12Q.

188. Madjid M, et al. Influenza and cardiovascular disease: is there a causal relationship? Tex Heart Inst J 2004;31:4–13.

CHAPTER 22

Photodynamic therapy

Ron Waksman & Pauline E McEwan

Photodynamic therapy (PDT) is an emergent treatment modality for numerous disease processes, which involves photosensitizing (light-sensitive) drugs, light, and tissue oxygen. Typically photosensitizing agents (photosensitizers) are porphyrins or chemicals of similar structure, which are administered locally or parenterally, and selectively absorbed or retained within the tissues targeted for therapy.[1] This differential selectivity or retention promotes selective damage when the target tissue is exposed to light of an appropriate wavelength; the surrounding normal tissue, containing little or no drug, absorbs little light and is thus spared injury.[1,2]

PDT clinical research has historically focused primarily and successfully on cancer treatment,[3–6] and is approved as a cytotoxic therapy for disease processes in dermatology, ophthalmology, and urology also. Any disease associated with rapidly growing tissue, including the formation of abnormal blood vessels, can potentially be treated with this technology. To this, PDT has recently revealed itself as an especially appealing approach in the treatment of cardiovascular diseases as well. Selectivity renders PDT particularly appealing in atherosclerotic illnesses such as coronary artery disease, in which a localized obstructive process leads to clinical ischemic syndromes. In typical treatment modalities for coronary artery disease, other catheter-based approaches are relatively nonselective and carry a substantial risk of damage to the normal arterial wall.[7] Preclinical and clinical studies have recently been targeted to examine the utility of PDT for vascular applications.

Mechanism of PDT action

The PDT response begins with a differential accumulation of a photosensitizer in the target tissue, the consequence of either selective uptake of the drug or of preferential retention caused by slower clearance from the abnormal tissue.[1,8–10] In atherosclerosis, drug lipophilicity and the high lipid content of vascular plaque both appear to predicate selective uptake.[7] Throughout the process, the drug serves simply as a catalyst for energy transfer, while light absorption leads to the release of cytotoxic singlet oxygen, a highly reactive, oxidizing agent with very short diffusion differences (≤ 0.1 μm).[11] The resultant photobiological response (direct, rapid cell apoptosis and delayed necrosis from neovascular damage) becomes maximal within several days.[1,8–10] Cell death is thus confined to those illuminated areas in which there is an adequate presence of the sensitized drug.[11]

To achieve optimal drug activation, light energy is delivered at a wavelength that matches the maximal absorption by the photosensitizer that is also able to penetrate efficiently through overlying blood and tissues.[7] For intravascular application, light is delivered to the treatment site directly with either balloon catheter-based illumination systems[12,13] or optical fibers with cylindrically emitting diffusing fibers. Light is usually in the form of red light derived from a laser, however it can originate from collimated or diffuse illuminators as well (e.g. high-power lamps and light-emitting diode panels).[7] While laser balloon systems have been purported to have therapeutic vascular effects,[14,15] the goal of illumination for PDT is to have no intrinsic biological activity due to thermal effects from the light source.

PDT has demonstrated in numerous trials and in different animal models the eradication potential of medial smooth muscle proliferation following endothelial denudation in the rat and rabbit model.

Over the long term, after PDT, a strong correlation exists between depletion of potential neointimal precursor cells at acute time points and inhibition of intimal hyperplasia.[16,17] This observation suggests that the main mechanisms of PDT action are by apoptosis and DNA fragmentation.

Photosensitizers and PDT systems

Early PDT agents were activated at wavelengths between 630 and 670 nm. At those wavelengths, blood and tissue substantially attenuated the delivery of light to target cells.[18] Tissue optics suggested that higher wavelengths were desired for penetration and photosensitizer activation, with a maximal absorption in the range of 700–800 or 950–1100 nm.[19] Although these early agents were available for clinical use in antineoplastic applications, the effectiveness of PDT of atherosclerosis in animal models was inconsistent, due in part to the inadequate penetration of shorter wavelengths of light through blood and vascular tissue.[20] Hematoporphyrin derivative (HpD) was the first of a number of photosensitizers with demostratable, selective accumulation within atherosclerotic plaque.[21]

Administration of the photosensitizing agent 5-aminolevulinic acid (ALA), a biological precursor for protoporphyrin IX, has been accomplished by topical, systemic, and local internal routes in a variety of malignant and dysplastic conditions.[11,22] However, its administration can elicit hemodynamic changes (depression of systemic and pulmonary pressures and pulmonary resistance) that could limit its ultimate utility in cardiovascular applications.[23]

The recent renewal of interest in the therapeutic potential of cardiovascular PDT has been prompted largely by the availability of expanded macrocycles known as the texaphyrins. Interest in the texaphyrin family of molecules as therapeutic agents for cardiovascular disease is based on tissue selectivity, cellular localization, and light activation properties. These drugs circumvent many of the physicochemical limitations of previously studied sensitizers. They localize in cancerous lesions, the neovasculature, and atheromatous plaque. Texaphyrins can disrupt the intracellular oxidation-reduction balance and alter bioenergetic processes within target cells; and when activated by various energy forms (e.g. ionizing radiation, chemotherapy, or light), they may also be able to reduce or eliminate diseased tissue targets.[7]

Biotechnology has developed a new generation of selective photosensitizers and catheter-based technological advances in light delivery, which have allowed the introduction of PDT into the vasculature. Two of these systems include Antrin phototherapy (Pharmacyclics, Inc., Sunnyvale, CA, USA) and PhotoPoint PDT (Miravant Medical Technologies, Santa Barbara, CA, USA).

Antrin phototherapy is a combination of endovascular illumination and motexafin lutetium (MLu, Antrin), an expanded porphyrin (texaphyrin) that accumulates in atherosclerotic plaque and, after activation by far-red light, produces cytotoxic singlet oxygen.[24] (Figure 22.1) Antrin is

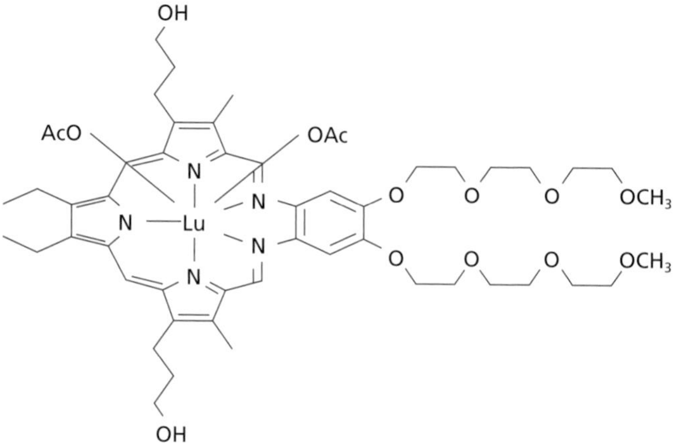

Figure 22.1 Motexafin lutetium (MLu) photosensitizer.

synthetic and water soluble and has a short plasma half-life.[25] Antrin phototherapy has been shown to reduce plaque in animal models and generates cytotoxic singlet oxygen that has been shown to induce apoptosis in macrophages and smooth muscle cells.[20]

A specialized diode laser (Figure 22.2) has been developed for use with MLu in the catheterization laboratory to produce a consistent 730-nm red light. It is approximately the size of a standard desk top PC with a touch screen control system that allows easy testing of the light fiber and calibration before endovascular illumination. The optical fiber involved, 0.018 inches in diameter (Figure 22.3), can be delivered through angioplasty balloon catheters and standard transfer catheters, and has been delivered to allow illumination at sites where standard interventional technologies can be delivered.[20]

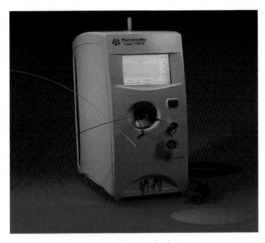

Figure 22.2 Antrin phototherapy diode laser.

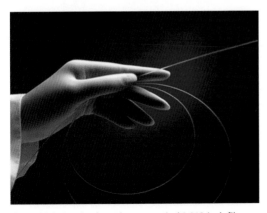

Figure 22.3 Antrin phototherapy optical 0.018-inch fiber.

PhotoPoint PDT is a newly developed proprietary catheter-based system involving photoselective delivery of a nonionizing, nonthermal energy source of visible light to activate a photosensitizer localized in the artery wall (Figure 22.4). The novel photosentsitizer molecule gallium chloride mesoporphyrin dimethyl ester (MV0611) was discovered through rational drug screening for use in cardiovascular applications (Miravant Pharmaceuticals Inc., Santa Barbara, CA, USA). The interaction between MV0611 and intravascular light generates reactive oxygen species, causing targeted medial smooth muscle cell apoptosis and depletion of neointimal precursor cells (Figure 22.5) in rat carotid and porcine coronary arteries.[16,26,27]

Photodynamic therapy and atherosclerotic plaque

Atherosclerosis, a vascular inflammatory disease, involves the pathologic development of fatty plaques in a heterogeneous cell matrix.[28] The complex polygenic cellular etiology of atherosclerotic plaque development has meant that single treatment modalities are limited in scope for reducing plaque inflammation and simultaneously limiting plaque cell proliferation. Interest in PDT as a possible therapy for atherosclerosis has therefore increased in recent years because of the advent of new photosensitive drugs with fewer side effects and more powerful, less expensive devices. PDT has the potential to provide safe debulking of the atheroma through elimination of the atherosclerosis-promoting cell types such as macrophage "foam" cells and proliferative smooth muscle cells (Figure 22.6). The potential of PDT to reduce plaque inflammation and proliferation whilst rendering plaques less sensitive to re-infiltration of inflammatory cells is of therapeutic value in limiting disease progression and promoting plaque stabilization. Given that acute coronary syndrome is frequently associated with focal atherosclerosis in remote locations from sites of rupture, the potential of PDT to stabilize such atherosclerotic lesions suggests a powerful preventative intervention for limiting future acute events. Current challenges, however, lie with the appropriate detection of such lesions and the identification of a "vulnerable" patient population. PDT may also be integrated

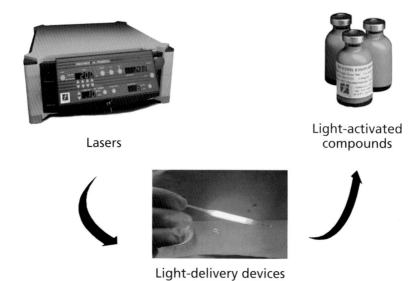

Lasers

Light-activated compounds

Light-delivery devices

Figure 22.4 PhotoPoint – an integrated system.

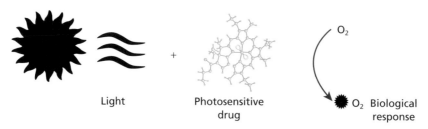

Light

Photosensitive drug

O_2

O_2 Biological response

- **Reactive Oxygen Species/Free Radicals**
  -Similar mechanism to brachytherapy

- **PDT Preferentially Induces Apoptosis**
  -No DNA strand breaks

Figure 22.5 PhotoPoint mechanism.

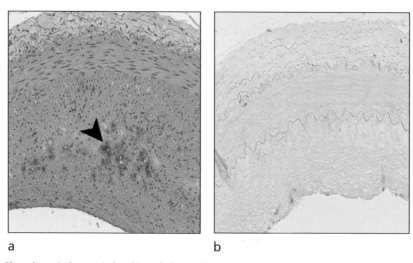

a

b

Figure 22.6 Photodynamic therapy-induced loss of "foam cell" macrophages (arrow in a): a, control; b, 7 days post-PDT treatment.

into traditional vascular procedures with or without stent implantation.[20]

While the precise mechanisms of PDT action remain unclear, Chen et al. explored the effect of altering the intracellular redox state on PDT-induced cell death by depleting intracellular glutathione stores with the use of L-buthionine [S,R]-sulfoximine (BSO), a specific inhibitor of γ-glutamyl cysteine synthetase. BSO alone had no effect on macrophage viability, however treatment of the cells with the antioxidant N-acetylcysteine (NAC) significantly reduced cell death induced by PDT. In contrast to PDT, macrophage apoptosis induced by exogenous C2-ceramide was largely unaffected by treatment with BSO or NAC. Investigators concluded that taken together, these observations suggested that apoptosis initiated by PDT is redox sensitive and that distinct signaling cascades may be operative in PDT compared with certain non-PDT pathways.[24]

Chen et al. also examined the mechanism of cell death induced by PDT with MLu by using annexin V staining of macrophages and smooth muscle cells. Annexin V binds membrane-associated phosphatidylserine (PS), which is located in the inner phospholipid bilayer but is externalized rapidly to the cell surface in the apoptotic process. Here, PDT increased the number of apoptotic macrophages 4.2 ± 1.2-fold (mean $\pm$ SD, $n = 4$) and the number of apoptotic smooth muscle cells 4.0 ± 1.9-fold ($n = 3$). The percentage of necrotic cells did not increase from baseline after PDT.[24]

In a vein-graft model, Yamaguchi et al. found that PDT significantly reduced the intima/media ratio in the early phase of vein graft disease by injecting inferior vena cava-grafted rats with MLu (10 mg/kg) 4 or 12 weeks after grafting. Biodistribution was assessed in a subgroup 24 hours after MLu administration. PDT at 4 weeks after surgery significantly reduced the intima/media ration, whereas treatment at 12 weeks did not reduce the intima/media ratio. Activated macrophages were observed 4 weeks after grafting; however, a significant reduction occurred in these cells by 12 weeks. Thus, it appeared that the mechanism by which PDT works may be related to the targeting of activated macrophages in these models of vascular disease.[20,29]

In their study, Waksman et al. examined the effects of the novel photosensitizing drug MV0611

to target entire plaque cell populations. Fifteen New Zealand White rabbits were fed a 1% cholesterol diet followed by bilateral iliac balloon endothelial denudation. At 5 weeks post denudation, rabbits received MV0611 (3 mg/kg IV) followed by light delivery using a Miravant catheter-based diode laser (15 J/cm^2) 4 hours post injection. PDT induced a significant reduction ($92 \pm 6\%$) in the population of nuclei of all cell types in plaques relative to controls ($P < 0.001$). Results indicated that PDT with MV0611 induces significant depletion of plaque cell populations, and programmed cell death of macrophages appeared to be an important component of plaque cell loss and subsequent lipid depletion.[28] All rabbits following PDT were devoid of thrombosis, necrosis, or aneurysm formation.

Photodynamic therapy for restenosis prevention

Restenosis, the major limitation of long-term success of percutaneous coronary interventions, is probably best treated with brachytherapy, which uses ionizing radiation. PDT, however, which in contrast to brachytherapy uses nonionizing radiation, has emerged as another possible strategy.[30] Smooth muscle cell migration and proliferation are the main mechanisms for restenosis following intervention. PDT has shown its ability to eradicate smooth muscle cells following injury in animal models and is known to increase collagen cross linkage in the extracellular matrix, creating a barrier to smooth muscle cell attachment, proliferation, and migration.[31]

Using the photosensitizer molecule MV0611, Waksman et al. examined the feasibility and efficacy of intracoronary PhotoPoint PDT in a porcine stented model of restenosis (Figure 22.7). MV0611 was given systemically followed by intravascular laser light, which was selectively delivered to porcine coronary arteries using a light diffuser centered with a balloon catheter. Bare metal stents were then implanted at the treatment site in the PDT ($n = 5$) or control ($n = 4$) arteries (Figure 22.8). At 30 days after stenting, the percent area occlusion in the PDT group was significantly reduced compared to controls ($39 \pm 3\%$ vs. $55 \pm 4\%$, $P < 0.01$). Mean intimal thickness was also reduced in PDT stents compared to controls ($P < 0.05$). Luminal

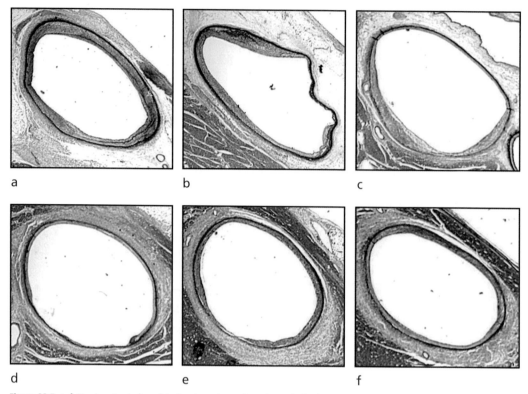

Figure 22.7 a–f, Porcine stented model of restenosis: sections through single artery 14 days post treatment.

area was increased with PDT, 5.8 ± 0.3 mm² vs. controls 3.6 ± 0.3 mm² ($P < 0.01$) and a maximal reendothelialization score was observed by gross histology in all PDT and control stents. No cases of aneurysm formation or thrombosis presented. Here, intracoronary PDT inhibited vascular neointima formation without impairing endothelial regeneration in the 30-day porcine model of in-stent restenosis.[32]

Further studies with the use of the same system of balloon overstretch injury in the porcine model demonstrated significant inhibition of neointima formation, with vascular remodeling and absence of fibrin deposition or thrombus formation. Other studies using PDT on arteriovenous grafts demonstrated depletion of neointimal precursor cells in the vessel wall. These observations support the idea that PDT can be selectively targeted to smooth muscle cells and fibroblasts, and can attenuate the restenosis process following intervention.

Clinical trials

Rockson et al. designed a phase I trial to evaluate the safety and tolerability of Antrin in the endovascular treatment of atherosclerosis. This was an open-label, single-dose, escalating drug- and light-dose study that originally was not designed to examine clinical efficacy; however, several secondary end points suggested a favorable therapeutic effect. Clinical evaluation, serial quantitative angiography, and intravascular ultrasonography were performed on a study population, which consisted of patients with symptomatic claudication and objectively documented peripheral arterial insufficiency ($n = 47$, 51 procedures). There was no angiographic or ultrasonographic evidence of embolization, vascular trauma, or disease progression that could be ascribed to the experimental treatment. The standardized classification of clinical outcomes (based on the Rutherford–Becker classification[33]) for the 47 patients at follow-up

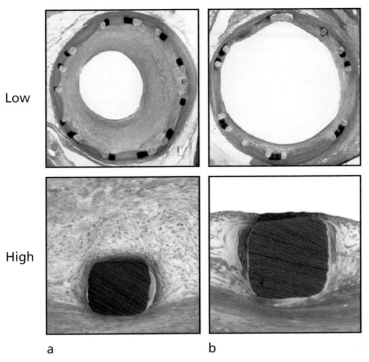

Figure 22.8 Bare metal stents implanted in control (a) and at treatment site in photodynamic therapy treated arteries (b).

showed improvement in 29 (62%), no change in 17 (36%), and moderate worsening in one (2%), demonstrating that photoangioplasty with Antrin is well tolerated and safe in the endovascular treatment of atherosclerosis.[34]

Bisaccia et al., in their initial evaluation using photopheresis, an immunomodulatory therapy, suggests that early use of this therapy in patients undergoing percutaneous transluminal coronary angioplasty (PTCA) with or without stent deployment may result in a reduction in clinical restenosis. A total of 78 patients with single-vessel coronary artery disease were enrolled, 41 in the control group and 37 in the photopheresis group. Clinical restenosis occurred in significantly less photopheresis patients than control patients (8 vs. 27%; $P = 0.04$), with a relative risk of 0.30 (95% confidence interval, 0.09–1.00). A multicenter clinical trial following a protocol recommended by the US Food and Drug Administration is currently underway to better determine what, if any, impact photopheresis has in preventing restenosis.[35]

In 1999 a pilot clinical study of adjuvant PDT in patients undergoing repeat superficial femoral angioplasty for restenosis was conducted.[36] The original study included seven patients with symptomatic restenosis of the superficial femoral artery within 6 months of angioplasty (one with two lesions in the same artery). In a follow-up, long-term study, Mansfield et al. determined that at 48 (mean) months after PDT, no patients developed critical limb ischemia or ulceration and there were no arterial complications. Only one of eight lesions treated by angioplasty with adjuvant PDT developed symptomatic restenosis at the treated site over a 4-year interval. Although the study was uncontrolled and had a small number of patients, the authors reported that adjunctive PDT seems to hold considerable promise as a new strategy to prevent restenosis after angioplasty.[37]

Kereiakes et al., in an open-label, phase I, drug andlight dose-escalation clinical trial of MLu phototherapy, enrolled 80 patients undergoing de novo coronary stent deployment. MLu was

Table 22.1 Quantitative coronary angiography (QCA) at follow-up by study stage and segment analyzed.[25]

	Stent	Injury	Illumination	Entire analysis
Stage 1				
Late loss (mm)				
Median	1.1	0.8	0.6	0.6
Mean (SD)	1.1 (0.59)	0.9 (0.64)	0.6 (0.48)	0.6 (0.55)
95% CI	0.9, 1.3	0.7, 1.1	0.5, 0.8	0.4, 0.8
Binary restenosis >50% (%)	39.5	42.1	42.1	44.7
Stage 2				
Late loss (mm)				
Median	1.0	0.9	0.6	0.4
Mean (SD)	0.9 (0.62)	0.9 (0.64)	0.6 (0.58)	0.6 (0.59)
95% CI	0.7–1.2	0.7–1.2	0.4–0.8	0.4–0.8
Binary restenosis >50% (%)	27.3	30.3	30.3	30.3

administered to 79 patients by intravenous infusion 18–24 hours before the procedure, and photoactivation was performed after balloon predilatation and before stent deployment. Clinical evaluation, serial quantitative angiography, and intravascular ultrasound were performed periprocedurally and at 6 months follow-up. Beyond 30 days (range 71–189 days), 15 (19%) patients experienced adverse outcomes, including non-Q-wave myocardial infarction ($n = 6$) and symptomatic target lesion revascularization ($n = 11$), with two patients experiencing both infarction and revascularization. MLu phototherapy was well tolerated without serious dose-limiting toxicities, and side effects (paresthesia and rash) were minor. No adverse angiographic outcomes were attributed to phototherapy.[25] QCA at follow-up by study stage and segment analyzed is depicted in Table 22.1.

Conclusions

Photodynamic therapy for vascular applications is promising and is expected to play a role in the prevention of restenosis, as a modality to attenuate atherosclerotic plaques, and perhaps to pacify vulnerable plaques. Nevertheless, the challenge lies in finding the optimal dose for both the drug (photosensitizer) and the light energy source to achieve these targets safely without affecting the integrity of the vessel or exposing the patients to additional risk. If this technology is proven in clinical trials, catheter-based photodynamic therapy will play a pivotal role in interventional cardiology.

Acknowledgments

The authors would like to acknowledge Ian Leitch and Robert Scott of Miravant Medical Technologies.

References

1. Henderson B, Dougherty T. How does photodynamic therapy work? Photochem Photobiol 1992;55:145–57.
2. Dougherty T. Photosensitizers: therapy and detection of malignant tumors. Photochem Photobiol 1987;45: 879–89.
3. Dougherty TJ, Gomer CJ, Henderson BW, et al. Photodynamic therapy. J Natl Cancer Inst 1998;90:889–905.
4. Pass Hi. Photodynamic therapy in oncology: mechanisms and clinical use. J Natl Cancer Inst 1993;85:443–56.
5. Prewitt TW, Pass HI. Photodynamic therapy for thoracic cancer: biology and applications. Sem Thorac Cardiovasc Surg 1993;5:229–37.
6. Woodburn KW, Fan Q, Kessel D, et al. Phototherapy of cancer and atheromatous plaque with texaphyrins. J Clin Laser Med Surg 1996;14:343–8.
7. Rockson SG, Lorenz DP, Cheong W-F, et al. Photoangioplasty: an emerging clinical cardiovascular role

for photodynamic therapy. Circulation 2000;102:591–6.

8. Kessel D, Luo Y, Deng Y, et al. The role of subcellular localization in initiation of apoptosis by photodynamic therapy. Photochem Photobiol 1997;65:422–6.

9. Sluiter W, de Vree W, Pietersma A, et al. Prevention of late lumen loss after coronary angioplasty by photodynamic therapy: role of activated neutrophils. Mol Cell Biochem 1996;157:233–8.

10. Reed M, Miller F, Wieman T, et al. The effect of photodynamic therapy on the microcirculation. J Surg Res 1988;45:452–9.

11. Nyamekye I, Anglin S, McEwan J, et al. Photodynamic therapy of normal and balloon-injured rat carotid arteries using 5-amino-levulinic acid. Circulation 1995;91:417–5.

12. Spears JR. Percutaneous laser treatment of atherosclerosis: an overview of emerging techniques. Cardiovasc Intervent Radiol 1986;9:303–12.

13. Jenkins MP, Buonaccorsi GA, Mansfield R, et al. Reduction in the response to coronary and iliac artery injury with photodynamic therapy using 5-aminolaevulinic acid. Cardiovasc Res 2000;45:478–85.

14. Spears JR, James LM, Leonard BM, et al. Plaque-media rewelding with reversible tissue optical property changes during receptive cw Nd: YAG laser exposure. Laser Surg Med 1988;8:477–85.

15. Cheong WF, Spears JR, Welch AJ. Laser balloon angioplasty. Crit Rev Biomed Engineer 1991;19:113–46.

16. Grove RI, Leitch I, Rychnovsky S, et al. Current status of photodynamic therapy for the prevention of restenosis. In: Waksman R, ed. Vascular brachytherapy, 3rd edn. New York: Futura Publishing, 2002:339–45.

17. Barton JM, Nielsen HV, Rychnovsky S, et al. PhotoPoint™ PDT Inhibits Intimal Hyperplasia in Arteriovenous Grafts. Presented at CRT 2003, January 26–29. Washington, DC.

18. Vincent GM, Fox J, Charlton G, et al. Presence of blood significantly decreases transmission of 630 nm laser light. Lasers Surg Med 1991;11:399–403.

19. Doiron DR, Keller GS. Porphyrin photodynamic therapy: principles and clinical applications. Curr Prob Dermatol 1986;15:85–93.

20. Chou TM, Woodburn KW, Cheong W-F, et al. Photodynamic therapy: applications in atherosclerotic vascular disease with motexafin lutetium. Catheter Cardiov Interv 2002;57:387–94.

21. Spears J, Serur J, Shropshire D, et al. Fluorescence of experimental atheromatous plaques with hematoporphyrin derivative. J Clin Invest 1983;71:395–9.

22. Kennedy J, Marcus S, Pottier R. Photodynamic therapy (PDT) and photodiagnosis (PD) using endogenous photosensitization induced by 5-aminolevulinic acid (ALA):

mechanisms and clinical results. J Clin Laser Med Surg 1996;14:289–304.

23. Herman M, Webber J, Fromm D, et al. Hemodynamic effects of 5-aminolevulinic acid in humans. J Photochem Photobiol B 1998;43:61–5.

24. Chen Z, Woodburn KW, Shi C, et al. Photodynamic therapy with motexafin lutetium induces redox-sensitive apoptosis of vascular cells. Arterioscler Thromb Vasc Biol 2001;21:759–64.

25. Kereiakes DJ, Szyniszewski AM, Wahr D, et al. Phase I drug and light dose-escalation trial of motexafin lutetium and far red light activation (phototherapy) in subjects with coronary artery disease undergoing percutaneous coronary intervention and stent deployment: procedural and long-term results. Circulation 2003;108:1310–15.

26. Wilson A, Leitch IM, Diaz E, et al. Endovascular photodynamic therapy with the new photosensitizer MV0611 reduces neo-intimal cell content in a rodent arterial injury model. Circulation 2001;104(suppl II) abstract 3133:II-663.

27. Yazdi H, Kim H-S, Seabron R, et al. Cellular effects of intracoronary photodynamic therapy with the new photosensitizer MV0611 in normal and balloon-injured porcine coronary arteries. Acute and long term effects. Circulation 2001;104(suppl II) abstract 1849:II-388.

28. Waksman R, Leborgne L, Seabron R, et al. Novel Photopoint photodynamic therapy for the treatment of atherosclerotic plaques. J Am Coll Cardiol 2003;41(suppl A):259A.

29. Yamaguchi A, Woodburn KW, Hayase M, et al. Reduction of vein graft disease using photodynamic therapy with monotexafin lutetium in a rodent isograft model. Circulation 2000;102:III275–80.

30. Mansfield R, Bown S, McEwan J. Photodynamic therapy: shedding light on restenosis. Heart 2001;86:612–18.

31. Overhaus M, Heckenkamp J, Kossodo S, et al. Photodynamic therapy generates a matrix barrier to invasive vascular cell migration. Circ Res 2000;86:334–40.

32. Waksman R, Leitch I, Roessler J, et al. Intracoronary PhotoPoint photodynamic therapy reduces neointimal growth without suppressing re-endothelialization in a porcine model of restenosis. Heart 2006;17 [Epub ahead of print].

33. Rutherford RB, Becker GJ. Standards for evaluating and reporting the results of surgical and percutaneous therapy for peripheral artery disease. J Vasc Interv Radiol 1991;181:277–81.

34. Rockson SG, Kramer P, Razavi M, et al. Photoangioplasty for human peripheral atherosclerosis: results of a phase I trial of photodynamic therapy with motexafin lutetium (antrin). Circulation 2000;102:2322–4.

35. Bisaccia E, Palangio M, Gonzalez J, et al. Photopheresis: therapeutic potential in preventing restenosis after percutaneous transluminal coronary angioplasty. Am J Cardiovasc Drugs 2003;3:43–51.

36. Jenkins MP, Buonaccorsi GA, Raphael M, et al. Clinical study of adjuvant photodynamic therapy to reduce restenosis following femoral angioplasty. Br J Surg 1999;86:1258–63.

37. Mansfield RJR, Jenkins MP, Pai ML, et al. Long-term safety and efficacy of superficial femoral artery angioplasty with adjuvant photodynamic therapy to prevent restenosis. Br J Surg 2002;89:1538–9.

CHAPTER 23

Thermal stabilization of vulnerable plaques

Samuel Ward Casscells, Birendra N Lal, Mohammad Madjid,
Tarun Tewatia, Ibrahim Aboshady, Yong-Jian Geng &
James T Willerson

As a major determinant of the progression and clinical outcome of atherosclerotic disease, inflammation is mediated through the action of monocytes, macrophages, T-lymphocytes, cytokines, interleukins, and the complement system.[1,3] The initial stage of the atherosclerotic lesion, the so-called fatty streak, which usually arises during the first decade of life, is a typical inflammatory lesion, consisting of monocyte-derived foamy macrophages and T-lymphocytes.[4]

As the lesion progresses, monocyte-derived macrophages, smooth muscle cells (SMCs), and T-lymphocytes replicate within it. Regulatory factors include tumor necrosis factor alpha (TNF-α), interleukin 6 (IL-6), interleukin 1 (IL-1), transforming growth factor beta (TGF-β), and proteolytic enzymes, particularly matrix metalloproteinases (MMPs) produced by macrophages, growth factors such as platelet-derived growth factor (PDGF) and insulin-like growth factor 1 (ILGF-1) produced by SMCs, and interferon γ (IFN-γ), IL-6, and interleukin-10 (IL-10) produced by T-cells.[1–3,5] Continued activation and infiltration of macrophages, as well as matrix degradation, can eventually cause erosion or rupture of the lesion's overlying fibrous cap.[6]

Rupture of the fibrous cap is likely to involve four processes: (i) proteolytic degradation of the matrix, mainly by macrophage enzymes; (ii) failure of vascular SMCs (VSMCs) to form a new matrix; (iii) failure of VSMCs to replicate after injury; and (iv) death of VSMCs in the fibrous cap.[2,7–9]

Cellular apoptosis in atherosclerosis

Apoptosis represents a model of genetically programmed cell death and is a major mechanism by which tissue removes unwanted, aged, or damaged cells.[10] Cells of mammalian tissues, despite their extensive broad diversity, undergo similar morphologic alterations during apoptosis, including chromatin compaction and margination, nuclear condensation and fragmentation, and cell body shrinkage and blebbing.[11]

Apoptosis is initiated through a complex interaction between external stimuli and internal gene expression. Once activated, the apoptotic process can progress in the absence of external stimuli. Apoptosis of vascular smooth muscle cells (SMCs), endothelial cells (ECs), and inflammatory cells or atheroma has been described in advanced human atherosclerosis.[7–9]

The main cellular components of the atherosclerotic lesions (i.e. SMCs, ECs, and MQs) are exposed to a broad variety of biologically active environmental factors which may induce or inhibit apoptosis (Table 23.1). Thus, apoptosis plays a critical role in atherosclerosis. It may contribute to a loss of luminal endothelial cells in response to cytokines, microbes, oxidants, or toxins. Apoptosis of macrophages and smooth muscle cells may have diverse impacts on the stability of the atherosclerotic lesions. Macrophage-derived cytokines and nitric oxide (NO) can inhibit SMC respiration and even

Table 23.1 Inducers and inhibitors of apoptosis in atherosclerosis. (Adapted from Geng YJ. Curr Atheroscler Rep 2001;3:234–42.[10])

Inducers

Oxidized low density lipoproteins

Oxysterols

Reactive oxygen species

Reactive nitrogen species (nitric oxide at high levels)

X-, gamma, and ultraviolet radiation

Heat

Cytokines

Fas ligand

Microorganisms

Inhibitors

Shear stress

Nitric oxide at low levels

Vascular endothelial growth factor

Basic fibroblast growth factor

Cowpox virus CremA

Baculovirus protein p35

The IAP protein family

lead to SMC apoptosis.[12] Therefore, macrophages, in addition to digesting the fibrous cap, are believed to prevent regeneration of the cap by SMCs.

SMC apoptosis appears to be involved in remodeling of the artery to compensate for reduced collagen production. More marked SMC apoptosis may contribute to formation of an aneurysm.[13]

Production of apoptosis-promoting cytotoxic substances by activated inflammatory cells or immune cells may induce death of vascular SMCs, which leads to the weakening of the fibrous cap and destabilization of the plaques. In addition, both apoptotic ECs and SMCs are highly pro-coagulative and may contribute to thrombus formation over the vulnerable plaques.[14–16]

Similarly, in the core of the plaque, macrophages undergo frequent apoptosis. This process presumably prevents them from exporting cholesterol and debris from the core, and it also protects against macrophage-derived cytokines and proteases.[17]

Role of nuclear factor-kappa B in atherosclerosis

The transcription factor known as nuclear factor-kappa B (NF-κB) plays an important role in inflammatory, immune, and proliferative processes and is activated in atherosclerotic lesions, e.g. in monocytic cells.[18–20] NF-κB comprises dimers, commonly p50/p65, that are trapped in the cytosol by inhibitory proteins, including IκB-α.[21] NF-κB is modulated by numerous conditions, including cytokines, bacterial products, oxidized lipoproteins, growth factors, platelets, and cellular stress.[22–24] Such modulation involves the phosphorylation of IκB, which subsequently undergoes ubiquitin-dependent proteasomal degradation. IκB phosphorylation is achieved by a high-molecular-weight kinase termed the IκB kinase (IKK) complex, with IKK-β and potentially IKK-α serving as the IκB phosphorylating components and IKK-α serving as a regulatory adaptor.[25,26] After stimulation, NF-κB translocates to the nucleus, where it may be involved in the coordinated expression of NF-κB target gene products within the lesion (e.g. cytokines, chemokines, adhesion molecules, proteases, growth factors, and procoagulatory molecules).[27]

Like cell proliferation, matrix synthesis, inflammation, and thrombosis, apoptosis is regulated in part by cytokines and NF-κB. TNF-α and IL-6, produced by both macrophages and SMCs, are multipotent mediators of inflammation and immunity in atherosclerotic plaques. These autocrine and paracrine mediators regulate the expression of vascular cell adhesion molecule 1 (VCAM-1), monocyte chemoattractant protein 1 (MCP-1), C-reactive protein (CRP), and fibrinogen, as well as the production of macrophage colony-stimulating factor (M-CSF) by vascular cells.[28,29] Activated T-cells may secrete interferon γ (IFN-γ), an inhibitor of SMC proliferation. Besides influencing arterial vasomotor tone by activating protein kinase C and NO synthase, cytokines also modulate endothelial functions that govern the formation and stability of thrombi.[30–33]

These diverse processes do not proceed uniformly within the arterial tree; plaques are histologically heterogeneous and, even in the same individual, adjacent plaques may be histologically different: some may be fibrous and muscular, whereas others may have large lipid cores with varying amounts of hemorrhage, calcification, and inflammation. The latter types – especially if thin-capped – are thought to be involved in the majority of plaque ruptures.[34] We have been able to show this heterogeneity at a functional level by demonstrating temperature heterogeneity and pH in adjacent plaques in the same artery.[35,36]

Heating and atherosclerosis

Gentle (fever-range) heating is known to have anti-proliferative, anti-inflammatory, and apoptosis-inducing capabilities.[35,37]

In vitro studies have shown that gentle heating enhances the cytotoxicity of chemotherapeutic agents.[38,39] Gentle heating reduces lipopolysaccharide (LPS) levels, stimulates secretion of TNF-α, IL-1β, and IL-6 by adult macrophages,[40] and, in isolated perfusion of the limb or liver, reduces cytokine production in endothelial cells.[41] We have previously shown that gentle heating downregulates pro-inflammatory genes (Table 23.2).

Consistent with the well-established heterogeneity of plaque histology (e.g. acellular regions, foci of apoptosis, and foci of inflammation), some areas of plaques are warmer than others.[35] This finding led us to determine whether heat influences the plaque or is just a metabolic byproduct.

A review of the literature yields ample evidence that heat can trigger apoptosis of malignant cells[42,43] and that thermal sensitivity varies among cell types,

Table 23.2 Heat (41°C/15 min) downregulates mRNA abundance for inflammation-related genes.

Target gene	Folds change in expression
Heat shock 27-kDa protein 1	3.5
Heat shock 70-kDa protein 1	3.2
Heat shock protein 86	2.2
Dad-1 (defender against cell death)	0.6
Cytokine receptor common gamma chain	0.6
Integrin alpha m	0.6
Intercellular adhesion molecule	0.6
Leukocyte adhesion protein (Ifa-1)	0.6
Map kinase-activated protein kinase	0.4
Interleukin 8	0.4
Glutathione peroxidase	0.3
Monocyte chemotactic protein	0.3
Interleukin 1 beta	0.3

being increased in highly active cells and in oxidized, hypoxic, and acidic environments.[43,44] These reports led us to hypothesize that plaque macrophages would be especially vulnerable to thermal apoptosis. Furthermore, in light of reports that heat can destabilize TNF-α m-RNA in cultured monocytes,[40] we also hypothesized that mild heat can inhibit the expression of inflammatory signals and genes.

Gentle thermal stimulation induces macrophage apoptosis in atherosclerotic lesions in human carotid plaques

We studied the effect of gentle heating on fresh atherectomy specimens collected from patients undergoing carotid artery endarterectomy at the Texas Heart Institute. Specimens were obtained in the operating room immediately after being inspected by the pathologist. To study inflamed plaques, we selected those with a temperature heterogeneity of >0.8°C. The tissues were placed in Dulbecco's modified eagle medium (DMEM; JRH Biosciences, Lenexa, KS, USA), which had been prewarmed at 37°C. Each specimen was cut into random pieces, which were heated in prewarmed DMEM at 36°C, 37°C, 38°C, 39°C, 40°C, 41°C, 42°C, and 43°C, respectively, for 15 minutes and were then transferred to an incubator, where they were kept for 6 hours.

All the plaque samples showed numerous TUNEL-positive nuclei characterized by a condensed, marginalized brown nucleus (Figure 23.1). Double staining with combined TUNEL and anti-SMC or macrophage staining revealed that the majority of apoptotic SMCs were located in the plaque intima and few were located in the media. In plaques incubated at 37°C, the percentages of TUNEL-positive SMCs and macrophages (Figure 23.1b, 23.2b, 23.3) were 4% and 8%, respectively. At higher temperatures, the number of apoptotic macrophages increased markedly compared to the number of SMCs. At 42°C, the percentages of apoptotic SMCs and macrophages were 10% and 46%, respectively (Figures 23.2b, 23.3).

In summary, at higher temperatures, there is a marked increase in the number of apoptotic macrophages but only a slight increase in the number of apoptotic SMCs. The results of TUNEL

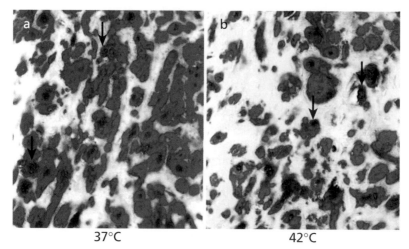

Figure 23.1 Results from TUNEL study. Note the dark brown TUNEL-positive nucleus: a, before heating (i.e. 37°C); b, after heating (i.e. 42°C for 15 minutes). The pink vector red areas represent α-actin-positive cells. The number of TUNEL-SMCs was insignificantly increased (4% at 37°C vs. 10% at 42°C).

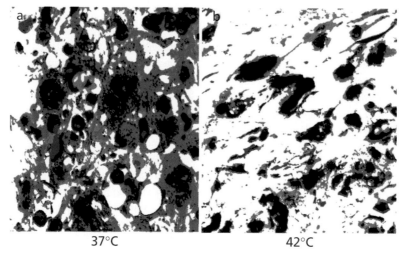

Figure 23.2 Results from the TUNEL study. a, Before heating (i.e. 37°C); b, after heating (i.e. 42°C for 15 minutes). The pink vector red areas represent HAM-56-positive cells. There was a significant increase in the number of TUNEL-positive macrophages (8% at 37°C vs. 46% at 42°C).

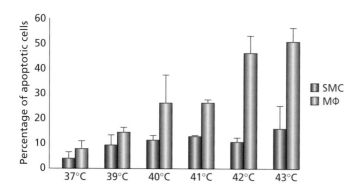

Figure 23.3 Temperature-response effects of heat on apoptosis in plaque macrophages (MΦ) and smooth muscle cells (SMCs). At 37°C, the proportion of apoptotic SMCs and macrophages was 4% and 8%, respectively. At 42°C, these proportions increased to 10% and 46%, respectively.

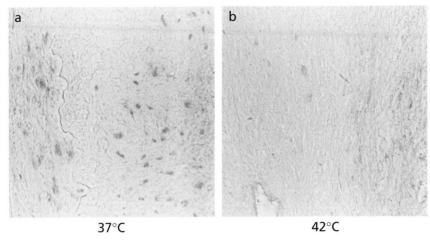

37°C   **42°C**

Figure 23.4 Immunohistochemical results showing expression of interleukin 6 (IL-6) in human carotid plaques. Paraffinized sections of plaques obtained during carotid endarterectomy were deparaffinized and stained with antibody to IL-6. Immunoreactive IL-6 in human specimens is shown: a, before heating (37°C); b, after heating (at 42°C for 15 minutes). Note the decrease in the total immunoreactive area after heating.

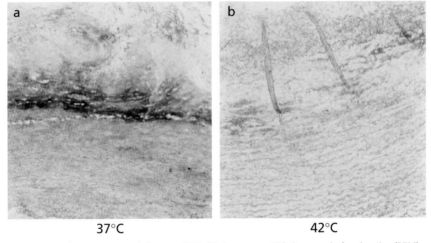

37°C   **42°C**

Figure 23.5 Immunoreactive tumor necrosis factor α (TNF-α) in human carotid plaque: a, before heating (37°C); b, after heating (at 42°C for 15 minutes). Note the decrease in the total immunoreactive area after heating.

staining of plaques were corroborated by electron microscopy.

Heating did not alter the morphology of the plaques. In plaques heated to 43°C, a large number of cells had disrupted membranes indicating necrosis. After thermal treatment, there was no significant change in the total area of immunoreactive myocyte enhancer factor 2 (MEF-2), a transcription factor, present only in living cells, indicating that different cell types in plaques are still viable after being heated up to 42°C.

Gentle heating reduces expression of proinflammatory cytokines

Thermal treatment reduced the amount of immunoreactive IL-6 by 50% (Figures 23.4a,b, 23.6a) and reduced the amount of immunoreactive TNF-β in human carotid plaques by 70% (Figures 23.5a,b, 23.6b). The average IL-6-stained area was 6.9% in untreated plaques versus 3.4% in treated ones. The lack of a significant change in the number of MEF-2-positive cells after heating indicates that the cells remain active and viable.

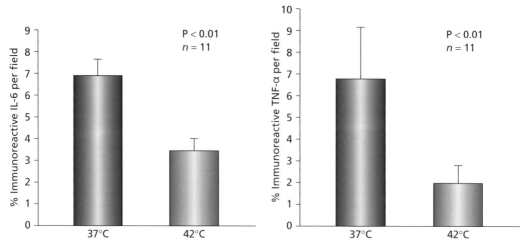

Figure 23.6 Results of manometric analysis of immunoreactive areas of interleukin 6 (IL-6) and tumor necrosis factor α (TNF-α) in human carotid plaques specimens. Heating at 42°C for 15 minutes reduced the IL-6 levels by 50% (a) and the TNF-α levels by 70% (b).

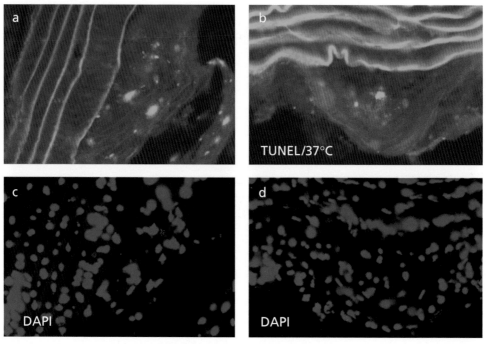

Figure 23.7 In situ labeling (TUNEL) of DNA fragments in the aortic tissue sections of apoE-null mice with and without gentle heating. Cryosections of aortas were labeled with terminal transferase and biotin-dUTP, and developed with FITC-Avidin (Intergen). Nuclear counterstaining was performed with DAPI. a, TUNEL of aorta with 42°C heating; b, TUNEL of aorta at 37°C; c and d, Images for total nuclear staining with DAPI in the same fields as a and b, respectively.

In situ end-labeling of DNA, DNA-ladder, and caspase studies in mice

Compared to heating at 37°C, ex vivo heating at 42°C for 15 minutes significantly increased the number of TUNEL-positive nuclei in the intima of the living aortas of apoE$^{-/-}$ mice ($n = 7$ in each group), as shown in Figure 23.7. The percentage of TUNEL-positive cells was approximately 15%

WILD TYPE APO-E^{−/−}

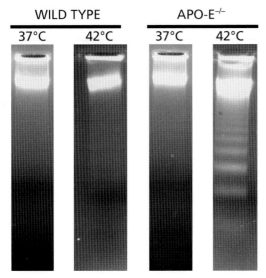

Figure 23.8 Internucleosomal DNA fragmentation in apoE-null aorta after gentle heating. Genomic DNA (2 μg/lane) was loaded into 2% agarose gels. After electrophoresis, DNA bands were documented by using a Kodak Image Station.

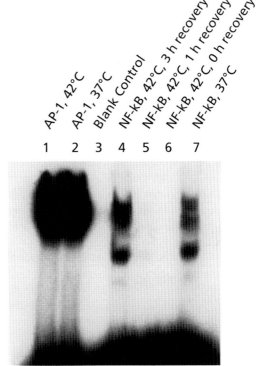

Figure 23.9 Electrophoretic mobility-shift assay detection of active NF-κB. Lanes 4 through 6 represent binding of NF-κB obtained from heat-treated (42°C) THP-1 cells at different recovery times. Lane 7 represents binding of NK-κB obtained from untreated (37°C) THP-1 cells.

in the 37°C apoE^{−/−} aortas versus >30% in the 42°C aortas. Most of the cells with TUNEL-positive nuclei were located in the lipid core regions of the plaques. Few or no TUNEL-positive nuclei were found in the medial layer.

To verify the occurrence of apoptosis, genomic DNA was isolated for electrophoresis. We detected a marked increase in internucleosomal DNA fragmentation in the apoE^{−/−} heated aortas but not the wild-type control specimens (Figure 23.8). At 37°C, no such "laddering" was found in the aortas of either the apoE^{−/−} or the wild-type mice. Double-labeling histochemistry showed that the majority of apoptotic cells were immunoreactive to antibodies against Mac3, a marker for macrophages, as well as to antibodies against caspase 3.

Gentle heating inactivates transcription factor NF-κB

The gel-shift assays demonstrated that heating can both prevent and reverse activation of NF-κB. There was almost total loss of the labeled NF-κB oligonucleotide shift with extracted THP-1 cells that were heated at 42°C but that were not incubated because nuclear extraction was done just after heating (Figure 23.9). The activity (shift) of

NF-κB recovered gradually over 3 hours. By contrast, heating had little effect on the gel shift assay using AP-1 oligonucleotides labeled with [γ-³²P] ATP as an internal control.

In summary, in human atherosclerotic tissues, gentle heat therapy (42 °C for 15 minutes) can suppress the inflammatory cytokines TNF-α and IL-6 by 70% and 50%, respectively. We measured the effect of heat on NF-κB activity to see whether TNF-α and IL-6 are downregulated by some biologic mechanism other than heat. Gentle heat had a direct inhibitory effect on NF-κB in THP-1 cells and was recovered completely after 3 hours. We used ATP-labeled γ-³²P AP-1 as an internal control. The fact that AP-1 activity was not affected by heating indicated that the heating specifically affected NF-κB activity.

However, inflammatory cells are not the sole contributors to plaque rupture. Apoptosis of

vascular SMCs is enhanced in atherosclerotic plaques compared to a normal arterial wall.[8] Plaque
vulnerability is better indicated by increased localization of macrophages and increased apoptosis of
cells in the plaque shoulders than by the integrity
of the fibrous cap that protects the highly thrombogenic necrotic core.[7]

In addition, the thin cap that overlies the atherosclerotic plaque has relatively small amounts of
collagen, and a large percentage of atheroma within
the plaque may predispose the plaque to rupture.[45]
In patients with high-grade internal carotid artery
stenosis, several groups have observed a significant
correlation between the extent of inflammatory
pathology and the development of plaque-related
ischemic complications.[46–48]

Plaque macrophages generate heat.[35] Because
heat is closely regulated in vivo and is capable of
causing apoptosis in cancer cells and other proliferating cells,[49] we hypothesized that plaque heat might
contribute to apoptosis of plaque macrophages.

Apoptosis in macrophages and smooth muscle cells

At 37 °C, the proportion of apoptotic SMCs and
macrophages was 4% and 8%, respectively. At 42
°C, the proportion increased to 10% and 46%. Also,
the viability of nonapoptotic cells in the plaque was
suggested by the fact that the results of MEF-2
immunostaining did not change significantly with
heat. Confirmatory findings were obtained with
transmission electron microscopy.

Gentle heat induced macrophage apoptosis at
high levels, which might protect the fibrous cap
since apoptosis of SMCs did not increase significantly with thermal treatment (Figure 23.10).

In untreated plaques, SMCs show apoptosis
but low levels of DNA synthesis and repair. By
contrast, macrophages show both apoptosis and
high levels of DNA synthesis and repair. Moreover, plaque macrophages express inducible nitric
oxygen synthase (iNOS) and may inactivate their
caspases by means of nitrosylation.[50] However, the
production of nitric oxide (NO) is inhibited
(although transiently) by heat, which is mediated
by a heat shock response.[51] Heating, superimposed
onto an already stressed plaque environment,
inhibits NO synthesis, decreases inactivation of
caspases, and, therefore, presumably increases

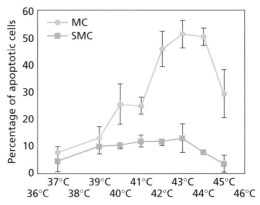

Figure 23.10 Plaque macrophages (MC) are more sensitive
to heat-induced apoptosis than smooth muscle cells (SMC).

apoptosis in macrophages. But, as mentioned
above, plaque SMCs show low levels of DNA synthesis and repair, so heating does not affect these
cells significantly. According to Hamuro and
coworkers,[52] induction of mild heat stress (42°C)
has enormous potential to inhibit SMC proliferation, thereby suppressing neointimal growth in vivo.

Effect of heat on cytokines

Heat is known to reduce the production of TNF-α
and IL-6.[40] Heat-induced heat shock proteins
(HSPs) also inhibit the DNA-binding activity of
NF-κB,[51] which, in turn, decreases TNF-α and IL-6
levels.

TNF-α provides cytoprotection to macrophages
and is known to be a survival factor for macrophages but not for SMCs. Thus, when heat
downregulates TNF-α, the natural protection for
macrophages is diminished, making plaque
macrophages vulnerable to death by apoptosis. By
contrast, SMCs are relatively unaffected because
their survival is not dependent on TNF-α.

Heating, crystallization, and macrophage apoptosis

Cholesterol crystals are abundant in atherosclerotic
lesions. Oxidized LDL cholesterol in foam cells is
originally in a solid state but melts after being heated
to 42°C. Human THP-1 macrophages treated with
the cholesterol oxide, 7-ketocholesterol, demonstrate a concentration- and time-dependent increase
in formation of cholesterol crystals in the cells.[53]
In experiments conducted under the normal cell

culture condition (i.e. 5% CO_2 and 37°C), incubation of macrophages with 7-ketocholesterol induced moderate levels of apoptosis. Increasing the temperature from 37°C to 40°C melts the crystals in the macrophages.[53] At high temperatures, significantly increased numbers of apoptotic cells can be detected in the cells treated with 7-ketocholesterol but not in those with native free cholesterol. These experiments by Geng et al. suggest that hyperthermia melts cholesterol crystals and promotes apoptotic effects of oxysterols on macrophages. The large number of crystals in foamy macrophages (compared to less foamy SMCs) may contribute to the greater sensitivity of plaque macrophages (compared to plaque SMCs) to thermal apoptosis.

Potential clinical relevance

Ten or 15 minutes of heating plaques to 40−42°C may prove useful as an adjunct to therapy to prevent restenosis and/or to decrease the amount of inflammation in an inflamed, thin-capped plaque. Inflammation is well established as a promoter of plaque progression and plaque rupture, and superficial inflammation is thought to promote thrombosis in the setting of denuded (eroded) plaque. Given the costs of drug-eluting stents and the increasing recognition that some patients have a second or even a third vulnerable plaque in a given coronary artery, a warm infusion could potentially reduce the risk of acute coronary events and be more cost-effective than the placement of multiple stents.

Obvious drawbacks include the fact that such a treatment would not remove cholesterol and would only increase the amount of necrotic debris. Whereas apoptosis is a natural, efficient and "clean" method of removing unwanted cells during embryogenesis and subsequent remodeling and wound healing, atherosclerotic plaques seem to "heal poorly." Compared to other wounds, plaques have a tendency to calcify and to scar rather than to regenerate the normal architecture. Most importantly, plaques accumulate cholesterol and necrotic cells, suggesting a failure of the usual clearance process for apoptotic and necrotic cells. The fact that clearance of apoptotic cells is mediated by the same scavenger receptor that takes up oxidized LDL suggests the hypothesis that large amounts of oxidized LDL competitively prevent the uptake of apoptotic cells. This may contribute to the "junkyard appearance" of advanced plaques. Obviously, the creation of more apoptotic macrophages would only add to this problem, even if it protected, for a short while, the plaque from being digested by living macrophages.

Fuster and colleagues have also offered the objection that apoptotic therapies might be nonselective, eliminating the smooth muscle cells required for regeneration of the fibrous cap and/or the antithrombotic vasorelaxing luminal endothelial cells. A second objection has been that in the process of apoptosis, cells flip the phosphatidylserine polarity of the membrane, and in so doing may release tissue factor. Apoptosis in general is not a process that leads to thrombosis, inflammation, or scarring, but conceivably could do so in the advanced, complex plaque.

The importance of this concern is hard to gauge, particularly if thermal apoptosis of macrophages is conducted in a cath lab setting with antithrombotic and anticoagulant treatments and careful monitoring. The concept would be akin to angioplasty and stenting, where significant damage is done under close monitoring to produce a long-term benefit. Since most of the macrophages are in fact located beneath the lumen, it is not at all certain that any transient release of tissue factor would be exposed to the circulating blood, and at any rate there is some logic to eliminating macrophages so that they can no longer divide and continue to release basal amounts of tissue factor and cytokines.

Other potential concerns include the possibility of a rebound after the gentle heating is terminated. Another drawback could be coagulation from the placement of a heating element in the bloodstream. Other studies have shown that a heating element above 55°C causes some platelet activation and red-cell hemolysis in a flowing artery. Warming strategies would have to use heating elements below that temperature or use other methods, such as the infusion of prewarmed saline, external warming as by ultrasound or radiofrequency, etc.

Still another drawback might be the activation of latent viruses, and this could be particularly problematic if it is combined with a reduction in macrophages, which could partially immunocompromise the plaque in the face of an activated virus.

Finally, there is a concern that the rapid melting of oxidized cholesterol crystals could create toxicity not only for the macrophages but for nearby smooth muscle or endothelial cells. On the plus side, gentle warming is likely to be vasodilating and could exert some myocardial benefit by means of heat-shock preconditioning, thereby improving the tolerance of any subsequent ischemic insult.

Suffice it to say that thermal therapy has strong potential benefits and drawbacks, and only careful experimentation can determine whether it might have some adjunctive role in the prevention of plaque progression, plaque rupture, thrombosis, or restenosis.

Conclusions

Gentle heating (42°C for 15 minutes) increases macrophage apoptosis, probably by inactivation of NF-κB, melting of crystal of oxidized cholesterol, and reduced expression of proinflammatory cytokines, TNF-α and IL-6. In the clinical setting, this method may prove useful to decrease inflammation in coronary plaques and "buy time" until systemic treatment can have an effect.

Acknowledgments

This work was supported in part by the United States Army's Disaster Relief and Emergency Medical Services (DREAMS) Grant #DAMD 17-98-1-8002. Authors wish to express their gratitude to John J Schwartz, PhD, Keith Youker, PhD, Mark Entman, MD, and Bruce Kone, MD for their help with selected experiments.

References

1. Ross R. Atherosclerosis – an inflammatory disease. N Engl J Med 1999;340:115–26.
2. Shah PK. Mechanisms of plaque vulnerability and rupture. J Am Coll Cardiol 2003;41:15S–22S.
3. Libby P, Aikawa M. Stabilization of atherosclerotic plaques: new mechanisms and clinical targets. Nat Med 2002;8:1257–62.
4. Stary HC, Chandler AB, Dinsmore RE, et al. A definition of advanced types of atherosclerotic lesions and a histological classification of atherosclerosis: a report from the Committee on Vascular Lesions of the Council on Arteriosclerosis, American Heart Association. 1995;15:1512–31.
5. Hansson GK. Regulation of immune mechanisms in atherosclerosis. Ann NY Acad Sci 2001;947:157–65; discussion 165–6.
6. Virmani R, Burke AP, Kolodgie FD, Farb A. Pathology of the thin-cap fibroatheroma: a type of vulnerable plaque. J Interv Cardiol 2003;16:267–72.
7. Geng YJ, Libby P. Evidence for apoptosis in advanced human atheroma. Colocalization with interleukin-1 beta-converting enzyme. Am J Pathol 1995;147:251–66.
8. Han DK, Haudenschild CC, Hong MK, Tinkle BT, Leon MB, Liau G. Evidence for apoptosis in human atherogenesis and in a rat vascular injury model. Am J Pathol 1995;147:267–77.
9. Isner JM, Kearney M, Bortman S, Passeri J. Apoptosis in human atherosclerosis and restenosis. Circulation 1995;91:2703–11.
10. Geng YJ. Biologic effect and molecular regulation of vascular apoptosis in atherosclerosis. Curr Atheroscler Rep 2001;3:234–42.
11. Kerr JF, Wyllie AH, Currie AR. Apoptosis: a basic biological phenomenon with wide-ranging implications in tissue kinetics. Br J Cancer 1972;26:239–57.
12. Lau HK. Cytotoxicity of nitric oxide donors in smooth muscle cells is dependent on phenotype, and mainly due to apoptosis. Atherosclerosis 2003;166:223–32.
13. Prati F, Arbustini E, Labellarte A, et al. Eccentric atherosclerotic plaques with positive remodelling have a pericardial distribution: a permissive role of epicardial fat? A three-dimensional intravascular ultrasound study of left anterior descending artery lesions. Eur Heart J 2003;24:329–36.
14. Bombeli T, Karsan A, Tait JF, Harlan JM. Apoptotic vascular endothelial cells become procoagulant. Blood 1997;89:2429–42.
15. Flynn PD, Byrne CD, Baglin TP, Weissberg PL, Bennett MR. Thrombin generation by apoptotic vascular smooth muscle cells. Blood 1997;89:4378–84.
16. Greeno EW, Bach RR, Moldow CF. Apoptosis is associated with increased cell surface tissue factor procoagulant activity. Lab Invest 1996;75:281–9.
17. Takahashi K, Takeya M, Sakashita N. Multifunctional roles of macrophages in the development and progression of atherosclerosis in humans and experimental animals. Med Electron Microsc 2002;35:179–203.
18. Brand K, Page S, Rogler G, et al. Activated transcription factor nuclear factor-kappa B is present in the atherosclerotic lesion. J Clin Invest 1996;97:1715–22.
19. Collins T. Endothelial nuclear factor-kappa B and the initiation of the atherosclerotic lesion. Lab Invest 1993;68:499–508.
20. Baeuerle PA, Baltimore D. NF-kappa B: ten years after. Cell 1996;87:13–20.

21. Thanos D, Maniatis T. NF-kappa B: a lesson in family values. Cell 1995;80:529–32.

22. Page S, Fischer C, Baumgartner B, et al. 4-Hydroxynonenal prevents NF-kappa B activation and tumor necrosis factor expression by inhibiting I kappa B phosphorylation and subsequent proteolysis. J Biol Chem 1999;274:11611–18.

23. Brand K, Eisele T, Kreusel U, et al. Dysregulation of monocytic nuclear factor-kappa B by oxidized low-density lipoprotein. Arterioscler Thromb Vasc Biol 1997;17:1901–9.

24. Gawaz M, Neumann FJ, Dickfeld T, et al. Activated platelets induce monocyte chemotactic protein-1 secretion and surface expression of intercellular adhesion molecule-1 on endothelial cells. Circulation 1998;98: 1164–71.

25. Karin M, Ben-Neriah Y. Phosphorylation meets ubiquitination: the control of NF-[kappa]B activity. Annu Rev Immunol 2000;18:621–63.

26. Israel A. The IKK complex: an integrator of all signals that activate NF-[kappa]B? Trends Cell Biol 2000;10: 129–33.

27. Whiteside ST, Israel A. I[kappa]B proteins: structure, function and regulation. Semin Cancer Biol 1997;8: 75–82.

28. Mortensen RF. C-reactive protein, inflammation, and innate immunity. Immunol Res 2001;24:163–76.

29. Libby P, Sukhova G, Lee RT, Galis ZS. Cytokines regulate vascular functions related to stability of the atherosclerotic plaque. J Cardiovasc Pharmacol 1995;25(suppl 2): S9–12.

30. Lidington EA, Haskard DO, Mason JC. Induction of decay-accelerating factor by thrombin through a protease-activated receptor 1 and protein kinase C-dependent pathway protects vascular endothelial cells from complement-mediated injury. Blood 2000;96:2784–92.

31. Pahl HL. Activators and target genes of Rel/NF-kappa B transcription factors. Oncogene 1999;18:6853–66.

32. Park SH, Kim KE, Hwang HY, Kim TY. Regulatory effect of SOCS on NF-kappa B activity in murine monocytes/macrophages. DNA Cell Biol 2003;22:131–9.

33. Barkett M, Gilmore TD. Control of apoptosis by Rel/NF-kappa B transcription factors. Oncogene 1999;18: 6910–24.

34. Ritchie ME. Nuclear factor-kappa B is selectively and markedly activated in humans with unstable angina pectoris. Circulation 1998;98:1707–13.

35. Casscells W, Hathorn B, David M, et al. Thermal detection of cellular infiltrates in living atherosclerotic plaques: possible implications for plaque rupture and thrombosis. Lancet 1996;347:1447–51.

36. Naghavi M, John R, Naguib S, et al. pH Heterogeneity of human and rabbit atherosclerotic plaques;a new insight into detection of vulnerable plaque. Atherosclerosis 2002;164:27–35.

37. Zellner M, Hergovics N, Roth E, Jilma B, Spittler A, Oehler R. Human monocyte stimulation by experimental whole body hyperthermia. Wien Klin Wochenschr 2002;114:102–7.

38. Urano M, Ling CC. Thermal enhancement of melphalan and oxaliplatin cytotoxicity in vitro. Int J Hyperthermia 2002;18:307–15.

39. Sakurai H, Mitsuhashi N, Kitamoto Y, et al. Cytotoxic enhancement of low dose-rate irradiation in human lung cancer cells by mild hyperthermia. Anticancer Res 1998;18:2525–8.

40. Fairchild KD, Viscardi RM, Hester L, Singh IS, Hasday JD. Effects of hypothermia and hyperthermia on cytokine production by cultured human mononuclear phagocytes from adults and newborns. J Interferon Cytokine Res 2000;20:1049–55.

41. Gnant MF, Turner EM, Alexander HR, Jr. Effects of hyperthermia and tumour necrosis factor on inflammatory cytokine secretion and procoagulant activity in endothelial cells. Cytokine 2000;12:339–47.

42. Brade AM, Szmitko P, Ngo D, Liu FF, Klamut HJ. Heat-directed suicide gene therapy for breast cancer. Cancer Gene Ther 2003;10:294–301.

43. Xia W, Hardy L, Liu L, et al. Concurrent exposure to heat shock and H7 synergizes to trigger breast cancer cell apoptosis while sparing normal cells. Breast Cancer Res Treat 2003;77:233–43.

44. Masunaga S, Ono K, Takahashi A, et al. Usefulness of combined treatment with mild temperature hyperthermia and/or tirapazamine in the treatment of solid tumors: its independence of p53 status. Cancer Sci 2003;94:125–33.

45. Davies MJ, Richardson PD, Woolf N, Katz DR, Mann J. Risk of thrombosis in human atherosclerotic plaques: role of extracellular lipid, macrophage, and smooth muscle cell content. Br Heart J 1993;69:377–81.

46. Bassiouny HS, Sakaguchi Y, Mikucki SA, et al. Juxtalumenal location of plaque necrosis and neoformation in symptomatic carotid stenosis. J Vasc Surg 1997;26:585–94.

47. Jander S, Sitzer M, Schumann R, et al. Inflammation in high-grade carotid stenosis: a possible role for macrophages and T cells in plaque destabilization. Stroke 1998;29:1625–30.

48. Golledge J, Greenhalgh RM, Davies AH. The symptomatic carotid plaque. Stroke 2000;31:774–81.

49. Ohtsubo T, Igawa H, Saito T, et al. Acidic environment modifies heat- or radiation-induced apoptosis in human maxillary cancer cells. Int J Radiat Oncol Biol Phys 2001;49:1391–8.

50. Kockx MM, Herman AG. Apoptosis in atherosclerosis: beneficial or detrimental? Cardiovasc Res 2000;45: 736–46.

51. de Vera ME, Kim YM, Wong HR, Wang Q, Billiar TR, Geller DA. Heat shock response inhibits cytokine-inducible nitric oxide synthase expression in rat hepatocytes. Hepatology 1996;24:1238–45.

52. Hamuro M, Nakamura K, Yamada R, Matsuoka T, Kaminou T, Nishida N. Inhibition of neointimal hyperplasia by heat stress in an experimental model. J Vasc Interv Radiol 2002;13:1247–53.

53. Geng Y-J, Phillips JE, Mason RP, Casscells SW. Cholesterol crystallization and macrophage apoptosis: implication for atherosclerotic plaque instability and rupture. Biochem Pharmacol 2003;66:1485–92.

CHAPTER 24

An interventionalist's perspective

Aloke V Finn, Ronald Waksman & Herman Gold

Plaque rupture resulting in thrombotic occlusion is the major pathologic event initiating myocardial infarction. Thus far, interventional cardiologists have focused on developing techniques designed to restore flow in arteries possessing hemodynamically significant lesions causing cardiac ischemia or infarction. This reactive strategy does little to prevent future coronary events. Since most acute coronary syndromes result from plaques that are are modest in severity, coronary angiography is of limited utility in detecting these lesions before they rupture.[1,2] These rupture-prone or vulnerable plaques have been defined pathologically to possess a large lipid core, thin-fibrous cap and inflammatory cell, particularly macrophage, infiltration. While pharmacologic therapy with agents such as aspirin and statins do reduce risk of future myocardial infarction they do not eliminate this risk.[3,4] The real question for the interventionalist remains whether early identification and invasive treatment of these lesions will reduce significantly future risk of acute coronary syndromes.

Although there have been recent advances in in vivo imaging of coronary plaques with the use of intravascular ultrasound (IVUS), optical coherence tomography (OCT), magnetic reasonance (MR), and computerized tomography (CT), these technologies have yet to achieve the goal of characterizing plaque morphology to the degree necessary to correctly identify rupture-prone lesions according to pathologic criteria.[5] Limitations of currently available technology include inability to provide high-resolution circumferential characterization of the vascular wall, significant motion artifact, and inability to adequately penetrate into the arterial wall in order to visualize plaque characteristics.

Another important problem with the concept that invasive treatment of vulnerable plaques will reduce cardiac morbidity and mortality is the lack of clear evidence between the presence of a pathologically defined vulnerable plaque and near-term risk of cardiac events.[6] The definition of vulnerable plaque stems from autopsy evidence from patients presenting with sudden cardiac death who had evidence of acute plaque rupture. These plaques were characterized by the presence of: (i) large necrotic core; (ii) thin fibrous cap overlying the core defined as <65 μm thick; and (iii) inflammatory cells, particularly macrophages within the cap itself especially in the shoulder regions.[7]

The major limitation to this current paradigm is lack of a prospective animal or human model of plaque rupture. As a result, no in vivo evidence exists to confirm that these pathologically defined vulnerable plaques consistently rupture leading to major cardiac events. Indeed, autopsy studies demonstrate that plaque rupture is often clinically silent and that repeated ruptures with or without associated thrombi may occur within the same plaque.[8,9] In patients dying of sudden cardiac death both Davies and Burke have demonstrated that healed ruptures occur frequently without occlusive or sub-occlusive thrombus and that these ruptures are a form of wound healing that progressively result in luminal narrowing without acute clinical effect. Therefore, even if the technology were adequate to correctly identify vulnerable plaques by the currently available rigorous pathology criteria, it is unclear whether percutaneous intervention by standard balloon angioplasty or stenting will result in fewer cardiac events.

Given these limitations, a more realistic strategy

is to identify by means of clinical, laboratory and angiographic criteria patients who are at high risk for recurrent cardiac events. Since these patients possess plaques whose near-term risk of causing acute coronary syndromes is high, these so called "vulnerable patients" may benefit from percutaneous coronary intervention (PCI) and adjunctive pharmacotherapy delivered either locally or systemically to stabilize high risk lesions. Goldstein et al. have shown that patients presenting with acute ST-elevation myocardial infarction (MI) may harbor multiple complex coronary plaques in addition to the culprit lesion and that nonculprit plaques are associated with adverse cardiac clinical outcomes within 1 year.[10] These complex plaques were defined angiographically as lesions >50% in diameter associated with an intraluminal filling defect consistent with thrombus and plaque ulceration or irregularity either in a different artery from the artery containing the infarct-related plaque or in the same artery containing the infarct-related artery but in a different branch (Figure 24.1). Patients were divided by whether they had one or multiple complex plaques and were followed clinically for 12 months. Those with multiple complex plaques had an increased frequency of recurrent acute coronary syndromes (19.0%) versus those

with a single complex plaque (2.0%, $P < 0.001$) and required more frequent revascularization within the next year. The authors postulated that acute MI reflected a diffuse pathophysiologic process resulting in multifocal plaque instability and rapid plaque progression associated with clinical instability. Patients presenting with acute MI who demonstrate multiple complex coronary plaques at angiography are at high risk for recurrent coronary events even after successful PCI of the culprit lesion.

Other data confirm that in patients presenting with acute MI systemic coronary disease activity may lead to nonculprit lesion progression even in the very near term. As reported by Guazzi et al., 1 month follow-up coronary angiography of nonculprit lesions in patients who presented with ST-segment elevation demonstrated significant progression (reduction from 12% to 45% of the minimal lumen diameter) in the majority of nonculprit lesions, whereas there was essentially no change on follow-up angiography in patients who had presented with stable angina.[11] Some investigators have also reported evidence of multifocal plaque instability as seen by angioscopy in patients with acute MI.[12] Using IVUS, Rioufol et al. found at least one plaque rupture in a site different from

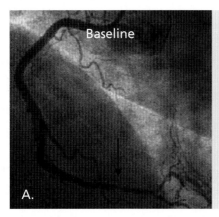
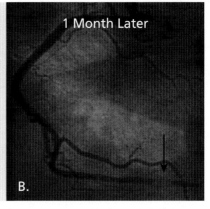

Figure 24.1 Rapid progression of nonculprit lesion in patients with type 2 diabetes mellitus. A 60-year-old female with a history of insulin treated type 2 diabetes mellitus, hypertension, and hyperlipidemia presented to our hospital with complaints of chest pain and shortness of breath. EKG revealed ST-segment elevation in I, L, V4–V6 and coronary angiography demonstrated acute occlusion of the mid left circumflex artery. Right coronary angiography revealed a moderate lesion in the distal vessel (A). The patient underwent stent placement to the circumflex with a good result and was discharged in good condition. She did well until 1 month later when she again complained of chest pain. Repeat coronary angiography demonstrated patent circumflex stent but significant progression of the distal right coronary artery lesion (B) which was felt to be the culprit. She underwent stent placement to this lesion and did well post PCI.

that of the culprit lesion in patients presenting with acute MI.[13]

In addition to patients with acute MI, those with diabetes mellitus also have significantly worse cardiac outcomes after coronary angioplasty of the culprit lesion and should be included as "vulnerable patients." It is commonly recognized that the increase in major adverse cardiac events seen in this patient population is in part due to the need for repeat revascularization of the stented lesion due to restenosis.[14,15] Another important factor underlying adverse outcomes seen in diabetic patients after PCI is the fact that a large number of these patients undergo repeat PCI at a site different from that of the initial treated lesion (Figure 24.2).[16] The Arterial Revascularization Therapy Study (ARTS) trial demonstrated a twofold high mortality in

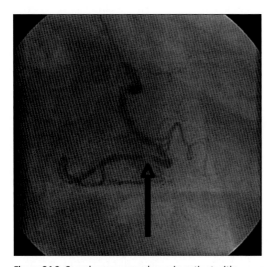

Figure 24.2 Complex coronary plaque in patient with anterior MI. A 75-year-old male with a history of hypertension and hyperlipidemia presented to our hospital complaining of chest pain. EKG revealed anterior ST segment elevation and he was taken to the cardiac catheterization lab. Left coronary angiography revealed acute occlusion of the proximal left anterior descending artery (LAD). Right coronary angiography demonstrated 65% stenosis of the mid right coronary artery (see arrow). The patient underwent stent placement to the proximal LAD and was discharged in good condition. Patients presenting with acute ST segment elevation MI who harbor complex nonculprit coronary lesions have been shown to be at high risk for recurrent coronary events.

diabetic patients with multivessel disease undergoing PCI versus coronary artery bypass surgery (CABG).[17] A significant reason for this was due to nonculprit lesion progression.[18] In the Prevention of REStenosis with Tranilast and its Outcomes (PRESTO) trial which examined the effect of tranilast on restenosis prevention after coronary stenting, diabetic patients had a 33% increase over nondiabetic patients in new lesion formation over the next 9 months.[19] Moreover, adverse clinical events including MI and death were more frequent in diabetic versus nondiabetic patients.

In these two groups of "vulnerable patients," there are a number of approaches available to the interventionalist with the idea of achieving coronary artery plaque stabilization, thereby preventing future coronary events. These include traditional mechanical approaches such as: (i) balloon angioplasty and stenting; (ii) new systemic therapies aimed at pharmacologic plaque passivation; and (iii) local catheter based drug delivery.

The use of traditional balloon angioplasty and stenting to prevent future cardiac events is an appealing concept. As eluded to earlier, multiple problems exist with this approach including inability to currently correctly identify vulnerable plaques and lack of an understanding of the natural history of vulnerable plaques in man or any animal model. Mercado et al. investigated the clinical and angiographic outcomes in patients with chronic stable angina and a single lesion with stenosis prior to PCI categorized into three groups (mild, moderate, and severe) who underwent either coronary balloon angioplasty or stenting.[20] The authors hypothesized that coronary intervention in patients with mild stenoses would prevent cardiac events as a consequence of "plaque sealing" (i.e. dilatation of angiographically nonsignificant lesions). Of the 3812 patients included in this study, 39% received balloon angioplasty alone and 61% were treated with stenting. One year mortality and rate of nonfatal MI did not differ in any of the three categories of lesion severity treated. The authors concluded that with current technology "plaque sealing" could not prevent death and future nonfatal MIs because 1-year event rates (in particular repeat revascularization) after PCI of nonsignificant stenosis remained unacceptably high when compared with the estimated probability of non-fatal MIs in lesions with <50% diameter stenosis. A similar result was seen in the DEFER trial which examined medical therapy or PCI based on fractional flow reserve for patients with angiographic stenoses, chest pain, but no ischemia on stress testing.[21] In conclusion, PCI of angiographically mild to moderate lesions in patients with stable coronary disease does not result in improved outcomes due to stabilization of these plaques. These results are not surprising given that the patient populations chosen in these two trials have not been identified to be at high risk for recurrent coronary events.

Recently the introduction of drug-eluting stents (DES) such as Cypher and Taxus for the treatment of coronary stenoses has resulted in a marked decrease in restenosis and target lesion revascularization when compared to bare metal stents.[22,23] They have been proposed as a superior alternative to the current generation of bare metal stents for treating angiographically mild to moderate lesions, since they would likely reduce the incidence of repeat revascularization. However, the major problem facing the use of DES to prophylactically treat lesions of mild to moderate severity is the fact that we lack the ability to correctly identify plaque morphology and predict the natural history of such lesions. Moreover, the risks associated with DES such as unpredictable stent thrombosis, hypersensitivity reactions, and possible late intimal rebound make such an approach less appealing but tenable.[24]

Another potential approach to treat vulnerable plaques is pharmacologic therapy based upon our understanding of the pathology and pathophysiology of coronary lesion development and progression. This concept has the advantage that is does not require direct identification of plaque morphology. Recently, data from the Pravastatin or Atorvastatin Evaluation and Infection Therapy (PROVE IT-TIMI 22) study demonstrated that an intensive lipid-lowering statin regimen provided greater protection against future death or major cardiovascular events than did a standard regimen in patients presenting with an acute coronary syndrome.[25] This study underscored the idea that systemic therapy with oral medications may be the best approach to preventing future cardiac events.

In addition to currently used therapies such as statins, aspirin, beta-blockers, and angiotensin converting enzyme inhibitors (ACEI), there is need for new medicines which target the multiple pathways thought to underlie coronary disease progression such as inflammation, smooth muscle cell migration and proliferation, insulin resistance, and defects in the endogenous fibrinolytic system. The glitazones are agonists of the peroxisomal proliferators-activated receptor gamma (PPARγ), have multiple beneficial effects on vascular cells, and are commercially available for the treatment of type 2 diabetes.[26] These drugs are known to: (i) inhibit smooth muscle cell growth and migration; (ii) limit the production of pro-inflammatory and pro-atherosclerotic cytokines; (iii) improve defects in fibrinolysis by decreasing fibrinogen and plasminogen activator inhibitor-1 (PAI-1) levels; and (iv) reduce insulin levels by improving insulin sensitivity in a variety of tissues.[27,28] Haffner et al. reported that in patients with type 2 diabetes treatment with 26 weeks of the PPARγ oral agonist rosiglitazone resulted in significantly lower levels of C-reactive protein (CRP) and matrix metalloproteinase-9 (MMP-9) compared to diabetic patients receiving pacebo.[29] These findings suggest a potential beneficial effect on overall atherosclerotic risk. Another study by Minamikawa et al. demonstrated that type 2 diabetic patients treated with the PPARγ agonist troglitazone demonstrated a significant decrease in common carotid intima to media ratio compared to control patients, suggesting a potent inhibitory effect on progression of early atherosclerosis.[30,31] We are currently conducting a trial (PROVIDENCE) to examine whether the PPARγ agonist rosiglitazone prevents stent restenosis and non-culprit lesion progression as indicated by 8 months quantitative coronary angiography (QCA) and IVUS in patients with type 2 diabetes mellitus undergoing coronary stent placement (Figure 24.3).

Another more invasive and targeted method of plaque stabilization might be local delivery of pharmacologic agents at plaque sites through a low pressure porous balloon. Potential drugs might include anti-angiogenic agents which would decrease plaque vascularity and thus the incidence of intraplaque hemorrhage, pro-fibrotic agents which would aim to increase smooth muscle and collagen content and thus the thickness of fibrous

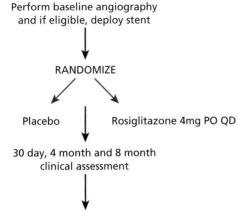

Perform baseline angiography
and if eligible, deploy stent

↓

RANDOMIZE

↙   ↘

Placebo   Rosiglitazone 4mg PO QD

↓

30 day, 4 month and 8 month
clinical assessment

↓

8-month follow-up angiogram and IVUS
(culprit and non culprit lesions)

Figure 24.3 PROVIDENCE Trial Schema. We are currently conducting a randomized double-blind placebo-controlled trial to examine the effects of rosiglitazone, a commercially available PPARγ agonist, on stent restenosis and nonculprit lesion progression in patients with type 2 diabetes undergoing coronary stent placement. The trial will randomize patients to 4 mg rosiglitazone or placebo per day and follow them for 8 months, at which time all patients will undergo repeat angiography and culprit vessel IVUS. The primary endpoint will be late lumen loss.

caps decreasing chances of rupture, and perhaps anti-inflammatory agents which would lower the inflammatory cell concentration of the cap itself which might stabilize plaques through a decrease in production of proteinases and other elements thought to be important in the genesis of plaque destabilization. As yet it is extremely difficult to know what the optimal agent might be, since no adequate animal model of prospective plaque rupture exists in which to tests these agents. Nonetheless, the concept of targeted treatment of vulnerable plaques is appealing. The goal might be to promote lesion stabilization by promoting accumulation of smooth muscle cell, collagen and matrix formation around a thin-fibrous cap with the idea of preventing cap rupture. As our technology improves to accurately locate vulnerable plaques, this might one day be a realistic approach.

Recently we have developed an animal model of plaque hemorrhage in which to test this idea. This model is based upon the hypothesis that intraplaque hemorrhage is a prerequisite for the development of a lipid core, a key feature of the vulnerable plaque. By injecting autologous red cells in a previously balloon-injured rabbit iliac artery, we demonstrated lesions with a significant increase in lipid as well as macrophage content that resembled advanced plaques seen in humans (Figure 24.4).[32] This model will be used to test the concept of whether interventional treatment of the vulnerable plaque will change the morphology in a favorable manner resulting in lesion stabilization.

In summary, the interventional treatment of vulnerable plaque is an appealing idea since it changes our focus from a reactive strategy of treating symptomatic coronary ischemia or infarction to preventing these events before they occur. However, the reality is that we currently do not have sufficient experimental or clinical information to justify such an approach. We need to understand better the relationship between our pathologic definition of vulnerable plaque and the actual progression of these plaques to clinical events. Moreover, we do not currently possess an imaging modality with enough resolution to allow us to visualize these plaques in vivo. In the meantime, we should concentrate on identifying patients known to be at high risk for disease progression, such as those with acute MI and evidence of other nonculprit lesions on coronary angiography as well as patients with diabetes mellitus. Treatment of these patients with agents known to decrease cardiac mortality and disease progression, such as beta-blockers, angiotensin converting enzyme inhibitors, statins, and perhaps PPARγ activators such as rosiglitazone or pioglitazone, should be our first priority. As our understanding of coronary disease grows, we may be able to make the interventional treatment of vulnerable plaque a reality.

References

1. Ambrose JA, Tannenbaum MA, Alexopoulos D, et al. Angiographic progression of coronary artery disease and the development of myocardial infarction. J Am Coll Cardiol 1988;12:56–62.
2. Falk E, Shah PK, Fuster V. Coronary plaque disruption. Circulation 1995;92:657–71.
3. MRC/BHF Heart Protection Study of cholesterol lowering with simvastatin in 20 536 high-risk individuals: a randomised placebo-controlled trial. Lancet 2002;360: 7–22.
4. Collaborative meta-analysis of randomised trials of antiplatelet therapy for prevention of death, myocardial

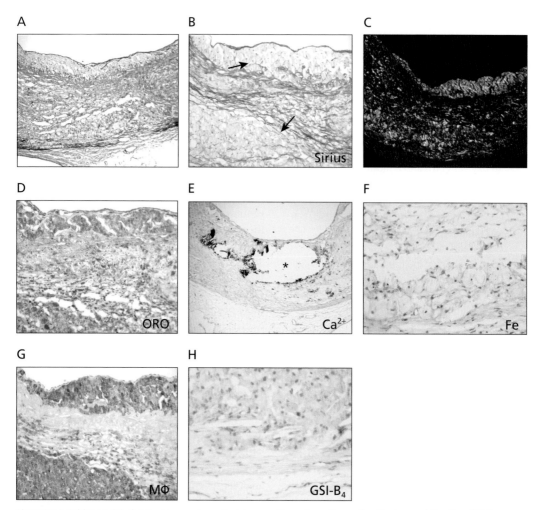

Figure 24.4 Rabbit model of plaque hemorrhage. Serial cryosections of an atherosclerotic plaque at the site of RBC injection. Autologous RBCs were injected into established plaques and arteries were harvested 6 weeks thereafter. A, High power view of an arterial section stained by Movat Pentachrome showing macrophage infiltration in the superficial and deep intima. B, Identification of interstitial collagen by Sirius red. A plane of dense connective tissue is seen separated by cellular-rich areas in the superficial and deep layers of the intima (arrows). C, The accumulation of strongly birefringent lipid. D, Oil red O staining demonstrating extensive lipid accumlation in the superficial and deep intima. E, Large calcified area (asterisk, von Kossa, ×100). F, Mallory's iron staining showing iron deposition in blue in an area of macrophage accumulation. G, Extensive macrophage (MΦ) accumulation at a site of injected red cells. H, Lectin staining of red cell membranes colocalized with numerous cholesterol crystals and macrophages (×400). (Figures A, D, F, G and H reproduced with permission from Kolodgie et al., New Eng J. 2003;349:2316–2325.)

infarction, and stroke in high risk patients. Br Med J 2002;324:71–86.

5. MacNeill BD, Lowe HC, Takano M, Fuster V, Jang IK. Intravascular modalities for detection of vulnerable plaque: current status. Arterioscler Thromb Vasc Biol 2003;23:1333–42.

6. Virmani R, Kolodgie FD, Burke AP, Farb A, Schwartz SM. Lessons from sudden coronary death: a comprehensive morphological classification scheme for atherosclerotic lesions. Arterioscler Thromb Vasc Biol 2000;20:1262–75.

7. Burke AP, Farb A, Malcom GT, Liang YH, Smialek J, Virmani R. Coronary risk factors and plaque morphology in men with coronary disease who died suddenly. N Engl J Med 1997;336:1276–82.

8. Mann J, Davies MJ. Mechanisms of progression in native coronary artery disease: role of healed plaque disruption. Heart 1999;82:265–8.

9. Burke AP, Kolodgie FD, Farb A, et al. Healed plaque ruptures and sudden coronary death: evidence that subclinical rupture has a role in plaque progression. Circulation 2001;103:934–40.

10. Goldstein JA, Demetriou D, Grines CL, Pica M, Shoukfeh M, O'Neill WW. Multiple complex coronary plaques in patients with acute myocardial infarction. N Engl J Med 2000;343:915–22.

11. Guazzi MD, Bussotti M, Grancini L, et al. Evidence of multifocal activity of coronary disease in patients with acute myocardial infarction. Circulation 1997;96: 1145–51.

12. Asakura M, Ueda Y, Yamaguchi O, et al. Extensive development of vulnerable plaques as a pan-coronary process in patients with myocardial infarction: an angioscopic study. J Am Coll Cardiol 2001;37:1284–8.

13. Rioufol G, Finet G, Ginon I, et al. Multiple atherosclerotic plaque rupture in acute coronary syndrome: a three-vessel intravascular ultrasound study. Circulation 2002;106:804–8.

14. Carrozza JP, Jr, Kuntz RE, Levine MJ, et al. Angiographic and clinical outcome of intracoronary stenting: immediate and long-term results from a large single-center experience. J Am Coll Cardiol 1992;20:328–37.

15. Kastrati A, Schomig A, Elezi S, et al. Predictive factors of restenosis after coronary stent placement. J Am Coll Cardiol 1997;30:1428–36.

16. Loutfi M, Mulvihill NT, Boccalatte M, Farah B, Fajadet J, Marco J. Impact of restenosis and disease progression on clinical outcome after multivessel stenting in diabetic patients. Catheter Cardiovasc Interv 2003;58:451–4.

17. Abizaid A, Costa MA, Centemero M, et al. Clinical and economic impact of diabetes mellitus on percutaneous and surgical treatment of multivessel coronary disease patients: insights from the Arterial Revascularization Therapy Study (ARTS) trial. Circulation 2001;104:533–8.

18. Kuntz RE. Importance of considering atherosclerosis progression when choosing a coronary revascularization strategy: the diabetes–percutaneous transluminal coronary angioplasty dilemma. Circulation 1999;99:847–51.

19. Mathew V, Gersh BJ, Williams BA, et al. Outcomes in patients with diabetes mellitus undergoing percutaneous coronary intervention in the current era: a report from the Prevention of REStenosis with Tranilast and its Outcomes (PRESTO) trial. Circulation 2004;109:476–80.

20. Mercado N, Maier W, Boersma E, et al. Clinical and angiographic outcome of patients with mild coronary lesions treated with balloon angioplasty or coronary stenting. Implications for mechanical plaque sealing. Eur Heart J 2003;24:541–51.

21. Bech GJ, De Bruyne B, Pijls NH, et al. Fractional flow reserve to determine the appropriateness of angioplasty in moderate coronary stenosis: a randomized trial. Circulation 2001;103:2928–34.

22. Moses JW, Leon MB, Popma JJ, et al. Sirolimus-eluting stents versus standard stents in patients with stenosis in a native coronary artery. N Engl J Med 2003;349:1315–23.

23. Stone GW, Ellis SG, Cox DA, et al. A polymer-based, paclitaxel-eluting stent in patients with coronary artery disease. N Engl J Med 2004;350:221–31.

24. Virmani R, Guagliumi G, Farb A, et al. Localized hypersensitivity and late coronary thrombosis secondary to a sirolimus-eluting stent: should we be cautious? Circulation 2004;109:701–5.

25. Cannon CP, Braunwald E, McCabe CH, et al. Intensive versus moderate lipid lowering with statins after acute coronary syndromes. N Engl J Med 2004;350:1495–504.

26. Duval C, Chinetti G, Trottein F, Fruchart JC, Staels B. The role of PPARs in atherosclerosis. Trends Mol Med 2002;8:422–30.

27. Law RE, Meehan WP, Xi XP, et al. Troglitazone inhibits vascular smooth muscle cell growth and intimal hyperplasia. J Clin Invest 1996;98:1897–905.

28. Haffner SM. Insulin resistance, inflammation, and the prediabetic state. Am J Cardiol 2003;92:18J–26J.

29. Haffner SM, Greenberg AS, Weston WM, Chen H, Williams K, Freed MI. Effect of rosiglitazone treatment on nontraditional markers of cardiovascular disease in patients with type 2 diabetes mellitus. Circulation 2002;106:679–84.

30. Minamikawa J, Tanaka S, Yamauchi M, Inoue D, Koshiyama H. Potent inhibitory effect of troglitazone on carotid arterial wall thickness in type 2 diabetes. J Clin Endocrinol Metab 1998;83:1818–20.

31. Sidhu JS, Kaski JC. Peroxisome proliferator activated receptor gamma: a potential therapeutic target in the management of ischaemic heart disease. Heart 2001;86: 255–8.

32. Kolodgie FD, Gold HK, Burke AP, et al. Intraplaque hemorrhage and progression of coronary atheroma. N Engl J Med 2003;349:2316–25.

CHAPTER 25

Genetic modulation of vulnerable plaques

Chunming Dong & Pascal J Goldschmidt-Clermont

Vulnerable atherosclerotic plaques were traditionally defined as those appearing ulcerative, fissured, and/or thrombotic and these are characterized histologically by a central lipid core, inflammatory infiltrate, and cap thinning. It is now recognized that this concept may be oversimplistic. Indeed, rupture of vulnerable plaques leading to acute atherothrombotic events involves multiple, diverse triggers and contributions of blood rheology and the coagulation cascade (high-risk blood).[1] In addition, various environmental cues, including mechanical stress, vasomotor tone, intercurrent infections, temperature extremes, blood viscosity, and coagulability, impact the interactions between anatomic (central lipid core, thin cap) and functional (intrinsic thrombogenicity, intraplaque inflammatory infiltrate) components of such plaques.[1,2] These facts underscore the notion that atherosclerosis itself is a multifactorial, polygenic, complex trait that involves gene–gene and gene–environment interactions.[3] Furthermore, the ulceration or rupture of plaques represents evidence of the failure of the constant repair process that involves circulatory endothelial and other vascular progenitor cells to maintain the homeostasis of the arterial wall. With aging and in the presence of constant injury, such progenitor cells from the bone marrow might become exhausted.[4]

Like many other common diseases that do not follow Mendelian inheritance patterns, the contribution of heredity to atherogenesis may be hard to pinpoint; its genetic determinants, however, are tractable, and knowledge of genetic predisposition will have broad consequences for preclinical diagnostics, preventive maneuvers, and therapeutic strategies. According to theories of inheritance of quantitative traits, disorders like atherosclerosis, including vulnerable plaques, involve a large number of genetic determinants, whose individual contribution can account for only a relatively small fraction of the variance.[5] Thus, delineation of the genetic modulation of vulnerable atherosclerotic plaques presents a much greater challenge than that of inherited Mendelian traits. The completion of the Human Genome Project and ongoing sequencing of mouse, rat, and other genomes has led to an explosion of genetics-related technologies that are finding their way into all areas of biological research, including cardiovascular research. These technologies, including cDNA microarray, genome-wide linkage mapping, single nucleotide polymorphism (SNP) search, and haplotype mapping, have already yielded useful information and will undoubtedly facilitate the dissection of the molecular mechanisms underlying the development of vulnerable plaques and their propensity to rupture. Proteomics and metabolomics approaches using vascular tissues and peripheral blood will help not only characterize the interactions between anatomic and functional plaque components, but also elucidate the impact of environmental cues on such interactions. Furthermore, advances in epigenetics have provided clues regarding the role of DNA methylation in the regulation of gene expression in atherosclerosis.[6] This chapter illustrates recent progress in these areas, focusing on SNP search and DNA methylation, and introduces the comparative genomic approaches undertaken by Duke investigators to dissect the molecular pathogenesis of atherosclerosis, including vulnerable plaques. Furthermore, using the cardiovascular system as a test-bed, the Duke approaches explore the use of multiple genomic methodologies and bioinformatics tools for gene expression profiling, molecular phenotyping and screening, and for relating large-scale SNP genotyping information to clinical outcomes and conditions, which may provide prototypic strategies for tackling complex traits. The integration of these genomic techniques is a process of genomic convergence, which represents the best opportunity to unravel the mystery of the genetic make-up of complex traits, such as atherosclerosis and its consequent thromboembolic complications.

SNP discovery – correlating genotypes with phenotypes

Any two randomly selected human genomes are 99.9% identical at the DNA level. The remaining 0.1% of DNA contains sequence variations. The most common type of such variation is called a single-nucleotide polymorphism, or SNP. SNPs are highly abundant, stable, and distributed throughout the genome. These variations are associated with diversity in the population, individuality, susceptibility to diseases, and individual response to environmental factors and to medicine. SNP genotyping can be used to identify and map complex, common diseases such as atherosclerosis, which may provide insight into the nature of human sequence variation in relation to disease pathogenesis. Indeed, many SNPs have been discovered in genes known to be involved in several aspects of atherogenesis.

SNPs and lipid metabolism

Hyperlipidemia represents a major risk factor for the development of vascular dysfunction and atherosclerosis. Various SNPs for apolipoprotein A-II (apoAII), apoAV, apoB, apoE, apoE2, very low density lipoprotein receptor (VLDLR), hepatic, endothelial and lipoprotein lipase, cholesteryl ester transfer protein, microsomal triglyceride transfer protein, beta-3-adrenergic receptor, paroxonase 1, PPAR, and calpain-10 have been identified that are associated with coronary artery disease in Caucasian, European, and Japanese populations.[7-32] ABCA1 protein belongs to a superfamily

of membrane transporters that bind and hydrolyze ATP to drive diverse substrates across membranes. ABCA1 stimulates cholesterol and phospholipid efflux to apo A-I and may also act as a cholesterol/phospholipid flippase at the plasma membrane level. This step is the first stage in reverse cholesterol transport (RCT), which mediates the movement of cholesterol from peripheral cells, including macrophage-derived foam cells in the arterial wall, back to the liver, where it is catabolized. This pathway is crucial to counteract deposition of cholesterol, by oxidized or otherwise modified LDL, in macrophages that have infiltrated the arterial wall; ineffective cholesterol efflux promotes the formation of foam cells, the precursors of arterial lesions. Several groups have identified a total of 179 SNPs in various regions of the ABCA1 gene. At least nine of them have shown reproducible association with atherosclerosis or altered lipid profiles.[33-36] These data support the role of SNPs in affecting lipid metabolism, and consequently atherogenesis, in particular the formation of central lipid core in vulnerable plaques.

SNPs in cytokines and adhesion molecules

Inflammation plays a pivotal role in the development of atherosclerosis and acute coronary syndromes. Coronary risk factors, particularly LDL cholesterol, injure the endothelium and decrease the bioavailability of nitric oxide, promoting the expression of proinflammatory genes, cellular adhesion molecules, cytokines, chemokines, and growth factors. Soluble markers of inflammation that are released into the blood, including C-reactive protein (CRP), interleukin 6 (IL-6), macrophage colony-stimulating factor (M-CSF), tumor necrosis factor alpha (TNFα), CD40 ligand (CD40-L), and vascular endothelial growth factor (VEGF), are highly predictive of the disease outcome.[37-45] In a genome-wide association study comprising 94 individuals with myocardial infarction (MI) and 658 individuals from the general Japanese population, Ozaki et al.[46] using high-throughput multiplex PCR-Invader assay for 92,788 randomly selected gene-based SNPs, identified a candidate locus on chromosome 6p21 associated with susceptibility to MI. Subsequent linkage-disequilibrium mapping and analyses of haplotype structure showed significant associations between MI and a single 50-kb halpotype composed of five SNPs in *LTA* (encoding lymphotoxin-α), *NFKBIL1* (encoding nuclear factor of κlight polypeptide gene enhancer in B cells, inhibitor-like 1), and *BAT1* (encoding HLA-B associated transcript 1). Remarkably, homozygosity with respect to each of the two SNPs in *LTA* was significantly associated with increased risk for MI (odds ratio = 1.78, $\chi^2 = 21.6$, $P = 0.00000033$). Using in vitro functional analyses, they demonstrated that one SNP in the coding region of *LTA*, which changed an amino acid residue from threonine to asparagine (Thr26Asn), induced a twofold increase in the induction of several cell adhesion molecules, including VCAM1, in vascular smooth muscle cells (SMCs) of human coronary arteries.[46] Using a chip-based MALDI-TOF mass spectrometry for multiplexed genotyping of SNPs associated with CAD, Nakai et al.[7] identified SNPs in multiple genes involved in inflammation and cell adhesion. Theses include CD36, CCR2, colony stimulating factor–2 (CSF2), Selectin P, Selectin E, ICAM1, MMP3, IL-1β, CD40L, and serotonin receptor 1A. Importantly, these findings were confirmed by conventional fluorescent dye-terminator cycle sequencing.[7] Together, these data indicate that genetic variants in genes involved in inflammation and cell adhesion are associated with increased risk for atherosclerosis and acute coronary syndromes, including myocardial infraction.

SNPs in the hemostatic system

The blood coagulation system plays an important role in determining the onset and outcome of atherosclerosis. The cleavage products from the coagulation system, e.g. thrombin, factor Xa, factor VIIa, and activated protein C, are thought to modulate the inflammatory responses of endothelial cells and leukocytes, which are crucial to the development of atherosclerosis and the pathogenesis of vulnerable plaques.[47] Indeed, the formation of blood clots represents a major event associated with the rupture of vulnerable plaques. Hence, the search for hemostatic candidate genes and polymorphisms involved in the predisposition to atherosclerosis and vulnerable plaques is a key step towards a more comprehensive understanding of the pathogenesis of the disease. Thus far, an impressive number of polymorphisms in genes coding for proteins of the hemostatic system have been identified. Due to the particular relevance of the hemostatic system to vulnerable plaques, a major portion of this chapter is devoted to SNPs identified in the genes involved in this system.

Gp Ia-IIa ($\alpha_2\beta_1$ integrin) is a major receptor on the platelet surface involved in platelet adhesion to collagens in the subendothelial matrix.[48] A silent dimorphism at nucleotide position 807 (C807T) of the GpIa-IIa gene was shown to affect $\alpha_2\beta_1$ integrin density on platelets and alter collagen receptor activity.[49] The 807T allele was associated with a 1.6-fold increase in the risk for myocardial infarction (MI) in male patients. The odds ratios for such an increased risk were more pronounced in young patients.[50] Several reports confirmed the 807T allele to be a risk factor for MI and stroke,[51–53] particularly in young patients, but others did not find any association between the 807T genotype and the clinical phenotype.[54–57] Therefore, additional studies with much larger patient cohorts are needed to determine the functional significance of this allele.

Gp IIb-IIIa ($\alpha_{IIb}III_a$ integrin) functions as a fibrinogen receptor on the platelets, mediating platelet aggregation. It also serves as a receptor for von Willebrand factor (vWF) and other soluble ligands. A number of polymorphisms of Gp IIb-IIIa have been described. The gene variant that has received particular attention is a T to C transition at nucleotide 1565, which results in a Pro to Leu substitution at amino acid position 33.[58] This polymorphism (PLA2 genotype) is known to exhibit a heterogeneous ethnic distribution and result in increased platelet aggregability. In some, but not all, studies, it was shown to be associated with increased risk of MI and early onset of coronary artery disease.[59–63] In an effort to establish the effects of PLA2 in atherosclerosis and vulnerable plaques, Chinese hamster ovary (CHO) cells overexpressing homozygous PLA1, PLA2, and GPIIb/IIIa receptors have been generated to elucidate the functional consequences of this polymorphism.[64] Another Gp IIb-IIIa polymorphism that has been investigated in its association with arterial thrombotic disease is the Gp IIb Ile-843Ser polymorphism, with most studies yielding negative results.[65–67] A recent study, however, suggested that the Ser-843 allele was associated with increased risk of MI in young women (aged <45 years) in the presence of other atherosclerosis risk factors, such as smoking, positive family history of MI, and high cholesterol levels.[68] Further studies are warranted to confirm these findings.

Gp Ib-V-IX is a platelet receptor for vWF that mediates platelet binding to VWF. Two polymorphisms in the gene coding for Gp Ibα were identified that affect the phenotype (HPA-2 and a variable number tandem repeat (VNTR)).[69–71] The HPA-2 alloantigen system is defined by the presence of a C to T substitution at nucleotide position 3550 resulting in a Thr-145Met substitution. The VNTR is a repeat of 39 basepairs (bp) in the macroglycopeptide region of the Gp Ibα, and the variant alleles include A (one repeat), B (two repeats), C (three repeats), and D (four repeats). Each repeat results in the addition of 13 amino acids to the protein, which modifies the distance between the vWF-binding domain and the platelet surface.[69–71] Both positive and negative findings were reported regarding the associations of HPA-2b and VNTR B allele with increased risk of MI and stroke. Recently, a gene polymorphism has been described in the Kozak sequence of the Gp Ibα receptor. This variation is a T/C dimorphism at nucleotide-5 located in the transcription initiation codon of the Gp Ibα gene.[72] The -5C allele is associated with enhanced mRNA transcription and increased levels of the Ibα receptor on the platelet surface. This Kozak polymorphism, however, was shown to have a neutral effect on the risk of stroke and a paradoxical trend towards protection against MI (odds ratio 0.53).[73] Further studies are needed to delineate the role of this polymorphism in thrombotic event associated with vulnerable plaques.

Fibrinogen levels influence platelet aggregation, blood viscosity, and endothelial cell injury, mechanisms that play important roles in influencing the outcome after vulnerable plaque rupture. The fibrinogen molecule is a glycoprotein containing two copies of three polypeptide chains (α, β, and γ) encoded by three distinct genes located on the long arm of chromosome 4 (q23–32). Various polymorphisms have been identified in all three genes, mainly in the locus coding for the β-chain of fibrinogen. Two dimorphisms in the β-chain gene: the *Hae*III polymorphism (a G to A substitution at position -455 in the 5′ promoter region) and the

*Bcl*I polymorphism in the 3′ untranslated region (UTR), have received considerable attention. These two polymorphisms are in linkage disequilibrium with each other.[74] The -455G/A substitution was found to be a determinant of plasma fibrinogen levels in different investigations, probably due to its close proximity to an IL-6 and a hepatocyte nuclear factor I-responsive element in the promoter region.[75–78] Conflicting results, however, were reported regarding the association between this polymorphism and the risk of arterial thrombosis.[79–82] Another fibrinogen gene variation that has drawn some attention is the α-chain Thr-312Ala polymorphism in the coding region.[83] The 312Ala allele was shown to increase clot stability. In the Etude Cas-Temoin de l'Infarctus du Myocarde (ECTIM) study, Thr-312Ala did not influence the risk of MI.[84] In another investigation, the 312Ala allele was associated with decreased survival after stroke and with increased risk of pulmonary embolism.[85] The exact role of Thr-312Ala in thrombotic events accompanying vulnerable plaques remains to be determined.

Plasminogen activator inhibitor 1 (PAI-1) is a member of the serine protease inhibitor (serpin) superfamily, which regulates fibrinolysis. Augmented PAI-1 mRNA and protein expression in macrophages and SMCs was found in human atheroma plaques and transplant arteriosclerosis.[86–89] Multiple variations have been discovered for the PAI-1 gene, including a variation at a CA(n) dinucleotide repeat in intron 3, a *Hind*III VNTR polymorphism in the 3′ UTR and a 4G/5G deletion/insertion promoter polymorphism. The 4G/5G polymorphism is known to determine PAI-1 levels, with the 4G genotype being associated with higher plasma concentrations.[90–93] The 4G/5G promoter polymorphism has been related to cardiovascular disease. A recent study has found that the 4G/5G genotype distribution was different across blacks, Hispanics, and non-Hispanic whites.[94] The allele frequencies for 4G and 5G, were 0.52 and 0.48 in non-Hispanic whites, 0.38 and 0.62 in Hispanics, and 0.28 and 0.72 in blacks, respectively. PAI-1 levels were lower in blacks than in non-Hispanic whites and Hispanics and lower in non-Hispanic whites than in Hispanics (all $P = 0.0001$). Moreover, subjects homozygous for the 4G allele had the highest plasma PAI-1, heterozygote subjects were intermediate, and 5G homozygotes had the lowest levels of PAI-1. These patterns remained unaffected by adjustments for age, gender, clinical center, glucose tolerance status, body mass index, waist, triglycerides, and insulin resistance. Multiple linear regression analyses showed that a weak but significant contribution of the 4G/5G genotype to the PAI-1 levels (0.63% in non-Hispanic whites, 0.99% in Hispanics, and 2.37% in blacks), and interaction analyses revealed no significant differences in the relation of circulating PAI-1 levels to the 4G/5G genotype by ethnicity.[94] Therefore, the association of the genotype with PAI-1 levels was consistent among different ethnic groups and was unaffected by metabolic covariates, including insulin resistance, indicating the independent predictability of the 4G/5G genotype for the phenotype.

Tissue-type plasminogen activator (t-PA) converts plasminogen to plasmin and mediates clot lysis. Increased plasma t-PA levels have been paradoxically associated with increased risk of coronary thrombotic disease, such as plaque rupture.[95–97] Numerous polymorphisms have been reported for the t-PA gene.[98] An Alu insertion/deletion polymorphism in the t-PA gene influences the release rates of total t-PA.[99] Homozygosity of the Alu insertion polymorphism has been associated with a twofold increase in the risk of MI in one study,[100] but this finding could not be confirmed in other investigations.[101,102] Thus, the role of this variation in atherosclerosis is uncertain. Recently, eight novel t-PA gene polymorphisms have been described. Three of these polymorphisms are in strong linkage disequilibrium with the Alu polymorphism and influence t-PA release rates. The other variations were silent and without apparent effect on t-PA release.[98] The functional significance of these polymorphisms is still unknown.

Thrombomodulin is an integral membrane protein of endothelial cells and monocytes. When thrombin binds to thrombomodulin, it loses its procoagulant activity but becomes capable of activating protein C, which inhibits the procoagulant activity of serine proteases in the coagulation cascade. Hence, polymorphisms/mutations of thrombomodulin might play a role as a risk factor for thrombotic events in vulnerable plaques. Several missense mutations have been identified

in the thrombomodulin gene.[103–108] It remains difficult, however, to determine the relationship between these mutations and the propensity for developing thrombosis. One reason for this is that simple functional assays are not available to study the impact of these mutations on thrombomodulin gene function. Indeed, in vitro data obtained with Asp-468Tyr genotype did not reveal any abnormality in production levels or functional activity.[109] An amino acid dimorphism, Ala-455Val, was shown to be more frequent in survivors of MI,[110] but was not confirmed by Norlund et al.[111] Interestingly, this allele was recently linked to a 6.1-fold increase in the risk of coronary heart disease in blacks but not in whites.[112,113] Another polymorphism in thrombomodulin is a G to A substitution at nucleotide position 127, resulting in an Ala-25Thr substitution in the protein. The 25Thr allele was found to be more prevalent among 560 male patients with MI than in 646 control subjects in the Study of Myocardial Infarctions Leiden (SMILE). A particularly high risk (6.5-fold increase) was observed in relatively young patients (aged below 50 years) and in the presence of additional risk factors such as smoking and metabolic risk factors (ninefold increased risk).[114] By contrast, in two subsequent investigations, the Ala-25Thr polymorphism was not found to be a risk factor for coronary artery disease or stroke.[115,116] A polymorphism (-33 G/A) located in the promoter region of thrombomodulin was recently identified that affected plasma soluble thrombomodulin levels and was linked to a 1.8-fold increased risk of coronary heart disease in the Chinese population.[117,118] A significant association between carriership of the -33A allele and a 2.4-fold increased risk of the occurrence of carotid atherosclerosis in subjects aged less than 60 years were also reported.[117,118] A frame-shift mutation of thrombomodulin gene was recently documented in a family with arterial disease, lending further support for the role of thrombomodulin mutations in MI.[119]

Various SNPs of genes that encode coagulation factors have been identified. These factors include factors II, V, VII, XIII, and tissue factor. Among them, a G to A transition at nucleotide position 20210 (G20210A) in the 3′ UTR of factor II gene, the Arg (R)-506 to Gln (Q) mutation in the factor V gene, the Arg-353Gln mutation in exon 8 of factor

VII, the G to T transition in exon 2 of the FXIII subunit A gene resulting in a Val to Leu substitution at amino acid position 34 (FXIII Val-34Leu) have received the most attention.[120–139] Data, however, were conflicting regarding the functional significance of these polymorphisms in affecting the plasma levels of the respective factors and their association with cardiac events, such as MI. Indeed, a recent study investigating the association between nine polymorphisms of genes encoding hemostasis factors, including G-455A beta-fibrinogen, G1691A factor V, G20210A factor II, G10976A factor VII, C807T glycoprotein Ia, C1565T glycoprotein IIIa, G185T factor XIII, C677T methylenetetrahydrofolate reductase, and 4G/5G PAI-1 and MI in a large sample of young patients provides no evidence supporting an association between these polymorphisms and the occurrence of premature MI or protection against it thereof.[140] Furthermore, no specific polymorphisms have been identified for factor VIII and vWF.

SNPs in thrombospondins

Thrombospondins are glycoproteins which constitute a family of at least five, structurally related, multidomain ECM proteins, of which three (THBS-1, -2, and -5) have been detected in vascular tissue.[141–143] While the primary function of THBS-1 as an anti-angiogenic factor has been established, the functions of THBS-2 and -5 in the extracellular matrix of the vessel wall are poorly understood. It is postulated that THBS-2 play a role as an adaptor and modulator of cell–matrix interactions through interaction with cell-surface receptors, cytokines, growth factors, proteases, and structural proteins. Gene knockout studies in fibroblasts have indicated that THBS-2 might influence the regulation of gelatinase A (MMP-2), a matrix metalloproteinase that is overexpressed in vulnerable atherosclerotic plaques.[144] Furthermore, THBS-2-deficient mice have a phenotype that would be expected to reduce the risk of MI.[145] Considering their potential significance for important cellular events in the arterial wall, thrombospondins have been regarded as candidate genes for vulnerable plaques and have served as targets for SNP search and genotype–phenotype association studies. Indeed, in the GeneQuest study comprising a total of 398 families, which were identified to fulfill the criteria of MI,

revascularization, or a significant coronary artery lesion diagnosed before 45 years in men or 50 years in women, Topol et al.[146] showed that SNPs in three members of the thrombospondin protein family were associated with premature coronary artery disease. A missense variant of thrombospondin 4 (A387P) showed the strongest association, with an adjusted odds ratio for MI of 1.89 ($P = 0.002$ adjusted for covariates) for individuals carrying the P allele. A variant in the 32′ untranslated region of thrombospondin-2 (change of thymidine to guanine) seemed to have a protective effect against MI in individuals homozygous for the variant. A missense variant in thrombospondin-1 (N700S) was associated with an adjusted odds ratio for coronary artery disease of 11.90 in homozygous individuals, who also had the lowest level of thrombospondin-1 by plasma assay. A subsequent study by Boekholdt et al.[147] provided further support for association of the homozygosity for the THBS-2 variant allele with reduced risk of premature MI. Contradicting to the GeneQuest study, however, these authors did not find any association between THBS-1 variant allele and an altered risk of premature CAD or MI. Furthermore, the THBS-4 variant (387P) allele was significantly associated with a reduced risk of premature MI compared with wild-type individuals, contrasting the GeneQuest report that showed the opposite. Hence, it appears that THBS-2 is an important candidate for further genetic and functional studies aimed at evaluating the functional properties of its putative regulatory regions in vitro and in relevant animal models, and family studies, which may allow the final confirmation that an association exists between the THBS-2 polymorphism and vulnerable plaques. Large-scale cohort studies are needed to establish the potential, modest risk ratios of THBS-1 and -4 in atherosclerosis.

In conclusion, results from association studies linking SNPs to atherosclerosis and cardiac events are generally inconsistent and conflicting, and positive results were more often than not found in post hoc subgroup analyses. Although diversity of study design may contribute to the discrepancies, making direct comparisons between studies complicated, many studies, however, suffer from a limited sample size that is frequently too small to confirm or rule out the presence of a relevant epidemiological association between specific polymorphisms and cardiovascular disease, which probably is the major contributor for the observed discrepancies among these studies. Furthermore, it is unlikely that a specific gene variation is, in isolation, a very strong risk factor for atherosclerosis and vulnerable plaques. More probable is the scenario in which many gene polymorphisms influence atherosclerosis or vulnerable plaque risk by interacting with each other and with environmental cues. Such interactions were not apparent in the above-cited investigations because of the influence of factors such as sample size and ethnicity (which may also affect the nature and magnitude of gene–gene and gene–environmental interactions). It is noteworthy that a biased approach was used to identify the above-described SNPs – all the genes are known players in atherosclerosis. Unbiased approaches, such as taken by investigators at Duke University as described below, are needed to fully characterize the molecular/genetic mechanisms underlying atherosclerosis/vulnerable plaques.

Epigenetic changes: potential therapeutic targets

While genomic information is uniform in the different cells of a complex organism, the programming of gene expression profiles is, to a large degree, affected by the epigenome, especially in complex diseases like atherosclerosis. Indeed, unlike cancer, in which gene mutation is a common phenomenon, and plays an important role in oncogenesis (genomitis), the pathogenesis of atherosclerosis is believed to involve mainly gene function changes, rather than mutations. Such functional changes can be due to either altered expression, or altered activity of the gene product, due to polymorphisms or epigenetic changes.

The epigenome is composed of two modules, covalent addition of a methyl group to the 5 position cytosines in the context of dinucleotide sequence CG and a noncovalent module, histone acetylation and chromatin condensation. Chromatin structure determines the state of activity of genes by gating the accessibility of the transcription machinery to transcriptional regulatory regions on genes.[148] Unlike genetic mutations, deletions, and

insertions, DNA methylation is an enzymatic process that can be measured, slowed, and possibly reversed using various strategies.[149] Therefore, investigation of gene-specific methylation changes may create new venues for the prevention and treatment of atherosclerosis.

Approximately 70% of CpG pairs in the mammalian genome are constitutively methylated.[150] These methylated regions are typical of the bulk chromatin that is responsible for the silencing of the overwhelming amount of noncoding DNA present in the mammalian genome, including introns, repetitive elements, and potentially active transposable elements.[151] In contrast to these constitutively methylated regions, there are short stretches of DNA sequences with an unusually high GC content and a high frequency of CpG dinucleotides, ranging from 0.5 to 5 kb and occurring on average every 100 kb, which are unmethylated. These unmethylated sequences are called CpG islands.[152] CpG islands are GC rich (60–70%), and have a ratio of CpG to GpC of at least 0.6.[153] Collectively, CpG islands account for 1–2% of the genome, and their location is primarily in the 5′ regulatory regions of all housekeeping genes as well as up to 40% of tissue-specific genes.[154] CpG islands have also been proposed to function as replication origins.[155] Although they are generally not methylated, CpG islands have been the focus of most investigations into the role of DNA methylation in biologic processes. Changes in methylation status of CpG islands are associated with increased expression of oncogenes and growth factors and decreased expression of tumor suppressor genes, leading to excess cell proliferation in carcinogenesis. Importantly, aberrant smooth muscle cell proliferation represents a key event in atherogenesis. Hence, it is possible that similar epigenetic mechanisms may, at least in part, account for the progression of atherosclerotic lesions. Indeed, recent evidence supports the notion that epigenetic events play an important role in the pathogenesis of atherosclerosis.[6]

DNA methylation profiling in atherosclerosis

Embryogenesis and differentiation are characterized by specific patterns of gene expression in specific tissues and organs, and proceed in the absence of any alterations in DNA sequences. Thus, the diversity of phenotypes in differentiated organs is not due to any genetic alterations, but to epigenetic changes. Furthermore, although individually genes do not have the capacity to auto-regulate themselves, the genome has developed epigenetic mechanisms, like DNA methylation, to silence gene expression. Keeping these facts in mind, we examined global DNA methylation patterns in atherosclerosis using Restriction Landmark Genomic Scanning (RLGS) – a 2D gel electrophoresis method capable of identifying genome-wide CpG island methylation changes.[155] The restriction landmark enzyme *Not*I in the *Not*I-*Eco*RV-*Hin*fI enzyme combination used for DNA digestion for RLGS is methylation-sensitive. If a genomic *Not*I site is methylated, the enzyme does not cut and the site will not be end-labeled with ^{32}P-labeled guanine and cytosine. On the other hand, if the *Not*I site is unmethylated, the site gets cut and the restriction ends are end-labeled. Remarkably, a highly

consistent methylation pattern, representing basal DNA methylation level, was observed in normal aortas. Nearly 2% spots showed marked intensity changes (decrease/increase or disappearance/reappearance), indicative of differential methylation of specific genes in atherosclerotic vessels relative to normal aortic tissues (Figure 25.1), suggesting a selective change in CpG island methylation during atherogenesis. Furthermore, in a rabbit model of atherosclerosis, 5′-methylcytosine content in the genome was decreased in atherosclerotic aortas, as compared with normal arteries, indicative of global hypomethylation.[156] Intriguingly, gene-specific hypermethylation and global hypomethylation have been observed with aging.[157] Considering that aging is the most important risk factor for atherosclerosis, these findings may suggest that epigenetic mechanisms may underlie the progressive drift of gene expression occurring with aging, leading to increased susceptibility to atherosclerosis in older individuals.

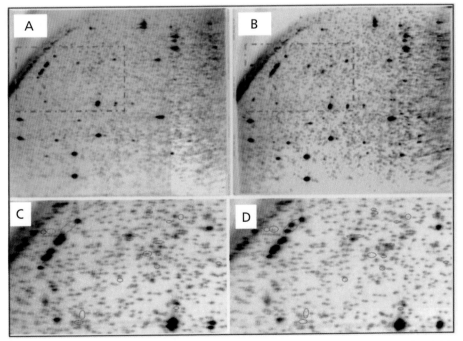

Figure 25.1 RLGS profile of aortas. RLGS was performed in a normal aorta (A) and an aorta with atherosclerosis (B). Comparative analysis in a designated area (red rectangle) between the two vessels reveals spots with marked alterations in intensity in the normal (C) and diseased vessel (D). Green circles indicate decrease in intensity or disappeared spots (methylation), whereas red circles represent increase in intensity or reappeared spots (demethylation).

Estrogen receptor-α methylation in proliferating SMCs

Detailed analysis of the RLGS profiles generated in normal versus atherosclerotic tissues revealed that one of the spots corresponded to the ERα gene. ERα was found to be present at normal diploid intensity in the RLGS profiles from normal aortas, but partly vanished from the RLGS profiles from atherosclerotic tissue. Considering that the de-differentiation of the contractile vascular SMCs within the media, which is required for their subsequent proliferation and migration into the intimal layer of the arterial wall, is a key step of the atherogenic process, and estrogen has been shown to control cell proliferation both in cancer cells and in vascular cells,[158–161] we examined the methylation status of ERα in a SMC dedifferentiation model, where cultured SMCs were used as surrogate for the proliferative and noncontractile SMC phenotype as occurring in atherosclerotic lesions in vivo. In this model, SMCs directly isolated from normal human aortas (representing contractile phenotype) were compared with the same cells explanted from the aorta and cultured in vitro (resembling the in vivo de-differentiated phenotype). Using Combined Bisulfite Restriction Analysis (COBRA) and Southern blot, we indeed demonstrated ERα methylation in the proliferative SMCs in a passage-dependent manner. By contrast, human aortic endothelial cells (HAECs) did not show any differential methylation in culture.[162] These data indicate that ERα methylation is a specific event in SMC dedifferentiation.

ERα methylation in atherosclerotic tissues

The methylation status of ERα was further investigated in multiple tissue specimens collected from patients undergoing coronary artery bypass surgery, and in atherosclerotic plaques collected from patients undergoing directional coronary atherectomy or carotid endotherectomy. DNA isolated from these tissues was treated with methylation-sensitive enzyme NotI, and subjected to Southern blot analysis, which revealed increased ERα gene methylation in all specimens showing atherosclerosis relative to normal aortic tissues.[163] These findings indicate that DNA methylation of ERα is associated with cardiovascular disease.

ERα, upon activation by estrogen, regulates a variety of cellular activities, including the inhibition of cell proliferation observed in cancer cells sensitive to estrogen. Such an antiproliferative effect could also slow the proliferation of SMCs that occurs within the blood vessel wall in response to injury. Moreover, activated ERα increases the expression/activity of nitric oxide synthase, resulting in enhanced nitric oxide (NO) production that, in turn, could inhibit SMC proliferation and platelet activation. These effects of ERα may account for the cardiovascular protection afforded by estrogen, contributing to the low incidence of atherosclerotic disease in premenopausal women, and accelerated atherosclerosis in postmenopausal women. The discovery of ERα methylation in atherosclerosis may help explain the failure of estrogen replacement therapy (HRT), as observed in the Heart and Estrogen/Progestin Replacement Study (HERS), in which women with pre-existing coronary artery disease were found to gain no clinical benefits following 4 years of HRT, in spite of improved lipid profile for the HRT recipients.[164] Methylation-induced silencing of the ERα gene associated with atherosclerosis in these women may render them resistant to the protective effects of estrogen.

DNA methylation, hyperhomocysteinemia, and atherosclerosis

Homocysteine exerts multiple deleterious effects on the cardiovascular system, including increased oxidant stress, impaired endothelial function, stimulation of mitogenesis, and induction of thrombosis. It serves as an independent risk factor for atherosclerosis, thrombosis, and hypertension. Homocysteine is a sulfur-containing amino acid, derived from methionine, which can be remethylated back to methionine as part of the methionine cycle. In this cycle, methionine is utilized for synthesis of S-adenosylmethionine (SAM), which is converted to homocysteine and S-adenosylhomocysteine (SAH), a potent methylation inhibitor. SAM is the methyl donor for >100 different transmethylation reactions, including DNA methylation. Mice deficient for methylenetetrahydrofolatereductase (MTHFR), which converts 5,10-methylenetetrahydrofolate to 5-methyltetrahydrofolate, a methyl donor for homocysteine remethylation to methionine, had significantly increased total plasma homocysteine levels (1.6-fold for heterozygotes, and 10-fold for homozygotes) compared with wild-type littermates. They also displayed either significantly decreased SAM levels or significantly increased SAH levels. These mice showed statistically significant increase in hypomethylated sites in DNA, suggestive of global hypomethylation. Interestingly, abnormal lipid deposition in the proximal portion of the aorta was present in older heterozygotes and homozygotes.[165] Moreover, Wang et al. found that clinically relevant concentrations of homocysteine (10–50 µmol), but not cysteine, inhibited DNA synthesis and growth in vascular endothelial cells, and such an inhibitory effect might be mediated through hypomethylation of proteins and genes.[166] Hence, global DNA hypomethylation may serve as a mechanistic link between hyperhomocysteinemia and atherosclerosis. Further work is warranted to characterize gene-specific hypermethylation as opposed to global hypomethylation in the presence of hyperhomocysteinemia and the significance of such hypermethylation in consequent atherosclerosis.

Comparative approaches to the identification of candidate genes for atherosclerosis

The human genome project and the technological breakthroughs it has brought about have moved the field of molecular medicine forward with breathtaking speed. Indeed, since the Human Genome Project Consortium presented the first near-complete draft of the human genome together with Celera Genetics in the year 2000, which marked the beginning of the so-called "post-genome era," many programs at academic and industry centers have proposed to identify candidate genes that are relevant to human diseases through different means, such as SNP search. Although candidate genes have been identified, and hundreds of thousands of variants within these genes have been registered, there is no consensus, nor established approach, for successfully translating the sequencing information of the human genome into information that can be used as a tool to prevent and/or treat disease. To effectively and fully characterize the molecular basis of atherosclerosis, investigators at Duke University Medical Center have carried out a multidisciplinary, large-scale investigation. The identification of candidate genes and their SNPs will involve the use of combinations of methods, including cDNA microarray gene expression profiling, metabolomic profiling, genome mapping, SNP search, and epigenetic investigation. For this purpose, we have collected in excess of 160 aortas from cardiac transplant donors (Figure 25.2) and thousands of blood samples from patients with early-onset cardiac disease and their relatives. Remarkably, atherosclerotic lesions display a symmetric pattern in their distributions in these aortas. For the aortic arch, the symmetry is distributed in a posterior/ventral fashion, whereas below the left subclavian, the symmetry becomes left/right along a symmetry line between the intercostal branches. Accordingly, all of the aortas collected thus far have been bisected longitudinally, along a sagittal plane for the proximal portion and along a parasternal plane for the portion below the left subclavian. One side will be used for genomic and epigenomic study and the other side will be utilized for histological analysis of disease burden. Such an approach allows for direct correlation between the molecular changes and disease phenotype. In addition, novel statistical modeling, such as Bayesian regression and Tree analyses, and bioinformatic approaches will be developed and utilized to analyze the massive amount of data generated to prioritize candidate genes. Importantly, the validity of classes of candidate genes and their polymorphisms identified using these multiple genome technology approaches will be tested in our unique cardiovascular database that includes in excess of 100,000 patients as sound clinical indicators. Hence, our substantial undertaking would allow us to compare approaches, such as expression arrays, genome-wide linkage association, or combination thereof, for their ability to identify genes and variants that can be used as useful diagnostic and prognostic tools. We envision that data generated from the substantial Approaches to Genomic Discovery for Atherosclerosis (AGENDA) project at Duke University Medical Center will deepen our understanding of the molecular/genomic pathogenesis of atherosclerosis. More important, our strategies will set the platform for using multiple genomic approaches to tackling other complex traits.

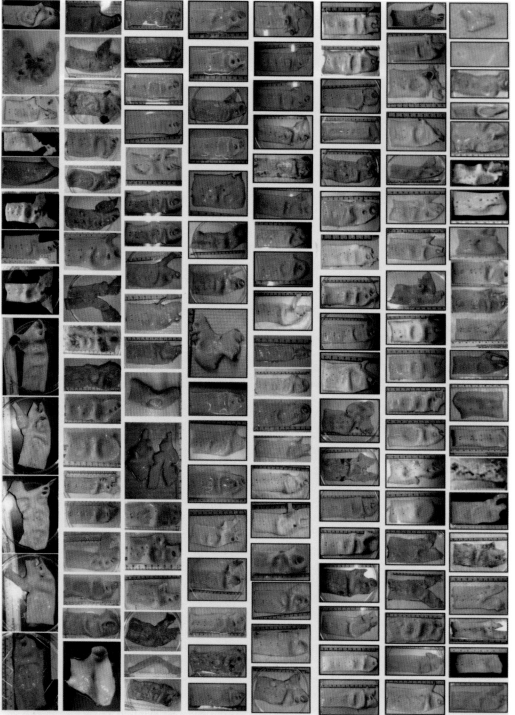

Figure 25.2 Aorta collection. Photographs of aortas collected from 136 transplant donors show various degree of atherosclerosis burden in these "healthy" donors. Multiple specimens exhibit ulcerations – characteristic of vulnerable plaques. These aortas are being used for genomic and epigenomic studies as part of the AGENDA project at Duke University Medical Center.

References

1. Maseri A, Fuster V. Is there a vulnerable plaque? Circulation 2003;107:2068–71.

2. Casscells W, Naghavi M, Willerson JT. Vulnerable atherosclerotic plaque: a multifocal disease. Circulation 2003;107:2072–5.

3. Dong C, Nevins JR, Goldschmidt-Clermont PJ. ABCA1 single nucleotide polymorphisms. Snipping at the pathogenesis of atherosclerosis. Circ Res 2001;88:855–7.

4. Rauscher FM, Goldschmidt-Clermont PJ, Davis BH, et al. Aging, progenitor cell exhaustion, and atherosclerosis. Circulation 2003;108:457–463.

5. McPeek MS. From mouse to human: fine mapping of quantitative trait loci in a model organism. Proc Natl Acad Sci USA 2000;97:12389–90.

6. Dong C, Yoon W, Goldschmidt-Clermont PJ. DNA methylation and atherosclerosis. J Nutr 2002;132: 2406S–9S.

7. Nakai K, Habano W, Fujita T, Nakai K, Schnackenberg J, Kawazoe K, Suwabe A, Itoh C. Highly multiplexed genotyping of coronary artery disease-associated SNPs using MALDI-TOF mass spectrometry. Hum Mutat 2002;20:133–8.

8. Mattu RK, Trevelyan J, Needham EW, et al. Lipoprotein lipase gene variants relate to presence and degree of microalbuminuria in Type II diabetes. Diabetologia 2002;45:905–13.

9. Clee SM, Loubser O, Collins J, Kastelein JJ, Hayden MR. The LPL S447X cSNP is associated with decreased blood pressure and plasma triglycerides, and reduced risk of coronary artery disease. Clin.Genet 2001;60: 293–300.

10. Couture P, Otvos JD, Cupples LA, Lahoz C, Wilson PW, Schaefer EJ, Ordovas JM. Association of the C-514T polymorphism in the hepatic lipase gene with variations in lipoprotein subclass profiles: The Framingham Offspring Study. Arterioscler Thromb Vasc Biol 2000;20:815–22.

11. Sass C, Herbeth B, Siest G, Visvikis S. Lipoprotein lipase (C/G)447 polymorphism and blood pressure in the Stanislas Cohort. J Hypertens 2000;18:1775–81.

12. Shimo-Nakanishi Y, Urabe T, Hattori N, et al. Polymorphism of the lipoprotein lipase gene and risk of atherothrombotic cerebral infarction in the Japanese. Stroke 2001;32:1481–6.

13. Wong WM, Hawe E, Li LK, et al. Apolipoprotein AIV gene variant S347 is associated with increased risk of coronary heart disease and lower plasma apolipoprotein AIV levels. Circ Res 2003;92:969–75.

14. Endo K, Yanagi H, Araki J, Hirano C, Yamakawa-Kobayashi K, Tomura S. Association found between the promoter region polymorphism in the apolipoprotein A-V gene and the serum triglyceride level in Japanese schoolchildren. Hum Genet 2002;111:570–2.

15. Talmud PJ, Hawe E, Martin S, et al. Relative contribution of variation within the APOC3/A4/A5 gene cluster in determining plasma triglycerides. Hum Mol Genet 2002;11:3039–46.

16. Pennacchio LA, Olivier M, Hubacek JA, Krauss RM, Rubin EM, Cohen JC. Two independent apolipoprotein A5 haplotypes influence human plasma triglyceride levels. Hum Mol Genet 2002;11:3031–8.

17. Nabika T, Nasreen S, Kobayashi S, Masuda J. The genetic effect of the apoprotein AV gene on the serum triglyceride level in Japanese. Atherosclerosis 2002;165: 201–4.

18. Jacobsen N, Bentzen J, Meldgaard M, Jakobsen MH, Fenger M, Kauppinen S, Skouv J. LNA-enhanced detection of single nucleotide polymorphisms in the apolipoprotein E. Nucleic Acids Res 2002;30:e100.

19. Stengard JH, Clark AG, Weiss KM, et al. Contributions of 18 additional DNA sequence variations in the gene encoding apolipoprotein E to explaining variation in quantitative measures of lipid metabolism. Am J Hum Genet 2002;71:501–17.

20. Elbein SC, Chu W, Ren Q, Wang H, Hemphill C, Hasstedt SJ. Evaluation of apolipoprotein A-II as a positional candidate gene for familial Type II diabetes, altered lipid concentrations, and insulin resistance. Diabetologia 2002;45:1026–33.

21. Fullerton SM, Clark AG, Weiss KM, et al. Sequence polymorphism at the human apolipoprotein AII gene (APOA2): unexpected deficit of variation in an African-American sample. Hum Genet 2002;111:75–87.

22. Yue P, Yuan B, Gerhard DS, Neuman RJ, Isley WL, Harris WS, Schonfeld G. Novel mutations of APOB cause ApoB truncations undetectable in plasma and familial hypobetalipoproteinemia. Hum Mutat 2002;20:110–16.

23. Roks G, Cruts M, Houwing-Duistermaat JJ, et al. Effect of the APOE-491A/T promoter polymorphism on apolipoprotein E levels and risk of Alzheimer disease: The Rotterdam Study. Am J Med Genet 2002;114:570–3.

24. Knoblauch H, Bauerfeind A, Krahenbuhl C, et al. Common haplotypes in five genes influence genetic variance of LDL and HDL cholesterol in the general population. Hum Mol Genet 2002;11:1477–85.

25. Copin B, Brezin AP, Valtot F, Dascotte JC, Bechetoille A, Garchon HJ. Apolipoprotein E-promoter single-nucleotide polymorphisms affect the phenotype of primary open-angle glaucoma and demonstrate interaction with the myocilin gene. Am J Hum Genet 2002;70:1575–81.

26. Bentzen J, Jorgensen T, Fenger M. The effect of six polymorphisms in the Apolipoprotein B gene on

parameters of lipid metabolism in a Danish population. Clin Genet 2002;61:126–34.

27. Bentzen J, Poulsen P, Vaag A, Beck-Nielsen H, Fenger M. The influence of the polymorphism in apolipoprotein B codon 2488 on insulin and lipid levels in a Danish twin population. Diabet Med 2002;19:12–18.

28. Schmidt S, Barcellos LF, DeSombre K, et al. Association of polymorphisms in the apolipoprotein E region with susceptibility to and progression of multiple sclerosis. Am J Hum Genet 2002;70:708–17.

29. Groenendijk M, Cantor RM, Funke H, Dallinga-Thie GM. Two newly identified SNPs in the APO AI-CIII intergenic region are strongly associated with familial combined hyperlipidaemia. Eur J Clin Invest 2001;31:852–9.

30. Ogorelkova M, Kraft HG, Ehnholm C, Utermann G. Single nucleotide polymorphisms in exons of the apo(a) kringles IV types 6 to 10 domain affect Lp(a) plasma concentrations and have different patterns in Africans and Caucasians. Hum Mol Genet 2001;10:815–24.

31. Orho-Melander M, Klannemark M, Svensson MK, Ridderstrale M, Lindgren CM, Groop L. Variants in the calpain-10 gene predispose to insulin resistance and elevated free fatty acid levels. Diabetes 2002;51:2658–64.

32. Ito T, Yasue H, Yoshimura M, et al. Paraoxonase gene Gln192Arg (Q192R) polymorphism is associated with coronary artery spasm. Hum Genet 2002;110:89–94.

33. Zwarts KY, Clee SM, Zwinderman AH, et al. ABCA1 regulatory variants influence coronary artery disease independent of effects on plasma lipid levels. Clin Genet 2002;61:115–25.

34. Iida A, Saito S, Sekine A, et al. High-density single-nucleotide polymorphism (SNP) map of the 150-kb region corresponding to the human ATP-binding cassette transporter A1 (ABCA1) gene. J Hum Genet 2001;46:522–8.

35. Clee SM, Zwinderman AH, Engert JC, et al. Common genetic variation in ABCA1 is associated with altered lipoprotein levels and a modified risk for coronary artery disease. Circulation 2001;103:1198–205.

36. Dvorakova L, Storkanova G, Unterrainer G, et al. Eight novel ABCD1 gene mutations and three polymorphisms in patients with X-linked adrenoleukodystrophy: the first polymorphism causing an amino acid exchange. Hum Mutat 2001;18:52–60.

37. Brasier AR, Recinos A, III, Eledrisi MS. Vascular inflammation and the renin-angiotensin system. Arterioscler Thromb Vasc Biol 2002;22:1257–66.

38. Lowe GD. The relationship between infection, inflammation, and cardiovascular disease: an overview. Ann Periodontol 2001;6:1–8.

39. Pfeilschifter J, Koditz R, Pfohl M, Schatz H. Changes in proinflammatory cytokine activity after menopause. Endocr Rev 2002;23:90–119.

40. Saadeddin SM, Habbab MA, Ferns GA. Markers of inflammation and coronary artery disease. Med Sci Monit 2002;8:RA5–12.

41. Plutzky J. Inflammatory pathways in atherosclerosis and acute coronary syndromes. Am J Cardiol 2001;88:10K–15K.

42. Mortensen RF. C-reactive protein, inflammation, and innate immunity. Immunol Res 2001;24:163–76.

43. Yamada DM, Topol EJ. Importance of microembolization and inflammation in atherosclerotic heart disease. Am Heart J 2000;140:S90–102.

44. Franceschi C, Bonafe M, Valensin S, Olivieri F, De Luca M, Ottaviani E, De Benedictis G. Inflamm-aging. An evolutionary perspective on immunosenescence. Ann NY Acad Sci 2000;908:244–54.

45. Yudkin JS, Kumari M, Humphries SE, Mohamed-Ali V. Inflammation, obesity, stress and coronary heart disease: is interleukin-6 the link? Atherosclerosis 2000;148:209–14.

46. Ozaki K, Ohnishi Y, Iida A, et al. Functional SNPs in the lymphotoxin-alpha gene that are associated with susceptibility to myocardial infarction. Nat.Genet 2002;32:650–4.

47. Esmon CT, Taylor FB, Jr, Snow TR. Inflammation and coagulation: linked processes potentially regulated through a common pathway mediated by protein C. Thromb Haemost 1991;66:160–5.

48. George JN. Platelets. Lancet 2000;355:1531–9.

49. Kritzik M, Savage B, Nugent DJ, Santoso S, Ruggeri ZM, Kunicki TJ. Nucleotide polymorphisms in the alpha2 gene define multiple alleles that are associated with differences in platelet alpha2 beta1 density. Blood 1998;92:2382–8.

50. Santoso S, Kunicki TJ, Kroll H, Haberbosch W, Gardemann A. Association of the platelet glycoprotein Ia C807T gene polymorphism with nonfatal myocardial infarction in younger patients. Blood 1999;93:2449–53.

51. Carlsson LE, Santoso S, Spitzer C, Kessler C, Greinacher A. The alpha2 gene coding sequence T807/A873 of the platelet collagen receptor integrin alpha2beta1 might be a genetic risk factor for the development of stroke in younger patients. Blood 1999;93:3583–6.

52. Reiner AP, Kumar PN, Schwartz SM, et al. Genetic variants of platelet glycoprotein receptors and risk of stroke in young women. Stroke 2000;31:1628–33.

53. Moshfegh K, Wuillemin WA, Redondo M, Lammle B, Beer JH, Liechti-Gallati S, Meyer BJ. Association of two silent polymorphisms of platelet glycoprotein Ia/IIa

receptor with risk of myocardial infarction: a case-control study. Lancet 1999;353:351–4.

54. Corral J, Gonzalez-Conejero R, Rivera J, Ortuno F, Aparicio P, Vicente V. Role of the 807 C/T polymorphism of the alpha2 gene in platelet GP Ia collagen receptor expression and function – effect in thromboembolic diseases. Thromb Haemost 1999;81:951–6.

55. Croft SA, Hampton KK, Sorrell JA, Steeds RP, Channer KS, Samani NJ, Daly ME. The GPIa C807T dimorphism associated with platelet collagen receptor density is not a risk factor for myocardial infarction. Br J Haematol 1999;106:771–6.

56. von Beckerath N, Koch W, Mehilli J, Bottiger C, Braun S, Schomig A, Kastrati A. Glycoprotein Ia C807T polymorphism and risk of restenosis following coronary stenting. Atherosclerosis 2001;156:463–8.

57. von Beckerath N, Koch W, Mehilli J, Bottiger C, Schomig A, Kastrati A. Glycoprotein Ia gene C807T polymorphism and risk for major adverse cardiac events within the first 30 days after coronary artery stenting. Blood 2000;95:3297–301.

58. Newman PJ, Derbes RS, Aster RH. The human platelet alloantigens, PlA1 and PlA2, are associated with a leucine33 proline33 amino acid polymorphism in membrane glycoprotein IIIa, and are distinguishable by DNA typing. J Clin Invest 1989;83:1778–81.

59. Feng D, Lindpaintner K, Larson MG, et al. Increased platelet aggregability associated with platelet GPIIIa PlA2 polymorphism: the Framingham Offspring Study. Arterioscler Thromb Vasc Biol 1999;19:1142–7.

60. Bray PF, Weiss EJ, Tayback M, Goldschmidt-Clermont PJ. PlA1/A2 polymorphism of platelet glycoprotein IIIa and risk of cardiovascular disease. Lancet 1997;349:1100–1.

61. Carter AM, Ossei-Gerning N, Wilson IJ, Grant PJ. Association of the platelet Pl(A) polymorphism of glycoprotein IIb/IIIa and the fibrinogen B beta 448 polymorphism with myocardial infarction and extent of coronary artery disease. Circulation 1997;96:1424–31.

62. Carter AM, Ossei-Gerning N, Grant PJ. Platelet glycoprotein IIIa PlA polymorphism and myocardial infarction. N Engl J Med 1996;335:1072–3.

63. Carter AM, Ossei-Gerning N, Grant PJ. Platelet glycoprotein IIIa PlA polymorphism in young men with myocardial infarction. Lancet 1996;348:485–6.

64. Frojmovic MM, O'Toole TE, Plow EF, Loftus JC, Ginsberg MH. Platelet glycoprotein IIb-IIIa (alpha IIb beta 3 integrin) confers fibrinogen- and activation-dependent aggregation on heterologous cells. Blood 1991;78:369–76.

65. Hato T, Minamoto Y, Fukuyama T, Fujita S. Polymorphisms of HPA-1 through 6 on platelet membrane glycoprotein receptors are not a genetic risk factor for myocardial infarction in the Japanese population. Am J Cardiol 1997;80:1222–4.

66. Bottiger C, Kastrati A, Koch W, et al. HPA-1 and HPA-3 polymorphisms of the platelet fibrinogen receptor and coronary artery disease and myocardial infarction. Thromb Haemost 2000;83:559–62.

67. Bottiger C, Kastrati A, Koch W, et al. Polymorphism of platelet glycoprotein IIb and risk of thrombosis and restenosis after coronary stent placement. Am J Cardiol 1999;84:987–91.

68. Reiner AP, Schwartz SM, Kumar PN, et al. Platelet glycoprotein IIb polymorphism, traditional risk factors and non-fatal myocardial infarction in young women. Br J Haematol 2001;112:632–6.

69. Lopez JA, Ludwig EH, McCarthy BJ. Polymorphism of human glycoprotein Ib alpha results from a variable number of tandem repeats of a 13-amino acid sequence in the mucin-like macroglycopeptide region. Structure/function implications. J Biol Chem 1992;267:10055–61.

70. Mazzucato M, de Pradella P, Steffan A, de Marco L. Frequency and functional relevance of genetic threonine145/methionine145 dimorphism in platelet glycoprotein Ib alpha in an Italian population. Transfusion 1996;36:891–4.

71. Li CQ, Garner SF, Davies J, Smethurst PA, Wardell MR, Ouwehand WH. Threonine-145/methionine-145 variants of baculovirus produced recombinant ligand binding domain of GPIb alpha express HPA-2 epitopes and show equal binding of von Willebrand factor. Blood 2000;95:205–11.

72. Afshar-Kharghan V, Li CQ, Khoshnevis-Asl M, Lopez, JA. Kozak sequence polymorphism of the glycoprotein (GP) Ib alpha gene is a major determinant of the plasma membrane levels of the platelet GP Ib-IX-V complex. Blood 1999;94:186–91.

73. Frank MB, Reiner AP, Schwartz SM, et al. The Kozak sequence polymorphism of platelet glycoprotein Ib alpha and risk of nonfatal myocardial infarction and nonfatal stroke in young women. Blood 2001;97:875–9.

74. Dalmon J, Laurent M, Courtois G. The human beta fibrinogen promoter contains a hepatocyte nuclear factor 1-dependent interleukin-6-responsive element. Mol Cell Biol 1993;13:1183–93.

75. Humphries SE, Ye S, Talmud P, Bara L, Wilhelmsen L, Tiret L. European Atherosclerosis Research Study: genotype at the fibrinogen locus (G-455-A beta-gene) is associated with differences in plasma fibrinogen levels in young men and women from different regions in Europe. Evidence for gender–genotype–environment interaction. Arterioscler Thromb Vasc Biol 1995;15:96–104.

76. Behague I, Poirier O, Nicaud V, et al. Beta fibrinogen gene polymorphisms are associated with plasma fibrinogen and coronary artery disease in patients with myocardial infarction. The ECTIM Study. Etude Cas-Temoins sur l'Infarctus du Myocarde. Circulation 1996;93:440–9.

77. Gardemann A, Schwartz O, Haberbosch W, et al. Positive association of the beta fibrinogen H1/H2 gene variation to basal fibrinogen levels and to the increase in fibrinogen concentration during acute phase reaction but not to coronary artery disease and myocardial infarction. Thromb Haemost 1997;77:1120–6.

78. Tybjaerg-Hansen A, Agerholm-Larsen B, Humphries SE, Abildgaard S, Schnohr P, Nordestgaard BG. A common mutation (G-455 → A) in the beta-fibrinogen promoter is an independent predictor of plasma fibrinogen, but not of ischemic heart disease. A study of 9127 individuals based on the Copenhagen City Heart Study. J Clin Invest 1997;99:3034–9.

79. Wang XL, Wang J, McCredie RM, Wilcken DE. Polymorphisms of factor V, factor VII, and fibrinogen genes. Relevance to severity of coronary artery disease. Arterioscler Thromb Vasc Biol 1997;17:246–51.

80. Zito F, Di Castelnuovo A, Amore C, D'Orazio A, Donati MB, Iacoviello L. Bcl I polymorphism in the fibrinogen beta-chain gene is associated with the risk of familial myocardial infarction by increasing plasma fibrinogen levels. A case-control study in a sample of GISSI-2 patients. Arterioscler Thromb Vasc Biol 1997; 17:3489–94.

81. de Maat MP, Kastelein JJ, Jukema JW, et al. -455G/A polymorphism of the beta-fibrinogen gene is associated with the progression of coronary atherosclerosis in symptomatic men: proposed role for an acute-phase reaction pattern of fibrinogen. REGRESS group. Arterioscler Thromb Vasc Biol 1998;18:265–71.

82. Folsom AR, Aleksic N, Ahn C, Boerwinkle E, Wu KK. Beta-fibrinogen gene -455G/A polymorphism and coronary heart disease incidence: the Atherosclerosis Risk in Communities (ARIC) Study. Ann Epidemiol 2001;11:166–70.

83. Baumann RE, Henschen AH. Human fibrinogen polymorphic site analysis by restriction endonuclease digestion and allele-specific polymerase chain reaction amplification: identification of polymorphisms at positions A alpha 312 and B beta 448. Blood 1993;82: 2117–24.

84. Curran JM, Evans A, Arveiler D, Luc G, Ruidavets JB, Humphries SE, Green FR. The alpha fibrinogen T/A312 polymorphism in the ECTIM study. Thromb Haemost 1998;79:1057–8.

85. Carter AM, Catto AJ, Grant PJ. Association of the alpha-fibrinogen Thr312Ala polymorphism with poststroke mortality in subjects with atrial fibrillation. Circulation 1999;99:2423–6.

86. Margaglione M, Di Minno G, Grandone E, et al. 1994. Abnormally high circulation levels of tissue plasminogen activator and plasminogen activator inhibitor-1 in patients with a history of ischemic stroke. Arterioscler Thromb 1999;14:1741–5.

87. Salomaa V, Stinson V, Kark JD, Folsom AR, Davis CE, Wu KK. Association of fibrinolytic parameters with early atherosclerosis. The ARIC Study. Atherosclerosis Risk in Communities Study. Circulation 1995;91: 284–90.

88. Cesari M, Rossi GP. Plasminogen activator inhibitor type 1 in ischemic cardiomyopathy. Arterioscler Thromb Vasc Biol 1999;19:1378–86.

89. Dong C, Zhu S, Wang T, Yoon W, Goldschmidt-Clermont P. Upregulation of PAI-1 is mediated through TGF-beta/Smad pathway in transplant arteriopathy. J Heart Lung Transplant. 2002;21:999.

90. Burzotta F, Di Castelnuovo A, Amore C, D'Orazio A, Donati MB, Iacoviello L. [The role of 4G/5G polymorphism in the regulation of plasma levels of PAI-1: a model of interaction between genetic and environmental factors.] Cardiologia 1998;43:83–8.

91. Burzotta F, Di Castelnuovo A, Amore C, D'Orazio A, Di Bitondo R, Donati MB, Iacoviello L. 4G/5G promoter PAI-1 gene polymorphism is associated with plasmatic PAI-1 activity in Italians: a model of gene–environment interaction. Thromb Haemost 1998;79:354–8.

92. Margaglione M, Cappucci G, d'Addedda M, et al. PAI-1 plasma levels in a general population without clinical evidence of atherosclerosis: relation to environmental and genetic determinants. Arterioscler Thromb Vasc Biol 1998;18:562–7.

93. Stegnar M, Uhrin P, Peternel P, Mavri A, Salobir-Pajnic B, Stare J, Binder BR. The 4G/5G sequence polymorphism in the promoter of plasminogen activator inhibitor-1 (PAI-1) gene: relationship to plasma PAI-1 level in venous thromboembolism. Thromb Haemost 1998;79:975–9.

94. Festa A, D'Agostino R, Jr, Rich SS, Jenny NS, Tracy RP, Haffner SM. Promoter (4G/5G) plasminogen activator inhibitor-1 genotype and plasminogen activator inhibitor-1 levels in blacks, Hispanics, and non-Hispanic whites: the Insulin Resistance Atherosclerosis Study. Circulation 2003;107:2422–7.

95. Ridker PM, Hennekens CH, Stampfer MJ, Manson JE, Vaughan DE. Prospective study of endogenous tissue plasminogen activator and risk of stroke. Lancet 1994;343:940–3.

96. Ridker PM, Vaughan DE, Stampfer MJ, Manson JE, Hennekens CH. Endogenous tissue-type plasminogen

activator and risk of myocardial infarction. Lancet 1993;341:1165–8.

97. Thompson SG, Kienast J, Pyke SD, Haverkate F, van de Loo JC. Hemostatic factors and the risk of myocardial infarction or sudden death in patients with angina pectoris. European Concerted Action on Thrombosis and Disabilities Angina Pectoris Study Group. N Engl J Med 1995;332:635–41.

98. Ladenvall P, Wall U, Jern S, Jern C. Eight single-nucleotide polymorphisms (SNPs) at the human tissue-type plasminogen activator (t-PA) locus. J Hum Genet 2001;46:737–8.

99. Jern C, Ladenvall P, Wall U, Jern S. Gene polymorphism of t-PA is associated with forearm vascular release rate of t-PA. Arterioscler Thromb Vasc Biol 1999;19:454–9.

100. van der Bom JG, de Knijff P, Haverkate F, et al. Tissue plasminogen activator and risk of myocardial infarction. The Rotterdam Study. Circulation 1997;95:2623–7.

101. Ridker PM, Baker MT, Hennekens CH, Stampfer MJ, Vaughan DE. Alu-repeat polymorphism in the gene coding for tissue-type plasminogen activator (t-PA) and risks of myocardial infarction among middle-aged men. Arterioscler Thromb Vasc Biol 1997;17:1687–90.

102. Steeds R, Adams M, Smith P, Channer K, Samani NJ. Distribution of tissue plasminogen activator insertion/deletion polymorphism in myocardial infarction and control subjects. Thromb Haemost 1998;79:980–4.

103. Norlund L, Holm J, Zoller B, Ohlin AK. The Ala25-Thr mutation in the thrombomodulin gene is not frequent in Swedish patients suffering from ischemic heart disease. Thromb Haemost 1999;82:1367–8.

104. Norlund L, Zoller B, Ohlin AK. A novel thrombomodulin gene mutation in a patient suffering from sagittal sinus thrombosis. Thromb Haemost 1997;78:1164–6.

105. Norlund L, Holm J, Zoller B, Ohlin AK. A common thrombomodulin amino acid dimorphism is associated with myocardial infarction. Thromb Haemost 1997;77:248–51.

106. Ohlin AK, Norlund L, Marlar RA. Thrombomodulin gene variations and thromboembolic disease. Thromb Haemost 1997;78:396–400.

107. Le Flem L, Mennen L, Aubry ML, Aiach M, Scarabin PY, Emmerich J, Alhenc-Gelas M. Thrombomodulin promoter mutations, venous thrombosis, and varicose veins. Arterioscler Thromb Vasc Biol 2001;21:445–1.

108. Le Flem L, Picard V, Emmerich J, Gandrille S, Fiessinger JN, Aiach M, Alhenc-Gelas M. 1999. Mutations in promoter region of thrombomodulin and venous thromboembolic disease. Arterioscler Thromb Vasc Biol 19:1098–1104.

109. Nakazawa F, Koyama T, Saito T, et al. Thrombomodulin with the Asp468Tyr mutation is expressed on the cell surface with normal cofactor activity for protein C activation. Br J Haematol 1999;106:416–20.

110. Ireland H, Kunz G, Kyriakoulis K, Stubbs PJ, Lane DA. Thrombomodulin gene mutations associated with myocardial infarction. Circulation 1997;96:15–18.

111. Norlund L, Holm J, Zoller B, Ohlin AK. The Ala25-Thr mutation in the thrombomodulin gene is not frequent in Swedish patients suffering from ischemic heart disease. Thromb Haemost 1999;82:1367–8.

112. Wu KK, Aleksic N, Ballantyne CM, Ahn C, Juneja H, Boerwinkle E. Interaction between soluble thrombomodulin and intercellular adhesion molecule-1 in predicting risk of coronary heart disease. Circulation 2003;107:1729–32.

113. Wu KK, Aleksic N, Ahn C, Boerwinkle E, Folsom AR, Juneja H. Thrombomodulin Ala455Val polymorphism and risk of coronary heart disease. Circulation 2001;103:1386–9.

114. Doggen CJ, Kunz G, Rosendaal FR, et al. A mutation in the thrombomodulin gene, 127G to A coding for Ala25Thr, and the risk of myocardial infarction in men. Thromb Haemost 1998;80:743–8.

115. Norlund L, Holm J, Zoller B, Ohlin AK. The Ala25-Thr mutation in the thrombomodulin gene is not frequent in Swedish patients suffering from ischemic heart disease. Thromb Haemost 1999;82:1367–8.

116. Warner D, Catto A, Kunz G, Ireland H, Grant PJ, Lane DA. The thrombomodulin gene mutation G(127)→A (Ala25Thr) and cerebrovascular disease. Cerebrovasc Dis 2000;10:359–63.

117. Li YH, Chen JH, Tsai WC, et al. Synergistic effect of thrombomodulin promoter -33G/A polymorphism and smoking on the onset of acute myocardial infarction. Thromb Haemost 2002;87:86–91.

118. Li YH, Chen JH, Wu HL, et al. G-33A mutation in the promoter region of thrombomodulin gene and its association with coronary artery disease and plasma soluble thrombomodulin levels. Am J Cardiol 2000;85:8–12.

119. Kunz G, Ireland HA, Stubbs PJ, et al. Identification and characterization of a thrombomodulin gene mutation coding for an elongated protein with reduced expression in a kindred with myocardial infarction. Blood 2000;95:569–76.

120. Schrijver I, Lay MJ, Zehnder JL. Diagnostic single nucleotide polymorphism analysis of factor V Leiden and prothrombin 20210G > A. A comparison of the Nanogen Electronic Microarray with restriction enzyme digestion and the Roche LightCycler. Am J Clin Pathol 2003;119:490–6.

121. Russell JA. Genetics of coagulation factors in acute lung injury. Crit Care Med 2003;31:S243–7.

122. Mannucci PM., Peyvandi F, Ardissino D. Risk of myocardial infarction and polymorphisms in candidate genes. N Engl J Med 2003;348:1176–7.

123. Endler G, Mannhalter C. Polymorphisms in coagulation factor genes and their impact on arterial and venous thrombosis. Clin Chim Acta 2003;330:31–55.

124. Leclerc JR. Hematology-neurology connection: association between Factor XIII and hemorrhagic stroke in young women through genetic polymorphism. Stroke 2001;32:2586–7.

125. Bloemenkamp KW, de Maat MP, Dersjant-Roorda MC, Helmerhorst FM, Kluft C. Genetic polymorphisms modify the response of factor VII to oral contraceptive use: an example of gene–environment interaction. Vascul Pharmacol 2002;39:131–6.

126. De Brasi CD, Rossetti LC, Larripa IB. Rapid genotyping of XbaI and MspI DNA polymorphisms of the human factor VIII gene: estimation of their combined heterozygosity in the Argentinean population. Haematologica 2003;88:232–4.

127. Donahue BS, Gailani D, Higgins MS, Drinkwater DC, George AL, Jr. Factor V Leiden protects against blood loss and transfusion after cardiac surgery. Circulation 2003;107:1003–8.

128. Mann KG. Factor VII-activating protease: coagulation, fibrinolysis, and atherothrombosis? Circulation 2003; 107:654–5.

129. De S, V, Rossi E, Paciaroni K, et al. Different circumstances of the first venous thromboembolism among younger or older heterozygous carriers of the G20210A polymorphism in the prothrombin gene. Haematologica 2003;88:61–6.

130. Endler G, Funk M, Haering D, et al. Is the factor XIII 34Val/Leu polymorphism a protective factor for cerebrovascular disease? Br J Haematol 2003;120:310–14.

131. Bi ZM, Hua BL, Yang RC, Wang HY, Wu WJ, Qian LS. [Sal I, Nru I and Mse I restriction fragment length polymorphisms of factor IX gene in Chinese Han people.] Zhongguo Shi Yan Xue Ye Xue Za Zhi 2002;10:247–50.

132. Schroeder V, Kohler HP. Factor XIII activation by thrombin depends on FXIIIVal34Leu genotype. Blood 2003;101:371–2.

133. Kang W, Wang H, Xiong L, et al. [Study on plasma coagulation factor VII (FVII) levels and polymorphisms of FVII gene in patients with coronary heart disease.] Zhonghua Xue Ye Xue Za Zhi 2002;23:457–9.

134. Finan RR, Tamim H, Ameen G, Sharida HE, Rashid M, Almawi WY. Prevalence of factor V G1691A (factor V-Leiden) and prothrombin G20210A gene mutations in a recurrent miscarriage population. Am J Hematol 2002;71:300–5.

135. Folsom AR, Cushman M, Tsai MY, Heckbert SR, Aleksic N. Prospective study of the G20210A polymor-phism in the prothrombin gene, plasma prothrombin concentration, and incidence of venous thromboembolism. Am J Hematol 2002;71:285–90.

136. Francis CW. Factor XIII polymorphisms and venous thromboembolism. Arch Pathol Lab Med 2002;126: 1391–3.

137. Zito F, Lowe GD, Rumley A, McMahon AD, Humphries SE. Association of the factor XII 46C > T polymorphism with risk of coronary heart disease (CHD) in the WOSCOPS study. Atherosclerosis 2002;165:153–8.

138. Ando R, Doi M, Yamauchi K, et al. Association of beta-fibrinogen and factor VII polymorphism with plasma fibrinogen and factor VII levels, and no association of PAI-1 polymorphism with plasma PAI-1 levels in hemodialysis patients. Clin Nephrol 2002;58:25–32.

139. Delahousse B, Gilbert M, Nicham F, Thirion C, Giraudeau B, Gruel Y. Comparative evaluation of five different methods for the measurement of plasma factor II levels in carriers of the 20210A prothrombin variant. Blood Coagul Fibrinolysis 2002;13:465–70.

140. Atherosclerosis, Thrombosis, and Vascular Biology Italian Study Group. No evidence of association between prothrombotic gene polymorphisms and the development of acute myocardial infarction at a young age. Circulation 2003;107:1117–22.

141. Wight TN, Raugi GJ, Mumby SM, Bornstein P. Light microscopic immunolocation of thrombospondin in human tissues. J Histochem Cytochem 1985;33:295–302.

142. Riessen R, Kearney M, Lawler J, Isner JM. Immunolocalization of thrombospondin-1 in human atherosclerotic and restenotic arteries. Am Heart J 1998;135:357–64.

143. Riessen R, Fenchel M, Chen H, Axel DI, Karsch KR, Lawler J. Cartilage oligomeric matrix protein (thrombospondin-5) is expressed by human vascular smooth muscle cells. Arterioscler Thromb Vasc Biol 2001;21:47–54.

144. Yang Z, Kyriakides TR, Bornstein P. Matricellular proteins as modulators of cell-matrix interactions: adhesive defect in thrombospondin 2-null fibroblasts is a consequence of increased levels of matrix metalloproteinase-2. Mol Biol Cell 2000;11:3353–64.

145. Kyriakides TR, Zhu YH, Smith LT, et al. Mice that lack thrombospondin 2 display connective tissue abnormalities that are associated with disordered collagen fibrillogenesis, an increased vascular density, and a bleeding diathesis. J Cell Biol 1998;140:419–30.

146. Topol EJ, McCarthy J, Gabriel S, et al. Single nucleotide polymorphisms in multiple novel thrombospondin genes may be associated with familial premature myocardial infarction. Circulation 2001;104:2641–4.

147. Boekholdt SM, Trip MD, Peters RJ, et al. Thrombospondin-2 polymorphism is associated with a reduced risk of premature myocardial infarction. Arterioscler Thromb Vasc Biol 2002;22:e24–7.

148. Thiagalingam S, Cheng KH, Lee HJ, Mineva N, Thiagalingam A, Ponte JF. Histone deacetylases: unique players in shaping the epigenetic histone code. Ann NY Acad Sci 2003;983:84–100.

149. Szyf M. Targeting DNA methylation in cancer. Ageing Res Rev 2003;2:299–328.

150. Cooper DN, Krawczak M. Cytosine methylation and the fate of CpG dinucleotides in vertebrate genomes. Hum Genet 1989;83:181–8.

151. Tazi J, Bird A. Alternative chromatin structure at CpG islands. Cell 1990;60:909–20.

152. Cross SH, Bird AP. CpG islands and genes. Curr Opin Genet Dev 1995;5:309–14.

153. Antequera F, Bird A. Number of CpG islands and genes in human and mouse. Proc Natl Acad Sci USA 1993;90:11995–9.

154. Delgado S, Gomez M, Bird A, Antequera F. Initiation of DNA replication at CpG islands in mammalian chromosomes. EMBO J 1998;17:2426–35.

155. Rush LJ, Plass C. Restriction landmark genomic scanning for DNA methylation in cancer: past, present, and future applications. Analyt Biochem 2002;307: 191–201.

156. Laukkanen MO, Mannermaa S, Hiltunen MO, Aittomaki S, Airenne K, Janne J, Yla-Herttuala S. Local hypomethylation in atherosclerosis found in rabbit ec-sod gene. Arterioscler Thromb Vasc Biol 1999;19: 2171–8.

157. Dunn BK. Hypomethylation: one side of a larger picture. Ann NY Acad Sci 2003;983:28–42.

158. Xu J, Attisano L. Mutations in the tumor suppressors Smad2 and Smad4 inactivate transforming growth factor beta signaling by targeting Smads to the ubiquitin-proteasome pathway. Proc Natl Acad Sci USA 2000;97:4820–5.

159. Zhu H, Kavsak P, Abdollah S, Wrana JL, Thomsen GH. A SMAD ubiquitin ligase targets the BMP pathway and affects embryonic pattern formation. Nature 1999; 400:687–93.

160. Lo RS, Massague J. Ubiquitin-dependent degradation of TGF-beta-activated smad2. Nat Cell Biol 1999;1: 472–8.

161. Ebisawa T, Fukuchi M, Murakami G, Chiba T, Tanaka K, Imamura T, Miyazono K. Smurf1 interacts with transforming growth factor-beta type I receptor through Smad7 and induces receptor degradation. J Biol Chem 2001;276:12477–80.

162. Ying AK, Hassanain HH, Roos CM, et al. Methylation of the estrogen receptor-alpha gene promoter is selectively increased in proliferating human aortic smooth muscle cells. Cardiovasc Res 2000;46:172–9.

163. Post WS, Goldschmidt-Clermont PJ, et al. Methylation of the estrogen receptor gene is associated with aging and atherosclerosis in the cardiovascular system. Cardiovasc Res 1999;43:985–91.

164. Hulley S, Grady D, Bush T, Furberg C, Herrington D, Riggs B, Vittinghoff E. Randomized trial of estrogen plus progestin for secondary prevention of coronary heart disease in postmenopausal women. Heart and Estrogen/progestin Replacement Study (HERS) Research Group. JAMA 1998;280:605–13.

165. Chen Z, Karaplis AC, Ackerman SL, et al. Mice deficient in methylenetetrahydrofolate reductase exhibit hyperhomocysteinemia and decreased methylation capacity, with neuropathology and aortic lipid deposition. Hum Mol Genet 2001;10:433–43.

166. Wang H, Yoshizumi M, Lai K, Tsai JC, Perrella MA, Haber E, Lee ME. Inhibition of growth and p21ras methylation in vascular endothelial cells by homocysteine but not cysteine. J Biol Chem 1997;272:25380–5.

Index